AF785095

1995

THE McGRAW-HILL

COMPLETE RBRVS

Disclaimer

THIS BOOK is designed to provide accurate and authoritative information on the subject matter covered. All information contained in this guide is based on the experiences of the editors and the recommendations are to be considered the opinion of the editors. It is sold with the understanding that neither the publisher nor editors are engaged in rendering legal, medical, accounting, or other professional service in specific situations. Although prepared for professionals, this publication should not be utilized as a substitute for professional service in specific situations. If legal or medical advice is required, the services of a professional should be sought. Neither the editors nor the publisher may be held liable for any misuse or misinterpretation of the guidelines in this text. All information provided is believed and intended to be reliable, but accuracy cannot be guaranteed by the editors or the publisher.

1995

THE McGRAW-HILL COMPLETE RBRVS

Relative Value Studies, Inc.

McGraw-Hill Inc.

New York St. Louis San Francisco Auckland Bogotá Caracas Lisbon
London Madrid Mexico Milan Montreal New Delhi Paris
San Juan Singapore Sydney Tokyo Toronto

A Product of McGraw-Hill, Inc.

THE McGRAW-HILL COMPLETE RBRVS

Copyright © 1995 by McGraw-Hill, Inc. All rights reserved. Printed in the United States of America. Except as permitted under the United States Copyright of 1976, no part of this publication may be reproduced or distributed in any form or by any means, electronic or mechanical, including photocopy and recording, or stored in a database or retrieval system, without prior written permission of the publisher.

1 2 3 4 5 6 7 8 9 0 SEM SEM 95

ISBN 0-07-600780-4

NOTICE:
Any five-digit numeric Physician's Current Procedural Terminology, Fourth Edition (CPT) codes, service descriptions, instructions and/or guidelines are Copyright © 1994 American Medical Association (AMA). All rights reserved.

CPT is a listing of descriptive terms and five-digit numeric identifying codes and modifiers for reporting medical services performed by physicians. This presentation includes only CPT descriptive terms, numeric identifying codes and modifiers for reporting medical services and procedures that were selected by McGraw-Hill, for inclusion in this Publication.

The most current CPT is available from the American Medical Association.

No fee schedules, basic unit values, relative value guides, conversion factors or scales are included in CPT. The AMA is not recommending that any specific relative values, fees, fee schedules, or related listings be attached to CPT. Any relative listings assigned to the CPT codes are not those of the AMA and such assignment should not be construed as a recommendation for use of these relative values by the AMA.

The AMA assumes no responsibility for the consequences attributable to or related to any use of interpretation of any information contained or not contained in this Publication.

NOTICE REGARDING COPYRIGHT DATES:
The AMA CPT for 1995 is published by the AMA in calendar year 1994 and carries a 1994 copyright. These are the valid CPT codes to be used for 1995.

This book was composed and set in Monotype Bulmer by C+S Gottfried.

Contents

Preface

Relative Values for Physicians (**RVP**) is the most accurate and comprehensive relative value system available. That said, you may be wondering why the developers of **RVP,** Relative Value Studies, Inc. (RVSI), have decided to get involved with a publication of the **Medicare Fee Schedule** (**RBRVS**). It was not an easy decision.

There was a time when the **Medicare Fee Schedule** was primarily utilized when physicians were treating patients within the Medicare program. Not true anymore. **RBRVS** is starting to see expanded use in the private sector, as well. How do we know?

Phone calls—lots of phone calls. Users of **RVP** (who have contracts in the private sector based on **RBRVS**) are calling us, hoping that even though **RBRVS** is not our product, we can help them: 1) find the Medicare code that best resembles the procedure performed, 2) determine what to do if the code they need has no unit value assigned to it, and 3) sift through the confusing rules and regulations. While addressing these questions, RVSI took a good look at the **RBRVS** system and what it could not provide to users in the private sector.

The **Medicare Fee Schedule** is not a complete schedule. By law, Medicare cannot pay for certain services. Services that are not covered may not have assigned unit values. Private sector users of the **RBRVS** then turn to the guidelines to see if there is any way to get reimbursed for these services. Unfortunately, the guidelines offer little help. Services that are not covered—are not covered.

It is precisely this incompleteness that caused RVSI to decide to become involved in the publication of **The Complete RBRVS.** This work includes unit values for covered services (taken directly from the Federal Register), as well as the insertion of values for those codes not valued in the **Medicare Fee Schedule.** (The methodology for development of noncovered services using **RVP** values as a base is described in the following section entitled **Development.**) It is *complete.* Unit values are listed for all procedures and user-friendly guidelines offer help in code use and interpretation.

The Complete RBRVS can be used in contract negotiation and reimbursement disputes. As it stands, **The Complete RBRVS** can assist those who are using (whether by choice or not) the **Medicare Fee Schedule** in the private sector. It is designed to provide a more fair way of determining reimbursement for services rendered. Because all users have access, it may also improve the trust between provider and payer. Having a *complete* system takes the guesswork out of reimbursement.

In addition to the development of unit values for the completion of the **Medicare Fee Schedule,** the staff at RVSI decided to limit its expertise to the interpretation of the rules and regulations as Medicare has written them in the federal register. Much thought was given to adopting the guidelines of McGraw-Hill's **RVP** into **The Complete RBRVS** publication. It was decided, however, that because the original work done by Dr. William Hsiao and the Relative Value Update Committee (RUC) was developed with concern for the Medicare rules and regulations, those rules and regulations would be reprinted in a user-friendly format in **The Complete RBRVS.** The guidelines are designed for use with the codes as they are designated in the update column. The update column was developed by HCFA to determine which conversion factor would be used for the fiscal year.

Relative Values for Physicians was developed with concern for actual relativity for each procedure. It is the most accurate and comprehensive relative value system available. Although the original work of Dr. Hsiao and RUC to develop a system (for use in the Medicare program) that would level the playing field between the specialist and the primary care physician was based on work values, federal government decisions made in regard to the values themselves (due to budgetary constraints) have skewed the numbers. In other words, the budget has become more important than the actual worth of the procedures. RVSI cannot change the Medicare system. What we can offer, however, is a *complete* study that is available, easier to understand and implement, and may be more fair to all parties.

If you are unable to use **RVP** in the private sector, **The Complete RBRVS** is the next best system.

Introduction

DEVELOPMENT

Much attention, both positive and negative, has been given to the development of the **Medicare Fee Schedule.** Because unit values for covered services will appear unchanged in this publication, RVSI will not concentrate on the development of the relative values for the Medicare study. Instead, our focus will be on the methodology used to develop unit values for those services that are not covered by Medicare (either by law or paid under Medicare Part A).

Unit values developed for McGraw-Hill's **Relative Values for Physicians** (**RVP**) are used as the base to provide values for those codes which do not currently have values in Medicare. **RVP** was developed through a physician survey process. Using a random sample of physicians (across the country), the physicians were asked to consider (based on an average case) time, skill, risk to the patient, risk to the provider, and severity of the illness for each of the procedures. This process, through extensive market testing, has been developed, refined, and used since 1983. The survey process and development of **RVP** is ongoing.

The data was first published for public use in 1984 and is currently used by tens of thousands of physicians and a majority of third-party payers. The full body of work in **RVP** can be obtained from McGraw-Hill.

Comparison

For purposes of comparison, the work values published in the **Medicare Fee Schedule** were found to be the most comparable to relative value units developed for use in **RVP.** [**Note:** A conversion factor is used in conjunction with the **RVP** database to account for practice expense and malpractice insurance. Major practice expenses such as rent, staff salaries, and malpractice are determined by specialty and geographic location and are not related to case mix. Therefore, unit values found in **RVP** reflect the value of work performed. The conversion factor is used to cost average the practice expense and malpractice.]

To align the **RVP** unit value scale to the current **RBRVS** work value scale, a comparison of work values to **RVP** values was used.

Percentages, by specialty, utilized by HCFA were used to impute practice expense and malpractice components. Remember, by law Medicare is required to break out practice expense and malpractice insurance values. The sum of the work, practice expense, and malpractice insurance percentages totals one hundred percent. (A detailed description of how the relative adjustment factor was created and applied follows this general explanation.)

Because data from **RVP** is developed using different value scales for Surgery, Radiology, Pathology, Medicine, and Evaluation and Management, it was necessary to compare each section separately to the **RBRVS** work values in order to establish comparative values for procedures that did not have or were not assigned values in **RBRVS.** Anesthesia values for both studies are based on the ASA Relative Value Guide and, therefore, did not require adjustment. This particular step in the comparative process is devised to eliminate any outliers that would skew the comparative values. To maintain a relationship to the work value within each section, the comparative values were then multiplied by the relative value units.

Once the work values were established, the methodology, used by HCFA for new procedures, was applied to develop the practice expense and malpractice values for each code.

CPT codes and descriptions only, © 1994 American Medical Association. Reimbursement information, © 1995 McGraw-Hill Inc.

DEVELOPMENT OF COMPARATIVE FACTORS

Comparative factors were developed by comparing current unit values from the 94.2 **Relative Values for Physicians' (RVP)** data set and the work units in the current **Medicare Fee Schedule.** Comparative factor development for surgery, radiology, medicine, and evaluation and management provided significant data for comparison. Due to the lack of data in the **Medicare Fee Schedule,** however, the data set for pathology was based on a much smaller data set.

Development of the comparative factors for surgery, medicine, and evaluation and management RVSI began by collecting and listing all codes (from each section) for which an **RVP** value and a **Medicare Fee Schedule** work value were published. The values for each group were totaled. The sum of the **Medicare Fee Schedule** work values was divided by the sum of the **RVP** values. This initial comparative factor was then multiplied by the existing **RVP** value for each code. The resulting converted **RVP** value for each code was then subracted from the current work values from the **Medicare Fee Schedule.** All codes with differences greater than two standard deviations from the mean were removed from the data sets. The comparative factor was then recalculated using the remaining data.

Because units in each section of **RVP** are based on separate scales, each section was analyzed separately. Statistical outliers were removed to prevent any skewing of the resultant data for final analysis. Frequency data were not used because the work relationship established for each scale is designed to measure clinical work and is therefore independent of frequency.

The comparative factor from the secondary analysis was then multiplied by the current **RVP** value for each code and the product used to establish work values for each code for which no value existed in the **Medicare Fee Schedule.**

The malpractice and practice expense components were then extrapolated from the resultant work value using percentages established by HCFA for similar usage. Rather than project the specialty-specific use of each code, the percentages established by HCFA for the primary specialty or the percentages for all physicians were used to extrapolate the practice expense and malpractice values. This methodology was found to be appropriate so as to eliminate unnecessary data extrapolation.

The radiology comparison factor for work values was developed in a similar manner. The **Medicare Fee Schedule** lists practice expense components for both the technical and professional components. **RVP** does not separate the technical component into these categories. For accuracy, it was determined that the technical component for radiology in **RVP** was equal to the global technical component in the **Medicare Fee Schedule.** An average practice expense ratio was ascertained and used to allocate practice expense for the professional and technical components. Malpractice components for the professional and technical components were similarly extrapolated using HCFA data and an average malpractice expense ratio.

The pathology section was developed using limited data. Given the percentages developed by HCFA, the data set did provide an acceptable analysis for global work, practice expense, and malpractice values. The analysis, however, did not provide acceptable ratios for the development of separate professional and technical components. We elected to publish only the global value data set. In the pathology section, the only professional and technical component values listed will be those which already had an established **Medicare Fee Schedule** value.

HOW TO USE THIS BOOK

The Complete RBRVS is a reference book on coding and reimbursement. It can be used for Medicare or private sector applications. The Medicare applications for **The Complete RBRVS** are taken from the **Federal Register** and interpreted for ease of use. The four-year phase-in may dictate payment differentials in some geographic areas. Medicare-specific applications, as well as the listing of 1995 Medicare conversion factors, are further explained in the *DESCRIPTION OF COLUMNS* section of this front matter. Medicare rules are explained where they differ from private sector application in each of the guideline sections.

Many have found that the **Medicare Fee Schedule** does not accurately cover the cost of practice and may find the implementation of this fee schedule difficult for private sector payments. The editors of **The Complete RBRVS** recommend that users make several adjustments when implementing this system for private sector use.

First, the editors have read, and agree with, many of the criticisms directed at the development of the geographic practice cost indices (GPCIs). One of the more relevant criticisms is the lack of medicine-specific data. For example, work values should not be area specific as they are designed for national comparison. In the case of private sector use, the editors recommend that GPCIs be disregarded. Instead, users should negotiate conversion factors based on relevant market data.

CPT codes and descriptions only, © 1994 American Medical Association. Reimbursement information, © 1995 McGraw-Hill Inc.

Secondly, the editors feel that the practice expense and malpractice values are not relevant to each procedure. Malpractice, rent, and staff salaries are not dependent upon case mix. Instead, these factors are specialty- and geography-dependent. Therefore, the editors recommend that, if indeed this schedule is desired or required, the work values be used as the relevant comparisons. Conversion factors should be negotiated and used with the work value only. Remember, your conversion factors should be developed using current market data or regulation.

In other words,

$$\text{Work Value} \times \text{Conversion Factor} = \$\ \text{Fee}$$

The following fictitious example, *Gross Conversion Factor Worksheet,* is provided for the development of a practice-specific conversion factor. Work values have been used to complete the conversion factor example. If a contract dictates use of the total value or the GPCI adjusted total value, these values should be used for the conversion factor analysis.

CPT codes and descriptions only, © 1994 American Medical Association. Reimbursement information, © 1995 McGraw-Hill Inc.

SURGERY EXAMPLE

GROSS CONVERSION FACTOR WORKSHEET

LIST YOUR MOST COMMON PROCEDURES

	DESCRIPTION	PROCEDURE CODE	WORK RELATIVE VALUE UNITS	YOUR BASE FEE ($)
1	TURP	52601	11.51	1900.00
2	Appendectomy	44950	6.06	950.00
3	Hernia	49500	4.41	740.00
4	Total Hip	27130	18.68	3600.00
5	Cholecystectomy	47600	10.68	1500.00
6	Total OB	59400	20.99	2100.00
7	Triple Bypass	33512	27.84	5200.00
8	Arthroscopy, Knee	29876	7.51	1750.00
9	Ethmoidectomy	31254	4.65	1000.00
10	Burr Hole	61140	14.84	2340.00
11	Breast reconstruction	19361	17.82	2400.00
12	Graft Trunk	15734	16.52	1700.00
13	Lesion	11604	2.53	310.00
14	Arthroplasty TMJ	21242	12.10	2500.00
15	Fracture	25560	2.29	250.00
16	Foreign Body Eye	65205	.78	65.00
17	Myringotomy	69420	1.28	89.00
18	Consult	99244	2.23	210.00
19	Office Visit	99203	1.14	98.00
20	Hospital Admit	99222	1.84	160.00
21				
22				
23				
24				
25				
		SUM TOTAL	185.70	28862.00

Divide the Total Fee by the Total Relative Value Units

$$\frac{28862.00 \text{ (Total fee)}}{185.7 \text{ (Total RVU)}} = \underline{\$155.42} \text{ Gross conversion factor}$$

CPT codes and descriptions only, © 1994 American Medical Association. Reimbursement information, © 1995 McGraw-Hill Inc.

GROSS CONVERSION FACTOR WORKSHEET FOR ____________________

LIST YOUR MOST COMMON PROCEDURES

	DESCRIPTION	PROCEDURE CODE	WORK RELATIVE VALUE UNITS	YOUR BASE FEE ($)
1				
2				
3				
4				
5				
6				
7				
8				
9				
10				
11				
12				
13				
14				
15				
16				
17				
18				
19				
20				
21				
22				
23				
24				
25				
		SUM TOTAL		

Divide the Total Fee by the Total Relative Value Units

$$\frac{\text{(Total fee)}}{\text{(Total RVU)}} = \$\_\_\_\_\_\_$$ Gross conversion factor

Note: Keep this form as a master copy for producing other worksheets.

CPT codes and descriptions only, © 1994 American Medical Association. Reimbursement information, © 1995 McGraw-Hill Inc.

DESCRIPTION OF COLUMNS

Code/CPT Column

The Code/CPT column lists the current numeric or alpha-numeric code designated in the **Medicare Fee Schedule** corresponding to the description in **CPT** developed by the American Medical Association (AMA) or the **HCPCS Level II** short description for the alpha-numeric codes developed by the Health Care Financing Administration (HCFA).

Modifier Column

The modifier column is listed to describe the services rendered.

- Modifier **00** indicates the total component value. It is the sum of the professional and technical components. This modifier indicates that both the professional services and the technical services (including the facility and personnel) are administered by the same physician group.
- Modifier **26** is used to describe the professional or physician services required for the performance of that service.
- Modifier **TC** is used to describe the personnel, equipment, and facility cost related to providing that particular service.

You'll notice that the **TC** codes have no work relative value units. Technical component values were compared to the technical relative value units from **RVP** and the values were adjusted appropriately using the current **RVP scale.**

The relative values corresponding to these codes have been a) developed by HCFA or b) imputed from the current **RVP scale.** Codes imputed from the current **RVP scale** are indicated by a (*) in the work relative value units column, a (#) sign in the practice expense column, and a (*) in the malpractice relative value units column.

The modifiers have been placed after the description to indicate those services provided for that description. We believe this format to be more user-friendly.

Status Column

The Status column denotes the payment methodology regardless of whether or not Medicare will pay for a particular code.

(A) An (A) in this column indicates that the corresponding code is an active code. These codes are paid under the **Medicare Fee Schedule.** The relative value units for these codes are developed by the HCFA process. An (A) status means that Medicare has made a national decision regarding the coverage of the service and it is payable under Medicare.

(B) A (B) in this column indicates that the service is always bundled in a payment for other services. If there is a (*) by the (B), relative value units indicated will be those imputed from the current **RVP scale.** Codes that show units are not used for Medicare payment. These codes may not be billed to Medicare.

(C) A (C) in this column indicates that Medicare allows the carrier to determine the payment level for these codes. The relative values indicated as having (C) status will be those values imputed by the current **RVP scale,** if applicable.

(D) A (D) in this column indicates that the codes have been deleted and are no longer effective in Medicare for the 1995 fiscal year. The values for these codes are imputed from the current **RVP scale,** when available.

(E) An (E) in this column indicates that these are excluded, by regulation, from the **Medicare Fee Schedule.** These codes may not be billed to Medicare. The relative values for these codes are imputed from the current **RVP scale.**

(G) A (G) in this column indicates that this code is not valued for Medicare purposes. Medicare requires the reporting of such codes under a separate code. Again, values for these codes are imputed by using the current **RVP scale.**

(H) An (H) in this column indicates a deleted modifier. These codes may not be used with a modifier for the 1995 fiscal year for Medicare. Where available, values for these codes are imputed using the current **RVP scale.**

(N) An (N) in this column indicates that this is a non-covered service. These services are not covered by Medicare. Medicare will not accept these codes for payment. If there is a (*) by the work value, relative value units indicated will be those imputed from the current **RVP scale.** Codes which do not include a (*) are included in the **Medicare Fee Schedule,** but still may not be reported to Medicare.

(P) A (P) in this column indicates codes that are considered to be bundled or excluded by Medicare. They may not be used to bill Medicare for these services. If a value is indicated for these services, the values have been imputed from the current **RVP scale.**

CPT codes and descriptions only, © 1994 American Medical Association. Reimbursement information, © 1995 McGraw-Hill Inc.

(R) An (R) in this column indicates codes that have restricted coverage. Medicare will apply special rules for payment. In Medicare these codes are carrier priced. Relative value units for these codes are imputed from the current **RVP scale.**

(T) A (T) in this column indicates a code for an injection. The relative value units and codes may be reported to Medicare if no other services are payable under the **Medicare Fee Schedule** or billed on the same date by the same provider. If any other services payable under the **Medicare Fee Schedule** are billed on the same date, these services may not be billed to Medicare. The values for these codes are established by the **Medicare Fee Schedule.**

(X) An (X) in this column indicates that these codes are not covered by law. Codes indicated as status (X) may not be billed to Medicare. Relative value units for these codes are imputed from the current **RVP scale.**

Description Column

The description column includes the full CPT description for each code as it appears in the American Medical Association's **Current Procedural Terminology** for 1995. These descriptions are reprinted by permission through an agreement that McGraw-Hill and the editors of **Relative Values for Physicians** have with the AMA.

Work Value Column

Work relative value units were either a) developed and determined by HCFA for the physician work for this service or b) imputed from the current **RVP scale.**

Codes which have a number sign (#) by the work unit indicate values included in the Medicare Fee Schedule that are not payable by Medicare.

Codes with a (*) by the work relative value unit indicate values that were imputed from the current **RVP scale.**

Practice Expense Column

This column indicates the practice expense relative value units for the 1995 fiscal year. These values were determined by the OBRA 1993 practice expense and are identified for 1995.

Codes that are subject to the OBRA 1993 practice expense reduction are identified, in this column, by a (*).

Codes for which the value was imputed using the current **RVP scale** and the percentage differential used by HCFA for other codes in that specialty are indicated by a number sign (#).

Malpractice Expense Column

This column indicates the malpractice expense relative value units for services calculated by final evaluation for HCFA for the 1995 fiscal year.

Codes with a (*) in this column are imputed using the HCFA methodology for computing malpractice expense for that specialty.

Total Value Column

The total relative value units column is the sum of the work, practice expense, and malpractice expense relative value units established for the 1995 fiscal year.

Values for codes with a (#) were imputed using the current **RVP scale.** These codes may not be applicable to your carrier. They have not been altered according to the GPCIs.

If using this schedule for Medicare, the units in the **total** column will differ from the units that will be used to calculate reimbursement in your area. (See GPCI.)

Global Period Column

This column indicates the number of days in the global period for which services directly related to the procedure are included. The majority of codes have a numerical designation (i.e., 000, 010, or 090).

- **MMM** codes describe services furnished in uncomplicated maternity care. This includes antepartum and postpartum care. The usual global surgery concept does not apply.
- **XXX** codes indicate that the global surgery concept does not apply.
- **YYY** codes indicate that the global period is to be set by the local carrier.
- **ZZZ** codes indicate that the code is an add-on service and therefore is treated in the global period of the other procedure which is billed in conjunction with a ZZZ code. Do not bill these codes with modifier -51. They should not be reduced.

Codes with a (*) in the global period column are adopted from the current **RVP scale.**

Update Indicator Column

The update indicator demonstrates which conversion factor is to be used with the given procedure. The following conversion factors are used with Medicare.

CPT codes and descriptions only, © 1994 American Medical Association. Reimbursement information, © 1995 McGraw-Hill Inc.

- **S** codes are surgical codes. The 1995 Medicare conversion factor for **S** codes is **$39.447.**
- **N** codes are other nonsurgical services. The 1995 Medicare conversion factor for **N** codes is **$34.616.**
- **P** codes are primary care codes. The 1995 Medicare conversion factor for **P** codes is **$36.382.**

If a (0) appears in this column the codes have either been deleted for 1995 or are not paid under Medicare part B.

If other payers are using the relative values listed, they may or may not use separate conversion factors dependent upon the update column.

GEOGRAPHIC PRACTICE COST INDICES

Chapter 8 contains a list of Geographic Practice Cost Indices (GPCIs) as they appear in the December 8, 1994 Federal Register for the 1995 fiscal year. GPCIs are developed for each location. The steps for setting a total GPCI are:

Step One: (*Multiply*)

$$\text{GPCI for work value} \times \text{work value} = A$$
$$\text{GPCI for practice expense} \times \text{practice expense value} = B$$
$$\text{GPCI for malpractice} \times \text{malpractice value} = C$$

Step Two: (*Add*)

$$A + B + C = \text{Total GPCI relative value}$$

Step Three: (*Multiply*)

$$\text{Total GPCI relative value} \times \begin{matrix}\text{conversion factor determined by}\\ \text{the update column}\end{matrix} = \textbf{Medicare Fee}$$

GPCIs were developed according to statute and are revised every three years according to statute. The revisions are implemented in a step fashion (reaching full change by the third year) in order to reduce the overall impact. [**Note:** There has been significant debate, given the available data used to compute these factors, as to the accuracy of GPCIs. Many payers do not use the GPCIs in the private sector. The editors recommend that the GPCIs be used only for Medicare payment calculation.]

COMPREHENSIVE LISTING OF MODIFIER CODES

Listed values may be modified under certain circumstances. When applicable, the modifying circumstance should be identified by the addition of the appropriate "modifier code number" (including the hyphen) after the usual procedure number. The modifier may also be listed using the modifier code along with 099 in front of the modifier (i.e. 09922 for -22). No hyphen is needed in this case. The fee should be listed as a single modified total for the procedure. Any modifier may be used in conjunction with any procedure, if appropriate.

CPT codes and descriptions only, © 1994 American Medical Association. Reimbursement information, © 1995 McGraw-Hill Inc.

Carriers will vary on the use and acceptance of modifiers. Some carriers will accept all modifiers listed here. Others may accept only CPT-compatible codes or some CPT-compatible codes. You may wish to determine which carriers will accept modifiers and which do not. Most carriers will accept "-22" with a report. This modifier may be used in place of unaccepted modifiers.

Modifer codes listing additional values show customary increases when available. Carriers may vary in actual reimbursement values.

When multiple modifiers are used, see modifier code -99.

CPT Compatible Modifiers

-20 Microsurgery: When the surgical procedures are performed using the techniques of microsurgery, requiring the use of an operating microscope, this modifier may be used. This modifier is not appropriate for use when a surgical loupe is used. Customary reimbursement warrants a value increase of 25% when this modifier is used. A report may be required to justify use of microsurgery. This modifier is not appropriate if a coded procedure for microsurgery exists. **Medicare will not pay.**

-21 Prolonged Evaluation and Management Services: When the service(s) provided is prolonged or otherwise greater than that usually required for the highest level of evaluation and management service within a given category, it (they) may be identified by adding this modifier to the evaluation and management code number. A report is also required.

-22 Unusual Services: When a service provided is greater than that usually provided for a listed procedure, use of this modifier is appropriate. A report is usually required when this modifier is used.

-23 Unusual Anesthesia: Sometimes a procedure which usually requires either no anesthesia (i.e., proctoscopy) or local anesthesia (i.e., skin biopsy or excision of subcutaneous tumor), because of unusual circumstances (i.e., age, noncooperation of patient), must be done under general anesthesia.

-24 Unrelated Evaluation and Management Service by the Same Physician During a Postoperative Period: The physician may need to indicate that an evaluation and management service was performed during a postoperative period for reason(s) unrelated to the original procedure. This circumstance may be reported by adding this modifier to the appropriate level of E/M service. Service should be substantiated by report and listed value should be allowed 100%. Most payers will require a new diagnosis when modifier -24 is used.

-25 Significant, Separately Identifiable Evaluation and Management Service by the Same Physician on the Day of a Procedure: The physician may need to indicate that on the day a procedure or service identified by a CPT code was performed, the patient's condition required a significant separately identifiable E/M service above and beyond the usual preoperative and postoperative care associated with the procedure that was performed. This circumstance may be reported by using this modifier to the appropriate level of E/M service. Service must be substantiated by report and listed value should be allowed 100%. **Medicare will accept this modifier for E/M services provided on the same day as a procedure with a 0 or 10 day global period only.**

-26 Professional Component: Under certain circumstances, the physician may wish to report a professional component.

-32 Mandated Services: Services related to mandated consultation and/or related services (i.e., PRO, third party payer) may be identified by adding this modifier.

-47 Anesthesia by Surgeon: When regional anesthesia is provided by the surgeon and not the anesthesiologist, use the "basic" anesthesia value without the added value for time. **Medicare will not pay.**

-50 Bilateral Procedure: When bilateral procedures which add significant time or complexity to patient care are provided at the same operative session, identify and value the first or major procedure as listed. Identify the secondary procedure by adding this modifier (-50) to the usual procedure number. Bill Medicare on one line of HCFA 1500 by listing the code used and modifier -50. Bill at 150% of allowable. Some carriers may require billing such that the first procedure and second procedure are valued the same and subsequently discounted. Other carriers may require billing for the first procedure at 100% and the second procedure valued at a discounted rate. Check the carrier for procedure. (Also see Surgery Value Guidelines.)

-51 Multiple Procedures: See Surgery Value Guidelines for rules.

-52 Reduced Values: Under certain circumstances, the listed value for a procedure is reduced or eliminated because of common practice, or at the physician's election. Use this modifier to identify such procedures.

-54 Surgical Procedure Only: When one physician performs the surgical procedure and another provides the follow-up care, the fee may be apportioned between them. Identify the surgeon's services by adding this modifier. The customary value should be listed at 70% of the value listed. **Medicare payment is dependent upon preestablished percentages.** (See Surgery Value

CPT codes and descriptions only, © 1994 American Medical Association. Reimbursement information, © 1995 McGraw-Hill Inc.

Guidelines for allowable payment rules.)

-55 Follow-up Care Only: When one physician performs the surgical procedure itself and another provides the follow-up care, the fee may be apportioned between them. Identify the services of the physician providing follow-up care by adding this modifier. The customary value should be listed at 30% of the value listed. **Medicare payment is dependent upon preestablished percentages.** (See Surgery Value Guidelines for allowable payment rules.)

-56 Preoperative Care Only: When one physician provides care up to the date of surgery, but another physician takes over the patient care. This should be billed under services rendered by the appropriate medical code. If the physician provides the total preoperative care (no pre-op by surgeon), the provider may bill using this code and is entitled to 10% of listed value. **Medicare will not pay.**

-57 Decision for Surgery: An evaluation and management service that resulted in the initial decision to perform the surgery may be identified by adding the modifier -57 to the appropriate level of E/M service. This modifier should allow 100% of listed value. **Medicare will accept this modifier for E/M services provided the day before or the day of surgeries with a 90 day global.**

-58 Staged or Related Procedure or Service by the Same Physician During the Postoperative Period: The physician may need to indicate that the performance of a procedure or service during the postoperative period was: a) planned prospectively at the time of the original procedure (staged); b) more extensive than the original procedure; or c) for therapy following a diagnostic surgical procedure. This circumstance may be reported by adding the modifier -58 to the staged or related procedure. Use of this modifier should be substantiated by a report and allow 100% of listed value.
Note: This modifier is not used to report the treatment of a complication related to the previous surgery.

-62 Two Surgeons: Under certain circumstances, the skills of two surgeons (usually with different skills) may be required in the management of a specific surgical problem (i.e., a urologist and a general surgeon in the creation of an ileal conduit, etc.). The value of the procedure (total value) should be valued at the customary value of 125% of the value listed. The total value (125%) may be apportioned in relation to the responsibility and work done, provided the patient is made aware of the arrangement. **Medicare will split the fee evenly between the co-surgeons.**

-66 Surgical Team: Under some circumstances, a highly complex procedure(s) may require the services of several physicians, often of different specialties plus other highly skilled, specially trained personnel and various types of complex equipment are denoted under the "surgical team" concept with a single, global value for the total service. These circumstances should be identified by adding this modifier. The value should be supported by a report to include itemization of the services, personnel, and equipment included in a "global" value.

-76 Repeat Procedure Done by Same Physician: For appropriate circumstance and value please refer to modifiers -58 and/or -78.

-77 Repeat Procedure Done by Another Physician: Use of this modifier should allow 100% of listed value.

-78 Return to Operating Room for a Related Procedure During the Postoperative Period: The physician may need to indicate that another procedure was performed during the postoperative period of the initial procedure. When this subsequent procedure is related to the first, and requires the use of the operating room, it may be reported by adding this modifier to the related procedure. (For repeat procedures on the same day, see -76.) Use of this modifier should allow 70% of the listed value. **Medicare payment is determined by use of the work value only.**

-79 Unrelated Procedure or Service by the Same Physician During the Postoperative Period: The physician needs to indicate that the performance of a procedure or service during the postoperative period was unrelated to the original procedure. This circumstance may be reported by using this modifier. An unrelated procedure or service should be allowed 100% of the listed value and should be substantiated by a different diagnosis and/or by report.

-80 Assistant Surgeon: Minimum surgical assistant services are identified by adding this modifier to the usual procedure number(s). A procedure with this modifier customarily warrants 20% of the value listed. **Medicare will pay 16%.**

-81 Minimum Assistant Surgeon: Minimum surgical assistant services are identified by adding this modifier. It is recommended that this modifier receive a value equal to 10% of the value listed. **Medicare will pay 16%.**

-82 Assistant Surgeon (When a Qualified Resident Surgeon Is Unavailable): The unavailability of a qualified resident surgeon is required for the use of this modifier. It is recommended that the physician receive 20% of the value listed. **Medicare will pay 16%.**

-90 Reference (Outside) Laboratory: When laboratory procedures are performed by other than the attending physician, the procedure(s) shall be identified by adding this modifier.

CPT codes and descriptions only, © 1994 American Medical Association. Reimbursement information, © 1995 McGraw-Hill Inc.

-99 Multiple Modifiers

Non-Compatible CPT Modifiers

(Medicare will not accept these modifiers. They are added here to assist in circumstances not covered in the current system.)

-TC Technical Component: Under certain circumstances a charge may be made for the technical component alone. **Medicare will pay for this modifier.**

-10 Endoscopic Surgery: When the surgical procedure is performed through any type of endoscope for which there is no endoscopic code, attach this modifier to the open surgery procedure code. Attachment of this modifier should warrant no reduction or increase in value for the interim.

-27 Technical Component: Under certain circumstances a charge may be made for the technical component alone.

-28 Debridement and/or Decontamination are considered of additional value when appreciable amounts of devitalized or contaminated tissue are removed. Report required.

-29 Services Provided by Other Than Physician: When a service is performed by a licensed physician assistant or personnel other than the physician under direct supervision of a physician.

-48 Reduced Anesthesia Value for Supervision: When the anesthesiologist is supervising the services of the nurse anesthetist and is involved in medical direction of the patient, including pre- and postoperative evaluation and care, but is not personally administering the anesthesia.

-59 Significant, Separately Identifiable Evaluation and Management Service by the Same Physician During a Preoperative Period and Prior to the Day of a Procedure: The physician may need to indicate that during a preoperative period and prior to the day of a procedure or service identified by a CPT code was performed, the patient's condition required a significant, separately identifiable E/M service above and beyond the usual preoperative care associated with the procedure that was performed. This circumstance may be reported by adding the modifier -59 to the appropriate level of E/M service. The use of the modifier requires substantiation by report and 100% of the listed value should be allowed.

-75 Concomitant Care: Services rendered by more than one physician. When the patient's condition requires the services of more than one physician, each physician may identify his or her services by adding this modifier to the basic service he or she performed.

CPT codes and descriptions only, © 1994 American Medical Association. Reimbursement information, © 1995 McGraw-Hill Inc.

CHAPTER 1

Anesthesia

The editors have elected to indicate that a relative value is not available for procedures with a "0" in the individual units column.

I. **General:** Values for anesthesia services are listed by CPT code in the anesthesia section. These values are to be used only when the anesthesia is legally administered by or under the responsible supervision of a licensed physician. These values include usual pre- and postoperative visits, the administration of the anesthetic, and administration of fluids and/or blood incident to the anesthesia or surgery. Discussion of values as derived from the base unit and time increment are discussed under Calculations of Total Anesthesia Values.

II. **Unlisted Service or Procedure:** When an unlisted service or procedure is provided, the value should be substantiated "by report" (BR).

III. **Procedures Listed without Specified Unit Values by Report "BR" Items:** "BR" in the value column indicates that the value of this service is to be determined "by report," because the service is too unusual or variable to be assigned a unit value. **A detailed clinical record is generally not necessary.**

IV. **Materials Supplied by Physician:** Identify as 99070. Supplies and materials provided by the physician (e.g., sterile trays, drugs, etc.) over and above those usually included with the office visit or other services.

V. **Stand-by Anesthesia:** When an anesthesiologist is requested by the attending physician to be present in the operating room to monitor vital signs and manage the patient from an anesthesia standpoint, even though the actual surgery is being done under local anesthesia, calculation will be the same as if the general anesthesia had been administered (time + base value). Medicare may not pay for Stand-by Anesthesia.

Stand-by anesthesia is generally accepted without justifying documentation for the following:

A. Deliveries;

B. Subdural hematomas;

C. Femoral or brachial arterial embolectomies;

D. Patients with physical status 4 or 5—the physician must document the patient's condition (e.g., severe systemic disease, moribund patient);

E. Insertion of a cardiac pacemaker;

F. Cataract extraction and/or lens implant;

G. Stand-by anesthesia for other than the above generally requires documentation.

VI. **More Than One Anesthesiologist:** When it is necessary to have a second anesthesiologist, the necessity should be substantiated "by report" (BR.) It is recommended that the second anesthesiologist receive 5.0 base units plus time units (calculation of total ANES value). Medicare may not pay.

CPT codes and descriptions only, © 1994 American Medical Association. Reimbursement information, © 1995 McGraw-Hill Inc.

VII. All anesthesia services are reported by use of the anesthesia five-digit procedure code (00100–01999) plus the addition of a physical status modifier. These modifying units may be added to the basic values. The use of other modifiers may be used if appropriate. A comprehensive listing of modifiers is provided in the introduction.

Physical status modifiers are represented by the letter P followed by a single digit defined below:

		Unit Values
1.	Healthy patient	0
2.	Patient with mild systemic disease	0
3.	Patient with severe systemic disease	1
4.	Patient with severe systemic disease that is a constant threat to life	2
5.	A moribund patient who is not expected to survive without the operation	3
6.	A declared brain-dead patient whose organs are being removed for donor purposes	0

The above six levels are consistent with the American Society of Anesthesiologists (ASA) ranking of patient physical status.

Examples: 00100-P1 or 11510-30-P1

VIII. Qualifying Circumstances: Some circumstances warrant additional value due to unusual events. The following list of CPT-4 codes and the corresponding anesthesia unit values may be listed if appropriate. More than one code may be necessary. The value listed is added to the existing anesthesia base.

CPT-4		Unit Values
99100	Anesthesia for patient of extreme age, under one year and over seventy	1
99116	Anesthesia complicated by utilization of total body hypothermia	5
99135	Anesthesia complicated by utilization of controlled hypotension	5
99140	Anesthesia complicated by emergency conditions (specify) (An emergency is defined as existing when delay in treatment of a patient would lead to a significant increase in the threat to life or body part.)	2

CALCULATIONS OF TOTAL ANESTHESIA VALUES

The total anesthesia value is calculated by adding the separately listed basic value and time value.

A basic value is listed for most procedures. This includes the value of all anesthesia services except the value of the actual time spent administering the anesthesia or in unusual detention with the patient. When multiple surgical procedures are performed during the same period of anesthesia, only the greater basic anesthesia value of the various surgical procedures will be used as the base.

The time value is computed by allowing 1.0 unit for each 15 minutes of anesthesia time. Five (5) minutes or greater is considered a significant portion of a time unit.

Anesthesia time begins when the anesthesiologist physically starts to prepare the patient for the induction of anesthesia in the operating room (or its equivalent) and ends when the anesthesiologist is no longer in constant attendance (when the patient may be safely placed under postoperative supervision).

The following examples illustrate the calculation of **total anesthesia values:**

CPT codes and descriptions only, © 1994 American Medical Association. Reimbursement information, © 1995 McGraw-Hill Inc.

1. Procedure Number + Anesthesia Modifier or Anesthesia Code

Basic Value
+ Time Value
Total Anesthesia Value
(sum of basic value and time value)

2. For a needle thyroid biopsy performed in 48 minutes (3 time units):

00322 Basic Value 3
+ Time Value 3
Total Anesthesia Value 6

Note: Modifiers and additional or reduced values should be used when appropriate.

CPT codes and descriptions only, © 1994 American Medical Association. Reimbursement information, © 1995 McGraw-Hill Inc.

ANESTHESIA VALUES

Code	Description	Work value
00100	Anesthesia for procedures on integumentary system of head and/or salivary glands, including biopsy; not otherwise specified	5
00102	Anesthesia for procedures on integumentary system of head and/or salivary glands, including biopsy; plastic repair of cleft lip	6
00103	Anesthesia for procedures on integumentary system of head and/or salivary glands, including biopsy; blepharoplasty	5
00104	Anesthesia for electroconvulsive therapy	4
00120	Anesthesia for procedures on external, middle, and inner ear including biopsy; not otherwise specified	5
00124	Anesthesia for procedures on external, middle, and inner ear including biopsy; otoscopy	4
00126	Anesthesia for procedures on external, middle, and inner ear including biopsy; tympanotomy	4
00140	Anesthesia for procedures on eye; not otherwise specified	5
00142	Anesthesia for procedures on eye; lens surgery	4
00144	Anesthesia for procedures on eye; corneal transplant	6
00145	Anesthesia for procedures on eye; vitrectomy	6
00147	Anesthesia for procedures on eye; iridectomy	4
00148	Anesthesia for procedures on eye; ophthalmoscopy	4
00160	Anesthesia for procedures on nose and accessory sinuses; not otherwise specified	5
00162	Anesthesia for procedures on nose and accessory sinuses; radical surgery	7
00164	Anesthesia for procedures on nose and accessory sinuses; biopsy, soft tissue	4
00170	Anesthesia for intraoral procedures, including biopsy; not otherwise specified	5
00172	Anesthesia for intraoral procedures, including biopsy; repair of cleft palate	6
00174	Anesthesia for intraoral procedures, including biopsy; excision of retropharyngeal tumor	6
00176	Anesthesia for intraoral procedures, including biopsy; radical surgery	7
00190	Anesthesia for procedures on facial bones; not otherwise specified	5
00192	Anesthesia for procedures on facial bones; radical surgery (including prognathism)	7
00210	Anesthesia for intracranial procedures; not otherwise specified	11
00212	Anesthesia for intracranial procedures; subdural taps	5
00214	Anesthesia for intracranial procedures; burr holes	9
00215	Anesthesia for intracranial procedures; elevation of depressed skull fracture, extradural (simple or compound)	9
00216	Anesthesia for intracranial procedures; vascular procedures	15
00218	Anesthesia for intracranial procedures; procedures in sitting position	13
00220	Anesthesia for intracranial procedures; spinal fluid shunting procedures	10
00222	Anesthesia for intracranial procedures; electrocoagulation of intracranial nerve	6
00300	Anesthesia for all procedures on integumentary system of neck, including subcutaneous tissue	5
00320	Anesthesia for all procedures on esophagus, thyroid, larynx, trachea and lymphatic system of neck; not otherwise specified	6
00322	Anesthesia for all procedures on esophagus, thyroid, larynx, trachea and lymphatic system of neck; needle biopsy of thyroid	3
00350	Anesthesia for procedures on major vessels of neck; not otherwise specified	10

CPT codes and descriptions only, © 1994 American Medical Association. Reimbursement information, © 1995 McGraw-Hill Inc.

Code	Description	Work value
00352	Anesthesia for procedures on major vessels of neck; simple ligation	5
00400	Anesthesia for procedures on anterior integumentary system of chest, including subcutaneous tissue; not otherwise specified	3
00402	Anesthesia for procedures on anterior integumentary system of chest, including subcutaneous tissue; reconstructive procedures on breast (eg, reduction or augmentation mammoplasty, muscle flaps)	5
00404	Anesthesia for procedures on anterior integumentary system of chest, including subcutaneous tissue; radical or modified radical procedures on breast	5
00406	Anesthesia for procedures on anterior integumentary system of chest, including subcutaneous tissue; radical or modified radical procedures on breast with internal mammary node dissection	13
00410	Anesthesia for procedures on anterior integumentary system of chest, including subcutaneous tissue; electrical conversion of arrhythmias	4
00420	Anesthesia for procedures on posterior integumentary system of chest, including subcutaneous tissue	5
00450	Anesthesia for procedures on clavicle and scapula; not otherwise specified	5
00452	Anesthesia for procedures on clavicle and scapula; radical surgery	6
00454	Anesthesia for procedures on clavicle and scapula; biopsy of clavicle	3
00470	Anesthesia for partial rib resection; not otherwise specified	6
00472	Anesthesia for partial rib resection; thoracoplasty (any type)	10
00474	Anesthesia for partial rib resection; radical procedures (eg, pectus excavatum)	13
00500	Anesthesia for all procedures on esophagus	15
00520	Anesthesia for closed chest procedures (including esophagoscopy, bronchoscopy, thoracoscopy); not otherwise specified	6
00522	Anesthesia for closed chest procedures (including esophagoscopy, bronchoscopy, thoracoscopy); needle biopsy of pleura	4
00524	Anesthesia for closed chest procedures (including esophagoscopy, bronchoscopy, thoracoscopy); pneumocentesis	4
00528	Anesthesia for closed chest procedures (including esophagoscopy, bronchoscopy, thoracoscopy); mediastinoscopy	8
00530	Anesthesia for transvenous pacemaker insertion	4
00532	Anesthesia for access to central venous circulation	4
00534	Anesthesia for transvenous insertion or replacement of cardioverter/defibrillator	7
00540	Anesthesia for thoracotomy procedures involving lungs, pleura, diaphragm, and mediastinum; not otherwise specified	13
00542	Anesthesia for thoracotomy procedures involving lungs, pleura, diaphragm, and mediastinum; decortication	15
00544	Anesthesia for thoracotomy procedures involving lungs, pleura, diaphragm, and mediastinum; pleurectomy	15
00546	Anesthesia for thoracotomy procedures involving lungs, pleura, diaphragm, and mediastinum; pulmonary resection with thoracoplasty	15
00548	Anesthesia for thoracotomy procedures involving lungs, pleura, diaphragm, and mediastinum; intrathoracic repair of trauma to trachea and bronchi	15
00560	Anesthesia for procedures on heart, pericardium, and great vessels of chest; without pump oxygenator	15
00562	Anesthesia for procedures on heart, pericardium, and great vessels of chest; with pump oxygenator	20
00580	Anesthesia for heart transplant or heart/lung transplant	20
00600	Anesthesia for procedures on cervical spine and cord; not otherwise specified	10
00604	Anesthesia for procedures on cervical spine and cord; posterior cervical laminectomy in sitting position	13
00620	Anesthesia for procedures on thoracic spine and cord; not otherwise specified	10
00622	Anesthesia for procedures on thoracic spine and cord; thoracolumbar sympathectomy	13
00630	Anesthesia for procedures in lumbar region; not otherwise specified	8
00632	Anesthesia for procedures in lumbar region; lumbar sympathectomy	7
00634	Anesthesia for procedures in lumbar region; chemonucleolysis	10
00670	Anesthesia for extensive spine and spinal cord procedures (eg, Harrington rod technique)	13
00700	Anesthesia for procedures on upper anterior abdominal wall; not otherwise specified	3

CPT codes and descriptions only, © 1994 American Medical Association. Reimbursement information, © 1995 McGraw-Hill Inc.

Code	Description	Work value
00702	Anesthesia for procedures on upper anterior abdominal wall; percutaneous liver biopsy	4
00730	Anesthesia for procedures on upper posterior abdominal wall	5
00740	Anesthesia for upper gastrointestinal endoscopic procedures	5
00750	Anesthesia for hernia repairs in upper abdomen; not otherwise specified	4
00752	Anesthesia for hernia repairs in upper abdomen; lumbar and ventral (incisional) hernias and/or wound dehiscence	6
00754	Anesthesia for hernia repairs in upper abdomen; omphalocele	7
00756	Anesthesia for hernia repairs in upper abdomen; transabdominal repair of diaphragmatic hernia	7
00770	Anesthesia for all procedures on major abdominal blood vessels	15
00790	Anesthesia for intraperitoneal procedures in upper abdomen including laparoscopy; not otherwise specified	7
00792	Anesthesia for intraperitoneal procedures in upper abdomen including laparoscopy; partial hepatectomy (excluding liver biopsy)	13
00794	Anesthesia for intraperitoneal procedures in upper abdomen including laparoscopy; pancreatectomy, partial or total (eg, Whipple procedure)	8
00796	Anesthesia for intraperitoneal procedures in upper abdomen including laparoscopy; liver transplant (recipient)	30
00800	Anesthesia for procedures on lower anterior abdominal wall; not otherwise specified	3
00802	Anesthesia for procedures on lower anterior abdominal wall; panniculectomy	5
00810	Anesthesia for intestinal endoscopic procedures	6
00820	Anesthesia for procedures on lower posterior abdominal wall	5
00830	Anesthesia for hernia repairs in lower abdomen; not otherwise specified	4
00832	Anesthesia for hernia repairs in lower abdomen; ventral and incisional hernias	6
00840	Anesthesia for intraperitoneal procedures in lower abdomen including laparoscopy; not otherwise specified	6
00842	Anesthesia for intraperitoneal procedures in lower abdomen including laparoscopy; amniocentesis	4
00844	Anesthesia for intraperitoneal procedures in lower abdomen including laparoscopy; abdominoperineal resection	7
00846	Anesthesia for intraperitoneal procedures in lower abdomen including laparoscopy; radical hysterectomy	8
00848	Anesthesia for intraperitoneal procedures in lower abdomen including laparoscopy; pelvic exenteration	8
00850	Anesthesia for intraperitoneal procedures in lower abdomen including laparoscopy; cesarean section	7
00855	Anesthesia for intraperitoneal procedures in lower abdomen including laparoscopy; cesarean hysterectomy	8
00857	Continuous epidural analgesia, for labor and cesarean section	7
00860	Anesthesia for extraperitoneal procedures in lower abdomen, including urinary tract; not otherwise specified	6
00862	Anesthesia for extraperitoneal procedures in lower abdomen, including urinary tract; renal procedures, including upper ⅓ of ureter, or donor nephrectomy	7
00864	Anesthesia for extraperitoneal procedures in lower abdomen, including urinary tract; total cystectomy	8
00866	Anesthesia for extraperitoneal procedures in lower abdomen, including urinary tract; adrenalectomy	10
00868	Anesthesia for extraperitoneal procedures in lower abdomen, including urinary tract; renal transplant (recipient)	10
00870	Anesthesia for extraperitoneal procedures in lower abdomen, including urinary tract; cystolithotomy	5
00872	Anesthesia for lithotripsy, extracorporeal shock wave; with water bath	7
00873	Anesthesia for lithotripsy, extracorporeal shock wave; without water bath	5
00880	Anesthesia for procedures on major lower abdominal vessels; not otherwise specified	15
00882	Anesthesia for procedures on major lower abdominal vessels; inferior vena cava ligation	10
00884	Anesthesia for procedures on major lower abdominal vessels; transvenous umbrella insertion	5
00900	Anesthesia for procedures on perineal integumentary system (including biopsy of male genital system); not otherwise specified	3
00902	Anesthesia for procedures on perineal integumentary system (including biopsy of male genital system); anorectal procedure (including endoscopy and/or biopsy)	4

CPT codes and descriptions only, © 1994 American Medical Association. Reimbursement information, © 1995 McGraw-Hill Inc.

Code	Description	Work value
00904	Anesthesia for procedures on perineal integumentary system (including biopsy of male genital system); radical perineal procedure	7
00906	Anesthesia for procedures on perineal integumentary system (including biopsy of male genital system); vulvectomy	4
00908	Anesthesia for procedures on perineal integumentary system (including biopsy of male genital system); perineal prostatectomy	6
00910	Anesthesia for transurethral procedures (including urethrocystoscopy); not otherwise specified	3
00912	Anesthesia for transurethral procedures (including urethrocystoscopy); transurethral resection of bladder tumor(s)	5
00914	Anesthesia for transurethral procedures (including urethrocystoscopy); transurethral resection of prostate	5
00916	Anesthesia for transurethral procedures (including urethrocystoscopy); post-transurethral resection bleeding	5
00918	Anesthesia for transurethral procedures (including urethrocystoscopy); with fragmentation and/or removal of ureteral calculus	5
00920	Anesthesia for procedures on male external genitalia; not otherwise specified	3
00922	Anesthesia for procedures on male external genitalia; seminal vesicles	6
00924	Anesthesia for procedures on male external genitalia; undescended testis, unilateral or bilateral	4
00926	Anesthesia for procedures on male external genitalia; radical orchiectomy, inguinal	4
00928	Anesthesia for procedures on male external genitalia; radical orchiectomy, abdominal	6
00930	Anesthesia for procedures on male external genitalia; orchiopexy, unilateral or bilateral	4
00932	Anesthesia for procedures on male external genitalia; complete amputation of penis	4
00934	Anesthesia for procedures on male external genitalia; radical amputation of penis with bilateral inguinal lymphadenectomy	6
00936	Anesthesia for procedures on male external genitalia; radical amputation of penis with bilateral inguinal and iliac lymphadenectomy	8
00938	Anesthesia for procedures on male external genitalia; insertion of penile prosthesis (perineal approach)	4
00940	Anesthesia for vaginal procedures (including biopsy of labia, vagina, cervix or endometrium); not otherwise specified	3
00942	Anesthesia for vaginal procedures (including biopsy of labia, vagina, cervix or endometrium); colpotomy, colpectomy, colporrhaphy	4
00944	Anesthesia for vaginal procedures (including biopsy of labia, vagina, cervix or endometrium); vaginal hysterectomy	6
00946	Anesthesia for vaginal procedures (including biopsy of labia, vagina, cervix or endometrium); vaginal delivery	5
00948	Anesthesia for vaginal procedures (including biopsy of labia, vagina, cervix or endometrium); cervical cerclage	4
00950	Anesthesia for vaginal procedures (including biopsy of labia, vagina, cervix or endometrium); culdoscopy	5
00952	Anesthesia for vaginal procedures (including biopsy of labia, vagina, cervix or endometrium); hysteroscopy	4
00955	Continuous epidural analgesia, for labor and vaginal delivery	5
01000	Anesthesia for procedures on anterior integumentary system of pelvis (anterior to iliac crest), except external genitalia	3
01110	Anesthesia for procedures on posterior integumentary system of pelvis (posterior to iliac crest), except perineum	5
01120	Anesthesia for procedures on bony pelvis	6
01130	Anesthesia for body cast application or revision	3
01140	Anesthesia for interpelviabdominal (hindquarter) amputation	15
01150	Anesthesia for radical procedures for tumor of pelvis, except hindquarter amputation	8
01160	Anesthesia for closed procedures involving symphysis pubis or sacroiliac joint	4
01170	Anesthesia for open procedures involving symphysis pubis or sacroiliac joint	8
01180	Anesthesia for obturator neurectomy; extrapelvic	3
01190	Anesthesia for obturator neurectomy; intrapelvic	4

CPT codes and descriptions only, © 1994 American Medical Association. Reimbursement information, © 1995 McGraw-Hill Inc.

Code	Description	Work value
01200	Anesthesia for all closed procedures involving hip joint	4
01202	Anesthesia for arthroscopic procedures of hip joint	4
01210	Anesthesia for open procedures involving hip joint; not otherwise specified	6
01212	Anesthesia for open procedures involving hip joint; hip disarticulation	10
01214	Anesthesia for open procedures involving hip joint; total hip replacement or revision	10
01220	Anesthesia for all closed procedures involving upper ⅔ of femur	4
01230	Anesthesia for open procedures involving upper ⅔ of femur; not otherwise specified	6
01232	Anesthesia for open procedures involving upper ⅔ of femur; amputation	5
01234	Anesthesia for open procedures involving upper ⅔ of femur; radical resection	8
01240	Anesthesia for all procedures on integumentary system of upper leg	3
01250	Anesthesia for all procedures on nerves, muscles, tendons, fascia, and bursa of upper leg	4
01260	Anesthesia for all procedures involving veins of upper leg, including exploration	3
01270	Anesthesia for procedures involving arteries of upper leg, including bypass graft; not otherwise specified	8
01272	Anesthesia for procedures involving arteries of upper leg, including bypass graft; femoral artery ligation	4
01274	Anesthesia for procedures involving arteries of upper leg, including bypass graft; femoral artery embolectomy	6
01300	Anesthesia for all procedures on integumentary system of knee and/or popliteal area	3
01320	Anesthesia for all procedures on nerves, muscles, tendons, fascia, and bursa of knee and/or popliteal area	4
01340	Anesthesia for all closed procedures on lower ⅓ of femur	4
01360	Anesthesia for all open procedures on lower ⅓ of femur	5
01380	Anesthesia for all closed procedures on knee joint	3
01382	Anesthesia for arthroscopic procedures of knee joint	3
01390	Anesthesia for all closed procedures on upper ends of tibia, fibula, and/or patella	3
01392	Anesthesia for all open procedures on upper ends of tibia, fibula, and/or patella	4
01400	Anesthesia for open procedures on knee joint; not otherwise specified	4
01402	Anesthesia for open procedures on knee joint; total knee replacement	7
01404	Anesthesia for open procedures on knee joint; disarticulation at knee	5
01420	Anesthesia for all cast applications, removal, or repair involving knee joint	3
01430	Anesthesia for procedures on veins of knee and popliteal area; not otherwise specified	3
01432	Anesthesia for procedures on veins of knee and popliteal area; arteriovenous fistula	5
01440	Anesthesia for procedures on arteries of knee and popliteal area; not otherwise specified	5
01442	Anesthesia for procedures on arteries of knee and popliteal area; popliteal thromboendarterectomy, with or without patch graft	8
01444	Anesthesia for procedures on arteries of knee and popliteal area; popliteal excision and graft or repair for occlusion or aneurysm	8
01460	Anesthesia for all procedures on integumentary system of lower leg, ankle, and foot	3
01462	Anesthesia for all closed procedures on lower leg, ankle, and foot	3
01464	Anesthesia for arthroscopic procedures of ankle joint	3
01470	Anesthesia for procedures on nerves, muscles, tendons, and fascia of lower leg, ankle, and foot; not otherwise specified	3
01472	Anesthesia for procedures on nerves, muscles, tendons, and fascia of lower leg, ankle, and foot; repair of ruptured Achilles tendon, with or without graft	5
01474	Anesthesia for procedures on nerves, muscles, tendons, and fascia of lower leg, ankle, and foot; gastrocnemius recession (eg, Strayer procedure)	5
01480	Anesthesia for open procedures on bones of lower leg, ankle, and foot; not otherwise specified	3
01482	Anesthesia for open procedures on bones of lower leg, ankle, and foot; radical resection	4
01484	Anesthesia for open procedures on bones of lower leg, ankle, and foot; osteotomy or osteoplasty of tibia and/or fibula	4
01486	Anesthesia for open procedures on bones of lower leg, ankle, and foot; total ankle replacement	7
01490	Anesthesia for lower leg cast application, removal, or repair	3

CPT codes and descriptions only, © 1994 American Medical Association. Reimbursement information, © 1995 McGraw-Hill Inc.

Code	Description	Work value
01500	Anesthesia for procedures on arteries of lower leg, including bypass graft; not otherwise specified	8
01502	Anesthesia for procedures on arteries of lower leg, including bypass graft; embolectomy, direct or catheter	6
01520	Anesthesia for procedures on veins of lower leg; not otherwise specified	3
01522	Anesthesia for procedures on veins of lower leg; venous thrombectomy, direct or catheter	5
01600	Anesthesia for all procedures on integumentary system of shoulder and axilla	3
01610	Anesthesia for all procedures on nerves, muscles, tendons, fascia, and bursa of shoulder and axilla	5
01620	Anesthesia for all closed procedures on humeral head and neck, sternoclavicular joint, acromioclavicular joint, and shoulder joint	4
01622	Anesthesia for arthroscopic procedures of shoulder joint	4
01630	Anesthesia for open procedures on humeral head and neck, sternoclavicular joint, acromioclavicular joint, and shoulder joint; not otherwise specified	5
01632	Anesthesia for open procedures on humeral head and neck, sternoclavicular joint, acromioclavicular joint, and shoulder joint; radical resection	6
01634	Anesthesia for open procedures on humeral head and neck, sternoclavicular joint, acromioclavicular joint, and shoulder joint; shoulder disarticulation	9
01636	Anesthesia for open procedures on humeral head and neck, sternoclavicular joint, acromioclavicular joint, and shoulder joint; interthoracoscapular (forequarter) amputation	15
01638	Anesthesia for open procedures on humeral head and neck, sternoclavicular joint, acromioclavicular joint, and shoulder joint; total shoulder replacement	10
01650	Anesthesia for procedures on arteries of shoulder and axilla; not otherwise specified	6
01652	Anesthesia for procedures on arteries of shoulder and axilla; axillary-brachial aneurysm	10
01654	Anesthesia for procedures on arteries of shoulder and axilla; bypass graft	8
01656	Anesthesia for procedures on arteries of shoulder and axilla; axillary-femoral bypass graft	10
01670	Anesthesia for all procedures on veins of shoulder and axilla	4
01680	Anesthesia for shoulder cast application, removal or repair; not otherwise specified	3
01682	Anesthesia for shoulder cast application, removal or repair; shoulder spica	4
01700	Anesthesia for all procedures on integumentary system of upper arm and elbow	3
01710	Anesthesia for procedures on nerves, muscles, tendons, fascia, and bursa of upper arm and elbow; not otherwise specified	3
01712	Anesthesia for procedures on nerves, muscles, tendons, fascia, and bursa of upper arm and elbow; tenotomy, elbow to shoulder, open	5
01714	Anesthesia for procedures on nerves, muscles, tendons, fascia, and bursa of upper arm and elbow; tenoplasty, elbow to shoulder	5
01716	Anesthesia for procedures on nerves, muscles, tendons, fascia, and bursa of upper arm and elbow; tenodesis, rupture of long tendon of biceps	5
01730	Anesthesia for all closed procedures on humerus and elbow	3
01732	Anesthesia for arthroscopic procedures of elbow joint	3
01740	Anesthesia for open procedures on humerus and elbow; not otherwise specified	4
01742	Anesthesia for open procedures on humerus and elbow; osteotomy of humerus	5
01744	Anesthesia for open procedures on humerus and elbow; repair of nonunion or malunion of humerus	5
01756	Anesthesia for open procedures on humerus and elbow; radical procedures	6
01758	Anesthesia for open procedures on humerus and elbow; excision of cyst or tumor of humerus	5
01760	Anesthesia for open procedures on humerus and elbow; total elbow replacement	7
01770	Anesthesia for procedures on arteries of upper arm and elbow; not otherwise specified	8
01772	Anesthesia for procedures on arteries of upper arm and elbow; embolectomy	6
01780	Anesthesia for procedures on veins of upper arm and elbow; not otherwise specified	3
01782	Anesthesia for procedures on veins of upper arm and elbow; phleborrhaphy	4
01784	Anesthesia for repair of arterio-venous (A-V) fistula, congenital or acquired	6
01800	Anesthesia for all procedures on integumentary system of forearm, wrist, and hand	3
01810	Anesthesia for all procedures on nerves, muscles, tendons, fascia, and bursa of forearm, wrist, and hand	3
01820	Anesthesia for all closed procedures on radius, ulna, wrist, or hand bones	3

CPT codes and descriptions only, © 1994 American Medical Association. Reimbursement information, © 1995 McGraw-Hill Inc.

Code	Description	Work value
01830	Anesthesia for open procedures on radius, ulna, wrist, or hand bones; not otherwise specified	3
01832	Anesthesia for open procedures on radius, ulna, wrist, or hand bones; total wrist replacement	6
01840	Anesthesia for procedures on arteries of forearm, wrist, and hand; not otherwise specified	6
01842	Anesthesia for procedures on arteries of forearm, wrist, and hand; embolectomy	6
01844	Anesthesia for vascular shunt, or shunt revision, any type (eg, dialysis)	6
01850	Anesthesia for procedures on veins of forearm, wrist, and hand; not otherwise specified	3
01852	Anesthesia for procedures on veins of forearm, wrist, and hand; phleborrhaphy	4
01860	Anesthesia for forearm, wrist, or hand cast application, removal, or repair	3
01900	Anesthesia for injection procedure for hysterosalpingography	3
01902	Anesthesia for burr hole(s) for ventriculography	9
01904	Anesthesia for injection procedure for pneumoencephalography	7
01906	Anesthesia for injection procedure for myelography; lumbar	5
01908	Anesthesia for injection procedure for myelography; cervical	5
01910	Anesthesia for injection procedure for myelography; posterior fossa	9
01912	Anesthesia for injection procedure for diskography; lumbar	5
01914	Anesthesia for injection procedure for diskography; cervical	6
01916	Anesthesia for arteriograms, needle; carotid, or vertebral	5
01918	Anesthesia for arteriograms, needle; retrograde, brachial or femoral	5
01920	Anesthesia for cardiac catheterization including coronary arteriography and ventriculography (not to include Swan-Ganz catheter)	7
01921	Anesthesia for angioplasty	7
01922	Anesthesia for non-invasive imaging or radiation therapy	7
01990	Physiological support for harvesting of organ(s) from brain-dead patient	7
01995	Regional IV administration of local anesthetic agent (upper or lower extremity)	5
01996	Daily management of epidural or subarachnoid drug administration	3
01999	Unlisted anesthesia procedure(s)	0

CPT codes and descriptions only, © 1994 American Medical Association. Reimbursement information, © 1995 McGraw-Hill Inc.

CHAPTER 2

Surgery

The editors have elected to indicate that a relative value is not available for procedures with a "0" in the individual units column.

I. Global Values:

A. The relative values for HCFA **therapeutic surgical procedures** are considered global and include:

1. The immediate preoperative care which starts after the decision for surgery has been made. [Medicare screens have been set so that modifiers must be used to indicate E/M services prior to preoperative care, under certain circumstances. These circumstances include decisions made either 1) the day of surgery for procedures in which the global period is 0 or 10 days, modifier -25 or 2) the day before and the day of surgery for procedures in which the global period is 90 days, modifier -57.]

   a. Additional value is warranted for preoperative services under the following circumstances:

   (1) Evaluation and Management services unrelated to the primary procedure.

   (2) Services required to stabilize the patient for the primary procedure.

   (3) When procedures not usually part of the basic surgical procedure (e.g., bronchoscopy prior to chest surgery) are provided during the immediate preoperative period.

2. The surgical procedure, including local infiltration, digital block, or topical anesthesia, when used.

3. Normal uncomplicated follow-up care for the period indicated: "Global."

   Additional value is warranted for care rendered during the follow-up period caused by an unusual circumstance complication (-75), unrelated care (-79, -24), or staged procedure (-58). (See also Comprehensive Modifiers.)

B. Care for diagnostic procedures (e.g., endoscopy, injection procedures for radiography, etc.) includes only that care related to the diagnostic procedure itself. Care of the condition for which the diagnostic procedure was performed or other concomitant conditions is not included, and may be listed separately. Follow-up care related to the diagnostic procedure is included for the period listed under "Global." Use appropriate modifiers to indicate same day or other global services.

C. When an additional surgical procedure(s) is carried out within the listed period of follow-up care for a previous surgery, the follow-up periods will continue concurrently to their normal terminations.

CPT codes and descriptions only, © 1994 American Medical Association.

Reimbursement information, © 1995 McGraw-Hill Inc.

II. Separate Procedures: Procedures identified as "separate procedures" are frequently included in the global value of other procedures. Listing of separate codes is not appropriate when a procedure is included in the global value of another (e.g., 29870 is not appropriate to list in conjunction with 29874 when performed on the same side).

III. Unusual Service or Procedure: A service may necessitate use of the skills and time of the physician over and above listed services and values. If substantiated "by report" (BR), additional values may be warranted. Use modifier -22 to indicate these procedures.

IV. Unlisted Service or Procedure: When a service or procedure provided is not adequately identified, use of the unlisted procedure code for the related anatomical area is appropriate. Most codes of this nature have 99 for the last two digits. Value should be substantiated "by report" (BR).

V. By Report (BR): Value of a procedure should be established for any "by report" (BR) circumstance by identifying a similar service and justifying value difference. When a report is indicated, the report should include the following:

A. Accurate procedure definition or description;

B. Operative report;

C. Justification for procedural variance, when appropriate;

D. Similar procedure and value comparisons; and

E. Justification for value difference.

VI. Reduced Values: Under some circumstances, value for a procedure may be reduced or eliminated. Use the modifier (-52) to identify reduced value services.

VII. Operating Microscope: When an operating microscope is used to perform a procedure, the use of modifier -20 is appropriate. An additional value of 25% is customarily added if the use of the microscope is medically beneficial and appropriate, and it requires increased skill and time. **Medicare will not pay.**

VIII. Anesthesia by Surgeon: Regional or general anesthesia provided by surgeon should be indicated using modifier -47. The surgeon may receive a value for the procedure equal to the base anesthesia value listed in the column of ANES. Anesthesia and surgery relative value units are based on different scales. Note: Customary conversion factors for anesthesia are approximately 25% of surgery conversion factors. **Medicare will not pay.**

IX. Preoperative, Surgery, and/or Postoperative Care Provided by Different Physicians: Medicare will pay for Post-op and Surgical Care Modifiers based on the following percentages:

Percent of total RVUs by procedure family applied after post hospital discharge

Family	Procedure codes	Surgery percentage	Postop percentage
Integumentary	10000–19499	81	19
Musculoskeletal	20000–29909	79	21
Respiratory	30000–32999	86	14
Cardiovascular	33010–37799	93	7
Hemic and Lymphatic	38100–38999	93	7
Mediastinum	39000–39599	93	7
Digestive	40490–49999	90	10
Urinary	50010–53899	91	9
Male Genital	54000–55980	90	10
Female Genital	56000–58999	86	14
Maternity	59000–59899	77	23
Endocrine	60000–60699	91	9
Nervous	61000–64999	87	13
Eye	65091–68899	80	20
Auditory	69000–69979	86	14

A. Surgical care only: When a physician provides only the surgical care and another physician provides preoperative and postoperative care, this circumstance should be indicated by the use of modifier -54. A customary 70% of the listed value is allowed for this circumstance.

CPT codes and descriptions only, © 1994 American Medical Association. Reimbursement information, © 1995 McGraw-Hill Inc.

B. Postoperative management only: If a physician provides the postoperative care only, the use of modifier -55 is warranted. A customary value of 30% of the listed value is appropriate.

C. Preoperative management only: If a physician provides the preoperative care only, the use of modifier -56 is warranted. A customary value of 10% of the listed value is appropriate. **Medicare will not pay.**

X. **Two Surgeons:** Under certain circumstances, the skills of two surgeons (usually with different skills) may be required in the management of a specific surgical problem (e.g., a urologist and a general surgeon in the creation of an ileal conduit, etc.). The procedure should be valued at the customary value of 125% of the value listed. Medicare will split this equally. If not used under Medicare rules, the total value (125%) may be apportioned in relation to the responsibility and work done, provided the patient is made aware of the arrangement. Such procedures should be marked using modifier -62.

XI. **Surgical Team:** Under some circumstances, a highly complex procedure(s) identified by a single code requires the services of more than two physicians, often of different specialties. These circumstances should be identified by adding modifier -66. The value should be supported by a report to include itemization of the services and personnel included in a "global" value. See CONCURRENT CARE and MULTIPLE PROCEDURES for help in determining the "global" value.

XII. **Surgical Assistants:**

A. Assistant Surgeon: When surgical assistance is provided by a qualified physician, the use of modifier -80 is appropriate. The use of this modifier customarily warrants 20% of the listed values. **Medicare only pays 16%.**

B. Minimum Assistant Surgeon: When minimal surgical assistance is provided, the use of modifier -81 is appropriate. The use of this modifier customarily warrants 10% of the listed value. **Medicare only pays up to 16%.**

C. Assistant Surgeon (when qualified resident surgeon not available): When a qualified resident surgeon is unavailable and a qualified nonresident surgeon provides surgical assistance, use of modifier -82 is appropriate. The use of this modifier customarily warrants 20% of the listed value. **Medicare only pays 16%.**

XIII. **Concurrent Care:** When separate procedures or services are provided by two or more physicians on the same date. Each physician should indicate his or her service(s) by appropriate procedure code(s). This circumstance does not warrant any increase or reduction in value. It is important to note that this circumstance can be used only if the procedures performed do not qualify for the use of modifiers -62 or -66. **Medicare will pay only one service, per diagnosis, per day provided it is not a multiple or bilateral procedure. Consults are the exception.**

XIV. **Multiple Procedures, Same Surgeon:**

A. Single Surgeon Incision: Procedures performed on the same date which significantly increase time and skill warrant the use of modifier -51. Modifier -51 should be added to the secondary, tertiary, etc. procedure(s) code(s). Multiple procedures should be listed according to value. (Multiple Procedure Guidelines do not apply to codes specifically identified as Add-on/Additional Procedures Global "ZZZ.") The primary procedure should reflect the greatest value and should not add modifier -51. All other procedures should be listed using modifier -51 in decreasing value. The values appropriate for each procedure are as follows:

1. Primary procedure	100% of listed value
2. Second, Third, and Fourth procedures	50% of listed value
3. Beyond Fifth procedure and each additional	BR

XV. **Bilateral Procedures:** Some procedures which are performed on both the left and right (bilateral procedures) warrant the use of modifier -50 for the second procedure. Follow appropriate rules of evaluation listed under MULTIPLE PROCEDURES. Bill Medicare on one line of HCFA 1500 by listing the code used and modifer -50. Bill at 150% of allowable.

XVI. **Multiple Modifiers:** If circumstances require the use of more than one modifier with any one procedure code, modifier -99 should be added to the procedure code. Other modifiers are then attached to the procedure code and listed separately with appropriate values for each.

XVII. **Materials Supplied By Physician:** Supplies and materials provided by the physician (i.e., sterile trays, drugs, etc.) are considered to be bundled by Medicare. Supplies should not be billed separately except for permanent condition supplies, home use, and surgical trays for designated procedures. For use within the private sector, identify supplies by using code 99070. Supplies and materials provided by the physician (i.e., sterile trays, drugs, etc.) over and above those usually indicated with the office visit or other services rendered may be listed separately. This rule varies by contract.

CPT codes and descriptions only, © 1994 American Medical Association. Reimbursement information, © 1995 McGraw-Hill Inc.

SURGERY VALUES

Code/ CPT	Mod- ifier	Status	Description	Work value	Practice expense	Mal- practice	Total value	Global period	Up- date
10040	00	A	Acne surgery (eg, marsupialization, opening or removal of multiple milia, comedones, cysts, pustules)	1.34	0.32	0.03	1.69	10	S
10060	00	A	Incision and drainage of abscess (eg, carbuncle, suppurative hidradenitis, cutaneous or subcutaneous abscess, cyst, furuncle, or paronychia); simple or single	1.12	0.44	0.04	1.60	10	S
10061	00	A	Incision and drainage of abscess (eg, carbuncle, suppurative hidradenitis, cutaneous or subcutaneous abscess, cyst, furuncle, or paronychia); complicated or multiple	2.48	0.64	0.06	3.18	10	S
10080	00	A	Incision and drainage of pilonidal cyst; simple	1.62	0.50	0.05	2.17	10	N
10081	00	A	Incision and drainage of pilonidal cyst; complicated	2.40	1.11	0.16	3.67	10	S
10120	00	A	Incision and removal of foreign body, subcutaneous tissues; simple	1.19	0.46	0.05	1.70	10	S
10121	00	A	Incision and removal of foreign body, subcutaneous tissues; complicated	2.64	1.00	0.12	3.76	10	S
10140	00	A	Incision and drainage of hematoma, seroma or fluid collection	1.48	0.48	0.05	2.01	10	S
10160	00	A	Puncture aspiration of abscess, hematoma, bulla, or cyst	1.15	0.38	0.05	1.58	10	S
10180	00	A	Incision and drainage, complex, postoperative wound infection	2.20	1.05	0.18	3.43	10	S
11000	00	A	Debridement of extensive eczematous or infected skin; up to 10% of body surface	0.91	0.40	0.04	1.35	0	S
11001	00	A	Debridement of extensive eczematous or infected skin; each additional 10% of the body surface	0.45	0.26	0.02	0.73	ZZZ	S
11040	00	A	Debridement; skin, partial thickness	0.50	0.40	0.04	0.94	0	S
11041	00	A	Debridement; skin, full thickness	0.82	0.56	0.06	1.44	0	S
11042	00	A	Debridement; skin, and subcutaneous tissue	1.12	0.65	0.08	1.85	0	S
11043	00	A	Debridement; skin, subcutaneous tissue, and muscle	1.83	1.81	0.34	3.98	10	S
11044	00	A	Debridement; skin, subcutaneous tissue, muscle, and bone	2.28	2.82	0.49	5.59	10	S
11050	00	A	Paring or curettement of benign hyperkeratotic skin lesion with or without chemical cauterization (such as verrucae or clavi) not extending through the stratum corneum (eg, callus or wart) with or without local anesthesia; single lesion	0.43	0.37	0.03	0.83	0	S
11051	00	A	Paring or curettement of benign hyperkeratotic skin lesion with or without chemical cauterization (such as verrucae or clavi) not extending through the stratum corneum (eg, callus or wart) with or without local anesthesia; two to four lesions	0.66	0.50	0.05	1.21	0	S
11052	00	A	Paring or curettement of benign hyperkeratotic skin lesion with or without chemical cauterization (such as verrucae or clavi) not extending through the stratum corneum (eg, callus or wart) with or without local anesthesia; more than four lesions	0.86	0.41	0.04	1.31	0	S

CPT codes and descriptions only, © 1994 American Medical Association. Reimbursement information, © 1995 McGraw-Hill Inc.

Code/ CPT	Mod- ifier	Status	Description	Work value	Practice expense	Mal- practice	Total value	Global period	Up- date
11100	00	A	Biopsy of skin, subcutaneous tissue and/or mucous membrane (including simple closure), unless otherwise listed (separate procedure); single lesion	0.81	0.51	0.04	1.36	0	S
11101	00	A	Biopsy of skin, subcutaneous tissue and/or mucous membrane (including simple closure), unless otherwise listed (separate procedure); each separate/additional lesion	0.41	0.29	0.02	0.72	ZZZ	S
11200	00	A	Removal of skin tags, multiple fibrocutaneous tags, any area; up to and including 15 lesions	0.69	0.43	0.04	1.16	10	S
11201	00	A	Removal of skin tags, multiple fibrocutaneous tags, any area; each additional ten lesions	0.26	0.17	0.02	0.45	ZZZ	S
11300	00	A	Shaving of epidermal or dermal lesion, single lesion, trunk, arms or legs; lesion diameter 0.5 cm or less	0.51	0.53	0.05	1.09	0	S
11301	00	A	Shaving of epidermal or dermal lesion, single lesion, trunk, arms or legs; lesion diameter 0.6 to 1.0 cm	0.85	0.67	0.06	1.58	0	S
11302	00	A	Shaving of epidermal or dermal lesion, single lesion, trunk, arms or legs; lesion diameter 1.1 to 2.0 cm	1.05	0.89	0.09	2.03	0	S
11303	00	A	Shaving of epidermal or dermal lesion, single lesion, trunk, arms or legs; lesion diameter over 2.0 cm	1.24	1.36	0.17	2.77	0	S
11305	00	A	Shaving of epidermal or dermal lesion, single lesion, scalp, neck, hands, feet, genitalia; lesion diameter 0.5 cm or less	0.67	0.52	0.05	1.24	0	S
11306	00	A	Shaving of epidermal or dermal lesion, single lesion, scalp, neck, hands, feet, genitalia; lesion diameter 0.6 to 1.0 cm	0.99	0.71	0.07	1.77	0	S
11307	00	A	Shaving of epidermal or dermal lesion, single lesion, scalp, neck, hands, feet, genitalia; lesion diameter 1.1 to 2.0 cm	1.14	0.94	0.10	2.18	0	S
11308	00	A	Shaving of epidermal or dermal lesion, single lesion, scalp, neck, hands, feet, genitalia; lesion diameter over 2.0 cm	1.41	1.40	0.17	2.98	0	S
11310	00	A	Shaving of epidermal or dermal lesion, single lesion, face, ears, eyelids, nose, lips, mucous membrane; lesion diameter 0.5 cm or less	0.73	0.69	0.06	1.48	0	S
11311	00	A	Shaving of epidermal or dermal lesion, single lesion, face, ears, eyelids, nose, lips, mucous membrane; lesion diameter 0.6 to 1.0 cm	1.05	0.85	0.08	1.98	0	S
11312	00	A	Shaving of epidermal or dermal lesion, single lesion, face, ears, eyelids, nose, lips, mucous membrane; lesion diameter 1.1 to 2.0 cm	1.20	1.12	0.11	2.43	0	S
11313	00	A	Shaving of epidermal or dermal lesion, single lesion, face, ears, eyelids, nose, lips, mucous membrane; lesion diameter over 2.0 cm	1.62	1.49	0.15	3.26	0	S
11400	00	A	Excision, benign lesion, except skin tag (unless listed elsewhere), trunk, arms or legs; lesion diameter 0.5 cm or less	0.86	0.53	0.05	1.44	10	S
11401	00	A	Excision, benign lesion, except skin tag (unless listed elsewhere), trunk, arms or legs; lesion diameter 0.6 to 1.0 cm	1.27	0.67	0.06	2.00	10	S
11402	00	A	Excision, benign lesion, except skin tag (unless listed elsewhere), trunk, arms or legs; lesion diameter 1.1 to 2.0 cm	1.56	0.89	0.09	2.54	10	S
11403	00	A	Excision, benign lesion, except skin tag (unless listed elsewhere), trunk, arms or legs; lesion diameter 2.1 to 3.0 cm	1.87	1.17	0.13	3.17	10	S
11404	00	A	Excision, benign lesion, except skin tag (unless listed elsewhere), trunk, arms or legs; lesion diameter 3.1 to 4.0 cm	2.15	1.38	0.17	3.70	10	S
11406	00	A	Excision, benign lesion, except skin tag (unless listed elsewhere), trunk, arms or legs; lesion diameter over 4.0 cm	2.71	1.88	0.33	4.92	10	S

CPT codes and descriptions only, © 1994 American Medical Association. Reimbursement information, © 1995 McGraw-Hill Inc.

Code/ CPT	Mod- ifier	Status	Description	Work value	Practice expense	Mal- practice	Total value	Global period	Up- date
11420	00	A	Excision, benign lesion, except skin tag (unless listed elsewhere), scalp, neck, hands, feet, genitalia; lesion diameter 0.5 cm or less	1.01	0.52	0.05	1.58	10	S
11421	00	A	Excision, benign lesion, except skin tag (unless listed elsewhere), scalp, neck, hands, feet, genitalia; lesion diameter 0.6 to 1.0 cm	1.48	0.71	0.07	2.26	10	S
11422	00	A	Excision, benign lesion, except skin tag (unless listed elsewhere), scalp, neck, hands, feet, genitalia; lesion diameter 1.1 to 2.0 cm	1.71	0.94	0.10	2.75	10	S
11423	00	A	Excision, benign lesion, except skin tag (unless listed elsewhere), scalp, neck, hands, feet, genitalia; lesion diameter 2.1 to 3.0 cm	2.12	1.31	0.15	3.58	10	S
11424	00	A	Excision, benign lesion, except skin tag (unless listed elsewhere), scalp, neck, hands, feet, genitalia; lesion diameter 3.1 to 4.0 cm	2.57	1.39	0.16	4.12	10	S
11426	00	A	Excision, benign lesion, except skin tag (unless listed elsewhere), scalp, neck, hands, feet, genitalia; lesion diameter over 4.0 cm	3.73	1.83	0.29	5.85	10	S
11440	00	A	Excision, other benign lesion (unless listed elsewhere), face, ears, eyelids, nose, lips, mucous membrane; lesion diameter 0.5 cm or less	1.10	0.69	0.06	1.85	10	S
11441	00	A	Excision, other benign lesion (unless listed elsewhere), face, ears, eyelids, nose, lips, mucous membrane; lesion diameter 0.6 to 1.0 cm	1.56	0.85	0.08	2.49	10	S
11442	00	A	Excision, other benign lesion (unless listed elsewhere), face, ears, eyelids, nose, lips, mucous membrane; lesion diameter 1.1 to 2.0 cm	1.82	1.12	0.11	3.05	10	S
11443	00	A	Excision, other benign lesion (unless listed elsewhere), face, ears, eyelids, nose, lips, mucous membrane; lesion diameter 2.1 to 3.0 cm	2.44	1.45	0.15	4.04	10	S
11444	00	A	Excision, other benign lesion (unless listed elsewhere), face, ears, eyelids, nose, lips, mucous membrane; lesion diameter 3.1 to 4.0 cm	3.37	1.47	0.14	4.98	10	S
11446	00	A	Excision, other benign lesion (unless listed elsewhere), face, ears, eyelids, nose, lips, mucous membrane; lesion diameter over 4.0 cm	4.44	1.78	0.18	6.40	10	S
11450	00	A	Excision of skin and subcutaneous tissue for hidradenitis, axillary; with simple or intermediate repair	2.58	2.68	0.44	5.70	90	S
11451	00	A	Excision of skin and subcutaneous tissue for hidradenitis, axillary; with complex repair	3.80	2.90	0.46	7.16	90	S
11462	00	A	Excision of skin and subcutaneous tissue for hidradenitis, inguinal; with simple or intermediate repair	2.36	2.41	0.36	5.13	90	S
11463	00	A	Excision of skin and subcutaneous tissue for hidradenitis, inguinal; with complex repair	3.80	2.00	0.34	6.14	90	S
11470	00	A	Excision of skin and subcutaneous tissue for hidradenitis, perianal, perineal, or umbilical; with simple or intermediate repair	3.10	2.78	0.45	6.33	90	S
11471	00	A	Excision of skin and subcutaneous tissue for hidradenitis, perianal, perineal, or umbilical; with complex repair	4.26	2.46	0.48	7.20	90	S
11600	00	A	Excision, malignant lesion, trunk, arms, or legs; lesion diameter 0.5 cm or less	1.36	1.13	0.10	2.59	10	S
11601	00	A	Excision, malignant lesion, trunk, arms, or legs; lesion diameter 0.6 to 1.0 cm	1.88	1.39	0.12	3.39	10	S
11602	00	A	Excision, malignant lesion, trunk, arms, or legs; lesion diameter 1.1 to 2.0 cm	2.04	1.82	0.16	4.02	10	S
11603	00	A	Excision, malignant lesion, trunk, arms, or legs; lesion diameter 2.1 to 3.0 cm	2.30	2.25	0.21	4.76	10	S

CPT codes and descriptions only, © 1994 American Medical Association. Reimbursement information, © 1995 McGraw-Hill Inc.

Code/ CPT	Mod-ifier	Status	Description	Work value	Practice expense	Mal-practice	Total value	Global period	Up-date
11604	00	A	Excision, malignant lesion, trunk, arms, or legs; lesion diameter 3.1 to 4.0 cm	2.53	2.59	0.26	5.38	10	S
11606	00	A	Excision, malignant lesion, trunk, arms, or legs; lesion diameter over 4.0 cm	3.38	3.11	0.49	6.98	10	S
11620	00	A	Excision, malignant lesion, scalp, neck, hands, feet, genitalia; lesion diameter 0.5 cm or less	1.29	1.34	0.12	2.75	10	S
11621	00	A	Excision, malignant lesion, scalp, neck, hands, feet, genitalia; lesion diameter 0.6 to 1.0 cm	1.92	1.75	0.16	3.83	10	S
11622	00	A	Excision, malignant lesion, scalp, neck, hands, feet, genitalia; lesion diameter 1.1 to 2.0 cm	2.29	2.20	0.19	4.68	10	S
11623	00	A	Excision, malignant lesion, scalp, neck, hands, feet, genitalia; lesion diameter 2.1 to 3.0 cm	2.88	2.58	0.25	5.71	10	S
11624	00	A	Excision, malignant lesion, scalp, neck, hands, feet, genitalia; lesion diameter 3.1 to 4.0 cm	3.38	3.21	0.32	6.91	10	S
11626	00	A	Excision, malignant lesion, scalp, neck, hands, feet, genitalia; lesion diameter over 4.0 cm	4.20	3.41	0.51	8.12	10	S
11640	00	A	Excision, malignant lesion, face, ears, eyelids, nose, lips; lesion diameter 0.5 cm or less	1.48	1.65	0.15	3.28	10	S
11641	00	A	Excision, malignant lesion, face, ears, eyelids, nose, lips; lesion diameter 0.6 to 1.0 cm	2.39	2.09	0.18	4.66	10	S
11642	00	A	Excision, malignant lesion, face, ears, eyelids, nose, lips; lesion diameter 1.1 to 2.0 cm	2.88	2.57	0.23	5.68	10	S
11643	00	A	Excision, malignant lesion, face, ears, eyelids, nose, lips; lesion diameter 2.1 to 3.0 cm	3.45	3.01	0.28	6.74	10	S
11644	00	A	Excision, malignant lesion, face, ears, eyelids, nose, lips; lesion diameter 3.1 to 4.0 cm	4.50	3.51	0.33	8.34	10	S
11646	00	A	Excision, malignant lesion, face, ears, eyelids, nose, lips; lesion diameter over 4.0 cm	5.85	4.32	0.60	10.77	10	S
11700	00	A	Debridement of nails, manual; five or less	0.32	0.32	0.03	0.67	0	S
11701	00	A	Debridement of nails, manual; each additional, five or less	0.23	0.23	0.02	0.48	ZZZ	S
11710	00	A	Debridement of nails, electric grinder; five or less	0.32	0.32	0.03	0.67	0	S
11711	00	A	Debridement of nails, electric grinder; each additional, five or less	0.20	0.19	0.02	0.41	ZZZ	S
11730	00	A	Avulsion of nail plate, partial or complete, simple; single	1.13	0.45	0.04	1.62	0	S
11731	00	A	Avulsion of nail plate, partial or complete, simple; second nail plate	0.55	0.51	0.05	1.11	ZZZ	S
11732	00	A	Avulsion of nail plate, partial or complete, simple; each additional nail plate	0.38	0.25	0.02	0.65	ZZZ	S
11740	00	A	Evacuation of subungual hematoma	0.37	0.39	0.04	0.80	0	S
11750	00	A	Excision of nail and nail matrix, partial or complete, (eg, ingrown or deformed nail) for permanent removal;	1.66	2.10	0.19	3.95	10	S
11752	00	A	Excision of nail and nail matrix, partial or complete, (eg, ingrown or deformed nail) for permanent removal; with amputation of tuft of distal phalanx	2.37	2.82	0.36	5.55	10	S
11755	00	A	Biopsy of nail unit, any method (eg, plate, bed, matrix, hyponychium, proximal and lateral nail folds) (separate procedure)	1.31	0.99	0.12	2.42	0	S
11760	00	A	Repair of nail bed	1.53	0.93	0.09	2.55	10	S
11762	00	A	Reconstruction of nail bed with graft	2.84	2.57	0.24	5.65	10	S
11765	00	A	Wedge excision of skin of nail fold (eg, for ingrown toenail)	0.64	0.51	0.05	1.20	10	S
11770	00	A	Excision of pilonidal cyst or sinus; simple	2.56	2.67	0.44	5.67	10	S
11771	00	A	Excision of pilonidal cyst or sinus; extensive	5.15	4.52	0.92	10.59	90	S
11772	00	A	Excision of pilonidal cyst or sinus; complicated	6.36	4.82	1.01	12.19	90	S
11900	00	A	Injection, intralesional; up to and including seven lesions	0.52	0.25	0.02	0.79	0	S

CPT codes and descriptions only, © 1994 American Medical Association. Reimbursement information, © 1995 McGraw-Hill Inc.

Code/ CPT	Mod-ifier	Status	Description	Work value	Practice expense	Mal-practice	Total value	Global period	Up-date
11901	00	A	Injection, intralesional; more than seven lesions	0.80	0.41	0.03	1.24	0	S
11920	00	R	Tattooing, intradermal introduction of insoluble opaque pigments to correct color defects of skin, including micropigmentation; 6.0 sq cm or less	1.61	1.18	0.23	3.02	0	S
11921	00	R	Tattooing, intradermal introduction of insoluble opaque pigments to correct color defects of skin, including micropigmentation; 6.1 to 20.0 sq cm	1.93	1.40	0.28	3.61	0	S
11922	00	R	Tattooing, intradermal introduction of insoluble opaque pigments to correct color defects of skin, including micropigmentation; each additional 20.0 sq cm	0.49	0.36	0.07	0.92	ZZZ	S
11950	00	R	Tattooing, intradermal introduction of insoluble opaque pigments to correct color defects of skin, including micropigmentation; Subcutaneous injection of filling material (eg, collagen); 1 cc or less	0.84	1.19	0.11	2.14	0	S
11951	00	R	Tattooing, intradermal introduction of insoluble opaque pigments to correct color defects of skin, including micropigmentation; 1.1 to 5.0 cc	1.19	1.19	0.11	2.49	0	S
11952	00	R	Tattooing, intradermal introduction of insoluble opaque pigments to correct color defects of skin, including micropigmentation; 5.1 to 10.0 cc	1.69	1.19	0.11	2.99	0	S
11954	00	R	Tattooing, intradermal introduction of insoluble opaque pigments to correct color defects of skin, including micropigmentation; over 10.0 cc	1.85	1.19	0.11	3.15	0	S
11960	00	A	Insertion of tissue expander(s) for other than breast, including subsequent expansion	6.04	7.73	1.48	15.25	90	S
11970	00	A	Replacement of tissue expander with permanent prosthesis	6.65	8.51	1.61	16.77	90	S
11971	00	A	Removal of tissue expander(s) without insertion of prosthesis	1.51	3.11	0.82	5.44	90	S
11975	00	N	Insertion, implantable contraceptive capsules	1.48	1.06	0.25	2.79	XXX	0
11976	00	R	Removal, implantable contraceptive capsules	1.78	1.28	0.30	3.36	XXX	N
11977	00	N	Removal with reinsertion, implantable contraceptive capsules	2.52	1.80	0.42	4.74	XXX	0
12001	00	A	Simple repair of superficial wounds of scalp, neck, axillae, external genitalia, trunk and/or extremities (including hands and feet); 2.5 cm or less	1.65	0.57	0.05	2.27	10	N
12002	00	A	Simple repair of superficial wounds of scalp, neck, axillae, external genitalia, trunk and/or extremities (including hands and feet); 2.6 cm to 7.5 cm	1.81	0.79	0.07	2.67	10	N
12004	00	A	Simple repair of superficial wounds of scalp, neck, axillae, external genitalia, trunk and/or extremities (including hands and feet); 7.6 cm to 12.5 cm	2.19	1.14	0.10	3.43	10	N
12005	00	A	Simple repair of superficial wounds of scalp, neck, axillae, external genitalia, trunk and/or extremities (including hands and feet); 12.6 cm to 20.0 cm	2.81	1.47	0.14	4.42	10	N
12006	00	A	Simple repair of superficial wounds of scalp, neck, axillae, external genitalia, trunk and/or extremities (including hands and feet); 20.1 cm to 30.0 cm	3.62	1.78	0.19	5.59	10	N
12007	00	A	Simple repair of superficial wounds of scalp, neck, axillae, external genitalia, trunk and/or extremities (including hands and feet); over 30.0 cm	4.07	1.80	0.19	6.06	10	S
12011	00	A	Simple repair of superficial wounds of face, ears, eyelids, nose, lips and/or mucous membranes; 2.5 cm or less	1.71	0.74	0.06	2.51	10	N
12013	00	A	Simple repair of superficial wounds of face, ears, eyelids, nose, lips and/or mucous membranes; 2.6 cm to 5.0 cm	1.94	1.03	0.08	3.05	10	N
12014	00	A	Simple repair of superficial wounds of face, ears, eyelids, nose, lips and/or mucous membranes; 5.1 cm to 7.5 cm	2.41	1.19	0.10	3.70	10	N

CPT codes and descriptions only, © 1994 American Medical Association. Reimbursement information, © 1995 McGraw-Hill Inc.

Code/ CPT	Mod- ifier	Status	Description	Work value	Practice expense	Mal- practice	Total value	Global period	Up- date
12015	00	A	Simple repair of superficial wounds of face, ears, eyelids, nose, lips and/or mucous membranes; 7.6 cm to 12.5 cm	3.14	1.62	0.14	4.90	10	N
12016	00	A	Simple repair of superficial wounds of face, ears, eyelids, nose, lips and/or mucous membranes; 12.6 cm to 20.0 cm	3.88	2.26	0.19	6.33	10	N
12017	00	A	Simple repair of superficial wounds of face, ears, eyelids, nose, lips and/or mucous membranes; 20.1 cm to 30.0 cm	4.66	3.36	0.31	8.33	10	N
12018	00	A	Simple repair of superficial wounds of face, ears, eyelids, nose, lips and/or mucous membranes; over 30.0 cm	5.48	5.15	0.48	11.11	10	S
12020	00	A	Treatment of superficial wound dehiscence; simple closure	2.57	1.19	0.18	3.94	10	S
12021	00	A	Treatment of superficial wound dehiscence; with packing	1.79	0.62	0.11	2.52	10	S
12031	00	A	Layer closure of wounds of scalp, axillae, trunk and/or extremities (excluding hands and feet); 2.5 cm or less	2.10	0.72	0.07	2.89	10	S
12032	00	A	Layer closure of wounds of scalp, axillae, trunk and/or extremities (excluding hands and feet); 2.6 cm to 7.5 cm	2.42	1.05	0.10	3.57	10	S
12034	00	A	Layer closure of wounds of scalp, axillae, trunk and/or extremities (excluding hands and feet); 7.6 cm to 12.5 cm	2.87	1.47	0.15	4.49	10	S
12035	00	A	Layer closure of wounds of scalp, axillae, trunk and/or extremities (excluding hands and feet); 12.6 cm to 20.0 cm	3.38	1.92	0.23	5.53	10	S
12036	00	A	Layer closure of wounds of scalp, axillae, trunk and/or extremities (excluding hands and feet); 20.1 cm to 30.0 cm	4.00	2.32	0.37	6.69	10	S
12037	00	A	Layer closure of wounds of scalp, axillae, trunk and/or extremities (excluding hands and feet); over 30.0 cm	4.62	3.09	0.48	8.19	10	S
12041	00	A	Layer closure of wounds of neck, hands, feet and/or external genitalia; 2.5 cm or less	2.32	0.84	0.08	3.24	10	N
12042	00	A	Layer closure of wounds of neck, hands, feet and/or external genitalia; 2.6 cm to 7.5 cm	2.69	1.17	0.12	3.98	10	N
12044	00	A	Layer closure of wounds of neck, hands, feet and/or external genitalia; 7.6 cm to 12.5 cm	3.09	1.62	0.17	4.88	10	N
12045	00	A	Layer closure of wounds of neck, hands, feet and/or external genitalia; 12.6 cm to 20.0 cm	3.59	2.13	0.23	5.95	10	N
12046	00	A	Layer closure of wounds of neck, hands, feet and/or external genitalia; 20.1 cm to 30.0 cm	4.20	2.82	0.37	7.39	10	S
12047	00	A	Layer closure of wounds of neck, hands, feet and/or external genitalia; over 30.0 cm	4.60	4.02	0.56	9.18	10	N
12051	00	A	Layer closure of wounds of face, ears, eyelids, nose, lips and/or mucous membranes; 2.5 cm or less	2.42	1.01	0.10	3.53	10	S
12052	00	A	Layer closure of wounds of face, ears, eyelids, nose, lips and/or mucous membranes; 2.6 cm to 5.0 cm	2.72	1.47	0.14	4.33	10	S
12053	00	A	Layer closure of wounds of face, ears, eyelids, nose, lips and/or mucous membranes; 5.1 cm to 7.5 cm	3.07	1.76	0.17	5.00	10	S
12054	00	A	Layer closure of wounds of face, ears, eyelids, nose, lips and/or mucous membranes; 7.6 cm to 12.5 cm	3.41	2.60	0.25	6.26	10	S
12055	00	A	Layer closure of wounds of face, ears, eyelids, nose, lips and/or mucous membranes; 12.6 cm to 20.0 cm	4.38	3.24	0.37	7.99	10	S
12056	00	A	Layer closure of wounds of face, ears, eyelids, nose, lips and/or mucous membranes; 20.1 cm to 30.0 cm	5.19	4.74	0.52	10.45	10	S
12057	00	A	Layer closure of wounds of face, ears, eyelids, nose, lips and/or mucous membranes; over 30.0 cm	5.91	5.57	0.48	11.96	10	S
13100	00	A	Repair, complex, trunk; 1.1 cm to 2.5 cm	3.07	1.14	0.13	4.34	10	S
13101	00	A	Repair, complex, trunk; 2.6 cm to 7.5 cm	3.87	2.08	0.21	6.16	10	S
13120	00	A	Repair, complex, scalp, arms, and/or legs; 1.1 cm to 2.5 cm	3.25	1.35	0.17	4.77	10	S
13121	00	A	Repair, complex, scalp, arms, and/or legs; 2.6 cm to 7.5 cm	4.28	2.65	0.33	7.26	10	S
13131	00	A	Repair, complex, forehead, cheeks, chin, mouth, neck, axillae, genitalia, hands and/or feet; 1.1 cm to 2.5 cm	3.74	1.98	0.23	5.95	10	S

CPT codes and descriptions only, © 1994 American Medical Association. Reimbursement information, © 1995 McGraw-Hill Inc.

Code/ CPT	Mod-ifier	Status	Description	Work value	Practice expense	Mal-practice	Total value	Global period	Up-date
13132	00	A	Repair, complex, forehead, cheeks, chin, mouth, neck, axillae, genitalia, hands and/or feet; 2.6 cm to 7.5 cm	4.21	4.57	0.44	9.22	10	S
13150	00	A	Repair, complex, eyelids, nose, ears and/or lips; 1.0 cm or less	3.76	1.76	0.23	5.75	10	S
13151	00	A	Repair, complex, eyelids, nose, ears and/or lips; 1.1 cm to 2.5 cm	4.40	2.45	0.35	7.20	10	S
13152	00	A	Repair, complex, eyelids, nose, ears and/or lips; 2.6 cm to 7.5 cm	6.28	5.13	0.68	12.09	10	S
13160	00	A	Secondary closure of surgical wound or dehiscence, extensive or complicated	9.53	3.33	0.58	13.44	90	S
13300	00	A	Repair, unusual, complicated, over 7.5 cm, any area	5.11	5.71	0.86	11.68	10	S
14000	00	A	Adjacent tissue transfer or rearrangement, trunk; defect 10 sq cm or less	5.43	3.41	0.38	9.22	90	S
14001	00	A	Adjacent tissue transfer or rearrangement, trunk; defect 10.1 sq cm to 30.0 sq cm	7.78	4.75	0.76	13.29	90	S
14020	00	A	Adjacent tissue transfer or rearrangement, scalp, arms and/or legs; defect 10 sq cm or less	6.08	4.90	0.49	11.47	90	S
14021	00	A	Adjacent tissue transfer or rearrangement, scalp, arms and/or legs; defect 10.1 sq cm to 30.0 sq cm	9.37	6.21	0.94	16.52	90	S
14040	00	A	Adjacent tissue transfer or rearrangement, forehead, cheeks, chin, mouth, neck, axillae, genitalia, hands and/or feet; defect 10 sq cm or less	7.18	6.77	0.65	14.60	90	S
14041	00	A	Adjacent tissue transfer or rearrangement, forehead, cheeks, chin, mouth, neck, axillae, genitalia, hands and/or feet; defect 10.1 sq cm to 30.0 sq cm	10.74	7.88	1.02	19.64	90	S
14060	00	A	Adjacent tissue transfer or rearrangement, eyelids, nose, ears and/or lips; defect 10 sq cm or less	8.05	7.75	1.04	16.84	90	S
14061	00	A	Adjacent tissue transfer or rearrangement, eyelids, nose, ears and/or lips; defect 10.1 sq cm to 30.0 sq cm	11.42	10.49	1.27	23.18	90	S
14300	00	A	Adjacent tissue transfer or rearrangement, more than 30 sq cm, unusual or complicated, any area	10.76	11.31	1.84	23.91	90	S
14350	00	A	Filleted finger or toe flap, including preparation of recipient site	9.05	6.07	1.05	16.17	90	S
15000	00	A	Excisional preparation or creation of recipient site by excision of essentially intact skin (including subcutaneous tissues), scar, or other lesion prior to repair with free skin graft (list as separate service in addition to skin graft)	1.95	2.55	0.53	5.03	ZZZ	S
15050	00	A	Pinch graft, single or multiple, to cover small ulcer, tip of digit, or other minimal open area (except on face), up to defect size 2 cm diameter	3.90	1.79	0.30	5.99	90	S
15100	00	A	Split graft, trunk, scalp, arms, legs, hands, and/or feet (except multiple digits); 100 sq cm or less, or each one percent of body area of infants and children (except 15050)	8.05	4.54	0.89	13.48	90	S
15101	00	A	Split graft, trunk, scalp, arms, legs, hands, and/or feet (except multiple digits); each additional 100 sq cm, or each one percent of body area of infants and children, or part thereof	1.72	1.59	0.33	3.64	ZZZ	S
15120	00	A	Split graft, face, eyelids, mouth, neck, ears, orbits, genitalia, and/or multiple digits; 100 sq cm or less, or each one percent of body area of infants and children (except 15050)	9.14	6.05	0.94	16.13	90	S
15121	00	A	Split graft, face, eyelids, mouth, neck, ears, orbits, genitalia, and/or multiple digits; each additional 100 sq cm, or each one percent of body area of infants and children, or part thereof	2.67	2.91	0.53	6.11	ZZZ	S
15200	00	A	Full thickness graft, free, including direct closure of donor site, trunk; 20 sq cm or less	7.46	4.13	0.69	12.28	90	S

CPT codes and descriptions only, © 1994 American Medical Association. Reimbursement information, © 1995 McGraw-Hill Inc.

Code/ CPT	Mod- ifier	Status	Description	Work value	Practice expense	Mal- practice	Total value	Global period	Up- date
15201	00	A	Full thickness graft, free, including direct closure of donor site, trunk; each additional 20 sq cm	1.32	2.06	0.50	3.88	ZZZ	S
15220	00	A	Full thickness graft, free, including direct closure of donor site, scalp, arms, and/or legs; 20 sq cm or less	7.42	4.84	0.85	13.11	90	S
15221	00	A	Full thickness graft, free, including direct closure of donor site, scalp, arms, and/or legs; each additional 20 sq cm	1.19	1.99	0.50	3.68	ZZZ	S
15240	00	A	Full thickness graft, free, including direct closure of donor site, forehead, cheeks, chin, mouth, neck, axillae, genitalia, hands, and/or feet; 20 sq cm or less	8.30	6.10	1.03	15.43	90	S
15241	00	A	Full thickness graft, free, including direct closure of donor site, forehead, cheeks, chin, mouth, neck, axillae, genitalia, hands, and/or feet; each additional 20 sq cm	1.86	2.64	0.58	5.08	ZZZ	S
15260	00	A	Full thickness graft, free, including direct closure of donor site, nose, ears, eyelids, and/or lips; 20 sq cm or less	9.56	7.46	0.99	18.01	90	S
15261	00	A	Full thickness graft, free, including direct closure of donor site, nose, ears, eyelids, and/or lips; each additional 20 sq cm	2.23	3.34	0.60	6.17	ZZZ	S
15350	00	A	Application of allograft, skin	3.89	2.15	0.42	6.46	90	S
15400	00	A	Application of xenograft, skin	4.91	1.06	0.17	6.14	90	S
15570	00	A	Formation of direct or tubed pedicle, with or without transfer; trunk	3.75	7.26	2.08	13.09	90	S
15572	00	A	Formation of direct or tubed pedicle, with or without transfer; scalp, arms, or legs	3.80	6.95	1.86	12.61	90	S
15574	00	A	Formation of direct or tubed pedicle, with or without transfer; forehead, cheeks, chin, mouth, neck, axillae, genitalia, hands or feet	3.85	6.95	1.66	12.46	90	S
15576	00	A	Formation of direct or tubed pedicle, with or without transfer; eyelids, nose, ears, lips, or intraoral	4.27	3.12	0.60	7.99	90	S
15580	00	A	Cross finger flap, including free graft to donor site	3.30	5.32	1.30	9.92	90	S
15600	00	A	Delay of flap or sectioning of flap (division and inset); at trunk	1.70	3.31	0.88	5.89	90	S
15610	00	A	Delay of flap or sectioning of flap (division and inset); at scalp, arms, or legs	2.21	3.19	0.80	6.20	90	S
15620	00	A	Delay of flap or sectioning of flap (division and inset); at forehead, cheeks, chin, neck, axillae, genitalia, hands (except 15625), or feet	2.69	3.96	0.86	7.51	90	S
15625	00	A	Delay of flap or sectioning of flap (division and inset); section pedicle of cross finger flap	1.81	3.04	0.78	5.63	90	S
15630	00	A	Delay of flap or sectioning of flap (division and inset); at eyelids, nose, ears, or lips	3.02	4.26	0.90	8.18	90	S
15650	00	A	Transfer, intermediate, of any pedicle flap (eg, abdomen to wrist, "Walking" tube), any location	3.61	4.62	0.93	9.16	90	S
15732	00	A	Muscle, myocutaneous, or fasciocutaneous flap; head and neck (eg, temporalis, masseter, sternocleidomastoid, levator scapulae)	12.10	15.79	3.46	31.35	90	S
15734	00	A	Muscle, myocutaneous, or fasciocutaneous flap; trunk	16.52	19.01	3.24	38.77	90	S
15736	00	A	Muscle, myocutaneous, or fasciocutaneous flap; upper extremity	15.26	16.21	3.02	34.49	90	S
15738	00	A	Muscle, myocutaneous, or fasciocutaneous flap; lower extremity	10.07	13.60	3.29	26.96	90	S
15740	00	A	Flap; island pedicle	9.45	10.39	1.62	21.46	90	S
15750	00	A	Flap; neurovascular pedicle	10.61	11.96	2.03	24.60	90	S
15755	00	A	Free flap (microvascular transfer)	28.33	30.09	5.33	63.75	90	S
15760	00	A	Graft; composite (eg, full thickness of external ear or nasal ala), including primary closure, donor area	8.28	7.29	1.11	16.68	90	S

CPT codes and descriptions only, © 1994 American Medical Association. Reimbursement information, © 1995 McGraw-Hill Inc.

Code/ CPT	Mod-ifier	Status	Description	Work value	Practice expense	Mal-practice	Total value	Global period	Up-date
15770	00	A	Graft; derma-fat-fascia	6.85	7.46	0.95	15.26	90	S
15775	00	R	Punch graft for hair transplant; 1 to 15 punch grafts	3.96	2.88	0.56	7.40	0	S
15776	00	R	Punch graft for hair transplant; more than 15 punch grafts	5.54	4.03	0.79	10.36	0	S
15780	00	A	Dermabrasion; total face (eg, for acne scarring, fine wrinkling, rhytids, general keratosis)	6.73	1.53	0.13	8.39	90	S
15781	00	A	Dermabrasion; segmental, face	4.67	3.77	0.39	8.83	90	S
15782	00	A	Dermabrasion; regional, other than face	4.19	1.19	0.13	5.51	90	S
15783	00	A	Dermabrasion; superficial, any site, (eg, tattoo removal)	4.16	1.85	0.19	6.20	90	S
15786	00	A	Abrasion; single lesion (eg, keratosis, scar)	1.98	0.62	0.06	2.66	10	S
15787	00	A	Abrasion; each additional four lesions or less	0.33	0.23	0.03	0.59	ZZZ	S
15788	00	A	Chemical peel, facial; epidermal	1.96	1.48	0.12	3.56	90	S
15789	00	A	Chemical peel, facial; dermal	4.69	1.48	0.12	6.29	90	S
15792	00	A	Chemical peel, nonfacial; epidermal	1.73	0.50	0.05	2.28	90	S
15793	00	A	Chemical peel, nonfacial; dermal	3.51	0.50	0.05	4.06	90	S
15810	00	A	Salabrasion; 20 sq cm or less	4.49	3.80	0.29	8.58	90	S
15811	00	A	Salabrasion; over 20 sq cm	5.14	3.74	0.73	9.61	90	S
15819	00	A	Cervicoplasty	8.87	8.01	0.87	17.75	90	S
15820	00	A	Blepharoplasty, lower eyelid;	4.80	6.14	0.64	11.58	90	S
15821	00	A	Blepharoplasty, lower eyelid; with extensive herniated fat pad	5.37	6.87	0.68	12.92	90	S
15822	00	A	Blepharoplasty, upper eyelid;	4.27	5.73	0.56	10.56	90	S
15823	00	A	Blepharoplasty, upper eyelid; with excessive skin weighting down lid	6.65	7.71	0.61	14.97	90	S
15824	00	R	Rhytidectomy; forehead	8.30*	6.03#	1.18*	15.51#	XXX	S
15825	00	R	Rhytidectomy; neck with platysmal tightening (platysmal flap, "P-flap")	7.17*	5.21#	1.02*	13.40#	XXX	S
15826	00	R	Rhytidectomy; glabellar frown lines	5.98*	4.35#	0.85*	11.18#	XXX	S
15828	00	R	Rhytidectomy; cheek, chin, and neck	20.40*	14.83#	2.9*	38.13#	XXX	S
15829	00	R	Rhytidectomy; superficial musculoaponeurotic system (SMAS) flap	20.40*	14.83#	2.90*	38.13#	XXX	S
15831	00	A	Excision, excessive skin and subcutaneous tissue (including lipectomy); abdomen (abdominoplasty)	11.66	9.84	2.01	23.51	90	S
15832	00	A	Excision, excessive skin and subcutaneous tissue (including lipectomy); thigh	10.97	8.29	1.33	20.59	90	S
15833	00	A	Excision, excessive skin and subcutaneous tissue (including lipectomy); leg	10.02	6.22	1.12	17.36	90	S
15834	00	A	Excision, excessive skin and subcutaneous tissue (including lipectomy); hip	10.16	7.18	1.22	18.56	90	S
15835	00	A	Excision, excessive skin and subcutaneous tissue (including lipectomy); buttock	10.98	7.00	1.22	19.20	90	S
15836	00	A	Excision, excessive skin and subcutaneous tissue (including lipectomy); arm	8.83	5.80	1.10	15.73	90	S
15837	00	A	Excision, excessive skin and subcutaneous tissue (including lipectomy); forearm or hand	8.08	5.97	0.85	14.90	90	S
15838	00	A	Excision, excessive skin and subcutaneous tissue (including lipectomy); submental fat pad	6.78	5.88	0.73	13.39	90	S
15839	00	A	Excision, excessive skin and subcutaneous tissue (including lipectomy); other area	8.92	2.44	0.46	11.82	90	S
15840	00	A	Graft for facial nerve paralysis; free fascia graft (including obtaining fascia)	12.26	15.54	2.28	30.08	90	S
15841	00	A	Graft for facial nerve paralysis; free muscle graft (including obtaining graft)	21.53	16.87	2.76	41.16	90	S

CPT codes and descriptions only, © 1994 American Medical Association. Reimbursement information, © 1995 McGraw-Hill Inc.

Code/ CPT	Mod- ifier	Status	Description	Work value	Practice expense	Mal- practice	Total value	Global period	Up- date
15842	00	A	Graft for facial nerve paralysis; free muscle graft by microsurgical technique	35.98	29	2.68	67.66	90	S
15845	00	A	Graft for facial nerve paralysis; regional muscle transfer	11.80	15.10	2.54	29.44	90	S
15850	00	B	Removal of sutures under anesthesia (other than local), same surgeon	0.78	0.36	0.04	1.18	XXX	0
15851	00	A	Removal of sutures under anesthesia (other than local), other surgeon	0.86	0.30	0.03	1.19	0	N
15852	00	A	Dressing change (for other than burns) under anesthesia (other than local)	0.86	0.44	0.07	1.37	0	N
15860	00	A	Intravenous injection of agent (eg, fluorescein) to test blood flow in flap or graft	1.95	1.35	0.25	3.55	0	S
15876	00	R	Suction assisted lipectomy; head and neck	4.92*	3.58#	0.70*	9.20#	XXX	S
15877	00	R	Suction assisted lipectomy; trunk	8.79*	6.39#	1.25*	16.43#	XXX	S
15878	00	R	Suction assisted lipectomy; upper extremity	4.92*	3.58#	0.70*	9.20#	XXX	S
15879	00	R	Suction assisted lipectomy; lower extremity	8.79*	6.39#	1.25*	16.43#	XXX	S
15920	00	A	Excision, coccygeal pressure ulcer, with coccygectomy; with primary suture	7.37	2.95	0.63	10.95	90	S
15922	00	A	Excision, coccygeal pressure ulcer, with coccygectomy; with flap closure	9.17	5.98	1.19	16.34	90	S
15931	00	A	Excision, sacral pressure ulcer, with primary suture;	8.13	2.93	0.55	11.61	90	S
15933	00	A	Excision, sacral pressure ulcer, with primary suture; with ostectomy	9.64	6.92	1.43	17.99	90	S
15934	00	A	Excision, sacral pressure ulcer, with skin flap closure;	11.40	7.46	1.50	20.36	90	S
15935	00	A	Excision, sacral pressure ulcer, with skin flap closure; with ostectomy	13.05	11.24	2.27	26.56	90	S
15936	00	A	Excision, sacral pressure ulcer, with muscle or myocutaneous flap closure;	11.31	10.27	2.05	23.63	90	S
15937	00	A	Excision, sacral pressure ulcer, with muscle or myocutaneous flap closure; with ostectomy	12.98	13.47	2.67	29.12	90	S
15940	00	A	Excision, ischial pressure ulcer, with primary suture;	8.19	3.55	0.73	12.47	90	S
15941	00	A	Excision, ischial pressure ulcer, with primary suture; with ostectomy (ischiectomy)	10.15	7.05	1.39	18.59	90	S
15944	00	A	Excision, ischial pressure ulcer, with skin flap closure;	10.18	9.26	1.82	21.26	90	S
15945	00	A	Excision, ischial pressure ulcer, with skin flap closure; with ostectomy	11.32	11.14	2.09	24.55	90	S
15946	00	A	Excision, ischial pressure ulcer, with ostectomy, with muscle or myocutaneous flap closure	19.81	16.61	3.24	39.66	90	S
15950	00	A	Excision, trochanteric pressure ulcer, with primary suture;	6.79	3.01	0.58	10.38	90	S
15951	00	A	Excision, trochanteric pressure ulcer, with primary suture; with ostectomy	9.57	7.65	1.58	18.80	90	S
15952	00	A	Excision, trochanteric pressure ulcer, with skin flap closure;	10.18	7.13	1.37	18.68	90	S
15953	00	A	Excision, trochanteric pressure ulcer, with skin flap closure; with ostectomy	11.39	9.08	1.87	22.34	90	S
15956	00	A	Excision, trochanteric pressure ulcer, with muscle or myocutaneous flap closure;	13.93	17.17	3.39	34.49	90	S
15958	00	A	Excision, trochanteric pressure ulcer, with muscle or myocutaneous flap closure; with ostectomy	13.89	17.77	3.76	35.42	90	S
15999	00	C	Unlisted procedure, excision pressure ulcer	0	0	0	0	YYY	S
16000	00	A	Initial treatment, first degree burn, when no more than local treatment is required	0.89	0.35	0.03	1.27	0	N
16010	00	A	Dressings and/or debridement, initial or subsequent; under anesthesia, small	0.87	0.32	0.03	1.22	0	N

CPT codes and descriptions only, © 1994 American Medical Association. Reimbursement information, © 1995 McGraw-Hill Inc.

Code/ CPT	Mod- ifier	Status	Description	Work value	Practice expense	Mal- practice	Total value	Global period	Up- date
16015	00	A	Dressings and/or debridement, initial or subsequent; under anesthesia, medium or large, or with major debridement	2.35	2.04	0.38	4.77	0	S
16020	00	A	Dressings and/or debridement, initial or subsequent; without anesthesia, office or hospital, small	0.80	0.34	0.03	1.17	0	N
16025	00	A	Dressings and/or debridement, initial or subsequent; without anesthesia, medium (eg, whole face or whole extremity)	1.85	0.45	0.05	2.35	0	S
16030	00	A	Dressings and/or debridement, initial or subsequent; without anesthesia, large (eg, more than one extremity)	2.08	0.52	0.08	2.68	0	S
16035	00	A	Escharotomy	4.53	1.88	0.34	6.75	90	S
16040	00	A	Excision burn wound, without skin grafting, employing alloplastic dressing (eg, synthetic mesh), any anatomic site; up to one percent total body surface area	1.02	2.10	0.53	3.65	0	S
16041	00	A	Excision burn wound, without skin grafting, employing alloplastic dressing (eg, synthetic mesh), any anatomic site; greater than one percent and up to nine percent total body surface area	2.70	3.16	0.53	6.39	0	S
16042	00	A	Excision burn wound, without skin grafting, employing alloplastic dressing (eg, synthetic mesh), any anatomic site; each additional nine percent total body surface area, or part thereof	2.35	3.02	0.53	5.90	0	S
17000	00	A	Destruction by any method, including laser, with or without surgical curettement, all benign facial lesions or premalignant lesions in any location, or benign lesions other than cutaneous vascular proliferative lesions, including local anesthesia; one lesion	0.64	0.42	0.03	1.09	10	S
17001	00	A	Destruction by any method, including laser, with or without surgical curettement, all benign facial lesions or premalignant lesions in any location, or benign lesions other than cutaneous vascular proliferative lesions, including local anesthesia; second and third lesions, each	0.19	0.19	0.02	0.40	ZZZ	S
17002	00	A	Destruction by any method, including laser, with or without surgical curettement, all benign facial lesions or premalignant lesions in any location, or benign lesions other than cutaneous vascular proliferative lesions, including local anesthesia; over three lesions, each additional lesion	0.19	0.10	0.01	0.30	ZZZ	S
17010	00	A	Destruction by any method, including laser, with or without surgical curettement, all benign facial lesions or premalignant lesions in any location, or benign lesions other than cutaneous vascular proliferative lesions, including local anesthesia; complicated lesion(s)	1.01	0.48	0.04	1.53	10	S
17100	00	A	Destruction by any method, including laser, of benign skin lesions other than cutaneous vascular proliferative lesions on any area other than the face, including local anesthesia; one lesion	0.53	0.37	0.03	0.93	10	S
17101	00	A	Destruction by any method, including laser, of benign skin lesions other than cutaneous vascular proliferative lesions on any area other than the face, including local anesthesia; second lesion	0.11	0.18	0.02	0.31	ZZZ	S
17102	00	A	Destruction by any method, including laser, of benign skin lesions other than cutaneous vascular proliferative lesions on any area other than the face, including local anesthesia; over two lesions, each additional lesion up to 15 lesions	0.11	0.08	0.01	0.20	ZZZ	S

CPT codes and descriptions only, © 1994 American Medical Association. Reimbursement information, © 1995 McGraw-Hill Inc.

Code/ CPT	Mod-ifier	Status	Description	Work value	Practice expense	Mal-practice	Total value	Global period	Up-date
17104	00	A	Destruction by any method, including laser, of benign skin lesions other than cutaneous vascular proliferative lesions on any area other than the face, including local anesthesia; 15 or more lesions	2.01	0.07	0.01	2.09	10	S
17105	00	A	Destruction by any method, including laser, of benign skin lesions other than cutaneous vascular proliferative lesions on any area other than the face, including local anesthesia; complicated or extensive lesions	0.76	0.31	0.03	1.10	10	S
17106	00	A	Destruction of cutaneous vascular proliferative lesions (eg, laser technique); less than 10 sq cm	4.54	1.93	0.18	6.65	90	S
17107	00	A	Destruction of cutaneous vascular proliferative lesions (eg, laser technique); 10.0–50.0 sq cm	9.06	3.70	0.39	13.15	90	S
17108	00	A	Destruction of cutaneous vascular proliferative lesions (eg, laser technique); over 50.0 sq cm	13.10	9.32	0.69	23.11	90	S
17110	00	A	Destruction by any method of flat (plane, juvenile) warts or molluscum contagiosum, milia, up to 15 lesions	0.55	0.40	0.03	0.98	10	S
17200	00	A	Electrosurgical destruction of multiple fibrocutaneous tags; up to 15 lesions	0.59	0.41	0.04	1.04	10	S
17201	00	A	Electrosurgical destruction of multiple fibrocutaneous tags; each additional ten lesions	0.38	0.15	0.01	0.54	ZZZ	S
17250	00	A	Chemical cauterization of granulation tissue (proud flesh, sinus or fistula)	0.50	0.34	0.04	0.88	0	S
17260	00	A	Destruction, malignant lesion, any method, trunk, arms or legs; lesion diameter 0.5 cm or less	0.86	1.13	0.10	2.09	10	S
17261	00	A	Destruction, malignant lesion, any method, trunk, arms or legs; lesion diameter 0.6 to 1.0 cm	1.12	1.39	0.12	2.63	10	S
17262	00	A	Destruction, malignant lesion, any method, trunk, arms or legs; lesion diameter 1.1 to 2.0 cm	1.53	1.82	0.16	3.51	10	S
17263	00	A	Destruction, malignant lesion, any method, trunk, arms or legs; lesion diameter 2.1 to 3.0 cm	1.74	2.25	0.21	4.20	10	S
17264	00	A	Destruction, malignant lesion, any method, trunk, arms or legs; lesion diameter 3.1 to 4.0 cm	1.89	2.59	0.26	4.74	10	S
17266	00	A	Destruction, malignant lesion, any method, trunk, arms or legs; lesion diameter over 4.0 cm	2.29	3.11	0.49	5.89	10	S
17270	00	A	Destruction, malignant lesion, any method, scalp, neck, hands, feet, genitalia; lesion diameter 0.5 cm or less	1.27	1.34	0.12	2.73	10	S
17271	00	A	Destruction, malignant lesion, any method, scalp, neck, hands, feet, genitalia; lesion diameter 0.6 to 1.0 cm	1.44	1.75	0.16	3.35	10	S
17272	00	A	Destruction, malignant lesion, any method, scalp, neck, hands, feet, genitalia; lesion diameter 1.1 to 2.0 cm	1.72	2.20	0.19	4.11	10	S
17273	00	A	Destruction, malignant lesion, any method, scalp, neck, hands, feet, genitalia; lesion diameter 2.1 to 3.0 cm	2.00	2.58	0.25	4.83	10	S
17274	00	A	Destruction, malignant lesion, any method, scalp, neck, hands, feet, genitalia; lesion diameter 3.1 to 4.0 cm	2.54	3.21	0.32	6.07	10	S
17276	00	A	Destruction, malignant lesion, any method, scalp, neck, hands, feet, genitalia; lesion diameter over 4.0 cm	3.15	3.41	0.51	7.07	10	S
17280	00	A	Destruction, malignant lesion, any method, face, ears, eyelids, nose, lips, mucous membrane; lesion diameter 0.5 cm or less	1.12	1.65	0.15	2.92	10	S
17281	00	A	Destruction, malignant lesion, any method, face, ears, eyelids, nose, lips, mucous membrane; lesion diameter 0.6 to 1.0 cm	1.67	2.09	0.18	3.94	10	S
17282	00	A	Destruction, malignant lesion, any method, face, ears, eyelids, nose, lips, mucous membrane; lesion diameter 1.1 to 2.0 cm	1.99	2.57	0.23	4.79	10	S

CPT codes and descriptions only, © 1994 American Medical Association. Reimbursement information, © 1995 McGraw-Hill Inc.

Code/ CPT	Mod- ifier	Status	Description	Work value	Practice expense	Mal- practice	Total value	Global period	Up- date
17283	00	A	Destruction, malignant lesion, any method, face, ears, eyelids, nose, lips, mucous membrane; lesion diameter 2.1 to 3.0 cm	2.59	3.01	0.28	5.88	10	S
17284	00	A	Destruction, malignant lesion, any method, face, ears, eyelids, nose, lips, mucous membrane; lesion diameter 3.1 to 4.0 cm	3.16	3.51	0.33	7.00	10	S
17286	00	A	Destruction, malignant lesion, any method, face, ears, eyelids, nose, lips, mucous membrane; lesion diameter over 4.0 cm	4.39	4.32	0.60	9.31	10	S
17304	00	A	Chemosurgery (Mohs' micrographic technique), including removal of all gross tumor, surgical excision of tissue specimens, mapping, color coding of specimens, microscopic examination of specimens by the surgeon, and complete histopathologic preparation; first stage, fresh tissue technique, up to 5 specimens	7.60	4.02	0.31	11.93	0	S
17305	00	A	Chemosurgery (Mohs' micrographic technique), including removal of all gross tumor, surgical excision of tissue specimens, mapping, color coding of specimens, microscopic examination of specimens by the surgeon, and complete histopathologic preparation; second stage, fixed or fresh tissue, up to 5 specimens	2.85	2.26	0.17	5.28	0	S
17306	00	A	Chemosurgery (Mohs' micrographic technique), including removal of all gross tumor, surgical excision of tissue specimens, mapping, color coding of specimens, microscopic examination of specimens by the surgeon, and complete histopathologic preparation; third stage, fixed or fresh tissue, up to 5 specimens	2.85	1.40	0.11	4.36	0	S
17307	00	A	Chemosurgery (Mohs' micrographic technique), including removal of all gross tumor, surgical excision of tissue specimens, mapping, color coding of specimens, microscopic examination of specimens by the surgeon, and complete histopathologic preparation; additional stage(s), up to 5 specimens, each stage	2.85	1.47	0.12	4.44	0	S
17310	00	A	Chemosurgery (Mohs' micrographic technique), including removal of all gross tumor, surgical excision of tissue specimens, mapping, color coding of specimens, microscopic examination of specimens by the surgeon, and complete histopathologic preparation; more than 5 specimens, fixed or fresh tissue, any stage	0.95	0.13	0.01	1.09	0	S
17340	00	A	Cryotherapy (CO_2 slush, liquid N_2) for acne	0.73	0.28	0.02	1.03	10	S
17360	00	A	Chemical exfoliation for acne (eg, acne paste, acid)	1.40	0.27	0.02	1.69	10	S
17380	00	R	Electrolysis epilation, each ½ hour	0.49*	0.35#	0.03*	0.87#	XXX	S
17999	00	C	Unlisted procedure, skin, mucous membrane and subcutaneous tissue	0	0	0	0	YYY	S
19000	00	A	Puncture aspiration of cyst of breast;	0.84	0.38	0.07	1.29	0	S
19001	00	A	Puncture aspiration of cyst of breast; each additional cyst	0.42	0.24	0.05	0.71	ZZZ	S
19020	00	A	Mastotomy with exploration or drainage of abscess, deep	3.37	1.40	0.28	5.05	90	S
19030	00	A	Injection procedure only for mammary ductogram or galactogram	1.53	0.49	0.04	2.06	0	N
19100	00	A	Biopsy of breast; needle core (separate procedure)	1.27	0.64	0.13	2.04	0	S
19101	00	A	Biopsy of breast; incisional	3.13	2.34	0.45	5.92	10	S
19110	00	A	Nipple exploration, with or without excision of a solitary lactiferous duct or a papilloma lactiferous duct	4.15	2.46	0.51	7.12	90	S
19112	00	A	Excision of lactiferous duct fistula	3.52	2.34	0.35	6.21	90	S

CPT codes and descriptions only, © 1994 American Medical Association. Reimbursement information, © 1995 McGraw-Hill Inc.

Code/ CPT	Mod-ifier	Status	Description	Work value	Practice expense	Mal-practice	Total value	Global period	Up-date
19120	00	A	Excision of cyst, fibroadenoma, or other benign or malignant tumor aberrant breast tissue, duct lesion or nipple lesion (except 19140), male or female, one or more lesions	4.84	2.90	0.60	8.34	90	S
19125	00	A	Excision of breast lesion identified by pre-operative placement of radiological marker; single lesion	5.85	2.90	0.60	9.35	0	S
19126	00	A	Excision of breast lesion identified by pre-operative placement of radiological marker; each additional lesion separately identified by a radiological marker	2.93	1.45	0.31	4.69	ZZZ	S
19140	00	A	Mastectomy for gynecomastia	4.90	4.29	0.91	10.10	90	S
19160	00	A	Mastectomy, partial;	6.65	4.13	0.88	11.66	90	S
19162	00	A	Mastectomy, partial; with axillary lymphadenectomy	12.81	9.38	1.96	24.15	90	S
19180	00	A	Mastectomy, simple, complete	8.15	5.61	1.17	14.93	90	S
19182	00	A	Mastectomy, subcutaneous	7.28	6.07	1.27	14.62	90	S
19200	00	A	Mastectomy, radical, including pectoral muscles, axillary lymph nodes	14.23	10.22	2.15	26.60	90	S
19220	00	A	Mastectomy, radical, including pectoral muscles, axillary and internal mammary lymph nodes (Urban type operation)	14.23	10.73	2.38	27.34	90	S
19240	00	A	Mastectomy, modified radical, including axillary lymph nodes, with or without pectoralis minor muscle, but excluding pectoralis major muscle	14.71	9.44	1.99	26.14	90	S
19260	00	A	Excision of chest wall tumor including ribs	13.91	5.05	1.04	20.00	90	S
19271	00	A	Excision of chest wall tumor involving ribs, with plastic reconstruction; without mediastinal lymphadenectomy	17.07	13.95	2.77	33.79	90	S
19272	00	A	Excision of chest wall tumor involving ribs, with plastic reconstruction; with mediastinal lymphadenectomy	19.47	12.60	2.56	34.63	90	S
19290	00	A	Preoperative placement of needle localization wire, breast;	1.27	0.44	0.07	1.78	0	S
19291	00	A	Preoperative placement of needle localization wire, breast; each additional lesion	0.63	0.25	0.04	0.92	ZZZ	S
19316	00	A	Mastopexy	10.07	12.84	2.43	25.34	90	S
19318	00	A	Reduction mammaplasty	11.08	14.18	3.23	28.49	90	S
19324	00	A	Mammaplasty, augmentation; without prosthetic implant	5.55	3.29	0.67	9.51	90	S
19325	00	A	Mammaplasty, augmentation; with prosthetic implant	8.05	5.87	1.13	15.05	90	S
19328	00	A	Removal of intact mammary implant	5.32	3.76	0.73	9.81	90	S
19330	00	A	Removal of mammary implant material	7.18	3.88	0.75	11.81	90	S
19340	00	A	Immediate insertion of breast prosthesis following mastopexy, mastectomy or in reconstruction	6.33	8.61	2.06	17.00	ZZZ	S
19342	00	A	Delayed insertion of breast prosthesis following mastopexy, mastectomy or in reconstruction	10.64	10.81	2.03	23.48	90	S
19350	00	A	Nipple/areola reconstruction	8.21	7.08	1.38	16.67	90	S
19355	00	A	Correction of inverted nipples	7.27	4.93	1.00	13.20	90	S
19357	00	A	Breast reconstruction, immediate or delayed, with tissue expander, including subsequent expansion	16.72	12.15	2.37	31.24	90	S
19361	00	A	Breast reconstruction with latissimus dorsi flap, with or without prosthetic implant	17.82	20.13	3.88	41.83	90	S
19362	00	D	Breast reconstruction	31.65*	23.01#	4.50*	59.16#	90	S
19364	00	A	Breast reconstruction with free flap	27.60	16.68	3.58	47.86	90	S
19366	00	A	Breast reconstruction with other technique	19.84	16.40	3.18	39.42	90	S
19367	00	A	Breast reconstruction with transverse rectus abdominis myocutaneous flap (TRAM), single pedicle, including closure of donor site;	24.73	20.13	3.88	48.74	90	S

CPT codes and descriptions only, © 1994 American Medical Association. Reimbursement information, © 1995 McGraw-Hill Inc.

Code/ CPT	Mod-ifier	Status	Description	Work value	Practice expense	Mal-practice	Total value	Global period	Up-date
19368	00	A	Breast reconstruction with transverse rectus abdominis myocutaneous flap (TRAM), single pedicle, including closure of donor site; with microvascular anastomosis (supercharging)	31.15	20.13	3.88	55.16	90	S
19369	00	A	Breast reconstruction with transverse rectus abdominis myocutaneous flap (TRAM), double pedicle, including closure of donor site	28.68	20.13	3.88	52.69	90	S
19370	00	A	Open periprosthetic capsulotomy, breast	7.59	6.17	1.19	14.95	90	S
19371	00	A	Periprosthetic capsulectomy, breast	8.84	7.91	1.54	18.29	90	S
19380	00	A	Revision of reconstructed breast	8.63	8.11	1.57	18.31	90	S
19396	00	A	Preparation of moulage for custom breast implant	2.17	1.57	0.31	4.05	0	S
19499	00	C	Unlisted procedure, breast	0	0	0	0	YYY	S
20000	00	A	Incision of soft tissue abscess (eg, secondary to osteomyelitis); superficial	1.85	0.85	0.08	2.78	10	S
20005	00	A	Incision of soft tissue abscess (eg, secondary to osteomyelitis); deep or complicated	3.02	1.83	0.28	5.13	10	S
20200	00	A	Biopsy, muscle; superficial	1.46	1.12	0.18	2.76	0	S
20205	00	A	Biopsy, muscle; deep	2.35	1.88	0.33	4.56	0	S
20206	00	A	Biopsy, muscle, percutaneous needle	0.99	0.96	0.14	2.09	0	S
20220	00	A	Biopsy, bone, trocar, or needle; superficial (eg, ilium, sternum, spinous process, ribs)	1.27	1.31	0.09	2.67	0	N
20225	00	A	Biopsy, bone, trocar, or needle; deep (vertebral body, femur)	1.87	2.39	0.28	4.54	0	N
20240	00	A	Biopsy, excisional; superficial (eg, ilium, sternum, spinous process, ribs, trochanter of femur)	3.07	1.88	0.18	5.13	10	S
20245	00	A	Biopsy, excisional; deep (eg, humerus, ischium, femur)	3.68	3.58	0.44	7.70	10	S
20250	00	A	Biopsy, vertebral body, open; thoracic	4.63	5.07	0.76	10.46	10	S
20251	00	A	Biopsy, vertebral body, open; lumbar or cervical	5.16	5.84	0.92	11.92	10	S
20500	00	A	Injection of sinus tract; therapeutic (separate procedure)	1.18	0.36	0.04	1.58	10	N
20501	00	A	Injection of sinus tract; diagnostic (sinogram)	0.76	0.30	0.02	1.08	0	N
20520	00	A	Removal of foreign body in muscle or tendon sheath; simple	1.80	0.71	0.08	2.59	10	S
20525	00	A	Removal of foreign body in muscle or tendon sheath; deep or complicated	3.23	2.23	0.33	5.79	10	S
20550	00	A	Injection, tendon sheath, ligament, trigger points or ganglion cyst	0.86	0.38	0.04	1.28	0	N
20600	00	A	Arthrocentesis, aspiration and/or injection; small joint, bursa or ganglion cyst (eg, fingers, toes)	0.66	0.47	0.05	1.18	0	S
20605	00	A	Arthrocentesis, aspiration and/or injection; intermediate joint, bursa or ganglion cyst (eg, temporomandibular, acromioclavicular, wrist, elbow or ankle, olecranon bursa)	0.68	0.45	0.05	1.18	0	S
20610	00	A	Arthrocentesis, aspiration and/or injection; major joint or bursa (eg, shoulder, hip, knee joint, subacromial bursa)	0.79	0.45	0.05	1.29	0	N
20615	00	A	Aspiration and injection for treatment of bone cyst	2.23	0.49	0.06	2.78	10	N
20650	00	A	Insertion of wire or pin with application of skeletal traction, including removal (separate procedure)	2.07	1.08	0.14	3.29	10	S
20660	00	A	Application of cranial tongs, caliper, or stereotactic frame, including removal (separate procedure)	2.51	1.56	0.21	4.28	0	S
20661	00	A	Application of halo, including removal; cranial	4.27	3.82	0.65	8.74	90	S
20662	00	A	Application of halo, including removal; pelvic	5.52	6.54	1.03	13.09	90	S
20663	00	A	Application of halo, including removal; femoral	4.88	4.64	0.76	10.28	90	S
20665	00	A	Removal of tongs or halo applied by another physician	1.26	0.50	0.07	1.83	10	S
20670	00	A	Removal of implant; superficial, (eg, buried wire, pin or rod) (separate procedure)	1.69	0.74	0.11	2.54	10	S

CPT codes and descriptions only, © 1994 American Medical Association. Reimbursement information, © 1995 McGraw-Hill Inc.

Code/ CPT	Mod- ifier	Status	Description	Work value	Practice expense	Mal- practice	Total value	Global period	Up- date
20680	00	A	Removal of implant; deep (eg, buried wire, pin, screw, metal band, nail, rod or plate)	3.25	3.33	0.51	7.09	90	S
20690	00	A	Application of a uniplane (pins or wires in one plane), unilateral, external fixation system	3.52	3.66	0.58	7.76	ZZZ	S
20692	00	A	Application of a multiplane (pins or wires in more than one plane), unilateral, external fixation system (eg, Ilizarov, Monticelli type)	6.41	5.51	0.89	12.81	ZZZ	S
20693	00	A	Adjustment or revision of external fixation system requiring anesthesia (eg, new pin(s) or wire(s) and/or new ring(s) or bar(s))	5.42	2.49	0.42	8.33	90	S
20694	00	A	Removal, under anesthesia, of external fixation system	3.81	2.60	0.41	6.82	90	S
20802	00	A	Replantation, arm (includes surgical neck of humerus through elbow joint); complete amputation	39.56	37.72	6.17	83.45	90	S
20804	00	C	Replantation, arm (includes surgical neck of humerus through elbow joint); incomplete amputation (devascularized extremity with soft tissue pedicle)	0	0	0	0	90	S
20805	00	A	Replantation, forearm (includes radius and ulna to radial carpal joint); complete amputation	48.41	46.17	7.56	102.14	90	S
20806	00	C	Replantation, forearm (includes radius and ulna to radial carpal joint); incomplete amputation (devascularized extremity with soft tissue pedicle)	0	0	0	0	90	S
20808	00	A	Replantation, hand (includes hand through metacarpophalangeal joints); complete amputation	60.19	57.40	9.40	126.99	90	S
20812	00	C	Replantation, hand (includes hand through metacarpophalangeal joints); incomplete amputation (devascularized extremity with soft tissue pedicle)	0	0	0	0	90	S
20816	00	A	Replantation, digit, excluding thumb (includes metacarpophalangeal joint to insertion of flexor sublimis tendon); complete amputation	29.67	28.30	4.63	62.60	90	S
20820	00	C	Replantation, digit, excluding thumb (includes metacarpophalangeal joint to insertion of flexor sublimis tendon); incomplete amputation (devascularized extremity with soft tissue pedicle)	0	0	0	0	90	S
20822	00	A	Replantation, digit, excluding thumb (includes distal tip to sublimis tendon insertion); complete amputation	24.53	23.39	3.83	51.75	90	S
20823	00	C	Replantation, digit, excluding thumb (includes distal tip to sublimis tendon insertion); incomplete amputation (devascularized extremity with soft tissue pedicle)	0	0	0	0	90	S
20824	00	A	Replantation, thumb (includes carpometacarpal joint to MP joint); complete amputation	29.67	28.30	4.63	62.60	90	S
20826	00	C	Replantation, thumb (includes carpometacarpal joint to MP joint); incomplete amputation (devascularized extremity with soft tissue pedicle)	0	0	0	0	90	S
20827	00	A	Replantation, thumb (includes distal tip to MP joint); complete amputation	25.22	24.05	3.94	53.21	90	S
20828	00	C	Replantation, thumb (includes distal tip to MP joint); incomplete amputation (devascularized extremity with soft tissue pedicle)	0	0	0	0	90	S
20832	00	C	Replantation, leg; complete amputation	49.24*	46.95#	7.69*	103.88#	90	S
20834	00	C	Replantation, leg; incomplete amputation (devascularized extremity with soft tissue pedicle)	0	0	0	0	90	S
20838	00	A	Replantation, foot; complete amputation	39.56	37.72	6.17	83.45	90	S
20840	00	C	Replantation, foot; incomplete amputation (devascularized extremity with soft tissue pedicle)	0	0	0	0	90	S
20900	00	A	Bone graft, any donor area; minor or small (eg, dowel or button)	5.03	2.80	0.45	8.28	90	S

CPT codes and descriptions only, © 1994 American Medical Association. Reimbursement information, © 1995 McGraw-Hill Inc.

Code/ CPT	Mod-ifier	Status	Description	Work value	Practice expense	Mal-practice	Total value	Global period	Up-date
21300	00	A	Closed treatment of skull fracture without operation	0.72	1.05	0.11	1.88	0	S
21310	00	A	Closed treatment of nasal bone fracture without manipulation	0.58	0.76	0.09	1.43	0	N
21315	00	A	Closed treatment of nasal bone fracture; without stabilization	1.41	1.81	0.21	3.43	10	S
21320	00	A	Closed treatment of nasal bone fracture; with stabilization	1.82	2.33	0.34	4.49	10	S
21325	00	A	Open treatment of nasal fracture; uncomplicated	3.52	4.09	0.52	8.13	90	S
21330	00	A	Open treatment of nasal fracture; complicated, with internal and/or external skeletal fixation	5.03	6.45	0.86	12.34	90	S
21335	00	A	Open treatment of nasal fracture; with concomitant open treatment of fractured septum	8.05	10.50	1.56	20.11	90	S
21336	00	A	Open treatment of nasal septal fracture, with or without stabilization	5.35	4.09	0.52	9.96	90	S
21337	00	A	Closed treatment of nasal septal fracture, with or without stabilization	2.52	2.82	0.38	5.72	90	S
21338	00	A	Open treatment of nasoethmoid fracture; without external fixation	6.04	5.01	0.66	11.71	90	S
21339	00	A	Open treatment of nasoethmoid fracture; with external fixation	7.56	7.09	0.70	15.35	90	S
21340	00	A	Percutaneous treatment of nasoethmoid complex fracture, with splint, wire or headcap fixation, including repair of canthal ligaments and/or the nasolacrimal apparatus	10.07	8.91	1.04	20.02	90	S
21343	00	A	Open treatment of depressed frontal sinus fracture	12.10	9.17	1.08	22.35	90	S
21344	00	A	Open treatment of complicated (eg, comminuted or involving posterior wall) frontal sinus fracture, via coronal or multiple approaches	18.43	9.17	1.08	28.68	90	S
21345	00	A	Closed treatment of nasomaxillary complex fracture (LeFort II type), with interdental wire fixation or fixation of denture or splint	7.63	7.90	0.81	16.34	90	S
21346	00	A	Open treatment of nasomaxillary complex fracture (LeFort II type); with wiring and/or local fixation	9.92	9.40	1.04	20.36	90	S
21347	00	A	Open treatment of nasomaxillary complex fracture (LeFort II type); requiring multiple open approaches	11.86	10.36	1.36	23.58	90	S
21348	00	A	Open treatment of nasomaxillary complex fracture (LeFort II type); with bone grafting (includes obtaining graft)	15.60	11.34	2.22	29.16	90	S
21355	00	A	Percutaneous treatment of fracture of malar area, including zygomatic arch and malar tripod, with manipulation	3.52	1.56	0.17	5.25	10	S
21356	00	A	Open treatment of depressed zygomatic arch fracture (eg, Gilles approach)	3.88	5.58	0.89	10.35	10	S
21360	00	A	Open treatment of depressed malar fracture, including zygomatic arch and malar tripod	6.04	7.28	0.89	14.21	90	S
21365	00	A	Open treatment of complicated (eg, comminuted or involving cranial nerve foramina) fracture(s) of malar area, including zygomatic arch and malar tripod; with internal fixation and multiple surgical approaches	13.97	12.35	1.63	27.95	90	S
21366	00	A	Open treatment of complicated (eg, comminuted or involving cranial nerve foramina) fracture(s) of malar area, including zygomatic arch and malar tripod; with bone grafting (includes obtaining graft)	16.61	12.08	2.36	31.05	90	S
21385	00	A	Open treatment of orbital floor "blowout" fracture; transantral approach (Caldwell-Luc type operation)	8.56	9.59	1.13	19.28	90	S
21386	00	A	Open treatment of orbital floor "blowout" fracture; periorbital approach	8.56	9.07	1.25	18.88	90	S
21387	00	A	Open treatment of orbital floor "blowout" fracture; combined approach	9.07	7.45	0.96	17.48	90	S

CPT codes and descriptions only, © 1994 American Medical Association. Reimbursement information, © 1995 McGraw-Hill Inc.

Code/ CPT	Mod- ifier	Status	Description	Work value	Practice expense	Mal- practice	Total value	Global period	Up- date
21390	00	A	Open treatment of orbital floor "blowout" fracture; periorbital approach, with alloplastic or other implant	9.47	11.89	1.37	22.73	90	S
21395	00	A	Open treatment of orbital floor "blowout" fracture; periorbital approach with bone graft (includes obtaining graft)	11.85	9.63	1.37	22.85	90	S
21400	00	A	Closed treatment of fracture of orbit, except "blowout"; without manipulation	1.31	1.67	0.17	3.15	90	N
21401	00	A	Closed treatment of fracture of orbit, except "blowout"; with manipulation	3.05	2.58	0.32	5.95	90	S
21406	00	A	Open treatment of fracture of orbit, except "blowout"; without implant	6.55	5.21	0.74	12.50	90	S
21407	00	A	Open treatment of fracture of orbit, except "blowout"; with implant	8.05	7.09	0.78	15.92	90	S
21408	00	A	Open treatment of fracture of orbit, except "blowout"; with bone grafting (includes obtaining graft)	11.57	8.49	0.99	21.05	90	S
21421	00	A	Closed treatment of palatal or maxillary fracture (LeFort I type), with interdental wire fixation or fixation of denture or splint	4.80	6.14	0.62	11.56	90	S
21422	00	A	Open treatment of palatal or maxillary fracture (LeFort I type);	7.78	9.80	1.19	18.77	90	S
21423	00	A	Open treatment of palatal or maxillary fracture (LeFort I type); complicated (comminuted or involving cranial nerve foramina), multiple approaches	9.72	9.80	1.19	20.71	90	S
21431	00	A	Closed treatment of craniofacial separation (LeFort III type) using interdental wire fixation of denture or splint	6.59	6.02	0.71	13.32	90	S
21432	00	A	Open treatment of craniofacial separation (LeFort III type); with wiring and/or internal fixation	8.05	6.76	0.84	15.65	90	S
21433	00	A	Open treatment of craniofacial separation (LeFort III type); complicated (eg, comminuted or involving cranial nerve foramina), multiple surgical approaches	23.69	17.96	2.10	43.75	90	S
21435	00	A	Open treatment of craniofacial separation (LeFort III type); complicated, utilizing internal and/or external fixation techniques (eg, head cap, halo device, and/or intermaxillary fixation)	16.12	13.25	1.88	31.25	90	S
21436	00	A	Open treatment of craniofacial separation (LeFort III type); complicated, multiple surgical approaches, internal fixation, with bone grafting (includes obtaining graft)	26.21	14.65	2.08	42.94	90	S
21440	00	A	Closed treatment of mandibular or maxillary alveolar ridge fracture (separate procedure)	2.52	3.07	0.28	5.87	90	S
21445	00	A	Open treatment of mandibular or maxillary alveolar ridge fracture (separate procedure)	5.03	6.11	0.56	11.70	90	S
21450	00	A	Closed treatment of mandibular fracture; without manipulation	2.78	2.84	0.26	5.88	90	S
21451	00	A	Closed treatment of mandibular fracture; with manipulation	4.55	6.05	0.74	11.34	90	S
21452	00	A	Percutaneous treatment of mandibular fracture, with external fixation	1.85	1.39	0.17	3.41	90	S
21453	00	A	Closed treatment of mandibular fracture with interdental fixation	5.18	6.64	0.55	12.37	90	S
21454	00	A	Open treatment of mandibular fracture with external fixation	6.04	10.34	1.42	17.80	90	S
21461	00	A	Open treatment of mandibular fracture; without interdental fixation	7.56	10.12	1.30	18.98	90	S
21462	00	A	Open treatment of mandibular fracture; with interdental fixation	9.15	11.71	1.34	22.20	90	S
21465	00	A	Open treatment of mandibular condylar fracture	11.13	8.44	0.99	20.56	90	S

CPT codes and descriptions only, © 1994 American Medical Association. Reimbursement information, © 1995 McGraw-Hill Inc.

Code/ CPT	Mod- ifier	Status	Description	Work value	Practice expense	Mal- practice	Total value	Global period	Up- date
21470	00	A	Open treatment of complicated mandibular fracture by multiple surgical approaches including internal fixation, interdental fixation, and/or wiring of dentures or splints	14.19	17.13	1.74	33.06	90	S
21480	00	A	Closed treatment of temporomandibular dislocation; initial or subsequent	0.61	0.83	0.09	1.53	0	S
21485	00	A	Closed treatment of temporomandibular dislocation; complicated (eg, recurrent requiring intermaxillary fixation or splinting), initial or subsequent	3.73	2.19	0.20	6.12	90	S
21490	00	A	Open treatment of temporomandibular dislocation	11.08	6.31	0.52	17.91	90	S
21493	00	A	Closed treatment of hyoid fracture; without manipulation	1.19	1.52	0.13	2.84	90	S
21494	00	A	Closed treatment of hyoid fracture; with manipulation	5.87	7.52	0.63	14.02	90	S
21495	00	A	Open treatment of hyoid fracture	5.32	4.82	0.51	10.65	90	S
21497	00	A	Interdental wiring, for condition other than fracture	3.61	3.97	0.38	7.96	90	S
21499	00	C	Unlisted musculoskeletal procedure, head	0	0	0	0	YYY	S
21501	00	A	Incision and drainage, deep abscess or hematoma, soft tissues of neck or thorax;	3.52	1.82	0.26	5.60	90	S
21502	00	A	Incision and drainage, deep abscess or hematoma, soft tissues of neck or thorax; with partial rib ostectomy	6.44	4.22	0.75	11.41	90	S
21510	00	A	Incision, deep, with opening of bone cortex (eg, for osteomyelitis or bone abscess), thorax	5.03	3.82	0.50	9.35	90	S
21550	00	A	Biopsy, soft tissue of neck or thorax	2.01	0.85	0.12	2.98	10	S
21555	00	A	Excision tumor, soft tissue of neck or thorax; subcutaneous	4.09	1.60	0.25	5.94	90	S
21556	00	A	Excision tumor, soft tissue of neck or thorax; deep, subfascial, intramuscular	5.28	3.80	0.64	9.72	90	S
21557	00	A	Radical resection of tumor (eg, malignant neoplasm), soft tissue of neck or thorax	8.56	8.50	1.41	18.47	90	S
21600	00	A	Excision of rib, partial	6.27	4.50	0.88	11.65	90	S
21610	00	A	Costotransversectomy (separate procedure)	8.54	5.17	0.76	14.47	90	S
21615	00	A	Excision first and/or cervical rib;	9.03	10.13	1.96	21.12	90	S
21616	00	A	Excision first and/or cervical rib; with sympathectomy	11.11	7.26	1.50	19.87	90	S
21620	00	A	Ostectomy of sternum, partial	6.04	6.85	1.23	14.12	90	S
21627	00	A	Sternal debridement	6.06	5.03	0.90	11.99	90	S
21630	00	A	Radical resection of sternum;	15.77	12.89	2.40	31.06	90	S
21632	00	A	Radical resection of sternum; with mediastinal lymphadenectomy	16.62	11.54	2.22	30.38	90	S
21633	00	D	Extensive sternum surgery	14.07*	13.42#	2.20*	29.69#	90	S
21700	00	A	Division of scalenus anticus; without resection of cervical rib	5.84	4.16	0.50	10.50	90	S
21705	00	A	Division of scalenus anticus; with resection of cervical rib	9.03	4.85	0.96	14.84	90	S
21720	00	A	Division of sternocleidomastoid for torticollis, open operation; without cast application	5.44	3.84	0.52	9.80	90	S
21725	00	A	Division of sternocleidomastoid for torticollis, open operation; with cast application	6.55	4.84	0.74	12.13	90	S
21740	00	A	Reconstructive repair of pectus excavatum or carinatum	15.42	8.99	1.64	26.05	90	S
21750	00	A	Closure of sternotomy separation with or without debridement (separate procedure)	10.07	7.33	1.43	18.83	90	S
21800	00	A	Closed treatment of rib fracture, uncomplicated, each	0.91	0.77	0.07	1.75	90	N
21805	00	A	Open treatment of rib fracture without fixation, each	2.62	1.35	0.17	4.14	90	S
21810	00	A	Treatment of rib fracture requiring external fixation ("flail chest")	6.68	7.33	0.61	14.62	90	N
21820	00	A	Closed treatment of sternum fracture	1.20	1.36	0.17	2.73	90	S
21825	00	A	Open treatment of sternum fracture with or without skeletal fixation	6.82	6.90	1.12	14.84	90	S

CPT codes and descriptions only, © 1994 American Medical Association. Reimbursement information, © 1995 McGraw-Hill Inc.

Code/ CPT	Mod- ifier	Status	Description	Work value	Practice expense	Mal- practice	Total value	Global period	Up- date
21899	00	C	Unlisted procedure, neck or thorax	0	0	0	0	YYY	S
21920	00	A	Biopsy, soft tissue of back or flank; superficial	2.01	0.79	0.11	2.91	10	S
21925	00	A	Biopsy, soft tissue of back or flank; deep	4.23	1.95	0.32	6.50	90	S
21930	00	A	Excision, tumor, soft tissue of back or flank	6.55	2.72	0.49	9.76	90	S
21935	00	A	Radical resection of tumor (eg, malignant neoplasm), soft tissue of back or flank	17.12	6.59	1.30	25.01	90	S
22100	00	A	Partial resection of vertebral component, spinous processes; cervical	8.19	6.37	0.83	15.39	90	S
22101	00	A	Partial resection of vertebral component, spinous processes; thoracic	8.19	6.57	1.19	15.95	90	S
22102	00	A	Partial resection of vertebral component, spinous processes; lumbar	8.78	4.38	0.62	13.78	90	S
22105	00	A	Partial resection of vertebral component for tumor (eg, partial facetectomy, without primary grafting); cervical	13.02	10.77	1.72	25.51	90	S
22106	00	A	Partial resection of vertebral component for tumor (eg, partial facetectomy, without primary grafting); thoracic	11.59	9.24	1.53	22.36	90	S
22107	00	A	Partial resection of vertebral component for tumor (eg, partial facetectomy, without primary grafting); lumbar	11.59	4.90	0.84	17.33	90	S
22110	00	A	Partial excision of vertebrae (eg, for osteomyelitis); cervical	11.59	9.72	1.64	22.95	90	S
22112	00	A	Partial excision of vertebrae (eg, for osteomyelitis); thoracic	11.59	9.90	1.63	23.12	90	S
22114	00	A	Partial excision of vertebrae (eg, for osteomyelitis); lumbar	11.59	7.25	1.17	20.01	90	S
22140	00	A	Reconstruction of spine with bone graft (autograft, allograft) and/or methylmethacrylate following resection of single vertebral body; cervical	22.19	16.92	2.73	41.84	90	S
22141	00	A	Reconstruction of spine with bone graft (autograft, allograft) and/or methylmethacrylate following resection of single vertebral body; thoracic	25.44	17.22	2.78	45.44	90	S
22142	00	A	Reconstruction of spine with bone graft (autograft, allograft) and/or methylmethacrylate following resection of single vertebral body; lumbar	25.44	21.57	3.20	50.21	90	S
22145	00	A	Reconstruction of spine following vertebral body resection, each additional vertebral body	6.71	6.85	1.09	14.65	ZZZ	S
22148	00	A	Harvesting of bone autograft for vertebral reconstruction following vertebral corpectomy	3.02	3.90	0.82	7.74	ZZZ	S
22150	00	A	Reconstruction of spine with prefabricated prosthetic replacement following resection of one or more vertebral bodies; cervical	22.15	17.55	2.76	42.46	90	S
22151	00	A	Reconstruction of spine with prefabricated prosthetic replacement following resection of one or more vertebral bodies; thoracic	22.15	17.64	3.24	43.03	90	S
22152	00	A	Reconstruction of spine with prefabricated prosthetic replacement following resection of one or more vertebral bodies; lumbar	22.15	18.34	3.25	43.74	90	S
22210	00	A	Osteotomy of spine, posterior approach, single segment; cervical	22.51	13.83	2.43	38.77	90	S
22212	00	A	Osteotomy of spine, posterior approach, single segment; thoracic	18.14	17.29	2.83	38.26	90	S
22214	00	A	Osteotomy of spine, posterior approach, single segment; lumbar	18.14	15.11	2.68	35.93	90	S
22220	00	A	Osteotomy of spine, anterior approach, single segment; cervical	20.15	16.64	2.63	39.42	90	S
22222	00	A	Osteotomy of spine, anterior approach, single segment; thoracic	20.15	13.61	1.58	35.34	90	S
22224	00	A	Osteotomy of spine, anterior approach, single segment; lumbar	20.15	14.68	2.66	37.49	90	S

CPT codes and descriptions only, © 1994 American Medical Association. Reimbursement information, © 1995 McGraw-Hill Inc.

Code/ CPT	Mod- ifier	Status	Description	Work value	Practice expense	Mal- practice	Total value	Global period	Up- date
22230	00	A	Osteotomy of spine, any approach, each additional segment	6.04	5.07	0.89	12.00	ZZZ	S
22305	00	A	Closed treatment of vertebral process fracture(s)	1.86	2.38	0.37	4.61	90	S
22310	00	A	Closed treatment of vertebral body fracture(s), without manipulation	1.86	3.19	0.69	5.74	90	S
22315	00	A	Closed treatment of vertebral fracture and/or dislocation requiring casting or bracing, with or without anesthesia, by manipulation or traction, each	8.36	5.51	0.86	14.73	90	S
22325	00	A	Open treatment of vertebral fracture and/or dislocation; lumbar, each	17.19	8.32	1.34	26.85	90	S
22326	00	A	Open treatment of vertebral fracture and/or dislocation; cervical, each	18.43	15.93	2.74	37.10	90	S
22327	00	A	Open treatment of vertebral fracture and/or dislocation; thoracic, each	17.56	15.95	2.35	35.86	90	S
22505	00	A	Manipulation of spine requiring anesthesia, any region	1.77	1.31	0.17	3.25	10	N
22548	00	A	Arthrodesis, anterior transoral or extraoral technique, clivus-C1-C2 (atlas-axis), with bone graft, with or without excision of odontoid process	24.08	22.74	3.82	50.64	90	S
22554	00	A	Arthrodesis, anterior interbody technique; cervical below C2, with bone graft	18.14	19.81	3.52	41.47	90	S
22556	00	A	Arthrodesis, anterior interbody technique; thoracic, with local bone (eg, rib) and/or bone allograft	23.17	21.68	3.58	48.43	90	S
22558	00	A	Arthrodesis, anterior interbody technique; lumbar, with bone graft	22.12	20.17	3.38	45.67	90	S
22585	00	A	Arthrodesis, anterior or anterolateral, each additional interspace (list separately in addition to single level arthrodesis)	5.53	5.40	0.93	11.86	ZZZ	S
22590	00	A	Arthrodesis, posterior technique, craniocervical (occiput-C2), with bone graft and/or internal fixation	18.96	21.57	3.44	43.97	90	S
22595	00	A	Arthrodesis, posterior technique, atlas-axis (C1-C2) with bone graft and/or internal fixation	19.24	22.46	3.87	45.57	90	S
22600	00	A	Arthrodesis, posterior technique, cervical below C2 segment, local bone or bone allograft and/or internal fixation	18.05	19.36	3.32	40.73	90	S
22610	00	A	Arthrodesis, posterior or posterolateral technique, with local bone or bone allograft and/or internal fixation; thoracic	15.11	17.87	2.75	35.73	90	S
22612	00	A	Arthrodesis, posterior or posterolateral technique, with local bone or bone allograft and/or internal fixation; lumbar	22.25	19.22	3.09	44.56	90	S
22625	00	A	Arthrodesis, lateral transverse process technique, with local bone or bone allograft and/or internal wire fixation, lumbar	19.91	21.93	3.56	45.40	90	S
22630	00	A	Arthrodesis, posterior interbody technique, with local bone or bone allograft and/or internal wire fixation, lumbar	20.93	18.44	3.15	42.52	90	S
22650	00	A	Arthrodesis, posterior, posterolateral or lateral transverse process technique, each additional interspace	6.44	5.65	0.92	13.01	ZZZ	S
22800	00	A	Arthrodesis, posterior, for spinal deformity, with or without cast, with bone graft; 6 or less vertebrae	16.92	21.66	3.58	42.16	90	S
22802	00	A	Arthrodesis, posterior, for spinal deformity, with or without cast, with bone graft; 7 or more vertebrae	31.31	28.32	4.61	64.24	90	S
22810	00	A	Arthrodesis, anterior, for spinal deformity, with or without cast, with bone graft; 4 to 7 vertebrae	29.00	18.41	3.15	50.56	90	S
22812	00	A	Arthrodesis, anterior, for spinal deformity, with or without cast, with bone graft; 8 or more vertebrae	27.20	25.93	4.24	57.37	90	S
22820	00	A	Harvesting of bone autograft through separate incision (eg, ilium, fibula) for spinal arthrodesis	2.79	3.64	0.74	7.17	ZZZ	S

CPT codes and descriptions only, © 1994 American Medical Association. Reimbursement information, © 1995 McGraw-Hill Inc.

Code/ CPT	Mod-ifier	Status	Description	Work value	Practice expense	Mal-practice	Total value	Global period	Up-date
22830	00	A	Exploration of spinal fusion	10.22	13.07	2.18	25.47	90	S
22840	00	A	Posterior instrumentation; without segmental fixation (eg, single Harrington rod technique)	12.54	17.61	3.63	33.78	0	S
22842	00	A	Posterior instrumentation; segmental fixation (eg, pedicle fixation, dual rods with multiple hooks and sublaminal wires)	14.42	19.62	4.02	38.06	0	S
22845	00	A	Anterior instrumentation	12.48	15.97	3.27	31.72	0	S
22849	00	A	Reinsertion of spinal fixation device	12.86	11.76	1.97	26.59	90	S
22850	00	A	Removal of posterior nonsegmental instrumentation (eg, Harrington rod)	8.98	9.17	1.50	19.65	90	S
22852	00	A	Removal of posterior segmental instrumentation	8.40	9.80	1.57	19.77	90	S
22855	00	A	Removal of anterior instrumentation	9.10	7.46	1.25	17.81	90	S
22899	00	C	Unlisted procedure, spine	0	0	0	0	YYY	S
22900	00	A	Excision, abdominal wall tumor, subfascial (eg, desmoid)	6.56	3.03	0.60	10.19	90	S
22999	00	C	Unlisted procedure, abdomen, musculoskeletal system	0	0	0	0	YYY	S
23000	00	A	Removal of subdeltoid (or intratendinous) calcareous deposits, open method	4.12	3.24	0.47	7.83	90	S
23020	00	A	Capsular contracture release (Sever type procedure)	8.25	7.27	1.09	16.61	90	S
23030	00	A	Incision and drainage, shoulder area; deep abscess or hematoma	3.16	2.16	0.35	5.67	10	S
23031	00	A	Incision and drainage, shoulder area; infected bursa	2.69	0.50	0.05	3.24	10	S
23035	00	A	Incision, deep, with opening of cortex (eg, for osteomyelitis or bone abscess), shoulder area	7.80	6.22	1.04	15.06	90	S
23040	00	A	Arthrotomy, glenohumeral joint, for infection, with exploration, drainage or removal of foreign body	8.39	9.27	1.47	19.13	90	S
23044	00	A	Arthrotomy, acromioclavicular, sternoclavicular joint, for infection, with exploration, drainage or removal of foreign body	6.40	6.91	1.18	14.49	90	S
23065	00	A	Biopsy, soft tissue of shoulder area; superficial	2.24	0.66	0.09	2.99	10	S
23066	00	A	Biopsy, soft tissue of shoulder area; deep	4.01	1.18	0.10	5.29	90	S
23075	00	A	Excision, tumor, shoulder area; subcutaneous	2.34	1.68	0.29	4.31	10	S
23076	00	A	Excision, tumor, shoulder area; deep, subfascial or intramuscular	7.12	3.54	0.65	11.31	90	S
23077	00	A	Radical resection of tumor (eg, malignant neoplasm), soft tissue of shoulder area	14.65	7.38	1.38	23.41	90	S
23100	00	A	Arthrotomy with biopsy, glenohumeral joint	5.63	7.20	1.24	14.07	90	S
23101	00	A	Arthrotomy with biopsy, or with excision of torn cartilage, acromioclavicular, sternoclavicular joint	5.21	6.68	1.21	13.10	90	S
23105	00	A	Arthrotomy with synovectomy; glenohumeral joint	7.74	9.91	1.73	19.38	90	S
23106	00	A	Arthrotomy with synovectomy; sternoclavicular joint	5.56	4.75	0.80	11.11	90	S
23107	00	A	Arthrotomy, glenohumeral joint, with joint exploration, with or without removal of loose or foreign body	8.13	9.59	1.60	19.32	90	S
23120	00	A	Claviculectomy; partial	6.65	4.61	0.74	12.00	90	S
23125	00	A	Claviculectomy; total	8.90	8.49	1.27	18.66	90	S
23130	00	A	Acromioplasty or acromionectomy, partial	7.10	7.05	1.14	15.29	90	S
23140	00	A	Excision or curettage of bone cyst or benign tumor of clavicle or scapula;	6.43	4.16	0.73	11.32	90	S
23145	00	A	Excision or curettage of bone cyst or benign tumor of clavicle or scapula; with autograft (includes obtaining graft)	8.54	8.13	1.33	18.00	90	S
23146	00	A	Excision or curettage of bone cyst or benign tumor of clavicle or scapula; with allograft	7.34	5.23	1.01	13.58	90	S
23150	00	A	Excision or curettage of bone cyst or benign tumor of proximal humerus;	7.80	6.64	1.01	15.45	90	S

CPT codes and descriptions only, © 1994 American Medical Association. Reimbursement information, © 1995 McGraw-Hill Inc.

Code/ CPT	Mod- ifier	Status	Description	Work value	Practice expense	Mal- practice	Total value	Global period	Up- date
23616	00	A	Open treatment of proximal humeral (surgical or anatomical neck) fracture, with or without internal or external fixation, with or without repair of tuberosity(-ies); with proximal humeral prosthetic replacement	19.88	22.32	3.54	45.74	90	S
23620	00	A	Closed treatment of greater tuberosity fracture; without manipulation	2.25	2.88	0.46	5.59	90	S
23625	00	A	Closed treatment of greater tuberosity fracture; with manipulation	3.64	3.82	0.60	8.06	90	S
23630	00	A	Open treatment of greater tuberosity fracture, with or without internal or external fixation	6.89	8.82	1.40	17.11	90	S
23650	00	A	Closed treatment of shoulder dislocation, with manipulation; without anesthesia	3.24	2.10	0.24	5.58	90	S
23655	00	A	Closed treatment of shoulder dislocation, with manipulation; requiring anesthesia	4.26	2.93	0.44	7.63	90	S
23660	00	A	Open treatment of acute shoulder dislocation	7.09	9.07	1.40	17.56	90	S
23665	00	A	Closed treatment of shoulder dislocation, with fracture of greater tuberosity, with manipulation	4.16	3.35	0.51	8.02	90	S
23670	00	A	Open treatment of shoulder dislocation, with fracture of greater tuberosity, with or without internal or external fixation	7.44	9.52	1.85	18.81	90	S
23675	00	A	Closed treatment of shoulder dislocation, with surgical or anatomical neck fracture, with manipulation	5.60	3.93	0.61	10.14	90	S
23680	00	A	Open treatment of shoulder dislocation, with surgical or anatomical neck fracture, with or without internal or external fixation	9.44	12.09	2.13	23.66	90	S
23700	00	A	Manipulation under anesthesia, shoulder joint, including application of fixation apparatus (dislocation excluded)	2.47	2.09	0.34	4.90	10	S
23800	00	A	Arthrodesis, shoulder joint; with or without local bone graft	13.32	16.35	2.63	32.30	90	S
23802	00	A	Arthrodesis, shoulder joint; with primary autogenous graft (includes obtaining graft)	14.67	14.07	2.24	30.98	90	S
23900	00	A	Interthoracoscapular amputation (forequarter)	18.40	12.57	2.40	33.37	90	S
23920	00	A	Disarticulation of shoulder;	13.60	13.85	2.54	29.99	90	S
23921	00	A	Disarticulation of shoulder; secondary closure or scar revision	5.03	4.27	0.74	10.04	90	S
23929	00	C	Unlisted procedure, shoulder	0	0	0	0	YYY	S
23930	00	A	Incision and drainage, upper arm or elbow area; deep abscess or hematoma	2.78	1.61	0.24	4.63	10	S
23931	00	A	Incision and drainage, upper arm or elbow area; infected bursa	1.63	0.75	0.11	2.49	10	S
23935	00	A	Incision, deep, with opening of bone cortex (eg, for osteomyelitis or bone abscess), humerus or elbow	5.56	4.69	0.78	11.03	90	S
24000	00	A	Arthrotomy, elbow, for infection, with exploration, drainage or removal of foreign body	5.32	7.10	1.44	13.86	90	S
24006	00	A	Arthrotomy of the elbow, with capsular excision for capsular release (separate procedure)	8.70	7.14	1.17	17.01	90	S
24065	00	A	Biopsy, soft tissue of upper arm or elbow area; superficial	2.03	0.79	0.10	2.92	10	S
24066	00	A	Biopsy, soft tissue of upper arm or elbow area; deep	4.95	2.71	0.41	8.07	90	S
24075	00	A	Excision, tumor, upper arm or elbow area; subcutaneous	3.79	1.98	0.35	6.12	90	S
24076	00	A	Excision, tumor, upper arm or elbow area; deep, subfascial or intramuscular	6.01	3.68	0.67	10.36	90	S
24077	00	A	Radical resection of tumor (eg, malignant neoplasm), soft tissue of upper arm or elbow area	11.18	9.79	1.87	22.84	90	S
24100	00	A	Arthrotomy, elbow; with synovial biopsy only	4.67	4.23	0.69	9.59	90	S
24101	00	A	Arthrotomy, elbow; with joint exploration, with or without biopsy, with or without removal of loose or foreign body	5.84	7.47	1.41	14.72	90	S

CPT codes and descriptions only, © 1994 American Medical Association. Reimbursement information, © 1995 McGraw-Hill Inc.

Code/ CPT	Mod- ifier	Status	Description	Work value	Practice expense	Mal- practice	Total value	Global period	Up- date
24102	00	A	Arthrotomy, elbow; with synovectomy	7.57	9.68	1.81	19.06	90	S
24105	00	A	Excision, olecranon bursa	3.43	3.77	0.63	7.83	90	S
24110	00	A	Excision or curettage of bone cyst or benign tumor, humerus;	7.08	7.69	1.22	15.99	90	S
24115	00	A	Excision or curettage of bone cyst or benign tumor, humerus; with autograft (includes obtaining graft)	8.88	7.68	1.33	17.89	90	S
24116	00	A	Excision or curettage of bone cyst or benign tumor, humerus; with allograft	11.13	9.72	1.47	22.32	90	S
24120	00	A	Excision or curettage of bone cyst or benign tumor of head or neck of radius or olecranon process;	6.36	6.02	0.98	13.36	90	S
24125	00	A	Excision or curettage of bone cyst or benign tumor of head or neck of radius or olecranon process; with autograft (includes obtaining graft)	7.40	5.79	0.61	13.80	90	S
24126	00	A	Excision or curettage of bone cyst or benign tumor of head or neck of radius or olecranon process; with allograft	7.76	7.40	1.21	16.37	90	S
24130	00	A	Excision, radial head	5.96	6.72	1.08	13.76	90	S
24134	00	A	Sequestrectomy (eg, for osteomyelitis or bone abscess), shaft or distal humerus	8.98	8.69	1.24	18.91	90	S
24136	00	A	Sequestrectomy (eg, for osteomyelitis or bone abscess), radial head or neck	7.33	8.78	0.92	17.03	90	S
24138	00	A	Sequestrectomy (eg, for osteomyelitis or bone abscess), olecranon process	7.36	6.39	1.06	14.81	90	S
24140	00	A	Partial excision (craterization, saucerization or diaphysectomy) of bone (eg, for osteomyelitis), humerus	8.56	8.77	1.45	18.78	90	S
24145	00	A	Partial excision (craterization, saucerization or diaphysectomy) of bone (eg, for osteomyelitis), radial head or neck	7.12	6.38	1.03	14.53	90	S
24147	00	A	Partial excision (craterization, saucerization or diaphysectomy) of bone (eg, for osteomyelitis), olecranon process	7.00	6.61	1.08	14.69	90	S
24150	00	A	Radical resection for tumor, shaft or distal humerus;	12.43	14.08	2.24	28.75	90	S
24151	00	A	Radical resection for tumor, shaft or distal humerus; with autograft (includes obtaining graft)	14.65	13.83	2.11	30.59	90	S
24152	00	A	Radical resection for tumor, radial head or neck;	9.51	6.80	1.16	17.47	90	S
24153	00	A	Radical resection for tumor, radial head or neck; with autograft (includes obtaining graft)	10.96	10.44	1.71	23.11	90	S
24155	00	A	Resection of elbow joint (arthrectomy)	11.11	10.75	1.72	23.58	90	S
24160	00	A	Implant removal; elbow joint	7.43	4.84	0.80	13.07	90	S
24164	00	A	Implant removal; radial head	5.79	5.53	0.90	12.22	90	S
24200	00	A	Removal of foreign body, upper arm or elbow area; subcutaneous	1.71	0.56	0.06	2.33	10	N
24201	00	A	Removal of foreign body, upper arm or elbow area; deep	4.30	3.06	0.49	7.85	90	S
24220	00	A	Injection procedure for elbow arthrography	1.31	0.51	0.05	1.87	0	N
24301	00	A	Muscle or tendon transfer, any type, upper arm or elbow, single (excluding 24320-24331)	9.78	7.90	1.23	18.91	90	S
24305	00	A	Tendon lengthening, upper arm or elbow, single, each	7.16	3.08	0.29	10.53	90	S
24310	00	A	Tenotomy, open, elbow to shoulder, single, each	5.72	2.95	0.48	9.15	90	S
24320	00	A	Tenoplasty, with muscle transfer, with or without free graft, elbow to shoulder, single (Seddon-Brookes type procedure)	10.01	9.20	1.29	20.50	90	S
24330	00	A	Flexor-plasty, elbow (eg, Steindler type advancement);	9.18	8.74	1.43	19.35	90	S
24331	00	A	Flexor-plasty, elbow (eg, Steindler type advancement); with extensor advancement	10.10	9.62	1.57	21.29	90	S
24340	00	A	Tenodesis of biceps tendon at elbow (separate procedure)	7.58	7.00	1.13	15.71	90	S

CPT codes and descriptions only, © 1994 American Medical Association. Reimbursement information, © 1995 McGraw-Hill Inc.

Code/ CPT	Mod- ifier	Status	Description	Work value	Practice expense	Mal- practice	Total value	Global period	Up- date
24342	00	A	Reinsertion or repair of ruptured or lacerated biceps or triceps tendon, distal, with or without tendon graft	10.13	10.38	1.76	22.27	90	S
24350	00	A	Fasciotomy, lateral or medial (eg, "tennis elbow" or epicondylitis);	5.05	4.23	0.69	9.97	90	S
24351	00	A	Fasciotomy, lateral or medial (eg, "tennis elbow" or epicondylitis); with extensor origin detachment	5.73	4.57	0.73	11.03	90	S
24352	00	A	Fasciotomy, lateral or medial (eg, "tennis elbow" or epicondylitis); with annular ligament resection	6.14	5.69	0.93	12.76	90	S
24354	00	A	Fasciotomy, lateral or medial (eg, "tennis elbow" or epicondylitis); with stripping	6.19	5.61	0.94	12.74	90	S
24356	00	A	Fasciotomy, lateral or medial (eg, "tennis elbow" or epicondylitis); with partial ostectomy	6.39	7.28	1.18	14.85	90	S
24360	00	A	Arthroplasty, elbow; with membrane	11.76	15.05	2.47	29.28	90	S
24361	00	A	Arthroplasty, elbow; with distal humeral prosthetic replacement	13.50	13.13	2.00	28.63	90	S
24362	00	A	Arthroplasty, elbow; with implant and fascia lata ligament reconstruction	14.41	13.14	0.80	28.35	90	S
24363	00	A	Arthroplasty, elbow; with distal humerus and proximal ulnar prosthetic replacement ("total elbow")	17.66	22.61	4.13	44.40	90	S
24365	00	A	Arthroplasty, radial head;	7.93	7.52	1.19	16.64	90	S
24366	00	A	Arthroplasty, radial head; with implant	8.67	11.05	1.80	21.52	90	S
24400	00	A	Osteotomy, humerus, with or without internal fixation	10.55	8.43	1.37	20.35	90	S
24410	00	A	Multiple osteotomies with realignment on intramedullary rod, humeral shaft (Sofield type procedure)	14.28	14.04	2.06	30.38	90	S
24420	00	A	Osteoplasty, humerus (eg, shortening or lengthening) (excluding 64876)	12.90	12.30	2.01	27.21	90	S
24430	00	A	Repair of nonunion or malunion, humerus; without graft (eg, compression technique)	12.26	14.66	2.34	29.26	90	S
24435	00	A	Repair of nonunion or malunion, humerus; with iliac or other autograft (includes obtaining graft)	12.19	15.61	2.84	30.64	90	S
24470	00	A	Hemiepiphyseal arrest (eg, for cubitus varus or valgus, distal humerus)	8.32	7.92	1.30	17.54	90	S
24495	00	A	Decompression fasciotomy, forearm, with brachial artery exploration	7.59	5.75	1.10	14.44	90	S
24498	00	A	Prophylactic treatment (nailing, pinning, plating or wiring), with or without methylmethacrylate, humerus	11.30	10.37	1.62	23.29	90	S
24500	00	A	Closed treatment of humeral shaft fracture; without manipulation	3.01	2.54	0.36	5.91	90	S
24505	00	A	Closed treatment of humeral shaft fracture; with manipulation, with or without skeletal traction	4.83	4.50	0.71	10.04	90	S
24515	00	A	Open treatment of humeral shaft fracture with plate/screws, with or without cerclage	10.92	9.65	1.54	22.11	90	S
24516	00	A	Open treatment of humeral shaft fracture, with insertion of intramedullary implant, with or without cerclage and/or locking screws	10.92	9.65	1.54	22.11	90	S
24530	00	A	Closed treatment of supracondylar or transcondylar humeral fracture, with or without intercondylar extension; without manipulation	3.30	2.73	0.42	6.45	90	S
24535	00	A	Closed treatment of supracondylar or transcondylar humeral fracture, with or without intercondylar extension; with manipulation, with or without skin or skeletal traction	6.51	4.85	0.78	12.14	90	S
24538	00	A	Percutaneous skeletal fixation of supracondylar or transcondylar humeral fracture, with or without intercondylar extension	8.85	7.98	1.26	18.09	90	S

CPT codes and descriptions only, © 1994 American Medical Association. Reimbursement information, © 1995 McGraw-Hill Inc.

Code/ CPT	Mod- ifier	Status	Description	Work value	Practice expense	Mal- practice	Total value	Global period	Up- date
24545	00	A	Open treatment of humeral supracondylar or transcondylar fracture, with or without internal or external fixation; without intercondylar extension	9.65	9.97	1.59	21.21	90	S
24546	00	A	Open treatment of humeral supracondylar or transcondylar fracture, with or without internal or external fixation; with intercondylar extension	14.66	9.97	1.59	26.22	90	S
24560	00	A	Closed treatment of humeral epicondylar fracture, medial or lateral; without manipulation	2.62	2.16	0.30	5.08	90	S
24565	00	A	Closed treatment of humeral epicondylar fracture, medial or lateral; with manipulation	5.22	3.45	0.54	9.21	90	S
24566	00	A	Percutaneous skeletal fixation of humeral epicondylar fracture, medial or lateral, with manipulation	7.17	6.06	0.96	14.19	90	S
24575	00	A	Open treatment of humeral epicondylar fracture, medial or lateral, with or without internal or external fixation	9.91	7.79	1.24	18.94	90	S
24576	00	A	Closed treatment of humeral condylar fracture, medial or lateral; without manipulation	2.66	2.16	0.33	5.15	90	S
24577	00	A	Closed treatment of humeral condylar fracture, medial or lateral; with manipulation	5.45	4.00	0.61	10.06	90	S
24579	00	A	Open treatment of humeral condylar fracture, medial or lateral, with or without internal or external fixation	10.85	8.37	1.35	20.57	90	S
24582	00	A	Percutaneous skeletal fixation of humeral condylar fracture, medial or lateral, with manipulation	7.83	6.62	1.06	15.51	90	S
24586	00	A	Open treatment of periarticular fracture and/or dislocation of the elbow (fracture distal humerus and proximal ulna and/or proximal radius);	14.37	14.72	2.36	31.45	90	S
24587	00	A	Open treatment of periarticular fracture and/or dislocation of the elbow (fracture distal humerus and proximal ulna and/or proximal radius); with implant arthroplasty	14.26	13.72	2.17	30.15	90	S
24600	00	A	Treatment of closed elbow dislocation; without anesthesia	4.08	1.95	0.26	6.29	90	S
24605	00	A	Treatment of closed elbow dislocation; requiring anesthesia	5.08	2.29	0.37	7.74	90	S
24615	00	A	Open treatment of acute or chronic elbow dislocation	8.76	9.29	1.48	19.53	90	S
24620	00	A	Closed treatment of Monteggia type of fracture dislocation at elbow (fracture proximal end of ulna with dislocation of radial head), with manipulation	6.62	3.78	0.57	10.97	90	S
24635	00	A	Open treatment of Monteggia type of fracture dislocation at elbow (fracture proximal end of ulna with dislocation of radial head), with or without internal or external fixation	12.42	11.06	1.78	25.26	90	S
24640	00	A	Closed treatment of radial head subluxation in child, nursemaid elbow with manipulation	1.15	1.01	0.08	2.24	10	N
24650	00	A	Closed treatment of radial head or neck fracture; without manipulation	2.01	2.25	0.33	4.59	90	S
24655	00	A	Closed treatment of radial head or neck fracture; with manipulation	4.17	3.01	0.45	7.63	90	S
24665	00	A	Open treatment of radial head or neck fracture, with or without internal fixation or radial head excision;	7.69	7.13	1.14	15.96	90	S
24666	00	A	Open treatment of radial head or neck fracture, with or without internal fixation or radial head excision; with radial head prosthetic replacement	8.87	10.27	1.60	20.74	90	S
24670	00	A	Closed treatment of ulnar fracture, proximal end (olecranon process); without manipulation	2.39	1.95	0.27	4.61	90	S
24675	00	A	Closed treatment of ulnar fracture, proximal end (olecranon process); with manipulation	4.52	3.51	0.54	8.57	90	S
24685	00	A	Open treatment of ulnar fracture proximal end (olecranon process), with or without internal or external fixation	8.34	8.40	1.34	18.08	90	S

CPT codes and descriptions only, © 1994 American Medical Association. Reimbursement information, © 1995 McGraw-Hill Inc.

Code/ CPT	Mod- ifier	Status	Description	Work value	Practice expense	Mal- practice	Total value	Global period	Up- date
24800	00	A	Arthrodesis, elbow joint; with or without local autograft or allograft	10.75	10.59	1.55	22.89	90	S
24802	00	A	Arthrodesis, elbow joint; with autograft (includes obtaining graft other than locally obtained)	12.79	12.18	1.99	26.96	90	S
24900	00	A	Amputation, arm through humerus; with primary closure	8.76	7.68	1.39	17.83	90	S
24920	00	A	Amputation, arm through humerus; open, circular (guillotine)	8.69	6.78	1.19	16.66	90	S
24925	00	A	Amputation, arm through humerus; secondary closure or scar revision	6.61	6.27	0.75	13.63	90	S
24930	00	A	Amputation, arm through humerus; re-amputation	9.40	8.16	1.17	18.73	90	S
24931	00	A	Amputation, arm through humerus; with implant	11.71	11.17	1.84	24.72	90	S
24935	00	A	Stump elongation, upper extremity	14.37	13.70	2.24	30.31	90	S
24940	00	C	Cineplasty, upper extremity, complete procedure	10.55*	10.06#	1.65*	22.26#	90	S
24999	00	C	Unlisted procedure, humerus or elbow	0	0	0	0	YYY	S
25000	00	A	Tendon sheath incision; at radial styloid (eg, for deQuervain's disease)	3.20	3.94	0.62	7.76	90	S
25005	00	D	Incision of tendon sheath	3.17*	3.02#	0.50*	6.69#	90	S
25020	00	A	Decompression fasciotomy, forearm and/or wrist; flexor or extensor compartment	5.55	4.35	0.77	10.67	90	S
25023	00	A	Decompression fasciotomy, forearm and/or wrist; with debridement of nonviable muscle and/or nerve	11.80	5.44	0.94	18.18	90	S
25028	00	A	Incision and drainage, forearm and/or wrist; deep abscess or hematoma	4.88	2.06	0.36	7.30	90	S
25031	00	A	Incision and drainage, forearm and/or wrist; infected bursa	3.90	0.66	0.09	4.65	90	S
25035	00	A	Incision, deep, with opening of bone cortex (eg, for osteomyelitis or bone abscess), forearm and/or wrist	6.83	6.30	1.01	14.14	90	S
25040	00	A	Arthrotomy, radiocarpal or midcarpal joint, with exploration, drainage, or removal of foreign body	6.61	5.69	0.90	13.20	90	S
25065	00	A	Biopsy, soft tissue of forearm and/or wrist; superficial	2.39	0.75	0.09	3.23	10	S
25066	00	A	Biopsy, soft tissue of forearm and/or wrist; deep	3.87	1.54	0.22	5.63	90	S
25075	00	A	Excision, tumor, forearm and/or wrist area; subcutaneous	3.61	2.19	0.37	6.17	90	S
25076	00	A	Excision, tumor, forearm and/or wrist area; deep, subfascial or intramuscular	4.77	3.77	0.67	9.21	90	S
25077	00	A	Radical resection of tumor (eg, malignant neoplasm), soft tissue of forearm and/or wrist area	9.25	8.48	1.67	19.40	90	S
25085	00	A	Capsulotomy, wrist (eg, for contracture)	5.13	4.62	0.71	10.46	90	S
25100	00	A	Arthrotomy, wrist joint; with biopsy	3.66	4.69	0.79	9.14	90	S
25101	00	A	Arthrotomy, wrist joint; with joint exploration, with or without biopsy, with or without removal of loose or foreign body	4.43	5.61	0.98	11.02	90	S
25105	00	A	Arthrotomy, wrist joint; with synovectomy	5.56	7.11	1.19	13.86	90	S
25107	00	A	Arthrotomy, distal radioulnar joint for repair of triangular cartilage complex	5.89	5.28	0.89	12.06	90	S
25110	00	A	Excision, lesion of tendon sheath, forearm and/or wrist	3.79	2.80	0.46	7.05	90	S
25111	00	A	Excision of ganglion, wrist (dorsal or volar); primary	3.24	3.22	0.55	7.01	90	S
25112	00	A	Excision of ganglion, wrist (dorsal or volar); recurrent	4.38	3.72	0.66	8.76	90	S
25115	00	A	Radical excision of bursa, synovia of wrist, or forearm tendon sheaths (eg, tenosynovitis, fungus, Tbc, or other granulomas, rheumatoid arthritis); flexors	6.26	7.14	1.23	14.63	90	S
25116	00	A	Radical excision of bursa, synovia of wrist, or forearm tendon sheaths (eg, tenosynovitis, fungus, Tbc, or other granulomas, rheumatoid arthritis); extensors, with or without transposition of dorsal retinaculum	6.44	8.17	1.38	15.99	90	S

CPT codes and descriptions only, © 1994 American Medical Association. Reimbursement information, © 1995 McGraw-Hill Inc.

Code/ CPT	Mod-ifier	Status	Description	Work value	Practice expense	Mal-practice	Total value	Global period	Up-date
25118	00	A	Synovectomy, extensor tendon sheath, wrist, single compartment;	4.11	5.26	1.02	10.39	90	S
25119	00	A	Synovectomy, extensor tendon sheath, wrist, single compartment; with resection of distal ulna	5.64	7.22	1.32	14.18	90	S
25120	00	A	Excision or curettage of bone cyst or benign tumor of radius or ulna (excluding head or neck of radius and olecranon process);	5.70	6.53	1.14	13.37	90	S
25125	00	A	Excision or curettage of bone cyst or benign tumor of radius or ulna (excluding head or neck of radius and olecranon process); with autograft (includes obtaining graft)	7.06	6.84	1.04	14.94	90	S
25126	00	A	Excision or curettage of bone cyst or benign tumor of radius or ulna (excluding head or neck of radius and olecranon process); with allograft	7.13	6.80	1.12	15.05	90	S
25130	00	A	Excision or curettage of bone cyst or benign tumor of carpal bones;	5.08	4.21	0.67	9.96	90	S
25135	00	A	Excision or curettage of bone cyst or benign tumor of carpal bones; with autograft (includes obtaining graft)	6.58	5.46	0.97	13.01	90	S
25136	00	A	Excision or curettage of bone cyst or benign tumor of carpal bones; with allograft	5.68	4.74	0.85	11.27	90	S
25145	00	A	Sequestrectomy (eg, for osteomyelitis or bone abscess), forearm and/or wrist	5.97	5.95	0.75	12.67	90	S
25150	00	A	Partial excision (craterization, saucerization or diaphysectomy) of bone (eg, for osteomyelitis); ulna	6.56	6.67	1.12	14.35	90	S
25151	00	A	Partial excision (craterization, saucerization or diaphysectomy) of bone (eg, for osteomyelitis); radius	6.86	5.75	1.02	13.63	90	S
25170	00	A	Radical resection for tumor, radius or ulna	10.45	9.79	1.51	21.75	90	S
25210	00	A	Carpectomy; one bone	5.55	4.88	0.80	11.23	90	S
25215	00	A	Carpectomy; all bones of proximal row	7.40	8.68	1.42	17.50	90	S
25230	00	A	Radial styloidectomy (separate procedure)	4.86	5.57	0.85	11.28	90	S
25240	00	A	Excision distal ulna partial or complete (eg, Darrach type or matched resection)	4.91	5.30	0.86	11.07	90	S
25246	00	A	Injection procedure for wrist arthrography	1.45	0.50	0.05	2.00	0	N
25248	00	A	Exploration with removal of deep foreign body, forearm or wrist	4.96	2.18	0.37	7.51	90	S
25250	00	A	Removal of wrist prosthesis; (separate procedure)	6.31	5.63	0.91	12.85	90	S
25251	00	A	Removal of wrist prosthesis; complicated, including "total wrist"	9.08	8.25	1.39	18.72	90	S
25260	00	A	Repair, tendon or muscle, flexor, forearm and/or wrist; primary, single, each tendon or muscle	7.33	4.61	0.78	12.72	90	S
25263	00	A	Repair, tendon or muscle, flexor, forearm and/or wrist; secondary, single, each tendon or muscle	7.37	5.77	1.03	14.17	90	S
25265	00	A	Repair, tendon or muscle, flexor, forearm and/or wrist; secondary, with free graft (includes obtaining graft), each tendon or muscle	9.54	7.93	1.41	18.88	90	S
25270	00	A	Repair, tendon or muscle, extensor, forearm and/or wrist; primary, single, each tendon or muscle	5.71	3.36	0.55	9.62	90	S
25272	00	A	Repair, tendon or muscle, extensor, forearm and/or wrist; secondary, single, each tendon or muscle	6.75	3.44	0.54	10.73	90	S
25274	00	A	Repair, tendon or muscle, extensor, secondary, with tendon graft (includes obtaining graft), forearm and/or wrist, each tendon or muscle	8.44	6.62	1.13	16.19	90	S
25280	00	A	Lengthening or shortening of flexor or extensor tendon, forearm and/or wrist, single, each tendon	6.82	4.22	0.69	11.73	90	S
25290	00	A	Tenotomy, open, flexor or extensor tendon, forearm and/or wrist, single, each tendon	5.03	2.47	0.41	7.91	90	S

CPT codes and descriptions only, © 1994 American Medical Association. Reimbursement information, © 1995 McGraw-Hill Inc.

Code/ CPT	Mod- ifier	Status	Description	Work value	Practice expense	Mal- practice	Total value	Global period	Up- date
25295	00	A	Tenolysis, flexor or extensor tendon, forearm and/or wrist, single, each tendon	6.26	3.05	0.52	9.83	90	S
25300	00	A	Tenodesis at wrist; flexors of fingers	8.46	7.36	1.19	17.01	90	S
25301	00	A	Tenodesis at wrist; extensors of fingers	8.09	6.77	1.18	16.04	90	S
25310	00	A	Tendon transplantation or transfer, flexor or extensor, forearm and/or wrist, single; each tendon	7.68	7.14	1.17	15.99	90	S
25312	00	A	Tendon transplantation or transfer, flexor or extensor, forearm and/or wrist, single; with tendon graft(s) (includes obtaining graft), each tendon	9.08	7.63	1.31	18.02	90	S
25315	00	A	Flexor origin slide (eg, for cerebral palsy, Volkmann contracture), forearm and/or wrist;	9.45	8.06	1.34	18.85	90	S
25316	00	A	Flexor origin slide (eg, for cerebral palsy, Volkmann contracture), forearm and/or wrist; with tendon(s) transfer	11.49	10.58	1.78	23.85	90	S
25317	00	D	Revise hand contracture	6.54*	6.24#	1.02*	13.80#	90	S
25318	00	D	Revise hand contracture	7.60*	7.25#	1.19*	16.04#	90	S
25320	00	A	Capsulorrhaphy or reconstruction, wrist, any method (eg, capsulodesis, ligament repair, tendon transfer or graft) (includes synovectomy, capsulotomy and open reduction) for carpal instability	9.89	8.60	1.45	19.94	90	S
25330	00	A	Arthroplasty, wrist;	10.85	9.23	1.50	21.58	90	S
25331	00	A	Arthroplasty, wrist; with implant	12.60	14.66	2.40	29.66	90	S
25332	00	A	Arthroplasty, wrist; pseudarthrosis type with internal fixation	10.83	9.98	1.61	22.42	90	S
25335	00	A	Centralization of wrist on ulna (eg, radial club hand)	12.11	11.41	1.56	25.08	90	S
25337	00	A	Reconstruction for stabilization of unstable distal ulna or distal radioulnar joint, secondary by soft tissue stabilization (eg, tendon transfer, tendon graft or weave, or tenodesis) with or without open reduction of distal radioulnar joint	9.10	8.60	1.45	19.15	90	S
25350	00	A	Osteotomy, radius; distal third	8.23	7.61	1.26	17.10	90	S
25355	00	A	Osteotomy, radius; middle or proximal third	9.55	9.12	1.49	20.16	90	S
25360	00	A	Osteotomy; ulna	7.88	6.41	0.99	15.28	90	S
25365	00	A	Osteotomy; radius and ulna	11.63	10.31	1.57	23.51	90	S
25370	00	A	Multiple osteotomies, with realignment on intramedullary rod (Sofield type procedure); radius OR ulna	12.34	11.76	1.92	26.02	90	S
25375	00	A	Multiple osteotomies, with realignment on intramedullary rod (Sofield type procedure); radius AND ulna	12.27	13.38	0.87	26.52	90	S
25390	00	A	Osteoplasty, radius OR ulna; shortening	9.85	8.82	1.50	20.17	90	S
25391	00	A	Osteoplasty, radius OR ulna; lengthening with autograft	12.75	11.25	1.93	25.93	90	S
25392	00	A	Osteoplasty, radius AND ulna; shortening (excluding 64876)	13.05	12.44	2.04	27.53	90	S
25393	00	A	Osteoplasty, radius AND ulna; lengthening with autograft	14.90	14.21	2.32	31.43	90	S
25400	00	A	Repair of nonunion or malunion, radius OR ulna; without graft (eg, compression technique)	10.30	10.78	1.75	22.83	90	S
25405	00	A	Repair of nonunion or malunion, radius OR ulna; with iliac or other autograft (includes obtaining graft)	13.48	12.42	2.02	27.92	90	S
25415	00	A	Repair of nonunion or malunion, radius AND ulna; without graft (eg, compression technique)	12.64	11.42	1.92	25.98	90	S
25420	00	A	Repair of nonunion or malunion, radius AND ulna; with iliac or other autograft (includes obtaining graft)	15.34	14.70	2.28	32.32	90	S
25425	00	A	Repair of defect with autograft; radius OR ulna	12.44	12.02	1.87	26.33	90	S
25426	00	A	Repair of defect with autograft; radius AND ulna	14.92	11.72	2.13	28.77	90	S
25440	00	A	Repair of nonunion, scaphoid (navicular) bone, with or without radial styloidectomy (includes obtaining graft and necessary fixation)	9.95	9.05	1.50	20.50	90	S

CPT codes and descriptions only, © 1994 American Medical Association. Reimbursement information, © 1995 McGraw-Hill Inc.

Code/ CPT	Mod-ifier	Status	Description	Work value	Practice expense	Mal-practice	Total value	Global period	Up-date
25441	00	A	Arthroplasty with prosthetic replacement; distal radius	12.26	11.36	1.89	25.51	90	S
25442	00	A	Arthroplasty with prosthetic replacement; distal ulna	10.34	7.06	1.22	18.62	90	S
25443	00	A	Arthroplasty with prosthetic replacement; scaphoid (navicular)	9.88	9.38	1.52	20.78	90	S
25444	00	A	Arthroplasty with prosthetic replacement; lunate	10.64	10.14	1.66	22.44	90	S
25445	00	A	Arthroplasty with prosthetic replacement; trapezium	9.27	10.36	1.72	21.35	90	S
25446	00	A	Arthroplasty with prosthetic replacement; distal radius and partial or entire carpus ("total wrist")	15.52	19.86	3.49	38.87	90	S
25447	00	A	Interposition arthroplasty, intercarpal or carpometacarpal joints	9.86	9.65	1.56	21.07	90	S
25449	00	A	Revision of arthroplasty, including removal of implant, wrist joint	13.78	7.84	1.16	22.78	90	S
25450	00	A	Epiphyseal arrest by epiphysiodesis or stapling; distal radius OR ulna	7.67	7.31	1.19	16.17	90	S
25455	00	A	Epiphyseal arrest by epiphysiodesis or stapling; distal radius AND ulna	9.15	8.71	1.42	19.28	90	S
25490	00	A	Prophylactic treatment (nailing, pinning, plating or wiring) with or without methylmethacrylate; radius	9.12	8.69	1.42	19.23	90	S
25491	00	A	Prophylactic treatment (nailing, pinning, plating or wiring) with or without methylmethacrylate; ulna	9.54	9.10	1.49	20.13	90	S
25492	00	A	Prophylactic treatment (nailing, pinning, plating or wiring) with or without methylmethacrylate; radius AND ulna	11.75	11.20	1.84	24.79	90	S
25500	00	A	Closed treatment of radial shaft fracture; without manipulation	2.30	2.33	0.29	4.92	90	S
25505	00	A	Closed treatment of radial shaft fracture; with manipulation	4.96	3.57	0.51	9.04	90	S
25515	00	A	Open treatment of radial shaft fracture, with or without internal or external fixation	8.63	7.63	1.22	17.48	90	S
25520	00	A	Closed treatment of radial shaft fracture, with dislocation of distal radio-ulnar joint (Galeazzi fracture/dislocation)	6.01	5.74	0.94	12.69	90	S
25525	00	A	Open treatment of radial shaft fracture, with internal and/or external fixation and closed treatment of dislocation of distal radio-ulnar joint (Galeazzi fracture/dislocation), with or without percutaneous skeletal fixation	11.69	11.15	1.83	24.67	90	S
25526	00	A	Open treatment of radial shaft fracture, with internal and/or external fixation and open treatment, with or without internal or external fixation of distal radio-ulnar joint (Galeazzi fracture/dislocation), includes repair of triangular cartilage	12.43	11.85	1.94	26.22	90	S
25530	00	A	Closed treatment of ulnar shaft fracture; without manipulation	1.94	2.44	0.35	4.73	90	S
25535	00	A	Closed treatment of ulnar shaft fracture; with manipulation	4.91	3.57	0.54	9.02	90	S
25545	00	A	Open treatment of ulnar shaft fracture, with or without internal or external fixation	8.35	7.58	1.20	17.13	90	S
25560	00	A	Closed treatment of radial and ulnar shaft fractures; without manipulation	2.29	2.27	0.27	4.83	90	S
25565	00	A	Closed treatment of radial and ulnar shaft fractures; with manipulation	5.29	4.66	0.70	10.65	90	S
25574	00	A	Open treatment of radial AND ulnar shaft fractures, with internal or external fixation; of radius or ulna	6.03	8.37	1.73	16.13	90	S
25575	00	A	Open treatment of radial AND ulnar shaft fractures, with internal or external fixation; of radius AND ulna	9.47	10.70	1.73	21.90	90	S
25600	00	A	Closed treatment of distal radial fracture (eg, Colles or Smith type) or epiphyseal separation, with or without fracture of ulnar styloid; without manipulation	2.48	2.84	0.42	5.74	90	S

CPT codes and descriptions only, © 1994 American Medical Association. Reimbursement information, © 1995 McGraw-Hill Inc.

Code/ CPT	Mod- ifier	Status	Description	Work value	Practice expense	Mal- practice	Total value	Global period	Up- date
25605	00	A	Closed treatment of distal radial fracture (eg, Colles or Smith type) or epiphyseal separation, with or without fracture of ulnar styloid; with manipulation	5.36	3.95	0.61	9.92	90	S
25611	00	A	Percutaneous skeletal fixation of distal radial fracture (eg, Colles or Smith type) or epiphyseal separation, with or without fracture of ulnar styloid, requiring manipulation, with or without external fixation	7.11	6.01	0.97	14.09	90	S
25620	00	A	Open treatment of distal radial fracture (eg, Colles or Smith type) or epiphyseal separation, with or without fracture of ulnar styloid, with or without internal or external fixation	8.15	7.13	1.14	16.42	90	S
25622	00	A	Closed treatment of carpal scaphoid (navicular) fracture; without manipulation	2.43	2.28	0.33	5.04	90	S
25624	00	A	Closed treatment of carpal scaphoid (navicular) fracture; with manipulation	4.28	3.67	0.57	8.52	90	S
25628	00	A	Open treatment of carpal scaphoid (navicular) fracture, with or without internal or external fixation	7.81	7.13	1.16	16.10	90	S
25630	00	A	Closed treatment of carpal bone fracture (excluding carpal scaphoid (navicular)); without manipulation, each bone	2.73	2.19	0.30	5.22	90	S
25635	00	A	Closed treatment of carpal bone fracture (excluding carpal scaphoid (navicular)); with manipulation, each bone	4.16	3.36	0.50	8.02	90	S
25645	00	A	Open treatment of carpal bone fracture (excluding carpal scaphoid (navicular)), each bone	6.85	6.68	0.95	14.48	90	S
25650	00	A	Closed treatment of ulnar styloid fracture	2.87	2.66	0.36	5.89	90	S
25660	00	A	Closed treatment of radiocarpal or intercarpal dislocation, one or more bones, with manipulation	4.53	1.82	0.26	6.61	90	S
25670	00	A	Open treatment of radiocarpal or intercarpal dislocation, one or more bones	7.52	7.08	1.12	15.72	90	S
25675	00	A	Closed treatment of distal radioulnar dislocation with manipulation	4.44	2.28	0.34	7.06	90	S
25676	00	A	Open treatment of distal radioulnar dislocation, acute or chronic	7.55	7.32	1.11	15.98	90	S
25680	00	A	Closed treatment of trans-scaphoperilunar type of fracture dislocation, with manipulation	5.63	2.44	0.36	8.43	90	S
25685	00	A	Open treatment of trans-scaphoperilunar type of fracture dislocation	9.23	8.79	1.44	19.46	90	S
25690	00	A	Closed treatment of lunate dislocation, with manipulation	5.16	4.89	0.73	10.78	90	S
25695	00	A	Open treatment of lunate dislocation	7.94	7.04	1.17	16.15	90	S
25800	00	A	Arthrodesis, wrist joint (including radiocarpal and/or ulnocarpal fusion); without bone graft	9.21	10.94	1.80	21.95	90	S
25805	00	A	Arthrodesis, wrist joint (including radiocarpal and/or ulnocarpal fusion); with sliding graft	10.57	12.85	2.09	25.51	90	S
25810	00	A	Arthrodesis, wrist joint (including radiocarpal and/or ulnocarpal fusion); with iliac or other autograft (includes obtaining graft)	9.79	12.53	2.06	24.38	90	S
25820	00	A	Intercarpal fusion; without bone graft	7.14	8.91	1.48	17.53	90	S
25825	00	A	Intercarpal fusion; with autograft (includes obtaining graft)	8.60	11.02	1.99	21.61	90	S
25830	00	A	Distal radioulnar joint arthrodesis and segmental resection of ulna (eg, Sauve-Kapandji procedure), with or without bone graft	9.10	8.60	1.45	19.15	90	S
25900	00	A	Amputation, forearm, through radius and ulna;	8.15	7.08	1.31	16.54	90	S
25905	00	A	Amputation, forearm, through radius and ulna; open, circular (guillotine)	8.40	7.11	1.15	16.66	90	S
25907	00	A	Amputation, forearm, through radius and ulna; secondary closure or scar revision	7.27	5.74	1.00	14.01	90	S

CPT codes and descriptions only, © 1994 American Medical Association. Reimbursement information, © 1995 McGraw-Hill Inc.

Code/ CPT	Mod- ifier	Status	Description	Work value	Practice expense	Mal- practice	Total value	Global period	Up- date
25909	00	A	Amputation, forearm, through radius and ulna; re-amputation	8.37	5.55	1.06	14.98	90	S
25915	00	A	Krukenberg procedure	16.61	15.83	2.59	35.03	90	S
25920	00	A	Disarticulation through wrist;	8.09	7.00	1.20	16.29	90	S
25922	00	A	Disarticulation through wrist; secondary closure or scar revision	6.96	5.55	1.02	13.53	90	S
25924	00	A	Disarticulation through wrist; re-amputation	7.87	7.50	1.22	16.59	90	S
25927	00	A	Transmetacarpal amputation;	8.27	6.29	1.22	15.78	90	S
25929	00	A	Transmetacarpal amputation; secondary closure or scar revision	7.13	4.74	0.96	12.83	90	S
25931	00	A	Transmetacarpal amputation; re-amputation	7.35	4.54	0.90	12.79	90	S
25999	00	C	Unlisted procedure, forearm or wrist	0	0	0	0	YYY	S
26010	00	A	Drainage of finger abscess; simple	1.49	0.48	0.05	2.02	10	N
26011	00	A	Drainage of finger abscess; complicated (eg, felon)	2.14	1.54	0.24	3.92	10	S
26020	00	A	Drainage of tendon sheath, one digit and/or palm	4.01	3.72	0.63	8.36	90	S
26025	00	A	Drainage of palmar bursa; single, ulnar or radial	4.32	4.51	0.76	9.59	90	S
26030	00	A	Drainage of palmar bursa; multiple or complicated	5.36	5.73	0.98	12.07	90	S
26034	00	A	Incision, deep, with opening of bone cortex (eg, for osteomyelitis or bone abscess), hand or finger	5.59	4.23	0.71	10.53	90	S
26035	00	A	Decompression fingers and/or hand, injection injury (eg, grease gun)	8.38	5.17	0.86	14.41	90	S
26037	00	A	Decompressive fasciotomy, hand (excludes 26035)	6.68	6.37	1.05	14.10	90	S
26040	00	A	Fasciotomy, palmar, for Dupuytren's contracture; closed (subcutaneous)	3.09	2.86	0.49	6.44	90	S
26045	00	A	Fasciotomy, palmar, for Dupuytren's contracture; open, partial	5.27	4.83	0.81	10.91	90	S
26055	00	A	Tendon sheath incision (eg, for trigger finger)	2.56	3.28	0.56	6.40	90	S
26060	00	A	Tenotomy, subcutaneous, single, each digit	2.71	1.13	0.17	4.01	90	S
26070	00	A	Arthrotomy, for infection, with exploration, drainage or removal of foreign body; carpometacarpal joint	3.34	2.76	0.42	6.52	90	S
26075	00	A	Arthrotomy, for infection, with exploration, drainage or removal of foreign body; metacarpophalangeal joint	3.44	3.78	0.62	7.84	90	S
26080	00	A	Arthrotomy, for infection, with exploration, drainage or removal of foreign body; interphalangeal joint, each	3.78	3.14	0.51	7.43	90	S
26100	00	A	Arthrotomy with synovial biopsy; carpometacarpal joint	3.54	2.99	0.45	6.98	90	S
26105	00	A	Arthrotomy with synovial biopsy; metacarpophalangeal joint	3.58	4.17	0.67	8.42	90	S
26110	00	A	Arthrotomy with synovial biopsy; interphalangeal joint, each	3.40	2.93	0.50	6.83	90	S
26115	00	A	Excision, tumor or vascular malformation, hand or finger; subcutaneous	3.68	2.01	0.34	6.03	90	S
26116	00	A	Excision, tumor or vascular malformation, hand or finger; deep, subfascial, intramuscular	5.19	3.71	0.62	9.52	90	S
26117	00	A	Radical resection of tumor (eg, malignant neoplasm), soft tissue of hand or finger	8.24	5.07	0.91	14.22	90	S
26121	00	A	Fasciectomy, palmar only, with or without z-plasty, other local tissue rearrangement, or skin grafting (includes obtaining graft);	7.34	9.40	1.61	18.35	90	S
26123	00	A	Fasciectomy, palmar only, with or without z-plasty, other local tissue rearrangement, or skin grafting (includes obtaining graft); partial palmar excision with release of single digit including proximal interphalangeal joint	8.64	9.10	1.53	19.27	90	S

CPT codes and descriptions only, © 1994 American Medical Association. Reimbursement information, © 1995 McGraw-Hill Inc.

Code/ CPT	Mod-ifier	Status	Description	Work value	Practice expense	Mal-practice	Total value	Global period	Up-date
26125	00	A	Fasciectomy, palmar only, with or without z-plasty, other local tissue rearrangement, or skin grafting (includes obtaining graft); partial excision with release of each additional digit, including proximal interphalangeal joint	4.61	2.62	0.45	7.68	ZZZ	S
26130	00	A	Synovectomy, carpometacarpal joint	5.13	5.01	0.86	11.00	90	S
26135	00	A	Synovectomy, metacarpophalangeal joint including intrinsic release and extensor hood reconstruction, each digit	6.67	4.86	0.82	12.35	90	S
26140	00	A	Synovectomy, proximal interphalangeal joint, including extensor reconstruction, each interphalangeal joint	5.88	4.40	0.75	11.03	90	S
26145	00	A	Synovectomy tendon sheath, radical (tenosynovectomy), flexor, palm or finger, single, each digit	6.03	4.71	0.80	11.54	90	S
26160	00	A	Excision of lesion of tendon sheath or capsule (eg, cyst, mucous cyst, or ganglion), hand or finger	3.00	2.32	0.40	5.72	90	S
26170	00	A	Excision of tendon, palm, flexor, single (separate procedure), each	4.62	2.83	0.45	7.90	90	S
26180	00	A	Excision of tendon, finger, flexor (separate procedure)	5.00	4.01	0.71	9.72	90	S
26200	00	A	Excision or curettage of bone cyst or benign tumor of metacarpal;	5.25	4.48	0.72	10.45	90	S
26205	00	A	Excision or curettage of bone cyst or benign tumor of metacarpal; with autograft (includes obtaining graft)	7.24	6.40	1.03	14.67	90	S
26210	00	A	Excision or curettage of bone cyst or benign tumor of proximal, middle or distal phalanx of finger;	4.97	3.90	0.64	9.51	90	S
26215	00	A	Excision or curettage of bone cyst or benign tumor of proximal, middle or distal phalanx of finger; with autograft (includes obtaining graft)	6.81	5.55	0.94	13.30	90	S
26230	00	A	Partial excision (craterization, saucerization, or diaphysectomy) of bone (eg, for osteomyelitis); metacarpal	5.96	4.26	0.69	10.91	90	S
26235	00	A	Partial excision (craterization, saucerization, or diaphysectomy) of bone (eg, for osteomyelitis); proximal or middle phalanx of finger	5.82	4.17	0.71	10.70	90	S
26236	00	A	Partial excision (craterization, saucerization, or diaphysectomy) of bone (eg, for osteomyelitis); distal phalanx of finger	4.95	3.86	0.66	9.47	90	S
26250	00	A	Radical resection (ostectomy) for tumor, metacarpal;	7.26	6.00	1.07	14.33	90	S
26255	00	A	Radical resection (ostectomy) for tumor, metacarpal; with autograft (includes obtaining graft)	11.66	8.94	1.54	22.14	90	S
26260	00	A	Radical resection (ostectomy) for tumor, proximal or middle phalanx of finger;	6.74	5.73	0.97	13.44	90	S
26261	00	A	Radical resection (ostectomy) for tumor, proximal or middle phalanx of finger; with autograft (includes obtaining graft)	8.54	7.70	1.31	17.55	90	S
26262	00	A	Radical resection (ostectomy) for tumor, distal phalanx of finger	5.41	4.75	0.76	10.92	90	S
26320	00	A	Removal of implant from finger or hand	3.74	3.54	0.57	7.85	90	S
26350	00	A	Flexor tendon repair or advancement, single, not in "no man's land"; primary or secondary without free graft, each tendon	5.76	5.74	0.99	12.49	90	S
26352	00	A	Flexor tendon repair or advancement, single, not in "no man's land"; secondary with free graft (includes obtaining graft), each tendon	7.26	6.60	1.10	14.96	90	S
26356	00	A	Flexor tendon repair or advancement, single, in "no man's land"; primary, each tendon	7.05	7.21	1.24	15.50	90	S
26357	00	A	Flexor tendon repair or advancement, single, in "no man's land"; secondary, each tendon	8.16	6.58	1.19	15.93	90	S

CPT codes and descriptions only, © 1994 American Medical Association. Reimbursement information, © 1995 McGraw-Hill Inc.

Code/ CPT	Mod- ifier	Status	Description	Work value	Practice expense	Mal- practice	Total value	Global period	Up- date
26358	00	A	Flexor tendon repair or advancement, single, in "no man's land"; secondary with free graft (includes obtaining graft), each tendon	8.69	7.40	1.27	17.36	90	S
26370	00	A	Profundus tendon repair or advancement, with intact sublimis; primary	6.71	6.71	1.13	14.55	90	S
26372	00	A	Profundus tendon repair or advancement, with intact sublimis; secondary with free graft (includes obtaining graft)	8.27	6.39	1.15	15.81	90	S
26373	00	A	Profundus tendon repair or advancement, with intact sublimis; secondary without free graft	7.67	6.85	1.11	15.63	90	S
26390	00	A	Flexor tendon excision, implantation of plastic tube or rod for delayed tendon graft, hand or finger	8.73	7.95	1.23	17.91	90	S
26392	00	A	Removal of tube or rod and insertion of flexor tendon graft (includes obtaining graft), hand or finger	9.77	8.61	1.26	19.64	90	S
26410	00	A	Extensor tendon repair, dorsum of hand, single, primary or secondary; without free graft, each tendon	4.37	3.29	0.51	8.17	90	S
26412	00	A	Extensor tendon repair, dorsum of hand, single, primary or secondary; with free graft (includes obtaining graft), each tendon	5.91	6.01	0.97	12.89	90	S
26415	00	A	Extensor tendon excision, implantation of plastic tube or rod for delayed extensor tendon graft, hand or finger	8.05	6.75	0.90	15.70	90	S
26416	00	A	Removal of tube or rod and insertion of extensor tendon graft (includes obtaining graft), hand or finger	9.06	8.64	1.41	19.11	90	S
26418	00	A	Extensor tendon repair, dorsum of finger, single, primary or secondary; without free graft, each tendon	4.02	3.58	0.59	8.19	90	S
26420	00	A	Extensor tendon repair, dorsum of finger, single, primary or secondary; with free graft (includes obtaining graft) each tendon	6.37	5.68	0.96	13.01	90	S
26426	00	A	Extensor tendon repair, central slip repair, secondary (boutonniere deformity); using local tissues	5.86	6.31	1.07	13.24	90	S
26428	00	A	Extensor tendon repair, central slip repair, secondary (boutonniere deformity); with free graft (includes obtaining graft)	6.90	5.50	1.00	13.40	90	S
26432	00	A	Extensor tendon repair, distal insertion ("mallet finger"), closed, splinting with or without percutaneous pinning	3.87	3.15	0.51	7.53	90	S
26433	00	A	Extensor tendon repair, distal insertion ("mallet finger"), open, primary or secondary repair; without graft	4.41	3.94	0.66	9.01	90	S
26434	00	A	Extensor tendon repair, distal insertion ("mallet finger"), open, primary or secondary repair; with free graft (includes obtaining graft)	5.80	4.95	0.84	11.59	90	S
26437	00	A	Extensor tendon realignment, hand	5.53	4.05	0.68	10.26	90	S
26440	00	A	Tenolysis, simple, flexor tendon; palm OR finger, single, each tendon	4.76	3.57	0.59	8.92	90	S
26442	00	A	Tenolysis, simple, flexor tendon; palm AND finger, each tendon	6.10	3.37	0.59	10.06	90	S
26445	00	A	Tenolysis, extensor tendon, dorsum of hand or finger; each tendon	4.16	3.25	0.54	7.95	90	S
26449	00	A	Tenolysis, complex, extensor tendon, dorsum of hand or finger, including hand and forearm	6.39	5.57	0.96	12.92	90	S
26450	00	A	Tenotomy, flexor, single, palm, open, each	3.54	2.28	0.36	6.18	90	S
26455	00	A	Tenotomy, flexor, single, finger, open, each	3.51	1.89	0.33	5.73	90	S
26460	00	A	Tenotomy, extensor, hand or finger, single, open, each	3.33	1.72	0.30	5.35	90	S
26471	00	A	Tenodesis; for proximal interphalangeal joint stabilization	5.55	4.15	0.67	10.37	90	S
26474	00	A	Tenodesis; for distal joint stabilization	5.14	4.61	0.75	10.50	90	S
26476	00	A	Tendon lengthening, extensor, hand or finger, single, each	5.00	2.89	0.27	8.16	90	S
26477	00	A	Tendon shortening, extensor, hand or finger, single, each	4.97	3.99	0.73	9.69	90	S

CPT codes and descriptions only, © 1994 American Medical Association. Reimbursement information, © 1995 McGraw-Hill Inc.

Code/ CPT	Mod- ifier	Status	Description	Work value	Practice expense	Mal- practice	Total value	Global period	Up- date
26478	00	A	Tendon lengthening, flexor, hand or finger, single, each	5.62	4.30	0.72	10.64	90	S
26479	00	A	Tendon shortening, flexor, hand or finger, single, each	5.56	5.29	0.86	11.71	90	S
26480	00	A	Tendon transfer or transplant, carpometacarpal area or dorsum of hand, single; without free graft, each	6.49	6.53	1.11	14.13	90	S
26483	00	A	Tendon transfer or transplant, carpometacarpal area or dorsum of hand, single; with free tendon graft (includes obtaining graft), each tendon	7.87	8.50	1.40	17.77	90	S
26485	00	A	Tendon transfer or transplant, palmar, single, each tendon; without free tendon graft	7.28	6.50	1.08	14.86	90	S
26489	00	A	Tendon transfer or transplant, palmar, single, each tendon; with free tendon graft (includes obtaining graft), each tendon	9.00	3.40	0.51	12.91	90	S
26490	00	A	Opponensplasty; sublimis tendon transfer type	7.99	7.80	1.28	17.07	90	S
26492	00	A	Opponensplasty; tendon transfer with graft (includes obtaining graft)	9.17	8.75	1.21	19.13	90	S
26494	00	A	Opponensplasty; hypothenar muscle transfer	8.05	7.28	1.23	16.56	90	S
26496	00	A	Opponensplasty; other methods	9.17	8.73	1.53	19.43	90	S
26497	00	A	Tendon transfer to restore intrinsic function; ring and small finger	9.15	8.02	1.38	18.55	90	S
26498	00	A	Tendon transfer to restore intrinsic function; all four fingers	13.55	11.78	2.04	27.37	90	S
26499	00	A	Correction claw finger, other methods	8.56	7.75	1.25	17.56	90	S
26500	00	A	Tendon pulley reconstruction; with local tissues (separate procedure)	5.67	3.49	0.60	9.76	90	S
26502	00	A	Tendon pulley reconstruction; with tendon or fascial graft (includes obtaining graft) (separate procedure)	6.74	5.27	0.95	12.96	90	S
26504	00	A	Tendon pulley reconstruction; with tendon prosthesis (separate procedure)	7.05	6.72	1.11	14.88	90	S
26508	00	A	Thenar muscle release for thumb contracture	5.61	4.15	0.72	10.48	90	S
26510	00	A	Cross intrinsic transfer	5.03	4.15	0.68	9.86	90	S
26516	00	A	Capsulodesis for M-P joint stabilization; single digit	6.75	4.16	0.67	11.58	90	S
26517	00	A	Capsulodesis for M-P joint stabilization; two digits	8.34	7.07	1.23	16.64	90	S
26518	00	A	Capsulodesis for M-P joint stabilization; three or four digits	8.53	6.51	1.22	16.26	90	S
26520	00	A	Capsulectomy or capsulotomy for contracture; metacarpophalangeal joint, single, each	5.01	4.48	0.71	10.20	90	S
26525	00	A	Capsulectomy or capsulotomy for contracture; interphalangeal joint, single, each	5.04	3.64	0.62	9.30	90	S
26527	00	D	Revise wrist joint	8.44*	8.05#	1.32*	17.81#	90	S
26530	00	A	Arthroplasty, metacarpophalangeal joint; single, each	6.38	5.16	0.85	12.39	90	S
26531	00	A	Arthroplasty, metacarpophalangeal joint; with prosthetic implant, single, each	7.57	6.65	1.11	15.33	90	S
26535	00	A	Arthroplasty interphalangeal joint; single, each	4.95	4.84	0.58	10.37	90	S
26536	00	A	Arthroplasty interphalangeal joint; with prosthetic implant, single, each	6.06	7.21	1.19	14.46	90	S
26540	00	A	Primary repair of collateral ligament, metacarpophalangeal joint;	6.03	6.64	1.12	13.79	90	S
26541	00	A	Primary repair of collateral ligament, metacarpophalangeal joint; with tendon or fascial graft (includes obtaining graft)	8.20	8.94	1.47	18.61	90	S
26542	00	A	Primary repair of collateral ligament, metacarpophalangeal joint; with local tissue (eg, adductor advancement)	6.38	5.67	0.97	13.02	90	S
26545	00	A	Reconstruction, collateral ligament, interphalangeal joint, single, including graft, each joint	6.50	5.27	0.94	12.71	90	S
26548	00	A	Repair and reconstruction, finger, volar plate, interphalangeal joint	7.61	5.79	1.00	14.40	90	S
26550	00	A	Pollicization of a digit	20.77	19.81	3.24	43.82	90	S

CPT codes and descriptions only, © 1994 American Medical Association. Reimbursement information, © 1995 McGraw-Hill Inc.

Code/ CPT	Mod- ifier	Status	Description	Work value	Practice expense	Mal- practice	Total value	Global period	Up- date
26552	00	C	Reconstruction thumb with toe	19.70*	18.79#	3.08*	41.57#	90	S
26555	00	A	Positional change of other finger	16.16	15.41	2.52	34.09	90	S
26557	00	C	Toe to finger transfer; first stage	5.63*	5.37#	0.88*	11.88#	90	S
26558	00	C	Toe to finger transfer; each delay	3.52*	3.36#	0.55*	7.43#	90	S
26559	00	C	Toe to finger transfer; second stage	7.03*	6.70#	1.1*	14.83#	90	S
26560	00	A	Repair of syndactyly (web finger) each web space; with skin flaps	5.23	4.65	0.66	10.54	90	S
26561	00	A	Repair of syndactyly (web finger) each web space; with skin flaps and grafts	10.50	8.89	1.56	20.95	90	S
26562	00	A	Repair of syndactyly (web finger) each web space; complex (eg, involving bone, nails)	9.23	10.97	0.82	21.02	90	S
26565	00	A	Osteotomy for correction of deformity; metacarpal	6.45	5.82	0.85	13.12	90	S
26567	00	A	Osteotomy for correction of deformity; phalanx of finger	6.53	4.28	0.67	11.48	90	S
26568	00	A	Osteoplasty for lengthening of metacarpal or phalanx	8.66	8.45	1.06	18.17	90	S
26580	00	A	Repair cleft hand	15.81	15.08	2.47	33.36	90	S
26585	00	A	Repair bifid digit	13.58	12.95	2.12	28.65	90	S
26587	00	C	Reconstruction of supernumerary digit, soft tissue and bone	4.57*	4.36#	0.71*	9.64#	90	S
26590	00	A	Repair macrodactylia	17.44	16.63	2.72	36.79	90	S
26591	00	A	Repair, intrinsic muscles of hand (specify)	2.90	2.29	0.39	5.58	90	S
26593	00	A	Release, intrinsic muscles of hand (specify)	4.89	4.12	0.70	9.71	90	S
26596	00	A	Excision of constricting ring of finger, with multiple Z-plasties	8.64	8.24	1.35	18.23	90	S
26597	00	A	Release of scar contracture, flexor or extensor, with skin grafts, rearrangement flaps, or Z-plasties, hand and/or finger	9.37	8.02	1.37	18.76	90	S
26600	00	A	Closed treatment of metacarpal fracture, single; without manipulation, each bone	1.81	1.54	0.22	3.57	90	S
26605	00	A	Closed treatment of metacarpal fracture, single; with manipulation, each bone	2.67	2.29	0.36	5.32	90	S
26607	00	A	Closed treatment of metacarpal fracture, with manipulation, with internal or external fixation, each bone	5.12	3.55	0.57	9.24	90	S
26608	00	A	Percutaneous skeletal fixation of metacarpal fracture, each bone	5.12	3.55	0.57	9.24	90	S
26615	00	A	Open treatment of metacarpal fracture, single, with or without internal or external fixation, each bone	5.18	4.87	0.80	10.85	90	S
26641	00	A	Closed treatment of carpometacarpal dislocation, thumb, with manipulation	3.74	1.11	0.14	4.99	90	S
26645	00	A	Closed treatment of carpometacarpal fracture dislocation, thumb (Bennett fracture), with manipulation	4.23	2.20	0.33	6.76	90	S
26650	00	A	Percutaneous skeletal fixation of carpometacarpal fracture dislocation, thumb (Bennett fracture), with manipulation, with or without external fixation	5.49	4.01	0.64	10.14	90	S
26665	00	A	Open treatment of carpometacarpal fracture dislocation, thumb (Bennett fracture), with or without internal or external fixation	7.14	6.39	1.09	14.62	90	S
26670	00	A	Closed treatment of carpometacarpal dislocation, other than thumb (Bennett fracture), single, with manipulation; without anesthesia	3.54	0.96	0.10	4.60	90	S
26675	00	A	Closed treatment of carpometacarpal dislocation, other than thumb (Bennett fracture), single, with manipulation; requiring anesthesia	4.44	4.34	0.60	9.38	90	S

CPT codes and descriptions only, © 1994 American Medical Association. Reimbursement information, © 1995 McGraw-Hill Inc.

Code/ CPT	Mod-ifier	Status	Description	Work value	Practice expense	Mal-practice	Total value	Global period	Up-date
26676	00	A	Percutaneous skeletal fixation of carpometacarpal dislocation, other than thumb (Bennett fracture), single, with manipulation	5.29	4.86	0.67	10.82	90	S
26685	00	A	Open treatment of carpometacarpal dislocation, other than thumb (Bennett fracture); single, with or without internal or external fixation	6.54	5.76	0.91	13.21	90	S
26686	00	A	Open treatment of carpometacarpal dislocation, other than thumb (Bennett fracture); complex, multiple or delayed reduction	7.48	6.31	1.04	14.83	90	S
26700	00	A	Closed treatment of metacarpophalangeal dislocation, single, with manipulation; without anesthesia	3.54	0.88	0.10	4.52	90	S
26705	00	A	Closed treatment of metacarpophalangeal dislocation, single, with manipulation; requiring anesthesia	3.99	1.78	0.27	6.04	90	S
26706	00	A	Percutaneous skeletal fixation of metacarpophalangeal dislocation, single, with manipulation	4.92	4.68	0.75	10.35	90	S
26715	00	A	Open treatment of metacarpophalangeal dislocation, single, with or without internal or external fixation	5.48	4.13	0.66	10.27	90	S
26720	00	A	Closed treatment of phalangeal shaft fracture, proximal or middle phalanx, finger or thumb; without manipulation, each	1.56	1.10	0.15	2.81	90	S
26725	00	A	Closed treatment of phalangeal shaft fracture, proximal or middle phalanx, finger or thumb; with manipulation, with or without skin or skeletal traction, each	3.18	1.54	0.23	4.95	90	S
26727	00	A	Percutaneous skeletal fixation of unstable phalangeal shaft fracture, proximal or middle phalanx, finger or thumb, with manipulation, each	4.92	2.45	0.38	7.75	90	S
26735	00	A	Open treatment of phalangeal shaft fracture, proximal or middle phalanx, finger or thumb, with or without internal or external fixation, each	5.72	3.73	0.61	10.06	90	S
26740	00	A	Closed treatment of articular fracture, involving metacarpophalangeal or interphalangeal joint; without manipulation, each	1.81	1.16	0.16	3.13	90	S
26742	00	A	Closed treatment of articular fracture, involving metacarpophalangeal or interphalangeal joint; with manipulation, each	3.70	1.98	0.32	6.00	90	S
26746	00	A	Open treatment of articular fracture, involving metacarpophalangeal or interphalangeal joint, with or without internal or external fixation, each	5.55	4.75	0.80	11.10	90	S
26750	00	A	Closed treatment of distal phalangeal fracture, finger or thumb; without manipulation, each	1.60	0.83	0.10	2.53	90	S
26755	00	A	Closed treatment of distal phalangeal fracture, finger or thumb; with manipulation, each	2.97	1.08	0.15	4.20	90	S
26756	00	A	Percutaneous skeletal fixation of distal phalangeal fracture, finger or thumb, each	4.19	1.90	0.33	6.42	90	S
26765	00	A	Open treatment of distal phalangeal fracture, finger or thumb, with or without internal or external fixation, each	4.04	2.66	0.45	7.15	90	S
26770	00	A	Closed treatment of interphalangeal joint dislocation, single, with manipulation; without anesthesia	2.89	0.76	0.08	3.73	90	S
26775	00	A	Closed treatment of interphalangeal joint dislocation, single, with manipulation; requiring anesthesia	3.51	1.13	0.17	4.81	90	S
26776	00	A	Percutaneous skeletal fixation of interphalangeal joint dislocation, single, with manipulation	4.60	2.08	0.35	7.03	90	S
26785	00	A	Open treatment of interphalangeal joint dislocation, with or without internal or external fixation, single	4.08	2.97	0.48	7.53	90	S
26820	00	A	Fusion in opposition, thumb, with autogenous graft (includes obtaining graft)	7.84	6.65	1.05	15.54	90	S

CPT codes and descriptions only, © 1994 American Medical Association. Reimbursement information, © 1995 McGraw-Hill Inc.

Code/ CPT	Mod- ifier	Status	Description	Work value	Practice expense	Mal- practice	Total value	Global period	Up- date
26841	00	A	Arthrodesis, carpometacarpal joint, thumb, with or without internal fixation;	6.79	6.17	1.00	13.96	90	S
26842	00	A	Arthrodesis, carpometacarpal joint, thumb, with or without internal fixation; with autograft (includes obtaining graft)	7.75	8.58	1.37	17.70	90	S
26843	00	A	Arthrodesis, carpometacarpal joint, digits, other than thumb;	7.21	6.37	1.10	14.68	90	S
26844	00	A	Arthrodesis, carpometacarpal joint, digits, other than thumb; with autograft (includes obtaining graft)	8.24	7.35	1.19	16.78	90	S
26850	00	A	Arthrodesis, metacarpophalangeal joint, with or without internal fixation;	6.57	4.63	0.76	11.96	90	S
26852	00	A	Arthrodesis, metacarpophalangeal joint, with or without internal fixation; with autograft (includes obtaining graft)	7.97	5.72	1.00	14.69	90	S
26860	00	A	Arthrodesis, interphalangeal joint, with or without internal fixation;	4.49	4.30	0.68	9.47	90	S
26861	00	A	Arthrodesis, interphalangeal joint, with or without internal fixation; each additional interphalangeal joint	1.74	2.23	0.43	4.40	ZZZ	S
26862	00	A	Arthrodesis, interphalangeal joint, with or without internal fixation; with autograft (includes obtaining graft)	7.06	5.16	0.85	13.07	90	S
26863	00	A	Arthrodesis, interphalangeal joint, with or without internal fixation; with autograft (includes obtaining graft), each additional joint	3.90	3.37	0.57	7.84	ZZZ	S
26910	00	A	Amputation, metacarpal, with finger or thumb (ray amputation), single, with or without interosseous transfer	7.18	5.16	0.93	13.27	90	S
26951	00	A	Amputation, finger or thumb, primary or secondary, any joint or phalanx, single, including neurectomies; with direct closure	4.41	2.87	0.49	7.77	90	S
26952	00	A	Amputation, finger or thumb, primary or secondary, any joint or phalanx, single, including neurectomies; with local advancement flaps (V-Y, hood)	6.02	4.00	0.69	10.71	90	S
26989	00	C	Unlisted procedure, hands or fingers	0	0	0	0	YYY	S
26990	00	A	Incision and drainage, pelvis or hip joint area; deep abscess or hematoma	6.76	3.10	0.51	10.37	90	S
26991	00	A	Incision and drainage, pelvis or hip joint area; infected bursa	6.05	1.81	0.29	8.15	90	S
26992	00	A	Incision, deep, with opening of bone cortex (eg, for osteomyelitis or bone abscess), pelvis and/or hip joint	13.97	6.38	1.05	21.40	90	S
27000	00	A	Tenotomy, adductor of hip, subcutaneous, closed (separate procedure)	5.27	1.85	0.24	7.36	90	S
27001	00	A	Tenotomy, adductor of hip, subcutaneous, open	7.70	2.34	0.38	10.42	90	S
27003	00	A	Tenotomy, adductor, subcutaneous, open, with obturator neurectomy	6.53	6.77	1.08	14.38	90	S
27005	00	A	Tenotomy, iliopsoas, open (separate procedure)	9.00	3.37	0.54	12.91	90	S
27006	00	A	Tenotomy, abductors of hip, open (separate procedure)	9.50	4.64	0.77	14.91	90	S
27025	00	A	Fasciotomy, hip or thigh, any type	10.16	6.12	1.02	17.30	90	S
27030	00	A	Arthrotomy, hip, for infection, with drainage	12.09	11.42	1.86	25.37	90	S
27033	00	A	Arthrotomy, hip, with exploration or removal of loose or foreign body	12.38	11.52	1.85	25.75	90	S
27035	00	A	Hip joint denervation, intrapelvic or extrapelvic intra-articular branches of sciatic, femoral or obturator nerves	15.72	11.86	2.21	29.79	90	S
27040	00	A	Biopsy, soft tissue of pelvis and hip area; superficial	3.26	0.72	0.11	4.09	10	N
27041	00	A	Biopsy, soft tissue of pelvis and hip area; deep	9.36	2.67	0.44	12.47	90	S
27047	00	A	Excision, tumor, pelvis and hip area; subcutaneous	7.16	1.89	0.32	9.37	90	S
27048	00	A	Excision, tumor, pelvis and hip area; deep, subfascial, intramuscular	5.70	4.33	0.82	10.85	90	S

CPT codes and descriptions only, © 1994 American Medical Association. Reimbursement information, © 1995 McGraw-Hill Inc.

Code/ CPT	Mod- ifier	Status	Description	Work value	Practice expense	Mal- practice	Total value	Global period	Up- date
27049	00	A	Radical resection of tumor (eg, malignant neoplasm), soft tissue of pelvis and hip area	12.52	10.14	1.87	24.53	90	S
27050	00	A	Arthrotomy, with biopsy; sacroiliac joint	3.73	4.78	0.90	9.41	90	S
27052	00	A	Arthrotomy, with biopsy; hip joint	5.45	7.78	1.59	14.82	90	S
27054	00	A	Arthrotomy with synovectomy, hip joint	7.60	10.74	2.26	20.60	90	S
27060	00	A	Excision; ischial bursa	4.73	3.93	0.68	9.34	90	S
27062	00	A	Excision; trochanteric bursa or calcification	4.74	4.23	0.70	9.67	90	S
27065	00	A	Excision of bone cyst or benign tumor; superficial (wing of ilium, symphysis pubis, or greater trochanter of femur) with or without autograft	4.98	5.59	0.90	11.47	90	S
27066	00	A	Excision of bone cyst or benign tumor; deep, with or without autograft	9.17	7.90	1.30	18.37	90	S
27067	00	A	Excision of bone cyst or benign tumor; with autograft requiring separate incision	12.64	11.63	1.93	26.20	90	S
27070	00	A	Partial excision (craterization, saucerization) (eg, for osteomyelitis); superficial (eg, wing of ilium, symphysis pubis or greater trochanter of femur)	9.58	7.41	1.21	18.20	90	S
27071	00	A	Partial excision (craterization, saucerization) (eg, for osteomyelitis); deep	10.23	8.50	1.45	20.18	90	S
27075	00	A	Radical resection of tumor or infection; wing of ilium, one pubic or ischial ramus or symphysis pubis	15.85	13.54	2.32	31.71	90	S
27076	00	A	Radical resection of tumor or infection; ilium, including acetabulum, both pubic rami, or ischium and acetabulum	17.93	16.37	2.61	36.91	90	S
27077	00	A	Radical resection of tumor or infection; innominate bone, total	21.29	18.98	3.24	43.51	90	S
27078	00	A	Radical resection of tumor or infection; ischial tuberosity and greater trochanter of femur	11.86	9.20	1.67	22.73	90	S
27079	00	A	Radical resection of tumor or infection; ischial tuberosity and greater trochanter of femur, with skin flaps	12.11	8.64	1.66	22.41	90	S
27080	00	A	Coccygectomy, primary	5.63	4.78	0.87	11.28	90	S
27086	00	A	Removal of foreign body, pelvis or hip; subcutaneous tissue	1.82	0.58	0.07	2.47	10	S
27087	00	A	Removal of foreign body, pelvis or hip; deep	8.01	3.62	0.60	12.23	90	S
27090	00	A	Removal of hip prosthesis; (separate procedure)	12.00	9.09	1.46	22.55	90	S
27091	00	A	Removal of hip prosthesis; complicated, including "total hip" and methylmethacrylate, when applicable	20.48	19.81	3.16	43.45	90	S
27093	00	A	Injection procedure for hip arthrography; without anesthesia	1.30	0.82	0.11	2.23	0	S
27095	00	A	Injection procedure for hip arthrography; with anesthesia	1.50	0.93	0.13	2.56	0	N
27097	00	A	Hamstring recession, proximal	8.08	7.71	1.26	17.05	90	S
27098	00	A	Adductor transfer to ischium	8.08	7.71	1.26	17.05	90	S
27100	00	A	Transfer external oblique muscle to greater trochanter including fascial or tendon extension (graft)	10.57	7.68	1.42	19.67	90	S
27105	00	A	Transfer paraspinal muscle to hip (includes fascial or tendon extension graft)	11.26	5.89	1.36	18.51	90	S
27110	00	A	Transfer iliopsoas; to greater trochanter	12.49	10.61	1.86	24.96	90	S
27111	00	A	Transfer iliopsoas; to femoral neck	11.44	11.63	1.65	24.72	90	S
27120	00	A	Acetabuloplasty; (eg, Whitman, Colonna, Haygroves, or cup type)	16.43	18.10	2.95	37.48	90	S
27122	00	A	Acetabuloplasty; resection femoral head (Girdlestone procedure)	13.56	17.36	2.94	33.86	90	S
27125	00	A	Partial hip replacement, prosthesis (eg, femoral stem prosthesis, bipolar arthroplasty)	13.21	16.91	3.01	33.13	90	S

CPT codes and descriptions only, © 1994 American Medical Association. Reimbursement information, © 1995 McGraw-Hill Inc.

Code/ CPT	Mod- ifier	Status	Description	Work value	Practice expense	Mal- practice	Total value	Global period	Up- date
27130	00	A	Arthroplasty, acetabular and proximal femoral prosthetic replacement (total hip replacement), with or without autograft or allograft	18.68	23.91	4.58	47.17	90	S
27132	00	A	Conversion of previous hip surgery to total hip replacement, with or without autograft or allograft	21.44	27.44	5.09	53.97	90	S
27134	00	A	Revision of total hip arthroplasty; both components, with or without autograft or allograft	24.54	31.41	5.96	61.91	90	S
27137	00	A	Revision of total hip arthroplasty; acetabular component only, with or without autograft or allograft	18.67	24.31	4.82	47.80	90	S
27138	00	A	Revision of total hip arthroplasty; femoral component only, with or without allograft	18.93	24.23	4.58	47.74	90	S
27140	00	A	Osteotomy and transfer of greater trochanter (separate procedure)	11.43	11.05	1.71	24.19	90	S
27146	00	A	Osteotomy, iliac, acetabular or innominate bone;	13.72	10.88	1.35	25.95	90	S
27147	00	A	Osteotomy, iliac, acetabular or innominate bone; with open reduction of hip	17.58	16.97	2.76	37.31	90	S
27151	00	A	Osteotomy, iliac, acetabular or innominate bone; with femoral osteotomy	18.58	17.71	2.90	39.19	90	S
27156	00	A	Osteotomy, iliac, acetabular or innominate bone; with femoral osteotomy and with open reduction of hip	20.16	18.32	3.08	41.56	90	S
27158	00	A	Osteotomy, pelvis, bilateral (eg, for congenital malformation)	18.10	14.42	2.64	35.16	90	S
27161	00	A	Osteotomy, femoral neck (separate procedure)	15.20	14.31	2.31	31.82	90	S
27165	00	A	Osteotomy, intertrochanteric or subtrochanteric including internal or external fixation and/or cast	16.20	16.76	2.63	35.59	90	S
27170	00	A	Bone graft, femoral head, neck, intertrochanteric or subtrochanteric area (includes obtaining bone graft)	14.90	16.41	2.65	33.96	90	S
27175	00	A	Treatment of slipped femoral epiphysis; by traction, without reduction	7.24	1.18	0.18	8.60	90	S
27176	00	A	Treatment of slipped femoral epiphysis; by single or multiple pinning, in situ	10.89	10.39	1.70	22.98	90	S
27177	00	A	Open treatment of slipped femoral epiphysis; single or multiple pinning or bone graft (includes obtaining graft)	13.76	12.39	2.05	28.20	90	S
27178	00	A	Open treatment of slipped femoral epiphysis; closed manipulation with single or multiple pinning	10.76	10.46	1.55	22.77	90	S
27179	00	A	Open treatment of slipped femoral epiphysis; osteoplasty of femoral neck (Heyman type procedure)	11.69	11.15	1.83	24.67	90	S
27181	00	A	Open treatment of slipped femoral epiphysis; osteotomy and internal fixation	13.80	13.14	2.16	29.10	90	S
27185	00	A	Epiphyseal arrest by epiphysiodesis or stapling, greater trochanter	8.30	2.77	0.87	11.94	90	S
27187	00	A	Prophylactic treatment (nailing, pinning, plating or wiring) with or without methylmethacrylate, femoral neck and proximal femur	12.57	16.09	2.76	31.42	90	S
27193	00	A	Closed treatment of pelvic ring fracture, dislocation, diastasis or subluxation; without manipulation	4.64	2.41	0.39	7.44	90	S
27194	00	A	Closed treatment of pelvic ring fracture, dislocation, diastasis or subluxation; with manipulation, requiring more than local anesthesia	8.73	3.90	0.50	13.13	90	S
27200	00	A	Closed treatment of coccygeal fracture	1.76	1.49	0.17	3.42	90	S
27202	00	A	Open treatment of coccygeal fracture	6.52	6.15	0.89	13.56	90	S
27215	00	A	Open treatment of iliac spine(s), tuberosity avulsion, or iliac wing fracture(s) (eg, pelvic fracture(s) which do not disrupt the pelvic ring), with internal fixation	9.39	12.02	2.33	23.74	90	S

CPT codes and descriptions only, © 1994 American Medical Association. Reimbursement information, © 1995 McGraw-Hill Inc.

Code/ CPT	Mod- ifier	Status	Description	Work value	Practice expense	Mal- practice	Total value	Global period	Up- date
27216	00	A	Percutaneous skeletal fixation of posterior pelvic ring fracture and/or dislocation (includes ilium, sacroiliac joint and/or sacrum)	14.20	4.30	0.66	19.16	90	S
27217	00	A	Open treatment of anterior ring fracture and/or dislocation with internal fixation, (includes pubic symphysis and/or rami)	13.19	14.55	2.33	30.07	90	S
27218	00	A	Open treatment of posterior ring fracture and/or dislocation with internal fixation (includes ilium, sacroiliac joint and/or sacrum)	18.83	14.55	2.33	35.71	90	S
27220	00	A	Closed treatment of acetabulum (hip socket) fracture(s); without manipulation	5.26	4.26	0.64	10.16	90	S
27222	00	A	Closed treatment of acetabulum (hip socket) fracture(s); with manipulation, with or without skeletal traction	10.95	6.37	1.03	18.35	90	S
27226	00	A	Open treatment of posterior or anterior acetabular wall fracture, with internal fixation	13.93	15.78	2.52	32.23	90	S
27227	00	A	Open treatment of acetabular fracture(s) involving anterior or posterior (one) column, or a fracture running transversely across the acetabulum, with internal fixation	15.39	19.70	3.20	38.29	90	S
27228	00	A	Open treatment of acetabular fracture(s) involving anterior and posterior (two) columns, includes T-fracture and both column fracture with complete articular detachment, or single column or transverse fracture with associated acetabular wall fracture, with internal fixation	17.90	19.95	3.20	41.05	90	S
27230	00	A	Closed treatment of femoral fracture, proximal end, neck; without manipulation	4.95	3.30	0.41	8.66	90	S
27232	00	A	Closed treatment of femoral fracture, proximal end, neck; with manipulation, with or without skeletal traction	9.32	8.98	1.46	19.76	90	S
27235	00	A	Percutaneous skeletal fixation of femoral fracture, proximal end, neck, undisplaced, mildly displaced, or impacted fracture	11.02	14.10	2.60	27.72	90	S
27236	00	A	Open treatment of femoral fracture, proximal end, neck, internal fixation or prosthetic replacement (direct fracture exposure)	14.14	16.91	2.71	33.76	90	S
27238	00	A	Closed treatment of intertrochanteric, pertrochanteric, or subtrochanteric femoral fracture; without manipulation	5.06	4.91	0.71	10.68	90	S
27240	00	A	Closed treatment of intertrochanteric, pertrochanteric, or subtrochanteric femoral fracture; with manipulation, with or without skin or skeletal traction	10.86	9.70	1.53	22.09	90	S
27244	00	A	Open treatment of intertrochanteric, pertrochanteric or subtrochanteric femoral fracture; with plate/screw type implant, with or without cerclage	14.35	16.30	2.62	33.27	90	S
27245	00	A	Open treatment of intertrochanteric, pertrochanteric or subtrochanteric femoral fracture; with intramedullary implant, with or without interlocking screws and/or cerclage	18.72	16.30	2.62	37.64	90	S
27246	00	A	Closed treatment of greater trochanteric fracture, without manipulation	4.36	3.87	0.60	8.83	90	S
27248	00	A	Open treatment of greater trochanteric fracture, with or without internal or external fixation	9.73	12.46	2.11	24.30	90	S
27250	00	A	Closed treatment of hip dislocation, traumatic; without anesthesia	6.31	3.19	0.45	9.95	90	S
27252	00	A	Closed treatment of hip dislocation, traumatic; requiring anesthesia	9.47	4.34	0.68	14.49	90	S
27253	00	A	Open treatment of hip dislocation, traumatic, without internal fixation	11.98	13.14	2.11	27.23	90	S

CPT codes and descriptions only, © 1994 American Medical Association. Reimbursement information, © 1995 McGraw-Hill Inc.

Code/ CPT	Mod- ifier	Status	Description	Work value	Practice expense	Mal- practice	Total value	Global period	Up- date
27254	00	A	Open treatment of hip dislocation, traumatic, with acetabular wall and femoral head fracture, with or without internal or external fixation	17.29	13.47	2.27	33.03	90	S
27256	00	A	Treatment of spontaneous hip dislocation (developmental, including congenital or pathological), by abduction, splint or traction; without anesthesia, without manipulation	3.72	1.88	0.31	5.91	10	S
27257	00	A	Treatment of spontaneous hip dislocation (developmental, including congenital or pathological), by abduction, splint or traction; with manipulation, requiring anesthesia	4.82	4.62	0.73	10.17	10	S
27258	00	A	Open treatment of spontaneous hip dislocation (developmental, including congenital or pathological), replacement of femoral head in acetabulum (including tenotomy, etc);	14.40	13.73	2.25	30.38	90	S
27259	00	A	Open treatment of spontaneous hip dislocation (developmental, including congenital or pathological), replacement of femoral head in acetabulum (including tenotomy, etc); with femoral shaft shortening	18.03	17.20	2.82	38.05	90	S
27265	00	A	Closed treatment of post hip arthroplasty dislocation; without anesthesia	5.58	3.46	0.54	9.58	90	S
27266	00	A	Closed treatment of post hip arthroplasty dislocation; requiring regional or general anesthesia	7.73	4.45	0.71	12.89	90	S
27275	00	A	Manipulation, hip joint, requiring general anesthesia	2.00	1.88	0.30	4.18	10	S
27280	00	A	Arthrodesis, sacroiliac joint (including obtaining graft)	11.81	10.06	1.77	23.64	90	S
27282	00	A	Arthrodesis, symphysis pubis (including obtaining graft)	10.57	9.01	1.69	21.27	90	S
27284	00	A	Arthrodesis, hip joint (includes obtaining graft);	15.62	14.50	2.40	32.52	90	S
27286	00	A	Arthrodesis, hip joint (includes obtaining graft); with subtrochanteric osteotomy	15.65	15.20	2.26	33.11	90	S
27290	00	A	Interpelviabdominal amputation (hindquarter amputation)	21.68	25.40	4.70	51.78	90	S
27295	00	A	Disarticulation of hip	17.32	16.54	2.95	36.81	90	S
27299	00	C	Unlisted procedure, pelvis or hip joint	0	0	0	0	YYY	S
27301	00	A	Incision and drainage of deep abscess, infected bursa, or hematoma, thigh or knee region	5.96	2.46	0.40	8.82	90	S
27303	00	A	Incision, deep, with opening of bone cortex (eg, for osteomyelitis or bone abscess), femur or knee	7.69	5.86	0.96	14.51	90	S
27305	00	A	Fasciotomy, iliotibial (tenotomy), open	5.42	3.80	0.68	9.90	90	S
27306	00	A	Tenotomy, subcutaneous, closed, adductor or hamstring, (separate procedure); single	4.27	1.99	0.32	6.58	90	S
27307	00	A	Tenotomy, subcutaneous, closed, adductor or hamstring, (separate procedure); multiple	5.30	3.01	0.48	8.79	90	S
27310	00	A	Arthrotomy, knee, for infection, with exploration, drainage or removal of foreign body	8.26	9.60	1.51	19.37	90	S
27315	00	A	Neurectomy, hamstring muscle	6.51	5.38	0.96	12.85	90	S
27320	00	A	Neurectomy, popliteal (gastrocnemius)	5.90	5.18	0.73	11.81	90	S
27323	00	A	Biopsy, soft tissue of thigh or knee area; superficial	2.67	0.91	0.13	3.71	10	S
27324	00	A	Biopsy, soft tissue of thigh or knee area; deep	4.53	2.63	0.45	7.61	90	S
27327	00	A	Excision, tumor, thigh or knee area; subcutaneous	4.32	2.29	0.40	7.01	90	S
27328	00	A	Excision, tumor, thigh or knee area; deep, subfascial, or intramuscular	5.31	4.07	0.73	10.11	90	S
27329	00	A	Radical resection of tumor (eg, malignant neoplasm), soft tissue of thigh or knee area	11.74	11.69	2.14	25.57	90	S
27330	00	A	Arthrotomy, knee; with synovial biopsy only	4.71	6.29	1.19	12.19	90	S
27331	00	A	Arthrotomy, knee; with joint exploration, with or without biopsy, with or without removal of loose or foreign bodies	5.51	7.45	1.49	14.45	90	S

CPT codes and descriptions only, © 1994 American Medical Association. Reimbursement information, © 1995 McGraw-Hill Inc.

Code/ CPT	Mod- ifier	Status	Description	Work value	Practice expense	Mal- practice	Total value	Global period	Up- date
27332	00	A	Arthrotomy, knee, with excision of semilunar cartilage (meniscectomy); medial OR lateral	7.85	10.05	1.73	19.63	90	S
27333	00	A	Arthrotomy, knee, with excision of semilunar cartilage (meniscectomy); medial AND lateral	6.81	11.23	2.52	20.56	90	S
27334	00	A	Arthrotomy, knee, with synovectomy; anterior OR posterior	7.95	10.18	1.77	19.90	90	S
27335	00	A	Arthrotomy, knee, with synovectomy; anterior AND posterior including popliteal area	9.19	11.76	2.05	23.00	90	S
27340	00	A	Excision, prepatellar bursa	3.92	3.85	0.62	8.39	90	S
27345	00	A	Excision of synovial cyst of popliteal space (Baker's cyst)	5.63	5.63	0.95	12.21	90	S
27350	00	A	Patellectomy or hemipatellectomy	7.42	9.49	1.54	18.45	90	S
27355	00	A	Excision or curettage of bone cyst or benign tumor of femur;	7.06	7.58	1.23	15.87	90	S
27356	00	A	Excision or curettage of bone cyst or benign tumor of femur; with allograft	8.60	8.20	1.34	18.14	90	S
27357	00	A	Excision or curettage of bone cyst or benign tumor of femur; with autograft (includes obtaining graft)	9.63	8.80	1.43	19.86	90	S
27358	00	A	Excision or curettage of bone cyst or benign tumor of femur; with internal fixation (list in addition to 27355, 27356, or 27357)	4.74	4.55	0.72	10.01	ZZZ	S
27360	00	A	Partial excision (craterization, saucerization, or diaphysectomy) of bone (eg, for osteomyelitis), femur, proximal tibia and/or fibula	9.23	8.56	1.40	19.19	90	S
27365	00	A	Radical resection of tumor, bone, femur or knee	13.84	13.94	2.43	30.21	90	S
27370	00	A	Injection procedure for knee arthrography	0.96	0.60	0.05	1.61	0	N
27372	00	A	Removal of foreign body, deep, thigh region or knee area	4.81	3.42	0.54	8.77	90	S
27380	00	A	Suture of infrapatellar tendon; primary	6.63	7.94	1.29	15.86	90	S
27381	00	A	Suture of infrapatellar tendon; secondary reconstruction, including fascial or tendon graft	9.66	11.27	1.82	22.75	90	S
27385	00	A	Suture of quadriceps or hamstring muscle rupture; primary	7.17	8.84	1.42	17.43	90	S
27386	00	A	Suture of quadriceps or hamstring muscle rupture; secondary reconstruction, including fascial or tendon graft	9.72	12.44	2.02	24.18	90	S
27390	00	A	Tenotomy, open, hamstring, knee to hip; single	4.89	4.36	0.71	9.96	90	S
27391	00	A	Tenotomy, open, hamstring, knee to hip; multiple, one leg	6.67	5.42	0.90	12.99	90	S
27392	00	A	Tenotomy, open, hamstring, knee to hip; multiple, bilateral	8.52	7.67	1.28	17.47	90	S
27393	00	A	Lengthening of hamstring tendon; single	5.95	5.67	0.93	12.55	90	S
27394	00	A	Lengthening of hamstring tendon; multiple, one leg	7.97	5.73	0.94	14.64	90	S
27395	00	A	Lengthening of hamstring tendon; multiple, bilateral	10.96	10.48	1.65	23.09	90	S
27396	00	A	Transplant, hamstring tendon to patella; single	7.33	7.06	1.11	15.50	90	S
27397	00	A	Transplant, hamstring tendon to patella; multiple	9.33	8.88	1.45	19.66	90	S
27400	00	A	Tendon or muscle transfer, hamstrings to femur (Eggers type procedure)	8.47	7.89	1.24	17.60	90	S
27403	00	A	Arthrotomy with open meniscus repair	7.80	8.79	1.44	18.03	90	S
27405	00	A	Repair, primary, torn ligament and/or capsule, knee; collateral	7.97	10.17	1.67	19.81	90	S
27407	00	A	Repair, primary, torn ligament and/or capsule, knee; cruciate	9.44	8.87	1.42	19.73	90	S
27409	00	A	Repair, primary, torn ligament and/or capsule, knee; collateral and cruciate ligaments	11.80	15.10	2.48	29.38	90	S
27418	00	A	Anterior tibial tubercleplasty (eg, for chondromalacia patellae)	9.82	12.23	1.85	23.90	90	S
27420	00	A	Reconstruction for recurrent dislocating patella; (Hauser type procedure)	9.15	10.99	1.74	21.88	90	S

CPT codes and descriptions only, © 1994 American Medical Association. Reimbursement information, © 1995 McGraw-Hill Inc.

Code/ CPT	Mod-ifier	Status	Description	Work value	Practice expense	Mal-practice	Total value	Global period	Up-date
27422	00	A	Reconstruction for recurrent dislocating patella; with extensor realignment and/or muscle advancement or release (Campbell, Goldwaite type procedure)	9.10	11.45	1.83	22.38	90	S
27424	00	A	Reconstruction for recurrent dislocating patella; with patellectomy	9.13	11.68	1.89	22.70	90	S
27425	00	A	Lateral retinacular release (any method)	5.04	6.46	1.08	12.58	90	S
27427	00	A	Ligamentous reconstruction (augmentation), knee; extra-articular	8.68	11.39	2.25	22.32	90	S
27428	00	A	Ligamentous reconstruction (augmentation), knee; intra-articular (open)	10.68	13.67	2.71	27.06	90	S
27429	00	A	Ligamentous reconstruction (augmentation), knee; intra-articular (open) and extra-articular	11.86	11.27	1.83	24.96	90	S
27430	00	A	Quadricepsplasty (Bennett or Thompson type)	8.92	9.36	1.50	19.78	90	S
27435	00	A	Capsulotomy, knee, posterior capsular release	8.74	7.03	1.13	16.90	90	S
27437	00	A	Arthroplasty, patella; without prosthesis	7.74	9.91	1.55	19.20	90	S
27438	00	A	Arthroplasty, patella; with prosthesis	10.29	13.13	2.14	25.56	90	S
27440	00	A	Arthroplasty, knee, tibial plateau;	9.49	11.83	2.10	23.42	90	S
27441	00	A	Arthroplasty, knee, tibial plateau; with debridement and partial synovectomy	9.81	9.14	1.51	20.46	90	S
27442	00	A	Arthroplasty, knee, femoral condyles or tibial plateaus;	11.14	14.98	3.05	29.17	90	S
27443	00	A	Arthroplasty, knee, femoral condyles or tibial plateaus; with debridement and partial synovectomy	10.18	15.27	3.34	28.79	90	S
27445	00	A	Arthroplasty, knee, constrained prosthesis (eg, Walldius type)	16.39	22.34	4.21	42.94	90	S
27446	00	A	Arthroplasty, knee, condyle and plateau; medial OR lateral compartment	15.03	19.79	3.87	38.69	90	S
27447	00	A	Arthroplasty, knee, condyle and plateau; medial AND lateral compartments with or without patella resurfacing ("total knee replacement")	19.69	25.31	4.95	49.95	90	S
27448	00	A	Osteotomy, femur, shaft or supracondylar; without fixation	10.25	12.87	2.09	25.21	90	S
27450	00	A	Osteotomy, femur, shaft or supracondylar; with fixation	13.08	14.84	2.36	30.28	90	S
27454	00	A	Osteotomy, multiple, femoral shaft, with realignment on intramedullary rod (Sofield type procedure)	12.26	15.70	2.82	30.78	90	S
27455	00	A	Osteotomy, proximal tibia, including fibular excision or osteotomy (includes correction of genu varus (bowleg) or genu valgus (knock-knee)); before epiphyseal closure	12.01	12.01	1.95	25.97	90	S
27457	00	A	Osteotomy, proximal tibia, including fibular excision or osteotomy (includes correction of genu varus (bowleg) or genu valgus (knock-knee)); after epiphyseal closure	12.60	13.30	2.14	28.04	90	S
27465	00	A	Osteoplasty, femur; shortening (excluding 64876)	12.84	12.24	2.00	27.08	90	S
27466	00	A	Osteoplasty, femur; lengthening	15.08	13.43	2.27	30.78	90	S
27468	00	A	Osteoplasty, femur; combined, lengthening and shortening with femoral segment transfer	17.65	16.84	2.75	37.24	90	S
27470	00	A	Repair, nonunion or malunion, femur, distal to head and neck; without graft (eg, compression technique)	14.82	16.67	2.60	34.09	90	S
27472	00	A	Repair, nonunion or malunion, femur, distal to head and neck; with iliac or other autogenous bone graft (includes obtaining graft)	16.40	19.87	3.16	39.43	90	S
27475	00	A	Epiphyseal arrest by epiphysiodesis or stapling; distal femur	8.11	7.74	1.27	17.12	90	S
27477	00	A	Epiphyseal arrest by epiphysiodesis or stapling; tibia and fibula, proximal	9.32	12.87	2.57	24.76	90	S
27479	00	A	Epiphyseal arrest by epiphysiodesis or stapling; combined distal femur, proximal tibia and fibula	12.18	11.63	1.89	25.70	90	S

CPT codes and descriptions only, © 1994 American Medical Association. Reimbursement information, © 1995 McGraw-Hill Inc.

Code/ CPT	Mod- ifier	Status	Description	Work value	Practice expense	Mal- practice	Total value	Global period	Up- date
27485	00	A	Arrest, hemiepiphyseal, distal femur or proximal leg (eg, for genu varus or valgus)	8.31	7.91	1.30	17.52	90	S
27486	00	A	Revision of total knee arthroplasty, with or without allograft; one component	16.63	21.74	4.26	42.63	90	S
27487	00	A	Revision of total knee arthroplasty, with or without allograft; all components	21.69	29.50	5.97	57.16	90	S
27488	00	A	Removal of knee prosthesis, including "total knee," methylmethacrylate and insertion of spacer, when applicable	14.48	16.16	2.58	33.22	90	S
27495	00	A	Prophylactic treatment (nailing, pinning, plating or wiring) with or without methylmethacrylate, femur	14.26	17.63	2.82	34.71	90	S
27496	00	A	Decompression fasciotomy, thigh and/or knee, one compartment (flexor or extensor or adductor);	4.75	4.53	0.74	10.02	90	S
27497	00	A	Decompression fasciotomy, thigh and/or knee, one compartment (flexor or extensor or adductor); with debridement of nonviable muscle and/or nerve	5.81	5.55	0.91	12.27	90	S
27498	00	A	Decompression fasciotomy, thigh and/or knee, multiple compartments;	6.63	6.32	1.04	13.99	90	S
27499	00	A	Decompression fasciotomy, thigh and/or knee, multiple compartments; with debridement of nonviable muscle and/or nerve	7.64	7.28	1.19	16.11	90	S
27500	00	A	Closed treatment of femoral shaft fracture, without manipulation	5.29	5.41	0.82	11.52	90	S
27501	00	A	Closed treatment of supracondylar or transcondylar femoral fracture with or without intercondylar extension, without manipulation	5.29	5.41	0.82	11.52	90	S
27502	00	A	Closed treatment of femoral shaft fracture, with manipulation, with or without skin or skeletal traction	9.51	7.67	1.21	18.39	90	S
27503	00	A	Closed treatment of supracondylar or transcondylar femoral fracture with or without intercondylar extension, with manipulation, with or without skin or skeletal traction	9.51	7.67	1.21	18.39	90	S
27506	00	A	Open treatment of femoral shaft fracture, with or without external fixation, with insertion of intramedullary implant, with or without cerclage and/or locking screws	15.93	16.02	2.56	34.51	90	S
27507	00	A	Open treatment of femoral shaft fracture with plate/screws, with or without cerclage	12.85	16.02	2.56	31.43	90	S
27508	00	A	Closed treatment of femoral fracture, distal end, medial or lateral condyle, without manipulation	5.21	4.22	0.65	10.08	90	S
27509	00	A	Percutaneous skeletal fixation of femoral fracture, distal end, medial or lateral condyle, or supracondylar or transcondylar, with or without intercondylar extension, or distal femoral epiphyseal separation	6.77	4.22	0.65	11.64	90	S
27510	00	A	Closed treatment of femoral fracture, distal end, medial or lateral condyle, with manipulation	8.19	6.82	1.09	16.10	90	S
27511	00	A	Open treatment of femoral supracondylar or transcondylar fracture without intercondylar extension, with or without internal or external fixation	12.50	16.00	2.56	31.06	90	S
27513	00	A	Open treatment of femoral supracondylar or transcondylar fracture with intercondylar extension, with or without internal or external fixation	16.78	16.02	2.56	35.36	90	S
27514	00	A	Open treatment of femoral fracture, distal end, medial or lateral condyle, with or without internal or external fixation	15.98	15.76	2.53	34.27	90	S
27516	00	A	Closed treatment of distal femoral epiphyseal separation; without manipulation	4.92	4.82	0.71	10.45	90	S
27517	00	A	Closed treatment of distal femoral epiphyseal separation; with manipulation, with or without skin or skeletal traction	8.20	7.82	1.28	17.30	90	S

CPT codes and descriptions only, © 1994 American Medical Association. Reimbursement information, © 1995 McGraw-Hill Inc.

Code/ CPT	Mod- ifier	Status	Description	Work value	Practice expense	Mal- practice	Total value	Global period	Up- date
27519	00	A	Open treatment of distal femoral epiphyseal separation, with or without internal or external fixation	13.82	12.68	2.05	28.55	90	S
27520	00	A	Closed treatment of patellar fracture, without manipulation	2.68	3.04	0.45	6.17	90	S
27524	00	A	Open treatment of patellar fracture, with internal fixation and/or partial or complete patellectomy and soft tissue repair	9.38	10.34	1.65	21.37	90	S
27530	00	A	Closed treatment of tibial fracture, proximal (plateau); without manipulation	3.23	3.40	0.51	7.14	90	S
27532	00	A	Closed treatment of tibial fracture, proximal (plateau); with or without manipulation, with skeletal traction	6.81	5.68	0.91	13.40	90	S
27535	00	A	Open treatment of tibial fracture, proximal (plateau); unicondylar, with or without internal or external fixation	10.36	11.69	1.88	23.93	90	S
27536	00	A	Open treatment of tibial fracture, proximal (plateau); bicondylar, with or without internal fixation	14.51	11.69	1.88	28.08	90	S
27538	00	A	Closed treatment of intercondylar spine(s) and/or tuberosity fracture(s) of knee, with or without manipulation	4.64	3.37	0.51	8.52	90	S
27540	00	A	Open treatment of intercondylar spine(s) and/or tuberosity fracture(s) of the knee, with or without internal or external fixation	12.38	10.95	1.74	25.07	90	S
27550	00	A	Closed treatment of knee dislocation; without anesthesia	5.53	2.57	0.36	8.46	90	S
27552	00	A	Closed treatment of knee dislocation; requiring anesthesia	7.39	3.43	0.53	11.35	90	S
27556	00	A	Open treatment of knee dislocation, with or without internal or external fixation; without primary ligamentous repair or augmentation/reconstruction	13.47	12.48	1.95	27.90	90	S
27557	00	A	Open treatment of knee dislocation, with or without internal or external fixation; with primary ligamentous repair	15.80	14.60	2.43	32.83	90	S
27558	00	A	Open treatment of knee dislocation, with or without internal or external fixation; with primary ligamentous repair, with augmentation/reconstruction	16.75	14.60	2.43	33.78	90	S
27560	00	A	Closed treatment of patellar dislocation; without anesthesia	3.64	1.43	0.16	5.23	90	S
27562	00	A	Closed treatment of patellar dislocation; requiring anesthesia	5.48	5.18	0.76	11.42	90	S
27566	00	A	Open treatment of patellar dislocation, with or without partial or total patellectomy	11.48	10.58	1.67	23.73	90	S
27570	00	A	Manipulation of knee joint under general anesthesia (includes application of traction or other fixation devices)	1.69	1.72	0.28	3.69	10	S
27580	00	A	Fusion of knee, any technique	12.26	15.70	2.56	30.52	90	S
27590	00	A	Amputation, thigh, through femur, any level;	10.24	9.11	1.80	21.15	90	S
27591	00	A	Amputation, thigh, through femur, any level; immediate fitting technique including first cast	11.09	11.77	2.11	24.97	90	S
27592	00	A	Amputation, thigh, through femur, any level; open, circular (guillotine)	8.75	8.11	1.61	18.47	90	S
27594	00	A	Amputation, thigh, through femur, any level; secondary closure or scar revision	6.30	3.65	0.68	10.63	90	S
27596	00	A	Amputation, thigh, through femur, any level; re-amputation	9.63	7.37	1.42	18.42	90	S
27598	00	A	Disarticulation at knee	9.56	10.04	1.78	21.38	90	S
27599	00	C	Unlisted procedure, femur or knee	0	0	0	0	YYY	S
27600	00	A	Decompression fasciotomy, leg; anterior and/or lateral compartments only	5.02	3.39	0.64	9.05	90	S
27601	00	A	Decompression fasciotomy, leg; posterior compartment(s) only	4.98	3.38	0.67	9.03	90	S
27602	00	A	Decompression fasciotomy, leg; anterior and/or lateral, and posterior compartment(s)	6.63	4.05	0.77	11.45	90	S

CPT codes and descriptions only, © 1994 American Medical Association. Reimbursement information, © 1995 McGraw-Hill Inc.

Code/ CPT	Mod- ifier	Status	Description	Work value	Practice expense	Mal- practice	Total value	Global period	Up- date
27603	00	A	Incision and drainage, leg or ankle; deep abscess or hematoma	4.41	2.38	0.41	7.20	90	S
27604	00	A	Incision and drainage, leg or ankle; infected bursa	4.23	1.02	0.14	5.39	90	S
27605	00	A	Tenotomy, Achilles tendon, subcutaneous (separate procedure); local anesthesia	2.82	1.18	0.14	4.14	10	S
27606	00	A	Tenotomy, Achilles tendon, subcutaneous (separate procedure); general anesthesia	3.87	2.12	0.35	6.34	10	S
27607	00	A	Incision, deep, with opening of bone cortex (eg, for osteomyelitis or bone abscess), leg or ankle	7.05	6.01	0.98	14.04	90	S
27610	00	A	Arthrotomy, ankle, for infection, with exploration, drainage or removal of foreign body	7.27	7.43	1.13	15.83	90	S
27612	00	A	Arthrotomy, ankle, posterior capsular release, with or without Achilles tendon lengthening	6.23	7.97	1.30	15.50	90	S
27613	00	A	Biopsy, soft tissue of leg or ankle area; superficial	2.12	0.67	0.10	2.89	10	S
27614	00	A	Biopsy, soft tissue of leg or ankle area; deep	5.29	2.26	0.38	7.93	90	S
27615	00	A	Radical resection of tumor (eg, malignant neoplasm), soft tissue of leg or ankle area	11.79	8.23	1.42	21.44	90	S
27618	00	A	Excision, tumor, leg or ankle area; subcutaneous	4.94	2.10	0.32	7.36	90	S
27619	00	A	Excision, tumor, leg or ankle area; deep, subfascial or intramuscular	7.98	4.13	0.67	12.78	90	S
27620	00	A	Arthrotomy, ankle, with joint exploration, with or without biopsy, with or without removal of loose or foreign body	5.69	6.03	0.96	12.68	90	S
27625	00	A	Arthrotomy, ankle, with synovectomy;	7.88	8.71	1.27	17.86	90	S
27626	00	A	Arthrotomy, ankle, with synovectomy; including tenosynovectomy	8.49	10.86	1.25	20.60	90	S
27630	00	A	Excision of lesion of tendon sheath or capsule (eg, cyst or ganglion), leg and/or ankle	4.65	3.10	0.46	8.21	90	S
27635	00	A	Excision or curettage of bone cyst or benign tumor, tibia or fibula;	7.29	8.04	1.27	16.60	90	S
27637	00	A	Excision or curettage of bone cyst or benign tumor, tibia or fibula; with autograft (includes obtaining graft)	9.14	8.47	1.40	19.01	90	S
27638	00	A	Excision or curettage of bone cyst or benign tumor, tibia or fibula; with allograft	9.89	9.15	1.52	20.56	90	S
27640	00	A	Partial excision (craterization, saucerization, or diaphysectomy) of bone (eg, for osteomyelitis or exostosis); tibia	10.21	9.81	1.57	21.59	90	S
27641	00	A	Partial excision (craterization, saucerization, or diaphysectomy) of bone (eg, for osteomyelitis or exostosis); fibula	8.36	7.13	1.18	16.67	90	S
27645	00	A	Radical resection of tumor, bone; tibia	13.14	11.64	1.98	26.76	90	S
27646	00	A	Radical resection of tumor, bone; fibula	11.69	10.75	1.71	24.15	90	S
27647	00	A	Radical resection of tumor, bone; talus or calcaneus	11.21	9.95	1.35	22.51	90	S
27648	00	A	Injection procedure for ankle arthrography	0.96	0.52	0.05	1.53	0	N
27650	00	A	Repair, primary, open or percutaneous, ruptured Achilles tendon;	9.07	8.98	1.41	19.46	90	S
27652	00	A	Repair, primary, open or percutaneous, ruptured Achilles tendon; with graft (includes obtaining graft)	9.62	10.41	1.56	21.59	90	S
27654	00	A	Repair, secondary, ruptured Achilles tendon, with or without graft	9.34	10.93	1.65	21.92	90	S
27656	00	A	Repair, fascial defect of leg	4.31	3.18	0.54	8.03	90	S
27658	00	A	Repair or suture of flexor tendon of leg; primary, without graft, single, each	4.61	4.02	0.60	9.23	90	S
27659	00	A	Repair or suture of flexor tendon of leg; secondary with or without graft, single tendon, each	6.28	5.87	0.86	13.01	90	S

CPT codes and descriptions only, © 1994 American Medical Association. Reimbursement information, © 1995 McGraw-Hill Inc.

Code/ CPT	Mod-ifier	Status	Description	Work value	Practice expense	Mal-practice	Total value	Global period	Up-date
27664	00	A	Repair or suture of extensor tendon of leg; primary, without graft, single, each	4.33	3.41	0.52	8.26	90	S
27665	00	A	Repair or suture of extensor tendon of leg; secondary with or without graft, single tendon, each	5.11	4.95	0.76	10.82	90	S
27675	00	A	Repair for dislocating peroneal tendons; without fibular osteotomy	6.78	6.40	0.94	14.12	90	S
27676	00	A	Repair for dislocating peroneal tendons; with fibular osteotomy	7.87	7.56	1.14	16.57	90	S
27680	00	A	Tenolysis, including tibia, fibula and ankle flexor; single	5.37	4.12	0.61	10.10	90	S
27681	00	A	Tenolysis, including tibia, fibula and ankle flexor; multiple (through same incision), each	6.36	5.97	0.86	13.19	90	S
27685	00	A	Lengthening or shortening of tendon, leg or ankle; single (separate procedure)	6.08	3.83	0.41	10.32	90	S
27686	00	A	Lengthening or shortening of tendon, leg or ankle; multiple (through same incision), each	6.93	6.56	0.90	14.39	90	S
27687	00	A	Gastrocnemius recession (eg, Strayer procedure)	5.84	5.45	0.76	12.05	90	S
27690	00	A	Transfer or transplant of single tendon (with muscle redirection or rerouting); superficial (eg, anterior tibial extensors into midfoot)	8.09	6.74	0.88	15.71	90	S
27691	00	A	Transfer or transplant of single tendon (with muscle redirection or rerouting); anterior tibial or posterior tibial through interosseous space	9.25	7.89	1.23	18.37	90	S
27692	00	A	Transfer or transplant of single tendon (with muscle redirection or rerouting); each additional tendon	1.87	2.03	0.29	4.19	ZZZ	S
27695	00	A	Suture, primary, torn, ruptured or severed ligament, ankle; collateral	6.09	7.79	1.32	15.20	90	S
27696	00	A	Suture, primary, torn, ruptured or severed ligament, ankle; both collateral ligaments	7.72	7.06	1.16	15.94	90	S
27698	00	A	Suture, secondary repair, torn, ruptured or severed ligament, ankle, collateral (eg, Watson-Jones procedure)	8.87	11.35	1.86	22.08	90	S
27700	00	A	Arthroplasty, ankle;	8.67	11.11	1.51	21.29	90	S
27702	00	A	Arthroplasty, ankle; with implant ("total ankle")	12.64	18.57	3.99	35.20	90	S
27703	00	A	Arthroplasty, ankle; secondary reconstruction, total ankle	14.49	13.82	2.25	30.56	90	S
27704	00	A	Removal of ankle implant	7.20	5.84	0.98	14.02	90	S
27705	00	A	Osteotomy; tibia	9.63	10.74	1.76	22.13	90	S
27707	00	A	Osteotomy; fibula	3.71	4.75	0.79	9.25	90	S
27709	00	A	Osteotomy; tibia and fibula	9.14	11.70	2.14	22.98	90	S
27712	00	A	Osteotomy; multiple, with realignment on intramedullary rod (Sofield type procedure)	11.81	10.99	1.63	24.43	90	S
27715	00	A	Osteoplasty, tibia and fibula, lengthening	12.97	12.61	1.88	27.46	90	S
27720	00	A	Repair of nonunion or malunion, tibia; without graft, (eg, compression technique)	10.95	13.97	2.25	27.17	90	S
27722	00	A	Repair of nonunion or malunion, tibia; with sliding graft	10.92	10.50	1.64	23.06	90	S
27724	00	A	Repair of nonunion or malunion, tibia; with iliac or other autograft (includes obtaining graft)	12.11	15.50	2.87	30.48	90	S
27725	00	A	Repair of nonunion or malunion, tibia; by synostosis, with fibula, any method	11.04	10.43	1.53	23.00	90	S
27727	00	A	Repair of congenital pseudarthrosis, tibia	12.89	9.38	1.84	24.11	90	S
27730	00	A	Epiphyseal arrest by epiphysiodesis or stapling; distal tibia	6.88	3.59	0.84	11.31	90	S
27732	00	A	Epiphyseal arrest by epiphysiodesis or stapling; distal fibula	5.06	4.84	0.79	10.69	90	S
27734	00	A	Epiphyseal arrest by epiphysiodesis or stapling; distal tibia and fibula	7.89	7.54	1.23	16.66	90	S
27740	00	A	Epiphyseal arrest by epiphysiodesis or stapling, combined, proximal and distal tibia and fibula;	8.75	8.36	1.36	18.47	90	S

CPT codes and descriptions only, © 1994 American Medical Association. Reimbursement information, © 1995 McGraw-Hill Inc.

Code/ CPT	Mod-ifier	Status	Description	Work value	Practice expense	Mal-practice	Total value	Global period	Up-date
27742	00	A	Epiphyseal arrest by epiphysiodesis or stapling, combined, proximal and distal tibia and fibula; and distal femur	9.72	9.29	1.52	20.53	90	S
27745	00	A	Prophylactic treatment (nailing, pinning, plating or wiring) with or without methylmethacrylate, tibia	9.39	8.97	1.39	19.75	90	S
27750	00	A	Closed treatment of tibial shaft fracture (with or without fibular fracture); without manipulation	2.90	3.45	0.50	6.85	90	S
27752	00	A	Closed treatment of tibial shaft fracture (with or without fibular fracture); with manipulation, with or without skeletal traction	5.16	5.09	0.81	11.06	90	S
27756	00	A	Percutaneous skeletal fixation of tibial shaft fracture (with or without fibular fracture) (eg, pins or screws)	5.84	8.21	1.70	15.75	90	S
27758	00	A	Open treatment of tibial shaft fracture, (with or without fibular fracture) with plate/screws, with or without cerclage	10.51	13.46	2.22	26.19	90	S
27759	00	A	Open treatment of tibial shaft fracture (with or without fibular fracture) by intramedullary implant, with or without interlocking screws and/or cerclage	12.60	13.74	2.22	28.56	90	S
27760	00	A	Closed treatment of medial malleolus fracture; without manipulation	2.81	2.58	0.37	5.76	90	S
27762	00	A	Closed treatment of medial malleolus fracture; with manipulation, with or without skin or skeletal traction	4.80	3.36	0.50	8.66	90	S
27766	00	A	Open treatment of medial malleolus fracture, with orwithout internal or external fixation	7.61	7.87	1.26	16.74	90	S
27780	00	A	Closed treatment of proximal fibula or shaft fracture; without manipulation	2.47	1.97	0.26	4.70	90	S
27781	00	A	Closed treatment of proximal fibula or shaft fracture; with manipulation	4.20	3.29	0.49	7.98	90	S
27784	00	A	Open treatment of proximal fibula or shaft fracture, with or without internal or external fixation	6.45	5.59	0.87	12.91	90	S
27786	00	A	Closed treatment of distal fibular fracture (lateral malleolus); without manipulation	2.66	2.52	0.38	5.56	90	S
27788	00	A	Closed treatment of distal fibular fracture (lateral malleolus); with manipulation	4.25	3.27	0.50	8.02	90	S
27792	00	A	Open treatment of distal fibular fracture (lateral malleolus), with or without internal or external fixation	7.04	7.38	1.17	15.59	90	S
27808	00	A	Closed treatment of bimalleolar ankle fracture, (including Potts); without manipulation	2.63	2.79	0.39	5.81	90	S
27810	00	A	Closed treatment of bimalleolar ankle fracture, (including Potts); with manipulation	4.82	5.05	0.80	10.67	90	S
27814	00	A	Open treatment of bimalleolar ankle fracture, with or without internal or external fixation	9.87	10.00	1.60	21.47	90	S
27816	00	A	Closed treatment of trimalleolar ankle fracture; without manipulation	2.71	3.47	0.55	6.73	90	S
27818	00	A	Closed treatment of trimalleolar ankle fracture; with manipulation	5.08	6.51	1.06	12.65	90	S
27822	00	A	Open treatment of trimalleolar ankle fracture, with or without internal or external fixation, medial and/or lateral malleolus; without fixation of posterior lip	8.39	10.73	1.88	21.00	90	S
27823	00	A	Open treatment of trimalleolar ankle fracture, with or without internal or external fixation, medial and/or lateral malleolus; with fixation of posterior lip	10.90	12.79	2.05	25.74	90	S
27824	00	A	Closed treatment of fracture of weight bearing articular portion of distal tibia (eg, pilon or tibial plafond), with or without anesthesia; without manipulation	2.71	3.47	0.55	6.73	90	S

CPT codes and descriptions only, © 1994 American Medical Association. Reimbursement information, © 1995 McGraw-Hill Inc.

Code/ CPT	Mod- ifier	Status	Description	Work value	Practice expense	Mal- practice	Total value	Global period	Up- date
27825	00	A	Closed treatment of fracture of weight bearing articular portion of distal tibia (eg, pilon or tibial plafond), with or without anesthesia; with skeletal traction and/or requiring manipulation	5.08	6.51	1.06	12.65	90	S
27826	00	A	Open treatment of fracture of weight bearing articular surface/portion of distal tibia (eg, pilon or tibial plafond), with internal or external fixation; of fibula only	7.43	9.57	1.88	18.88	90	S
27827	00	A	Open treatment of fracture of weight bearing articular surface/portion of distal tibia (eg, pilon or tibial plafond), with internal or external fixation; of tibia only	9.90	11.71	1.88	23.49	90	S
27828	00	A	Open treatment of fracture of weight bearing articular surface/portion of distal tibia (eg, pilon or tibial plafond), with internal or external fixation; of both tibia and fibula	12.33	12.79	2.05	27.17	90	S
27829	00	A	Open treatment of distal tibiofibular joint (syndesmosis) disruption, with or without internal or external fixation	4.87	6.74	1.37	12.98	90	S
27830	00	A	Closed treatment of proximal tibiofibular joint dislocation; without anesthesia	3.50	3.25	0.46	7.21	90	S
27831	00	A	Closed treatment of proximal tibiofibular joint dislocation; requiring anesthesia	4.27	3.98	0.59	8.84	90	S
27832	00	A	Open treatment of proximal tibiofibular joint dislocation, with or without internal or external fixation, or with excision of proximal fibula	5.96	5.70	0.89	12.55	90	S
27840	00	A	Closed treatment of ankle dislocation; without anesthesia	4.27	1.87	0.21	6.35	90	S
27842	00	A	Closed treatment of ankle dislocation; requiring anesthesia, with or without percutaneous skeletal fixation	5.72	2.22	0.34	8.28	90	S
27846	00	A	Open treatment of ankle dislocation, with or without percutaneous skeletal fixation; without repair or internal fixation	9.04	8.59	1.37	19.00	90	S
27848	00	A	Open treatment of ankle dislocation, with or without percutaneous skeletal fixation; with repair or internal or external fixation	10.45	8.36	1.32	20.13	90	S
27860	00	A	Manipulation of ankle under general anesthesia (includes application of traction or other fixation apparatus)	2.29	1.39	0.23	3.91	10	S
27870	00	A	Arthrodesis, ankle, any method	10.42	13.34	2.22	25.98	90	S
27871	00	A	Arthrodesis, tibiofibular joint, proximal or distal	8.55	7.79	1.21	17.55	90	S
27880	00	A	Amputation, leg, through tibia and fibula;	10.69	8.36	1.60	20.65	90	S
27881	00	A	Amputation, leg, through tibia and fibula; with immediate fitting technique including application of first cast	10.89	10.82	1.87	23.58	90	S
27882	00	A	Amputation, leg, through tibia and fibula; open, circular (guillotine)	7.80	7.36	1.42	16.58	90	S
27884	00	A	Amputation, leg, through tibia and fibula; secondary closure or scar revision	7.40	3.37	0.61	11.38	90	S
27886	00	A	Amputation, leg, through tibia and fibula; re-amputation	8.35	7.17	1.34	16.86	90	S
27888	00	A	Amputation, ankle, through malleoli of tibia and fibula (Syme, Pirogoff type procedures), with plastic closure and resection of nerves	8.70	9.49	1.65	19.84	90	S
27889	00	A	Ankle disarticulation	8.82	8.43	1.55	18.80	90	S
27892	00	A	Decompression fasciotomy, leg; anterior and/or lateral compartments only, with debridement of nonviable muscle and/or nerve	6.03	3.39	0.64	10.06	90	S
27893	00	A	Decompression fasciotomy, leg; posterior compartment(s) only, with debridement of nonviable muscle and/or nerve	5.99	3.38	0.67	10.04	90	S
27894	00	A	Decompression fasciotomy, leg; anterior and/or lateral, and posterior compartment(s), with debridement of nonviable muscle and/or nerve	7.64	4.05	0.77	12.46	90	S
27899	00	C	Unlisted procedure, leg or ankle	0	0	0	0	YYY	S

CPT codes and descriptions only, © 1994 American Medical Association. Reimbursement information, © 1995 McGraw-Hill Inc.

Code/ CPT	Mod- ifier	Status	Description	Work value	Practice expense	Mal- practice	Total value	Global period	Up- date
28001	00	A	Incision and drainage, infected bursa, foot	2.68	0.52	0.05	3.25	10	S
28002	00	A	Deep dissection below fascia, for deep infection of foot, with or without tendon sheath involvement; single bursal space, specify	3.76	2.25	0.33	6.34	10	S
28003	00	A	Deep dissection below fascia, for deep infection of foot, with or without tendon sheath involvement; multiple areas	7.49	3.50	0.59	11.58	90	S
28005	00	A	Incision, deep, with opening of bone cortex (eg, for osteomyelitis or bone abscess), foot	7.65	4.08	0.61	12.34	90	S
28008	00	A	Fasciotomy, foot and/or toe	4.19	2.68	0.29	7.16	90	S
28010	00	A	Tenotomy, subcutaneous, toe; single	2.97	3.62	0.33	6.92	90	S
28011	00	A	Tenotomy, subcutaneous, toe; multiple	3.99	1.77	0.19	5.95	90	S
28020	00	A	Arthrotomy, with exploration, drainage or removal of loose or foreign body; intertarsal or tarsometatarsal joint	4.75	4.40	0.56	9.71	90	S
28022	00	A	Arthrotomy, with exploration, drainage or removal of loose or foreign body; metatarsophalangeal joint	4.41	2.74	0.31	7.46	90	S
28024	00	A	Arthrotomy, with exploration, drainage or removal of loose or foreign body; interphalangeal joint	4.12	2.39	0.24	6.75	90	S
28030	00	A	Neurectomy of intrinsic musculature of foot	5.78	3.93	0.42	10.13	90	S
28035	00	A	Tarsal tunnel release (posterior tibial nerve decompression)	4.83	6.18	0.90	11.91	90	S
28043	00	A	Excision, tumor, foot; subcutaneous	3.41	1.73	0.20	5.34	90	S
28045	00	A	Excision, tumor, foot; deep, subfascial, intramuscular	4.46	3.99	0.46	8.91	90	S
28046	00	A	Radical resection of tumor (eg, malignant neoplasm), soft tissue of foot	9.41	5.35	0.79	15.55	90	S
28050	00	A	Arthrotomy for synovial biopsy; intertarsal or tarsometatarsal joint	3.99	3.84	0.53	8.36	90	S
28052	00	A	Arthrotomy for synovial biopsy; metatarsophalangeal joint	3.70	3.82	0.43	7.95	90	S
28054	00	A	Arthrotomy for synovial biopsy; interphalangeal joint	3.21	2.24	0.28	5.73	90	S
28060	00	A	Fasciectomy, excision of plantar fascia; partial (separate procedure)	5.05	4.22	0.53	9.80	90	S
28062	00	A	Fasciectomy, excision of plantar fascia; radical (separate procedure)	6.23	7.06	0.86	14.15	90	S
28070	00	A	Synovectomy; intertarsal or tarsometatarsal joint, each	4.73	4.48	0.48	9.69	90	S
28072	00	A	Synovectomy; metatarsophalangeal joint, each	4.32	3.21	0.42	7.95	90	S
28080	00	A	Excision of interdigital (Morton) neuroma, single, each	3.18	4.07	0.45	7.70	90	S
28086	00	A	Synovectomy, tendon sheath, foot; flexor	4.52	3.12	0.46	8.10	90	S
28088	00	A	Synovectomy, tendon sheath, foot; extensor	3.62	3.62	0.40	7.64	90	S
28090	00	A	Excision of lesion of tendon or fibrous sheath or capsule (including synovectomy) (cyst or ganglion); foot	4.26	3.02	0.29	7.57	90	S
28092	00	A	Excision of lesion of tendon or fibrous sheath or capsule (including synovectomy) (cyst or ganglion); toes	3.49	2.03	0.25	5.77	90	S
28100	00	A	Excision or curettage of bone cyst or benign tumor, talus or calcaneus;	5.37	4.58	0.56	10.51	90	S
28102	00	A	Excision or curettage of bone cyst or benign tumor, talus or calcaneus; with iliac or other autograft (includes obtaining graft)	7.31	6.84	0.85	15.00	90	S
28103	00	A	Excision or curettage of bone cyst or benign tumor, talus or calcaneus; with allograft	6.10	5.61	0.69	12.40	90	S
28104	00	A	Excision or curettage of bone cyst or benign tumor, tarsal or metatarsal bones, except talus or calcaneus;	4.86	4.33	0.49	9.68	90	S
28106	00	A	Excision or curettage of bone cyst or benign tumor, tarsal or metatarsal bones, except talus or calcaneus; with iliac or other autograft (includes obtaining graft)	6.74	6.42	0.79	13.95	90	S

CPT codes and descriptions only, © 1994 American Medical Association. Reimbursement information, © 1995 McGraw-Hill Inc.

Code/ CPT	Mod- ifier	Status	Description	Work value	Practice expense	Mal- practice	Total value	Global period	Up- date
28107	00	A	Excision or curettage of bone cyst or benign tumor, tarsal or metatarsal bones, except talus or calcaneus; with allograft	5.16	4.86	0.48	10.50	90	S
28108	00	A	Excision or curettage of bone cyst or benign tumor, phalanges of foot	4.01	4.20	0.38	8.59	90	S
28110	00	A	Ostectomy, partial excision, fifth metatarsal head (bunionette) (separate procedure)	3.82	3.48	0.39	7.69	90	S
28111	00	A	Ostectomy, complete excision; first metatarsal head	4.64	5.04	0.65	10.33	90	S
28112	00	A	Ostectomy, complete excision; other metatarsal head (second, third or fourth)	4.23	3.96	0.45	8.64	90	S
28113	00	A	Ostectomy, complete excision; fifth metatarsal head	4.09	4.44	0.48	9.01	90	S
28114	00	A	Ostectomy, complete excision; all metatarsal heads, with partial proximal phalangectomy, excluding first metatarsal (Clayton type procedure)	7.16	9.17	1.42	17.75	90	S
28116	00	A	Ostectomy, excision of tarsal coalition	6.17	5.48	0.57	12.22	90	S
28118	00	A	Ostectomy, calcaneus;	5.56	5.71	0.66	11.93	90	S
28119	00	A	Ostectomy, calcaneus; for spur, with or without plantar fascial release	5.10	5.44	0.57	11.11	90	S
28120	00	A	Partial excision (craterization, saucerization, sequestrectomy, or diaphysectomy) of bone (eg, for osteomyelitis or talar bossing), talus or calcaneus	4.81	5.04	0.67	10.52	90	S
28122	00	A	Partial excision (craterization, saucerization, or diaphysectomy) of bone (eg, for osteomyelitis or tarsal bossing), tarsal or metatarsal bone, except talus or calcaneus	6.62	4.48	0.54	11.64	90	S
28124	00	A	Partial excision (craterization, saucerization, or diaphysectomy) of bone (eg, for osteomyelitis or dorsal bossing), phalanx of toe	4.39	4.11	0.37	8.87	90	S
28126	00	A	Resection, partial or complete, phalangeal base, single toe, each	3.39	3.98	0.36	7.73	90	S
28130	00	A	Talectomy (astragalectomy)	7.33	7.03	0.88	15.24	90	S
28140	00	A	Metatarsectomy	6.45	4.93	0.62	12.00	90	S
28150	00	A	Phalangectomy of toe, single, each	3.83	3.29	0.38	7.50	90	S
28153	00	A	Resection, head of phalanx, toe	3.40	3.99	0.36	7.75	90	S
28160	00	A	Hemiphalangectomy or interphalangeal joint excision, toe, single, each	3.59	4.12	0.38	8.09	90	S
28171	00	A	Radical resection of tumor, bone; tarsal (except talus or calcaneus)	8.98	7.99	0.88	17.85	90	S
28173	00	A	Radical resection of tumor, bone; metatarsal	8.18	5.74	0.74	14.66	90	S
28175	00	A	Radical resection of tumor, bone; phalanx of toe	5.59	5.38	0.58	11.55	90	S
28190	00	A	Removal of foreign body, foot; subcutaneous	1.91	0.52	0.05	2.48	10	S
28192	00	A	Removal of foreign body, foot; deep	4.49	1.95	0.24	6.68	90	S
28193	00	A	Removal of foreign body, foot; complicated	5.44	2.38	0.30	8.12	90	S
28200	00	A	Repair or suture of tendon, foot, flexor, single; primary or secondary, without free graft, each tendon	4.45	5.06	0.50	10.01	90	S
28202	00	A	Repair or suture of tendon, foot, flexor, single; secondary with free graft, each tendon (includes obtaining graft)	6.38	5.82	0.77	12.97	90	S
28208	00	A	Repair or suture of tendon, foot, extensor, single; primary or secondary, each tendon	4.11	2.81	0.28	7.20	90	S
28210	00	A	Repair or suture of tendon, foot, extensor, single; secondary with free graft, each tendon (includes obtaining graft)	5.95	5.60	0.60	12.15	90	S
28220	00	A	Tenolysis, flexor, foot; single	4.27	3.87	0.43	8.57	90	S
28222	00	A	Tenolysis, flexor, foot; multiple (through same incision)	5.36	6.40	0.63	12.39	90	S

CPT codes and descriptions only, © 1994 American Medical Association. Reimbursement information, © 1995 McGraw-Hill Inc.

Code/ CPT	Mod- ifier	Status	Description	Work value	Practice expense	Mal- practice	Total value	Global period	Up- date
28225	00	A	Tenolysis, extensor, foot; single	3.42	2.37	0.25	6.04	90	S
28226	00	A	Tenolysis, extensor, foot; multiple (through same incision)	4.27	3.38	0.40	8.05	90	S
28230	00	A	Tenotomy, open, flexor; foot, single or multiple (separate procedure)	4.00	2.43	0.22	6.65	90	S
28232	00	A	Tenotomy, open, flexor; toe, single (separate procedure)	3.26	1.60	0.15	5.01	90	S
28234	00	A	Tenotomy, open, extensor, foot or toe	3.19	1.53	0.14	4.86	90	S
28236	00	A	Transfer of tendon, anterior tibial into tarsal bone	8.01	7.52	1.09	16.62	90	S
28238	00	A	Advancement of posterior tibial tendon with excision of accessory navicular bone (Kidner type procedure)	7.27	7.23	0.85	15.35	90	S
28240	00	A	Tenotomy, lengthening, or release, abductor hallucis muscle	4.12	2.13	0.23	6.48	90	S
28250	00	A	Division of plantar fascia and muscle ("Steindler stripping") (separate procedure)	5.66	4.46	0.50	10.62	90	S
28260	00	A	Capsulotomy, midfoot; medial release only (separate procedure)	7.50	4.43	0.48	12.41	90	S
28261	00	A	Capsulotomy, midfoot; with tendon lengthening	8.92	5.91	0.58	15.41	90	S
28262	00	A	Capsulotomy, midfoot; extensive, including posterior talotibial capsulotomy and tendon(s) lengthening as for resistant clubfoot deformity	12.19	11.91	1.44	25.54	90	S
28264	00	A	Capsulotomy, midtarsal (Heyman type procedure)	9.80	9.56	1.17	20.53	90	S
28270	00	A	Capsulotomy; metatarsophalangeal joint, with or without tenorrhaphy, single, each joint (separate procedure)	4.58	2.63	0.23	7.44	90	S
28272	00	A	Capsulotomy; interphalangeal joint, single, each joint (separate procedure)	3.67	2.04	0.18	5.89	90	S
28280	00	A	Webbing operation (create syndactylism of toes)(Kelikian type procedure)	4.93	2.22	0.30	7.45	90	S
28285	00	A	Hammertoe operation, one toe (eg, interphalangeal fusion, filleting, phalangectomy)	4.41	4.37	0.39	9.17	90	S
28286	00	A	Cock-up fifth toe operation with plastic skin closure (Ruiz-Mora type procedure)	4.41	3.58	0.38	8.37	90	S
28288	00	A	Ostectomy, partial, exostectomy or condylectomy, single, metatarsal head, first through fifth, each metatarsal head	3.73	3.75	0.43	7.91	90	S
28290	00	A	Hallux valgus (bunion) correction, with or without sesamoidectomy; simple exostectomy (Silver type procedure)	5.37	5.36	0.63	11.36	90	S
28292	00	A	Hallux valgus (bunion) correction, with or without sesamoidectomy; Keller, McBride or Mayo type procedure	6.24	7.05	0.74	14.03	90	S
28293	00	A	Hallux valgus (bunion) correction, with or without sesamoidectomy; resection of joint with implant	8.25	9.55	0.98	18.78	90	S
28294	00	A	Hallux valgus (bunion) correction, with or without sesamoidectomy; with tendon transplants (Joplin type procedure)	8.14	9.16	0.86	18.16	90	S
28296	00	A	Hallux valgus (bunion) correction, with or without sesamoidectomy; with metatarsal osteotomy (eg, Mitchell, Chevron, or concentric type procedures)	8.69	8.81	0.98	18.48	90	S
28297	00	A	Hallux valgus (bunion) correction, with or without sesamoidectomy; Lapidus type procedure	8.69	9.02	1.05	18.76	90	S
28298	00	A	Hallux valgus (bunion) correction, with or without sesamoidectomy; by phalanx osteotomy	7.52	8.89	0.79	17.20	90	S
28299	00	A	Hallux valgus (bunion) correction, with or without sesamoidectomy; by other methods (eg, double osteotomy)	8.46	10.14	1.08	19.68	90	S
28300	00	A	Osteotomy; calcaneus (Dwyer or Chambers type procedure), with or without internal fixation	9.12	6.52	0.79	16.43	90	S
28302	00	A	Osteotomy; talus	9.13	8.89	1.12	19.14	90	S
28304	00	A	Osteotomy, midtarsal bones, other than calcaneus or talus;	8.67	6.44	0.70	15.81	90	S

CPT codes and descriptions only, © 1994 American Medical Association. Reimbursement information, © 1995 McGraw-Hill Inc.

Code/ CPT	Mod- ifier	Status	Description	Work value	Practice expense	Mal- practice	Total value	Global period	Up- date
28305	00	A	Osteotomy, midtarsal bones, other than calcaneus or talus; with autograft (includes obtaining graft) (Fowler type)	9.99	9.85	1.03	20.87	90	S
28306	00	A	Osteotomy, metatarsal, base or shaft, single, with or without lengthening, for shortening or angular correction; first metatarsal	5.71	4.57	0.47	10.75	90	S
28307	00	A	Osteotomy, metatarsal, base or shaft, single, with or without lengthening, for shortening or angular correction; first metatarsal with autograft	6.04	5.87	0.76	12.67	90	S
28308	00	A	Osteotomy, metatarsal, base or shaft, single, with or without lengthening, for shortening or angular correction; other than first metatarsal	5.09	5.71	0.50	11.30	90	S
28309	00	A	Osteotomy, metatarsals, multiple, for cavus foot (Swanson type procedure)	8.83	6.87	1.00	16.70	90	S
28310	00	A	Osteotomy for shortening, angular or rotational correction; proximal phalanx, first toe (separate procedure)	5.06	4.17	0.42	9.65	90	S
28312	00	A	Osteotomy for shortening, angular or rotational correction; other phalanges, any toe	4.29	4.56	0.45	9.30	90	S
28313	00	A	Reconstruction, angular deformity of toe (overlapping second toe, fifth toe, curly toes), soft tissue procedures only	4.75	2.57	0.31	7.63	90	S
28315	00	A	Sesamoidectomy, first toe (separate procedure)	4.60	4.24	0.41	9.25	90	S
28320	00	A	Repair of nonunion or malunion; tarsal bones (eg, calcaneus, talus)	8.76	8.69	1.03	18.48	90	S
28322	00	A	Repair of nonunion or malunion; metatarsal, with or without bone graft (includes obtaining graft)	8.03	4.67	0.52	13.22	90	S
28340	00	A	Reconstruction, toe, macrodactyly; soft tissue resection	6.58	6.34	0.91	13.83	90	S
28341	00	A	Reconstruction, toe, macrodactyly; requiring bone resection	7.86	7.66	0.96	16.48	90	S
28344	00	A	Reconstruction, toe(s); polydactyly	3.89	3.70	0.60	8.19	90	S
28345	00	A	Reconstruction, toe(s); syndactyly, with or without skin graft(s), each web	5.52	5.34	0.73	11.59	90	S
28360	00	A	Reconstruction, cleft foot	12.49	11.91	1.95	26.35	90	S
28400	00	A	Closed treatment of calcaneal fracture; without manipulation	2.01	2.57	0.40	4.98	90	S
28405	00	A	Closed treatment of calcaneal fracture; with manipulation	4.28	3.90	0.58	8.76	90	S
28406	00	A	Percutaneous skeletal fixation of calcaneal fracture, with manipulation	5.82	6.09	0.93	12.84	90	S
28415	00	A	Open treatment of calcaneal fracture, with or without internal or external fixation;	13.28	9.02	1.39	23.69	90	S
28420	00	A	Open treatment of calcaneal fracture, with or without internal or external fixation; with primary iliac or other autogenous bone graft (includes obtaining graft)	15.80	10.89	1.63	28.32	90	S
28430	00	A	Closed treatment of talus fracture; without manipulation	1.96	2.45	0.35	4.76	90	S
28435	00	A	Closed treatment of talus fracture; with manipulation	3.25	3.36	0.50	7.11	90	S
28436	00	A	Percutaneous skeletal fixation of talus fracture, with manipulation	4.40	4.19	0.68	9.27	90	S
28445	00	A	Open treatment of talus fracture, with or without internal or external fixation	8.78	8.80	1.40	18.98	90	S
28450	00	A	Treatment of tarsal bone fracture (except talus and calcaneus); without manipulation, each	1.77	1.87	0.25	3.89	90	S
28455	00	A	Treatment of tarsal bone fracture (except talus and calcaneus); with manipulation, each	2.94	2.54	0.34	5.82	90	S
28456	00	A	Percutaneous skeletal fixation of tarsal bone fracture (except talus and calcaneus), with manipulation, each	2.39	2.27	0.38	5.04	90	S

CPT codes and descriptions only, © 1994 American Medical Association. Reimbursement information, © 1995 McGraw-Hill Inc.

Code/ CPT	Mod- ifier	Status	Description	Work value	Practice expense	Mal- practice	Total value	Global period	Up- date
28465	00	A	Open treatment of tarsal bone fracture (except talus and calcaneus), with or without internal or external fixation, each	6.55	5.54	0.81	12.90	90	S
28470	00	A	Closed treatment of metatarsal fracture; without manipulation, each	1.76	1.80	0.23	3.79	90	S
28475	00	A	Closed treatment of metatarsal fracture; with manipulation, each	2.74	2.34	0.30	5.38	90	S
28476	00	A	Percutaneous skeletal fixation of metatarsal fracture, with manipulation, each	3.15	3.37	0.45	6.97	90	S
28485	00	A	Open treatment of metatarsal fracture, with or without internal or external fixation, each	5.31	4.68	0.60	10.59	90	S
28490	00	A	Closed treatment of fracture great toe, phalanx or phalanges; without manipulation	1.01	0.90	0.10	2.01	90	S
28495	00	A	Closed treatment of fracture great toe, phalanx or phalanges; with manipulation	1.48	1.12	0.13	2.73	90	S
28496	00	A	Percutaneous skeletal fixation of fracture great toe, phalanx or phalanges, with manipulation	2.18	2.07	0.31	4.56	90	S
28505	00	A	Open treatment of fracture great toe, phalanx or phalanges, with or without internal or external fixation	3.55	2.99	0.43	6.97	90	S
28510	00	A	Closed treatment of fracture, phalanx or phalanges, other than great toe; without manipulation, each	1.01	0.89	0.09	1.99	90	S
28515	00	A	Closed treatment of fracture, phalanx or phalanges, other than great toe; with manipulation, each	1.36	1.12	0.11	2.59	90	S
28525	00	A	Open treatment of fracture, phalanx or phalanges, other than great toe, with or without internal or external fixation, each	3.08	2.06	0.29	5.43	90	S
28530	00	A	Closed treatment of sesamoid fracture	1.01	1.00	0.10	2.11	90	S
28531	00	A	Open treatment of sesamoid fracture, with or without internal fixation	2.01	1.91	0.32	4.24	90	S
28540	00	A	Closed treatment of tarsal bone dislocation, other than talotarsal; without anesthesia	1.89	0.60	0.06	2.55	90	S
28545	00	A	Closed treatment of tarsal bone dislocation, other than talotarsal; requiring anesthesia	2.19	1.31	0.14	3.64	90	S
28546	00	A	Percutaneous skeletal fixation of tarsal bone dislocation, other than talotarsal, with manipulation	2.89	2.74	0.45	6.08	90	S
28555	00	A	Open treatment of tarsal bone dislocation, with or without internal or external fixation	5.84	5.58	0.73	12.15	90	S
28570	00	A	Closed treatment of talotarsal joint dislocation; without anesthesia	1.56	1.59	0.17	3.32	90	S
28575	00	A	Closed treatment of talotarsal joint dislocation; requiring anesthesia	2.91	2.77	0.42	6.10	90	S
28576	00	A	Percutaneous skeletal fixation of talotarsal joint dislocation, with manipulation	3.75	2.77	0.42	6.94	90	S
28585	00	A	Open treatment of talotarsal joint dislocation, with or without internal or external fixation	7.46	4.96	0.55	12.97	90	S
28600	00	A	Closed treatment of tarsometatarsal joint dislocation; without anesthesia	1.76	0.68	0.08	2.52	90	S
28605	00	A	Closed treatment of tarsometatarsal joint dislocation; requiring anesthesia	2.42	2.26	0.34	5.02	90	S
28606	00	A	Percutaneous skeletal fixation of tarsometatarsal joint dislocation, with manipulation	4.48	3.49	0.55	8.52	90	S
28615	00	A	Open treatment of tarsometatarsal joint dislocation, with or without internal or external fixation	5.12	4.96	0.78	10.86	90	S
28630	00	A	Closed treatment of metatarsophalangeal joint dislocation; without anesthesia	1.65	1.03	0.11	2.79	10	S

CPT codes and descriptions only, © 1994 American Medical Association. Reimbursement information, © 1995 McGraw-Hill Inc.

Code/ CPT	Mod- ifier	Status	Description	Work value	Practice expense	Mal- practice	Total value	Global period	Up- date
28635	00	A	Closed treatment of metatarsophalangeal joint dislocation; requiring anesthesia	1.86	1.45	0.18	3.49	10	S
28636	00	A	Percutaneous skeletal fixation of metatarsophalangeal joint dislocation, with manipulation	2.67	2.56	0.42	5.65	10	S
28645	00	A	Open treatment of metatarsophalangeal joint dislocation, with or without internal or external fixation	3.96	3.24	0.38	7.58	90	S
28660	00	A	Closed treatment of interphalangeal joint dislocation; without anesthesia	1.18	0.63	0.06	1.87	10	S
28665	00	A	Closed treatment of interphalangeal joint dislocation; requiring anesthesia	1.87	0.98	0.11	2.96	10	S
28666	00	A	Percutaneous skeletal fixation of interphalangeal joint dislocation, with manipulation	2.56	2.44	0.40	5.40	10	S
28675	00	A	Open treatment of interphalangeal joint dislocation, with or without internal or external fixation	2.68	3.00	0.41	6.09	90	S
28705	00	A	Pantalar arthrodesis	14.23	15.11	2.35	31.69	90	S
28715	00	A	Triple arthrodesis	12.18	12.33	1.89	26.40	90	S
28725	00	A	Subtalar arthrodesis	10.86	9.44	1.44	21.74	90	S
28730	00	A	Arthrodesis, midtarsal or tarsometatarsal, multiple or transverse;	9.91	9.00	1.33	20.24	90	S
28735	00	A	Arthrodesis, midtarsal or tarsometatarsal, multiple or transverse; with osteotomy as for flatfoot correction	10.07	9.76	1.37	21.20	90	S
28737	00	A	Arthrodesis, midtarsal navicular-cuneiform, with tendon lengthening and advancement (Miller type procedure)	8.89	8.87	1.13	18.89	90	S
28740	00	A	Arthrodesis, midtarsal or tarsometatarsal, single joint	6.20	5.14	0.72	12.06	90	S
28750	00	A	Arthrodesis, great toe; metatarsophalangeal joint	4.77	5.32	0.82	10.91	90	S
28755	00	A	Arthrodesis, great toe; interphalangeal joint	4.48	3.69	0.45	8.62	90	S
28760	00	A	Arthrodesis, great toe, interphalangeal joint, with extensor hallucis longus transfer to first metatarsal neck (Jones type procedure)	5.47	5.40	0.65	11.52	90	S
28800	00	A	Amputation, foot; midtarsal (Chopart type procedure)	7.37	6.65	1.19	15.21	90	S
28805	00	A	Amputation, foot; transmetatarsal	7.55	6.32	1.21	15.08	90	S
28810	00	A	Amputation, metatarsal, with toe, single	5.53	3.91	0.75	10.19	90	S
28820	00	A	Amputation, toe; metatarsophalangeal joint	3.56	2.58	0.46	6.60	90	S
28825	00	A	Amputation, toe; interphalangeal joint	3.13	2.40	0.41	5.94	90	S
28899	00	C	Unlisted procedure, foot or toes	0	0	0	0	YYY	S
29000	00	A	Application of halo type body cast (see 20661-20663 for insertion)	2.25	1.85	0.21	4.31	0	S
29010	00	A	Application of Risser jacket, localizer, body; only	2.06	2.33	0.34	4.73	0	S
29015	00	A	Application of Risser jacket, localizer, body; including head	2.41	2.33	0.33	5.07	0	S
29020	00	A	Application of turnbuckle jacket, body; only	2.11	1.82	0.23	4.16	0	S
29025	00	A	Application of turnbuckle jacket, body; including head	2.40	0.75	0.14	3.29	0	S
29035	00	A	Application of body cast, shoulder to hips;	1.77	1.95	0.32	4.04	0	S
29040	00	A	Application of body cast, shoulder to hips; including head, Minerva type	2.22	2.02	0.30	4.54	0	S
29044	00	A	Application of body cast, shoulder to hips; including one thigh	2.12	2.09	0.34	4.55	0	S
29046	00	A	Application of body cast, shoulder to hips; including both thighs	2.41	2.23	0.36	5.00	0	S
29049	00	A	Application; plaster figure-of-eight	0.89	0.42	0.06	1.37	0	S
29055	00	A	Application; shoulder spica	1.78	1.20	0.17	3.15	0	S
29058	00	A	Application; plaster Velpeau	1.31	0.65	0.09	2.05	0	S
29065	00	A	Application; shoulder to hand (long arm)	0.87	0.80	0.13	1.80	0	S
29075	00	A	Application; elbow to finger (short arm)	0.77	0.61	0.10	1.48	0	S

CPT codes and descriptions only, © 1994 American Medical Association. Reimbursement information, © 1995 McGraw-Hill Inc.

Code/ CPT	Mod- ifier	Status	Description	Work value	Practice expense	Mal- practice	Total value	Global period	Up- date
29085	00	A	Application; hand and lower forearm (gauntlet)	0.87	0.50	0.08	1.45	0	S
29105	00	A	Application of long arm splint (shoulder to hand)	0.87	0.50	0.08	1.45	0	S
29125	00	A	Application of short arm splint (forearm to hand); static	0.59	0.37	0.05	1.01	0	S
29126	00	A	Application of short arm splint (forearm to hand); dynamic	0.77	0.40	0.06	1.23	0	S
29130	00	A	Application of finger splint; static	0.50	0.17	0.02	0.69	0	S
29131	00	A	Application of finger splint; dynamic	0.55	0.39	0.06	1.00	0	S
29200	00	A	Strapping; thorax	0.65	0.27	0.03	0.95	0	N
29220	00	A	Strapping; low back	0.64	0.38	0.05	1.07	0	S
29240	00	A	Strapping; shoulder (eg, Velpeau)	0.71	0.27	0.03	1.01	0	S
29260	00	A	Strapping; elbow or wrist	0.55	0.23	0.03	0.81	0	S
29280	00	A	Strapping; hand or finger	0.51	0.21	0.02	0.74	0	S
29305	00	A	Application of hip spica cast; one leg	2.03	1.88	0.31	4.22	0	S
29325	00	A	Application of hip spica cast; one and one-half spica or both legs	2.32	1.94	0.28	4.54	0	S
29345	00	A	Application of long leg cast (thigh to toes);	1.40	1.02	0.16	2.58	0	S
29355	00	A	Application of long leg cast (thigh to toes); walker or ambulatory type	1.53	1.10	0.17	2.80	0	S
29358	00	A	Application of long leg cast brace	1.43	1.84	0.33	3.60	0	S
29365	00	A	Application of cylinder cast (thigh to ankle)	1.18	0.86	0.14	2.18	0	S
29405	00	A	Application of short leg cast (below knee to toes);	0.86	0.79	0.12	1.77	0	S
29425	00	A	Application of short leg cast (below knee to toes); walking or ambulatory type	1.01	0.97	0.14	2.12	0	S
29435	00	A	Application of patellar tendon bearing (PTB) cast	1.18	1.18	0.18	2.54	0	S
29440	00	A	Adding walker to previously applied cast	0.57	0.23	0.03	0.83	0	S
29445	00	A	Application of rigid total contact leg cast	1.78	1.70	0.28	3.76	0	S
29450	00	A	Application of clubfoot cast with molding or manipulation, long or short leg	1.02	0.39	0.04	1.45	0	S
29505	00	A	Application of long leg splint (thigh to ankle or toes)	0.69	0.57	0.07	1.33	0	S
29515	00	A	Application of short leg splint (calf to foot)	0.73	0.47	0.06	1.26	0	S
29520	00	A	Strapping; hip	0.54	0.36	0.03	0.93	0	S
29530	00	A	Strapping; knee	0.57	0.35	0.05	0.97	0	S
29540	00	A	Strapping; ankle	0.51	0.30	0.03	0.84	0	S
29550	00	A	Strapping; toes	0.47	0.28	0.03	0.78	0	S
29580	00	A	Strapping; Unna boot	0.57	0.79	0.04	1.40	0	S
29590	00	A	Denis-Browne splint strapping	0.76	0.28	0.03	1.07	0	S
29700	00	A	Removal or bivalving; gauntlet, boot or body cast	0.88	0.32	0.05	1.25	0	S
29705	00	A	Removal or bivalving; full arm or full leg cast	1.12	0.35	0.05	1.52	0	S
29710	00	A	Removal or bivalving; shoulder or hip spica, Minerva, or Risser jacket, etc.	1.34	0.45	0.07	1.86	0	S
29715	00	A	Removal or bivalving; turnbuckle jacket	0.94	0.86	0.12	1.92	0	S
29720	00	A	Repair of spica, body cast or jacket	0.68	0.23	0.04	0.95	0	S
29730	00	A	Windowing of cast	0.75	0.26	0.04	1.05	0	S
29740	00	A	Wedging of cast (except clubfoot casts)	1.12	0.38	0.06	1.56	0	S
29750	00	A	Wedging of clubfoot cast	1.26	0.50	0.07	1.83	0	S
29799	00	C	Unlisted procedure, casting or strapping	0	0	0	0	YYY	S
29800	00	A	Arthroscopy, temporomandibular joint, diagnostic, with or without synovial biopsy (separate procedure)	5.28	4.01	0.46	9.75	90	S
29804	00	A	Arthroscopy, temporomandibular joint, surgical	7.99	11.75	1.46	21.20	90	S
29815	00	A	Arthroscopy, shoulder, diagnostic, with or without synovial biopsy (separate procedure)	5.74	4.84	0.76	11.34	90	S

CPT codes and descriptions only, © 1994 American Medical Association. Reimbursement information, © 1995 McGraw-Hill Inc.

Code/ CPT	Mod- ifier	Status	Description	Work value	Practice expense	Mal- practice	Total value	Global period	Up- date
29819	00	A	Arthroscopy, shoulder, surgical; with removal of loose body or foreign body	7.33	9.38	1.73	18.44	90	S
29820	00	A	Arthroscopy, shoulder, surgical; synovectomy, partial	6.81	8.72	1.73	17.26	90	S
29821	00	A	Arthroscopy, shoulder, surgical; synovectomy, complete	7.43	10.36	2.13	19.92	90	S
29822	00	A	Arthroscopy, shoulder, surgical; debridement, limited	7.14	9.14	1.74	18.02	90	S
29823	00	A	Arthroscopy, shoulder, surgical; debridement, extensive	7.86	11.10	2.32	21.28	90	S
29825	00	A	Arthroscopy, shoulder, surgical; with lysis and resection of adhesions, with or without manipulation	7.33	10.00	2.05	19.38	90	S
29826	00	A	Arthroscopy, shoulder, surgical; decompression of subacromial space with partial acromioplasty, with or without coracoacromial release	8.70	11.44	2.31	22.45	90	S
29830	00	A	Arthroscopy, elbow, diagnostic, with or without synovial biopsy (separate procedure)	5.63	5.32	0.83	11.78	90	S
29834	00	A	Arthroscopy, elbow, surgical; with removal of loose body or foreign body	6.13	5.84	0.96	12.93	90	S
29835	00	A	Arthroscopy, elbow, surgical; synovectomy, partial	6.33	6.03	0.99	13.35	90	S
29836	00	A	Arthroscopy, elbow, surgical; synovectomy, complete	7.37	7.03	1.15	15.55	90	S
29837	00	A	Arthroscopy, elbow, surgical; debridement, limited	6.72	6.40	1.06	14.18	90	S
29838	00	A	Arthroscopy, elbow, surgical; debridement, extensive	7.42	7.05	1.14	15.61	90	S
29840	00	A	Arthroscopy, wrist, diagnostic, with or without synovial biopsy (separate procedure)	5.39	3.29	0.54	9.22	90	S
29843	00	A	Arthroscopy, wrist, surgical; for infection, lavage and drainage	5.86	5.60	0.91	12.37	90	S
29844	00	A	Arthroscopy, wrist, surgical; synovectomy, partial	6.22	5.59	0.95	12.76	90	S
29845	00	A	Arthroscopy, wrist, surgical; synovectomy, complete	7.34	7.00	1.15	15.49	90	S
29846	00	A	Arthroscopy, wrist, surgical; excision and/or repair of triangular fibrocartilage and/or joint debridement	6.60	9.44	2.20	18.24	90	S
29847	00	A	Arthroscopy, wrist, surgical; internal fixation for fracture or instability	6.93	6.78	0.97	14.68	90	S
29848	00	A	Arthroscopy, wrist, surgical; with release of transverse carpal ligament	4.04	3.85	0.62	8.51	90	S
29850	00	A	Arthroscopically aided treatment of intercondylar spine(s) and/or tuberosity fracture(s) of the knee, with or without manipulation; without internal or external fixation (includes arthroscopy)	7.96	10.19	1.74	19.89	90	S
29851	00	A	Arthroscopically aided treatment of intercondylar spine(s) and/or tuberosity fracture(s) of the knee, with or without manipulation; with internal or external fixation (includes arthroscopy)	12.38	10.95	1.74	25.07	90	S
29855	00	A	Arthroscopically aided treatment of tibial fracture, proximal (plateau); unicondylar, with or without internal or external fixation (includes arthroscopy)	9.48	11.69	1.88	23.05	90	S
29856	00	A	Arthroscopically aided treatment of tibial fracture, proximal (plateau); bicondylar, with or without internal or external fixation (includes arthroscopy)	13.28	11.69	1.88	26.85	90	S
29870	00	A	Arthroscopy, knee, diagnostic, with or without synovial biopsy (separate procedure)	4.94	4.02	0.64	9.60	90	S
29871	00	A	Arthroscopy, knee, surgical; for infection, lavage and drainage	6.29	6.77	0.96	14.02	90	S
29874	00	A	Arthroscopy, knee, surgical; for removal of loose body or foreign body (eg, osteochondritis dissecans fragmentation, chondral fragmentation)	6.79	8.69	1.52	17.00	90	S
29875	00	A	Arthroscopy, knee, surgical; synovectomy, limited (eg, plica or shelf resection) (separate procedure)	6.16	8.10	1.61	15.87	90	S

CPT codes and descriptions only, © 1994 American Medical Association. Reimbursement information, © 1995 McGraw-Hill Inc.

Code/ CPT	Mod- ifier	Status	Description	Work value	Practice expense	Mal- practice	Total value	Global period	Up- date
29876	00	A	Arthroscopy, knee, surgical; synovectomy, major, two or more compartments (eg, medial or lateral)	7.51	9.78	1.95	19.24	90	S
29877	00	A	Arthroscopy, knee, surgical; debridement/shaving of articular cartilage (chondroplasty)	7.05	9.13	1.81	17.99	90	S
29879	00	A	Arthroscopy, knee, surgical; abrasion arthroplasty (includes chondroplasty where necessary) or multiple drilling	7.63	10.55	2.19	20.37	90	S
29880	00	A	Arthroscopy, knee, surgical; with meniscectomy (medial AND lateral, including any meniscal shaving)	8.09	10.95	2.22	21.26	90	S
29881	00	A	Arthroscopy, knee, surgical; with meniscectomy (medial OR lateral, including any meniscal shaving)	7.46	9.54	1.82	18.82	90	S
29882	00	A	Arthroscopy, knee, surgical; with meniscus repair (medial OR lateral)	8.24	10.54	1.90	20.68	90	S
29883	00	A	Arthroscopy, knee, surgical; with meniscus repair (medial AND lateral)	9.00	13.07	2.80	24.87	90	S
29884	00	A	Arthroscopy, knee, surgical; with lysis of adhesions, with or without manipulation (separate procedure)	6.92	8.86	1.56	17.34	90	S
29885	00	A	Arthroscopy, knee, surgical; drilling for osteochondritis dissecans with bone grafting, with or without internal fixation (including debridement of base of lesion)	8.63	8.23	1.35	18.21	90	S
29886	00	A	Arthroscopy, knee, surgical; drilling for intact osteochondritis dissecans lesion	7.13	6.80	1.12	15.05	90	S
29887	00	A	Arthroscopy, knee, surgical; drilling for intact osteochondritis dissecans lesion with internal fixation	8.58	10.52	1.71	20.81	90	S
29888	00	A	Arthroscopically aided anterior cruciate ligament repair/augmentation or reconstruction	13.28	17.00	3.18	33.46	90	S
29889	00	A	Arthroscopically aided posterior cruciate ligament repair/augmentation or reconstruction	10.76	10.26	1.68	22.70	90	S
29894	00	A	Arthroscopy, ankle (tibiotalar and fibulotalar joints), surgical; with removal of loose body or foreign body	6.95	8.90	1.47	17.32	90	S
29895	00	A	Arthroscopy, ankle (tibiotalar and fibulotalar joints), surgical; synovectomy, partial	6.73	8.60	1.51	16.84	90	S
29897	00	A	Arthroscopy, ankle (tibiotalar and fibulotalar joints), surgical; debridement, limited	6.92	8.90	1.77	17.59	90	S
29898	00	A	Arthroscopy, ankle (tibiotalar and fibulotalar joints), surgical; debridement, extensive	8.03	10.28	1.91	20.22	90	S
29909	00	C	Unlisted procedure, arthroscopy	0	0	0	0	YYY	S
30000	00	A	Drainage abscess or hematoma, nasal, internal approach	1.38	0.58	0.05	2.01	10	S
30020	00	A	Drainage abscess or hematoma, nasal septum	1.38	0.60	0.06	2.04	10	S
30100	00	A	Biopsy, intranasal	0.94	0.69	0.08	1.71	0	S
30110	00	A	Excision, nasal polyp(s), simple	1.58	1.29	0.14	3.01	10	S
30115	00	A	Excision, nasal polyp(s), extensive	4.25	2.81	0.30	7.36	90	S
30117	00	A	Excision or destruction, any method (including laser), intranasal lesion; internal approach	3.06	2.84	0.31	6.21	90	S
30118	00	A	Excision or destruction, any method (including laser), intranasal lesion; external approach (lateral rhinotomy)	9.23	8.01	0.92	18.16	90	S
30120	00	A	Excision or surgical planing of skin of nose for rhinophyma	5.14	6.59	1.00	12.73	90	S
30124	00	A	Excision dermoid cyst, nose; simple, skin, subcutaneous	3.00	1.34	0.16	4.50	90	S
30125	00	A	Excision dermoid cyst, nose; complex, under bone or cartilage	6.79	5.55	0.73	13.07	90	S
30130	00	A	Excision turbinate, partial or complete	3.17	1.67	0.17	5.01	90	S
30140	00	A	Submucous resection turbinate, partial or complete	3.28	3.04	0.34	6.66	90	S
30150	00	A	Rhinectomy; partial	8.48	7.92	1.07	17.47	90	S
30160	00	A	Rhinectomy; total	8.92	11.42	1.73	22.07	90	S
30200	00	A	Injection into turbinate(s), therapeutic	0.78	0.37	0.04	1.19	0	S

CPT codes and descriptions only, © 1994 American Medical Association. Reimbursement information, © 1995 McGraw-Hill Inc.

Code/ CPT	Mod- ifier	Status	Description	Work value	Practice expense	Mal- practice	Total value	Global period	Up- date
30210	00	A	Displacement therapy (Proetz type)	1.03	0.26	0.03	1.32	10	S
30220	00	A	Insertion, nasal septal prosthesis (button)	1.49	1.51	0.16	3.16	10	S
30300	00	A	Removal foreign body, intranasal; office type procedure	0.99	0.46	0.05	1.50	10	S
30310	00	A	Removal foreign body, intranasal; requiring general anesthesia	1.91	1.62	0.18	3.71	10	S
30320	00	A	Removal foreign body, intranasal; by lateral rhinotomy	4.39	4.29	0.43	9.11	90	S
30400	00	R	Rhinoplasty, primary; lateral and alar cartilages and/or elevation of nasal tip	9.24	9.97	1.36	20.57	90	S
30410	00	R	Rhinoplasty, primary; complete, external parts including bony pyramid, lateral and alar cartilages, and/or elevation of nasal tip	12.39	14.54	2.01	28.94	90	S
30420	00	R	Rhinoplasty, primary; including major septal repair	15.40	17.78	2.22	35.40	90	S
30430	00	R	Rhinoplasty, secondary; minor revision (small amount of nasal tip work)	6.73	6.09	0.66	13.48	90	S
30435	00	R	Rhinoplasty, secondary; intermediate revision (bony work with osteotomies)	11.23	10.17	1.10	22.50	90	S
30450	00	R	Rhinoplasty, secondary; major revision (nasal tip work and osteotomies)	18.06	11.24	0.91	30.21	90	S
30460	00	A	Rhinoplasty for nasal deformity secondary to congenital cleft lip and/or palate, including columellar lengthening; tip only	9.48	8.58	0.93	18.99	90	S
30462	00	A	Rhinoplasty for nasal deformity secondary to congenital cleft lip and/or palate, including columellar lengthening; tip, septum, osteotomies	18.98	17.16	1.87	38.01	90	S
30520	00	A	Septoplasty or submucous resection, with or without cartilage scoring, contouring or replacement with graft	5.55	7.13	0.96	13.64	90	S
30540	00	A	Repair choanal atresia; intranasal	7.46	6.63	0.70	14.79	90	S
30545	00	A	Repair choanal atresia; transpalatine	10.89	10.83	0.93	22.65	90	S
30560	00	A	Lysis intranasal synechia	1.21	0.55	0.06	1.82	10	S
30580	00	A	Repair fistula; oromaxillary (combine with 31030 if antrotomy is included)	6.49	6.24	0.57	13.30	90	S
30600	00	A	Repair fistula; oronasal	5.87	3.77	0.36	10.00	90	S
30620	00	A	Septal or other intranasal dermatoplasty (does not include obtaining graft)	5.55	7.61	1.10	14.26	90	S
30630	00	A	Repair nasal septal perforations	6.83	6.24	0.71	13.78	90	S
30801	00	A	Cauterization and/or ablation, mucosa of turbinates, unilateral or bilateral, any method, (separate procedure); superficial	1.02	0.47	0.05	1.54	10	S
30802	00	A	Cauterization and/or ablation, mucosa of turbinates, unilateral or bilateral, any method, (separate procedure); intramural	1.98	0.94	0.11	3.03	10	S
30901	00	A	Control nasal hemorrhage, anterior, simple (limited cautery and/or packing) any method	1.21	0.56	0.06	1.83	0	S
30903	00	A	Control nasal hemorrhage, anterior, complex (extensive cautery and/or packing) any method	1.54	0.85	0.08	2.47	0	S
30905	00	A	Control nasal hemorrhage, posterior, with posterior nasal packs and/or cauterization, any method; initial	1.97	1.79	0.17	3.93	0	S
30906	00	A	Control nasal hemorrhage, posterior, with posterior nasal packs and/or cauterization, any method; subsequent	2.45	1.08	0.11	3.64	0	S
30915	00	A	Ligation arteries; ethmoidal	6.72	4.95	0.52	12.19	90	S
30920	00	A	Ligation arteries; internal maxillary artery, transantral	7.46	9.85	1.32	18.63	90	S
30930	00	A	Fracture nasal turbinate(s), therapeutic	1.21	0.71	0.08	2.00	10	S
30999	00	C	Unlisted procedure, nose	0	0	0	0	YYY	N

CPT codes and descriptions only, © 1994 American Medical Association. Reimbursement information, © 1995 McGraw-Hill Inc.

Code/ CPT	Mod- ifier	Status	Description	Work value	Practice expense	Mal- practice	Total value	Global period	Up- date
31000	00	A	Lavage by cannulation; maxillary sinus (antrum puncture or natural ostium)	1.10	0.43	0.05	1.58	10	S
31002	00	A	Lavage by cannulation; sphenoid sinus	1.86	0.46	0.05	2.37	10	S
31020	00	A	Sinusotomy, maxillary (antrotomy); intranasal	2.81	2.66	0.29	5.76	90	S
31030	00	A	Sinusotomy, maxillary (antrotomy); radical (Caldwell-Luc) without removal of antrochoanal polyps	5.60	7.16	0.86	13.62	90	S
31032	00	A	Sinusotomy, maxillary (antrotomy); radical (Caldwell-Luc) with removal of antrochoanal polyps	6.22	7.96	0.99	15.17	90	S
31040	00	A	Pterygomaxillary fossa surgery, any approach	8.83	7.98	0.86	17.67	90	S
31050	00	A	Sinusotomy, sphenoid, with or without biopsy;	5.07	5.96	0.64	11.67	90	S
31051	00	A	Sinusotomy, sphenoid, with or without biopsy; with mucosal stripping or removal of polyp(s)	6.85	8.12	0.85	15.82	90	S
31070	00	A	Sinusotomy frontal; external, simple (trephine operation)	4.04	4.69	0.50	9.23	90	S
31071	00	D	Exploration of frontal sinus	8.44*	7.64#	0.83*	16.91#	90	S
31075	00	A	Sinusotomy frontal; transorbital, unilateral (for mucocele or osteoma, Lynch type)	8.57	10.51	1.10	20.18	90	S
31080	00	A	Sinusotomy frontal; obliterative without osteoplastic flap, brow incision (includes ablation)	10.73	9.21	1.12	21.06	90	S
31081	00	A	Sinusotomy frontal; obliterative, without osteoplastic flap, coronal incision (includes ablation)	11.93	10.32	1.30	23.55	90	S
31084	00	A	Sinusotomy frontal; obliterative, with osteoplastic flap, brow incision	12.69	14.79	1.62	29.10	90	S
31085	00	A	Sinusotomy frontal; obliterative, with osteoplastic flap, coronal incision	13.38	15.65	1.76	30.79	90	S
31086	00	A	Sinusotomy frontal; nonobliterative, with osteoplastic flap, brow incision	11.98	10.87	1.15	24.00	90	S
31087	00	A	Sinusotomy frontal; nonobliterative, with osteoplastic flap, coronal incision	12.14	10.39	1.33	23.86	90	S
31090	00	A	Sinusotomy combined, three or more sinuses	8.65	13.98	2.12	24.75	90	S
31200	00	A	Ethmoidectomy; intranasal, anterior	4.68	4.62	0.48	9.78	90	S
31201	00	A	Ethmoidectomy; intranasal, total	7.91	7.01	0.75	15.67	90	S
31205	00	A	Ethmoidectomy; extranasal, total	9.65	8.03	0.81	18.49	90	S
31225	00	A	Maxillectomy; without orbital exenteration	15.19	19.44	2.37	37	90	S
31230	00	A	Maxillectomy; with orbital exenteration (en bloc)	21.06	21.74	2.48	45.28	90	S
31231	00	A	Nasal endoscopy, diagnostic, unilateral or bilateral (separate procedure)	0.73	1.37	0.15	2.25	0	S
31233	00	A	Nasal/sinus endoscopy, diagnostic with maxillary sinusoscopy (via inferior meatus or canine fossa puncture)	1.56	2.00	0.31	3.87	0	S
31235	00	A	Nasal/sinus endoscopy, diagnostic with sphenoid sinusoscopy (via puncture of sphenoidal face or cannulation of ostium)	2.74	0.96	0.10	3.80	0	S
31237	00	A	Nasal/sinus endoscopy, surgical; with biopsy, polypectomy or debridement (separate procedure)	1.88	2.40	0.37	4.65	0	S
31238	00	A	Nasal/sinus endoscopy, surgical; with control of epistaxis	3.26	4.17	0.45	7.88	0	S
31239	00	A	Nasal/sinus endoscopy, surgical; with dacryocystorhinostomy	8.50	10.88	1.18	20.56	10	S
31240	00	A	Nasal/sinus endoscopy, surgical; with concha bullosa resection	2.61	3.34	0.37	6.32	0	S
31245	00	D	Nasal/sinus endoscopy, surgical; with osteomeatal complex (OMC) resection and/or anterior ethmoidectomy, with or without removal of polyp(s); (CCR 31254)	4.50*	4.08#	0.44*	9.02#	0	S

CPT codes and descriptions only, © 1994 American Medical Association. Reimbursement information, © 1995 McGraw-Hill Inc.

Code/ CPT	Mod- ifier	Status	Description	Work value	Practice expense	Mal- practice	Total value	Global period	Up- date
31246	00	D	Nasal/sinus endoscopy, surgical; with osteomeatal complex (OMC) resection and/or anterior ethmoidectomy, with or without removal of polyp(s); with antrostomy (CCR 31254 and 31256)	5.56*	5.04#	0.55*	11.15#	0	S
31247	00	D	Nasal/sinus endoscopy, surgical; with osteomeatal complex (OMC) resection and/or anterior ethmoidectomy, with or without removal of polyp(s); with antrostomy and removal of antral mucosal disease (CCR 31254 and 31267)	6.33*	5.74#	0.62*	12.69#	0	S
31248	00	D	Nasal/sinus endoscopy, surgical; with osteomeatal complex (OMC) resection and/or anterior ethmoidectomy, with or without removal of polyp(s); with frontal sinus exploration (CCR 31254 and 31276)	6.75*	6.12#	0.66*	13.53#	0	S
31249	00	D	Nasal/sinus endoscopy, surgical; with osteomeatal complex (OMC) resection and/or anterior ethmoidectomy, with or without removal of polyp(s); with frontal sinus exploration and antrostomy (CCR 31254, 31256, and 32176)	8.02*	7.26#	0.79*	16.07#	0	S
31250	00	D	Nasal endoscopy, diagnostic, with or without biopsy (includes examination of the medial meatus, infundibulum and sinus ostia) (separate procedure) (CCR 31231-31235)	0.77*	0.70#	0.08*	1.55#	0	S
31251	D		Nasal endoscopy, diagnostic, with or without biopsy (includes examination of the medial meatus, infundibulum and sinus ostia) (separate procedure) (CCR 31254, 31267, and 31276)						
	00		**Editor's Note:** The McGraw-Hill Code M 31251 has been deleted. To report see 92511	8.30*	7.52#	0.81*	16.63#	0	S
31252	00	D	Nasal endoscopy, surgical; with nasal polypectomy (CCR 31237)	2.25*	2.04#	0.22*	4.51#	0	S
31254	00	A	Nasal/sinus endoscopy, surgical; with ethmoidectomy, partial (anterior)	4.65	5.95	0.69	11.29	0	S
31255	00	A	Nasal/sinus endoscopy, surgical; with ethmoidectomy, total (anterior and posterior)	6.96	8.91	1.14	17.01	0	S
31256	00	A	Nasal/sinus endoscopy, surgical, with maxillary antrostomy;	3.29	3.77	0.41	7.47	0	S
31258	00	D	Nasal/sinus endoscopy, surgical, with maxillary antrostomy; with removal of foreign body(s) (CCR 31327)	1.13*	1.02#	0.11*	2.26#	0	S
31260	00	D	Maxillary sinus endoscopy, diagnostic, with or with biopsy (separate procedure) (CCR 31233)	0.91*	0.82#	0.09*	1.82#	0	S
31261	00	D	Nasal/sinus endoscopy, surgical, with anterior and posterior ethmoidectomy (APE), with or without removal of polyp(s); (CCR 31255)	7.25*	6.57#	0.71*	14.53#	0	S
31262	00	D	Nasal/sinus endoscopy, surgical, with anterior and posterior ethmoidectomy (APE), with or without removal of polyp(s); with antrostomy (CCR 31255 and 31256)	8.30*	7.52#	0.81*	16.63#	0	S
31263	00	D	Maxillary sinus endoscopy, surgical; with removal of foreign body(s) (CCR 31299)	2.25*	2.04#	0.22*	4.51#	0	S
31264	00	D	Maxillary sinus endoscopy, surgical; with removal of foreign body(s); with antrostomy and removal of antral mucosal disease (CCR 31255 and 31267)	8.93*	8.09#	0.88*	17.9#	0	S

CPT codes and descriptions only, © 1994 American Medical Association. Reimbursement information, © 1995 McGraw-Hill Inc.

Code/ CPT	Mod- ifier	Status	Description	Work value	Practice expense	Mal- practice	Total value	Global period	Up- date
31265	00	D	Maxillary sinus endoscopy, surgical; with removal of foreign body(s); with removal of cyst (CCR 31299)	3.94*	3.57#	0.39*	7.9#	0	S
31266	00	D	Maxillary sinus endoscopy, surgical; with removal of foreign body(s); with frontal sinus exploration (CCR 31255 and 31276)	9.57*	8.67#	0.94*	19.18#	0	S
31267	00	A	Nasal/sinus endoscopy, surgical, with maxillary antrostomy; with removal of tissue from maxillary sinus	5.46	5.23	0.81	11.50	0	S
31268	00	D	Maxillary sinus endoscopy, surgical; with removal of foreign body(s); with removal of fungus ball (CCR 31299)	7.88*	7.14#	0.77*	15.79#	0	S
31269	00	D	Maxillary sinus endoscopy, surgical; with removal of foreign body(s); with frontal sinus exploration and antrostomy (CCR 31255, 31256, and 31276)	10.62*	9.62#	1.04*	21.28#	0	S
31270	00	D	Sphenoid endoscopy, diagnostic, with or without biopsy (separate procedure) (CCR 31235)	1.27*	1.15#	0.12*	2.54#	0	S
31271	00	D	Sphenoid endoscopy, diagnostic, with or without biopsy (separate procedure); with frontal sinus exploration, antrostomy, and removal of antral mucosal disease (CCR 31255, 31267, and 31276)	11.04*	10.00#	1.08*	22.12#	0	S
31275	00	D	Sphenoid endoscopy, surgical	4.50*	4.08#	0.44*	9.02#	0	S
31276	00	A	Nasal/sinus endoscopy, surgical with frontal sinus exploration, with or without removal of tissue from frontal sinus	7.42	6.72	0.73	14.87	0	S
31277	00	D	Nasal/sinus endoscopy, surgical with frontal sinus exploration, with or without removal of tissue from frontal sinus; with removal of mucous membrane (CCR 31288)	8.16*	7.39#	0.80*	16.35#	0	S
31280	00	D	Nasal/sinus endoscopy, surgical, with anterior and posterior ethmoidectomy and sphenoidotomy (APS), with or without removal of polyp(s); (CCR 31255 and 31287 or 31288)	9.14*	8.28#	0.90*	18.32#	0	S
31281	00	D	Nasal/sinus endoscopy, surgical, with anterior and posterior ethmoidectomy and sphenoidotomy (APS), with or without removal of polyp(s); with antrostomy (CCR 31255, 31256 and 312287 or 31288)	10.27*	9.30#	1.01*	20.58#	0	S
31282	00	D	Nasal/sinus endoscopy, surgical, with anterior and posterior ethmoidectomy and sphenoidotomy (APS), with or without removal of polyp(s); with antrostomy and removal of antral mucosal disease (CCR 31255, 31267 and 31287 or 31288)	10.97*	9.93#	1.08*	21.98#	0	S
31283	00	D	Nasal/sinus endoscopy, surgical, with anterior and posterior ethmoidectomy and sphenoidotomy (APS), with or without removal of polyp(s); with frontal sinus exploration (CCR 31255, 31287 or 31288 and 31276)	11.04*	10.00#	1.08*	22.12#	0	S
31284	00	D	Nasal/sinus endoscopy, surgical, with anterior and posterior ethmoidectomy and sphenoidotomy (APS), with or without removal of polyp(s); with frontal sinus exploration and antrostomy (CCR 31255, 31256, 31257 or 31288 and 31276)	12.66*	11.47#	1.24*	25.37#	0	S
31285	00	D	Sinus endoscopy, two or more sinuses, unilateral (CCR 31231-31235)	11.61*	10.52#	1.14*	23.27#	0	S
31286	00	D	Sinus endoscopy, two or more sinuses, unilateral; with frontal sinus exploration, antrostomy and removal of antral mucosal disease (CCR 31255, 31267, 31287 or 31288 and 31276)	12.94*	11.72#	1.27*	25.93#	0	S

CPT codes and descriptions only, © 1994 American Medical Association. Reimbursement information, © 1995 McGraw-Hill Inc.

Code/ CPT	Mod- ifier	Status	Description	Work value	Practice expense	Mal- practice	Total value	Global period	Up- date
31287	00	A	Nasal/sinus endoscopy, surgical, with sphenoidotomy;	3.92	5.01	0.65	9.58	0	S
31288	00	A	Nasal/sinus endoscopy, surgical, with sphenoidotomy; with removal of tissue from the sphenoid sinus	4.58	5.86	0.78	11.22	0	S
31290	00	A	Nasal/sinus endoscopy, surgical, with repair of cerebrospinal fluid leak; ethmoid region	12.87	16.47	1.80	31.14	10	S
31291	00	A	Nasal/sinus endoscopy, surgical, with repair of cerebrospinal fluid leak; sphenoid region	13.52	17.31	1.88	32.71	10	S
31292	00	A	Nasal/sinus endoscopy, surgical; with medial or inferior orbital wall decompression	10.45	13.38	1.45	25.28	10	S
31293	00	A	Nasal/sinus endoscopy, surgical; with medial orbital wall and inferior orbital wall decompression	11.43	14.64	1.59	27.66	10	S
31294	00	A	Nasal/sinus endoscopy, surgical; with optic nerve decompression	13.06	16.72	1.83	31.61	10	S
31299	00	C	Unlisted procedure, accessory sinuses	0	0	0	0	YYY	S
31300	00	A	Laryngotomy (thyrotomy, laryngofissure); with removal of tumor or laryngocele, cordectomy	13.28	11.58	1.28	26.14	90	S
31320	00	A	Laryngotomy (thyrotomy, laryngofissure); diagnostic	4.54	3.87	0.48	8.89	90	S
31360	00	A	Laryngectomy; total, without radical neck dissection	15.19	19.36	2.19	36.74	90	S
31365	00	A	Laryngectomy; total, with radical neck dissection	21.83	27.14	3.10	52.07	90	S
31367	00	A	Laryngectomy; subtotal supraglottic, without radical neck dissection	18.98	17.22	1.88	38.08	90	S
31368	00	A	Laryngectomy; subtotal supraglottic, with radical neck dissection	23.72	26.76	3.06	53.54	90	S
31370	00	A	Partial laryngectomy (hemilaryngectomy); horizontal	18.50	17.18	1.88	37.56	90	S
31375	00	A	Partial laryngectomy (hemilaryngectomy); laterovertical	18.50	14.84	1.56	34.90	90	S
31380	00	A	Partial laryngectomy (hemilaryngectomy); anterovertical	18.50	17.27	1.88	37.65	90	S
31382	00	A	Partial laryngectomy (hemilaryngectomy); antero-latero-vertical	18.50	16.06	1.78	36.34	90	S
31390	00	A	Pharyngolaryngectomy, with radical neck dissection; without reconstruction	21.15	28.01	4.05	53.21	90	S
31395	00	A	Pharyngolaryngectomy, with radical neck dissection; with reconstruction	26.19	33.52	4.42	64.13	90	S
31400	00	A	Arytenoidectomy or arytenoidopexy, external approach	9.06	7.81	0.91	17.78	90	S
31420	00	A	Epiglottidectomy	9.06	8.08	0.84	17.98	90	S
31500	00	A	Intubation, endotracheal, emergency procedure	2.33	1.14	0.14	3.61	0	N
31502	00	A	Tracheotomy tube change prior to establishment of fistula tract	0.65	0.58	0.07	1.30	0	S
31505	00	A	Laryngoscopy, indirect (separate procedure); diagnostic	0.61	0.43	0.05	1.09	0	S
31510	00	A	Laryngoscopy, indirect (separate procedure); with biopsy	1.92	0.55	0.07	2.54	0	S
31511	00	A	Laryngoscopy, indirect (separate procedure); with removal of foreign body	2.16	0.96	0.10	3.22	0	S
31512	00	A	Laryngoscopy, indirect (separate procedure); with removal of lesion	2.07	1.79	0.20	4.06	0	S
31513	00	A	Laryngoscopy, indirect (separate procedure); with vocal cord injection	2.10	2.78	0.38	5.26	0	S
31515	00	A	Laryngoscopy direct, with or without tracheoscopy; for aspiration	1.80	1.13	0.14	3.07	0	S
31520	00	A	Laryngoscopy direct, with or without tracheoscopy; diagnostic, newborn	2.56	1.64	0.18	4.38	0	S
31525	00	A	Laryngoscopy direct, with or without tracheoscopy; diagnostic, except newborn	2.63	2.20	0.23	5.06	0	S
31526	00	A	Laryngoscopy direct, with or without tracheoscopy; diagnostic, with operating microscope	2.57	3.29	0.38	6.24	0	S

CPT codes and descriptions only, © 1994 American Medical Association. Reimbursement information, © 1995 McGraw-Hill Inc.

Code/ CPT	Mod- ifier	Status	Description	Work value	Practice expense	Mal- practice	Total value	Global period	Up- date
31527	00	A	Laryngoscopy direct, with or without tracheoscopy; with insertion of obturator	3.27	2.99	0.30	6.56	0	S
31528	00	A	Laryngoscopy direct, with or without tracheoscopy; with dilatation, initial	2.37	2.66	0.30	5.33	0	S
31529	00	A	Laryngoscopy direct, with or without tracheoscopy; with dilatation, subsequent	2.68	2.46	0.25	5.39	0	S
31530	00	A	Laryngoscopy, direct, operative, with foreign body removal;	3.39	3.63	0.39	7.41	0	S
31531	00	A	Laryngoscopy, direct, operative, with foreign body removal; with operating microscope	3.73	4.78	0.60	9.11	0	S
31535	00	A	Laryngoscopy, direct, operative, with biopsy;	3.16	4.01	0.45	7.62	0	S
31536	00	A	Laryngoscopy, direct, operative, with biopsy; with operating microscope	3.17	4.37	0.59	8.13	0	S
31540	00	A	Laryngoscopy, direct, operative, with excision of tumor and/or stripping of vocal cords or epiglottis;	4.13	5.29	0.61	10.03	0	S
31541	00	A	Laryngoscopy, direct, operative, with excision of tumor and/or stripping of vocal cords or epiglottis; with operating microscope	3.56	5.24	0.75	9.55	0	S
31560	00	A	Laryngoscopy, direct, operative, with arytenoidectomy;	5.46	4.99	0.51	10.96	0	S
31561	00	A	Laryngoscopy, direct, operative, with arytenoidectomy; with operating microscope	4.90	7.48	1.08	13.46	0	S
31570	00	A	Laryngoscopy, direct, with injection into vocal cord(s), therapeutic;	3.87	4.95	0.60	9.42	0	S
31571	00	A	Laryngoscopy, direct, with injection into vocal cord(s), therapeutic; with operating microscope	3.52	4.96	0.69	9.17	0	S
31575	00	A	Laryngoscopy, flexible fiberoptic; diagnostic	1.10	1.56	0.17	2.83	0	S
31576	00	A	Laryngoscopy, flexible fiberoptic; with biopsy	1.97	2.52	0.33	4.82	0	S
31577	00	A	Laryngoscopy, flexible fiberoptic; with removal of foreign body	2.47	3.16	0.37	6.00	0	S
31578	00	A	Laryngoscopy, flexible fiberoptic; with removal of lesion	2.84	3.73	0.48	7.05	0	S
31579	00	A	Laryngoscopy, flexible fiberoptic; with stroboscopy	2.26	2.33	0.26	4.85	0	S
31580	00	A	Laryngoplasty; for laryngeal web, two stage, with keel insertion and removal	11.01	14.09	1.63	26.73	90	S
31582	00	A	Laryngoplasty; for laryngeal stenosis, with graft or core mold, including tracheotomy	19.73	17.87	1.94	39.54	90	S
31584	00	A	Laryngoplasty; with open reduction of fracture	18.50	12.72	1.34	32.56	90	S
31585	00	A	Treatment of closed laryngeal fracture; without manipulation	4.40	3.77	0.40	8.57	90	S
31586	00	A	Treatment of closed laryngeal fracture; with closed manipulative reduction	7.24	6.55	0.71	14.50	90	S
31587	00	A	Laryngoplasty, cricoid split	7.98	7.21	0.79	15.98	90	S
31588	00	A	Laryngoplasty, not otherwise specified (eg, for burns, reconstruction after partial laryngectomy)	11.82	10.70	1.16	23.68	90	S
31590	00	A	Laryngeal reinnervation by neuromuscular pedicle	6.36	5.76	0.62	12.74	90	S
31595	00	A	Section recurrent laryngeal nerve, therapeutic (separate procedure), unilateral	7.58	6.84	0.74	15.16	90	S
31599	00	C	Unlisted procedure, larynx	0	0	0	0	YYY	S
31600	00	A	Tracheostomy, planned (separate procedure);	3.62	4.04	0.65	8.31	0	S
31601	00	A	Tracheostomy, planned (separate procedure); under two years	4.45	5.03	0.66	10.14	0	S
31603	00	A	Tracheostomy, emergency procedure; transtracheal	4.15	4.23	0.66	9.04	0	S
31605	00	A	Tracheostomy, emergency procedure; cricothyroid membrane	3.58	4.19	0.50	8.27	0	S
31610	00	A	Tracheostomy, fenestration procedure with skin flaps	7.87	6.67	0.92	15.46	90	S

CPT codes and descriptions only, © 1994 American Medical Association. Reimbursement information, © 1995 McGraw-Hill Inc.

Code/ CPT	Mod-ifier	Status	Description	Work value	Practice expense	Mal-practice	Total value	Global period	Up-date
31611	00	A	Construction of tracheoesophageal fistula and subsequent insertion of an alaryngeal speech prosthesis (eg, voice button, Blom-Singer prosthesis)	5.03	7.23	1.04	13.30	90	S
31612	00	A	Tracheal puncture, percutaneous with transtracheal aspiration and/or injection	0.91	1.17	0.12	2.20	0	S
31613	00	A	Tracheostoma revision; simple, without flap rotation	4.24	2.21	0.28	6.73	90	S
31614	00	A	Tracheostoma revision; complex, with flap rotation	6.11	6.74	0.73	13.58	90	S
31615	00	A	Tracheobronchoscopy through established tracheostomy incision	2.09	1.95	0.22	4.26	0	S
31622	00	A	Bronchoscopy; diagnostic, (flexible or rigid), with or without cell washing or brushing	2.80	3.57	0.34	6.71	0	N
31625	00	A	Bronchoscopy; with biopsy	3.37	3.83	0.35	7.55	0	N
31628	00	A	Bronchoscopy; with transbronchial lung biopsy, with or without fluoroscopic guidance	3.81	4.88	0.38	9.07	0	N
31629	00	A	Bronchoscopy; with transbronchial needle aspiration biopsy	3.37	4.31	0.34	8.02	0	N
31630	00	A	Bronchoscopy; with tracheal or bronchial dilation or closed reduction of fracture	3.82	3.72	0.50	8.04	0	S
31631	00	A	Bronchoscopy; with tracheal dilation and placement of tracheal stent	4.37	3.94	0.48	8.79	0	N
31635	00	A	Bronchoscopy; with removal of foreign body	3.68	4.53	0.53	8.74	0	S
31640	00	A	Bronchoscopy; with excision of tumor	4.94	5.02	0.67	10.63	0	S
31641	00	A	Bronchoscopy; with destruction of tumor or relief of stenosis by any method other than excision (eg, laser)	5.03	6.49	0.85	12.37	0	N
31645	00	A	Bronchoscopy; with therapeutic aspiration of tracheobronchial tree, initial (eg, drainage of lung abscess)	3.16	3.62	0.30	7.08	0	N
31646	00	A	Bronchoscopy; with therapeutic aspiration of tracheobronchial tree, subsequent	2.72	3.06	0.27	6.05	0	N
31656	00	A	Bronchoscopy; with injection of contrast material for segmental bronchography (fiberscope only)	2.17	2.77	0.31	5.25	0	N
31659	00	D	Bronchoscopic procedures	0	0	0	0	0	N
31700	00	A	Catheterization, transglottic (separate procedure)	1.34	1.38	0.17	2.89	0	N
31708	00	A	Instillation of contrast material for laryngography or bronchography, without catheterization	1.41	0.77	0.09	2.27	0	N
31710	00	A	Catheterization for bronchography, with or without instillation of contrast material	1.30	0.90	0.12	2.32	0	N
31715	00	A	Transtracheal injection for bronchography	1.11	0.48	0.04	1.63	0	N
31717	00	A	Catheterization with bronchial brush biopsy	2.12	0.73	0.06	2.91	0	N
31720	00	A	Catheter aspiration (separate procedure); nasotracheal	1.06	0.74	0.09	1.89	0	N
31725	00	A	Catheter aspiration (separate procedure); tracheobronchial with fiberscope, bedside	1.96	1.41	0.15	3.52	0	N
31730	00	A	Transtracheal (percutaneous) introduction of needle wire dilator/stent or indwelling tube for oxygen therapy	2.85	2.47	0.23	5.55	0	N
31750	00	A	Tracheoplasty; cervical	9.05	8.88	1.09	19.02	90	S
31755	00	A	Tracheoplasty; tracheopharyngeal fistulization, each stage	14.69	13.30	1.44	29.43	90	S
31760	00	A	Tracheoplasty; intrathoracic	20.89	10.92	2.55	34.36	90	S
31766	00	A	Carinal reconstruction	28.82	18.40	1.12	48.34	90	S
31770	00	A	Bronchoplasty; graft repair	21.15	15.07	2.08	38.30	90	S
31775	00	A	Bronchoplasty; excision stenosis and anastomosis	22.15	16.37	1.92	40.44	90	S
31780	00	A	Excision tracheal stenosis and anastomosis; cervical	16.14	17.33	2.08	35.55	90	S
31781	00	A	Excision tracheal stenosis and anastomosis; cervicothoracic	22.22	16.86	1.96	41.04	90	S
31785	00	A	Excision of tracheal tumor or carcinoma; cervical	16.14	8.92	1.17	26.23	90	S
31786	00	A	Excision of tracheal tumor or carcinoma; thoracic	22.54	13.30	2.24	38.08	90	S
31800	00	A	Suture of tracheal wound or injury; cervical	6.77	4.90	0.76	12.43	90	S

CPT codes and descriptions only, © 1994 American Medical Association. Reimbursement information, © 1995 McGraw-Hill Inc.

Code/ CPT	Mod- ifier	Status	Description	Work value	Practice expense	Mal- practice	Total value	Global period	Up- date
31805	00	A	Suture of tracheal wound or injury; intrathoracic	12.59	9.82	1.41	23.82	90	S
31820	00	A	Surgical closure tracheostomy or fistula; without plastic repair	4.10	3.58	0.46	8.14	90	S
31825	00	A	Surgical closure tracheostomy or fistula; with plastic repair	6.31	5.00	0.58	11.89	90	S
31830	00	A	Revision of tracheostomy scar	4.26	3.66	0.42	8.34	90	S
31899	00	C	Unlisted procedure, trachea, bronchi	0	0	0	0	YYY	S
32000	00	A	Thoracentesis, puncture of pleural cavity for aspiration, initial or subsequent	1.54	0.90	0.08	2.52	0	N
32002	00	A	Thoracentesis with insertion of tube with or without water seal (eg, for pneumothorax) (separate procedure)	2.19	1.34	0.22	3.75	0	N
32005	00	A	Chemical pleurodesis (eg, for recurrent or persistent pneumothorax)	2.19	1.09	0.15	3.43	0	S
32020	00	A	Tube thoracostomy with or without water seal (eg, for abscess, hemothorax, empyema) (separate procedure)	3.98	2.63	0.43	7.04	0	S
32035	00	A	Thoracostomy; with rib resection for empyema	6.55	6.76	1.25	14.56	90	S
32036	00	A	Thoracostomy; with open flap drainage for empyema	7.56	7.13	1.32	16.01	90	S
32095	00	A	Thoracotomy, limited, for biopsy of lung or pleura	7.13	8.25	1.45	16.83	90	S
32100	00	A	Thoracotomy, major; with exploration and biopsy	10.07	11.24	2.10	23.41	90	S
32110	00	A	Thoracotomy, major; with control of traumatic hemorrhage and/or repair of lung tear	11.76	11.51	2.01	25.28	90	S
32120	00	A	Thoracotomy, major; for postoperative complications	9.62	9.45	1.72	20.79	90	S
32124	00	A	Thoracotomy, major; with open intrapleural pneumonolysis	10.93	10.94	2.21	24.08	90	S
32140	00	A	Thoracotomy, major; with cyst(s) removal, with or without a pleural procedure	12.14	12.37	2.42	26.93	90	S
32141	00	A	Thoracotomy, major; with excision-plication of bullae, with or without any pleural procedure	12.14	13.42	2.53	28.09	90	S
32150	00	A	Thoracotomy, major; with removal of intrapleural foreign body or fibrin deposit	12.42	10.34	2.01	24.77	90	S
32151	00	A	Thoracotomy, major; with removal of intrapulmonary foreign body	12.42	9.15	1.37	22.94	90	S
32160	00	A	Thoracotomy, major; with cardiac massage	7.13	9.13	1.52	17.78	90	S
32200	00	A	Pneumonostomy, with open drainage of abscess or cyst	13.10	6.89	0.93	20.92	90	S
32215	00	A	Pleural scarification for repeat pneumothorax	10.07	7.62	1.28	18.97	90	S
32220	00	A	Decortication, pulmonary, (separate procedure); total	17.62	15.81	3.01	36.44	90	S
32225	00	A	Decortication, pulmonary, (separate procedure); partial	12.10	11.84	2.28	26.22	90	S
32310	00	A	Pleurectomy, parietal (separate procedure)	12.05	11.64	2.10	25.79	90	S
32315	00	D	Partial removal chest lining	9.85*	7.16#	1.40*	18.41#	90	S
32320	00	A	Decortication and parietal pleurectomy	19.15	18.10	3.40	40.65	90	S
32400	00	A	Biopsy, pleura; percutaneous needle	1.76	1.48	0.12	3.36	0	N
32402	00	A	Biopsy, pleura; open	6.55	7.58	1.34	15.47	90	S
32405	00	A	Biopsy, lung or mediastinum, percutaneous needle	1.93	2.12	0.18	4.23	0	N
32420	00	A	Pneumonocentesis, puncture of lung for aspiration	2.18	1.50	0.13	3.81	0	N
32440	00	A	Removal of lung, total pneumonectomy;	19.15	18.56	3.55	41.26	90	S
32442	00	A	Removal of lung, total pneumonectomy; with resection of segment of trachea followed by broncho-tracheal anastomosis (sleeve pneumonectomy)	24.68	17.94	3.50	46.12	90	S
32445	00	A	Removal of lung, total pneumonectomy; extrapleural	23.37	20.46	3.88	47.71	90	S
32480	00	A	Removal of lung, other than total pneumonectomy; single lobe (lobectomy)	16.84	17.15	3.23	37.22	90	S
32482	00	A	Removal of lung, other than total pneumonectomy; two lobes (bilobectomy)	18.54	17.15	3.23	38.92	90	S
32484	00	A	Removal of lung, other than total pneumonectomy; single segment (segmentectomy)	19.52	17.15	3.23	39.90	90	S

CPT codes and descriptions only, © 1994 American Medical Association. Reimbursement information, © 1995 McGraw-Hill Inc.

Code/ CPT	Mod- ifier	Status	Description	Work value	Practice expense	Mal- practice	Total value	Global period	Up- date
32485	00	A	Removal of lung, other than total pneumonectomy; with bronchoplasty	21.53	21.46	3.93	46.92	90	S
32486	00	A	Removal of lung, other than total pneumonectomy; with circumferential resection of segment of bronchus followed by broncho-bronchial anastomosis (sleeve lobectomy)	22.75	16.54	3.23	42.52	90	S
32488	00	A	Removal of lung, other than total pneumonectomy; all remaining lung following previous removal of a portion of lung (completion pneumonectomy)	24.41	17.74	3.46	45.61	90	S
32500	00	A	Removal of lung, other than total pneumonectomy; wedge resection, single or multiple	13.10	13.47	2.56	29.13	90	S
32520	00	A	Resection of lung; with resection of chest wall	19.42	20.67	3.93	44.02	90	S
32522	00	A	Resection of lung; with reconstruction of chest wall, without prosthesis	21.94	21.90	4.19	48.03	90	S
32525	00	A	Resection of lung; with major reconstruction of chest wall, with prosthesis	24.33	23.50	4.61	52.44	90	S
32540	00	A	Extrapleural enucleation of empyema (empyemectomy)	13.31	11.67	2.05	27.03	90	S
32601	00	A	Thoracoscopy, diagnostic (separate procedure); lungs and pleural space, without biopsy	5.46	3.47	0.57	9.50	0	S
32602	00	A	Thoracoscopy, diagnostic (separate procedure); lungs and pleural space, with biopsy	5.96	3.87	0.64	10.47	0	S
32603	00	A	Thoracoscopy, diagnostic (separate procedure); pericardial sac, without biopsy	7.81	3.47	0.57	11.85	0	S
32604	00	A	Thoracoscopy, diagnostic (separate procedure); pericardial sac, with biopsy	8.78	3.87	0.64	13.29	0	S
32605	00	A	Thoracoscopy, diagnostic (separate procedure); mediastinal space, without biopsy	6.93	3.47	0.57	10.97	0	S
32606	00	A	Thoracoscopy, diagnostic (separate procedure); mediastinal space, with biopsy	8.40	3.87	0.64	12.91	0	S
32650	00	A	Thoracoscopy, surgical; with pleurodesis, any method	10.07	7.62	1.28	18.97	90	S
32651	00	A	Thoracoscopy, surgical; with partial pulmonary decortication	12.10	11.84	2.28	26.22	90	S
32652	00	A	Thoracoscopy, surgical; with total pulmonary decortication, including intrapleural pneumonolysis	17.62	15.81	3.01	36.44	90	S
32653	00	A	Thoracoscopy, surgical; with removal of intrapleural foreign body or fibrin deposit	12.42	10.34	2.01	24.77	90	S
32654	00	A	Thoracoscopy, surgical; with control of traumatic hemorrhage	11.76	11.51	2.01	25.28	90	S
32655	00	A	Thoracoscopy, surgical; with excision-plication of bullae, including any pleural procedure	12.42	13.42	2.53	28.37	90	S
32656	00	A	Thoracoscopy, surgical; with parietal pleurectomy	12.10	13.36	2.36	27.82	90	S
32657	00	A	Thoracoscopy, surgical; with wedge resection of lung, single or multiple	13.10	13.47	2.56	29.13	90	S
32658	00	A	Thoracoscopy, surgical; with removal of clot or foreign body from pericardial sac	11.08	13.26	2.52	26.86	90	S
32659	00	A	Thoracoscopy, surgical; with creation of pericardial window or partial resection of pericardial sac for drainage	10.91	13.96	2.61	27.48	90	S
32660	00	A	Thoracoscopy, surgical; with total pericardiectomy	16.62	19.93	3.56	40.11	90	S
32661	00	A	Thoracoscopy, surgical; with excision of pericardial cyst, tumor, or mass	12.70	9.25	1.47	23.42	90	S
32662	00	A	Thoracoscopy, surgical; with excision of mediastinal cyst, tumor, or mass	15.76	14.55	2.74	33.05	90	S
32663	00	A	Thoracoscopy, surgical; with lobectomy, total or segmental	17.43	17.15	3.23	37.81	90	S
32664	00	A	Thoracoscopy, surgical; with thoracic sympathectomy	13.65	10.55	2.04	26.24	90	S
32665	00	A	Thoracoscopy, surgical; with esophagomyotomy (Heller type)	14.73	14.33	2.64	31.70	90	S

CPT codes and descriptions only, © 1994 American Medical Association. Reimbursement information, © 1995 McGraw-Hill Inc.

Code/ CPT	Mod-ifier	Status	Description	Work value	Practice expense	Mal-practice	Total value	Global period	Up-date
32800	00	A	Repair lung hernia through chest wall	12.10	8.28	1.58	21.96	90	S
32810	00	A	Closure of chest wall following open flap drainage for empyema (Clagett type procedure)	11.59	6.50	1.19	19.28	90	S
32815	00	A	Open closure of major bronchial fistula	21.36	15.22	2.62	39.20	90	S
32820	00	A	Major reconstruction, chest wall (post-traumatic)	19.78	19.01	3.24	42.03	90	S
32850	00	X	Donor pneumonectomy(ies) with preparation and maintenance of allograft (cadaver)	11.96*	8.70#	1.70*	22.36#	XXX	0
32851	00	A	Lung transplant, single; without cardiopulmonary bypass	35.14	25.55	4.99	65.68	90	S
32852	00	A	Lung transplant, single; with cardiopulmonary bypass	38.11	27.71	5.41	71.23	90	S
32853	00	A	Lung transplant, double (bilateral sequential or en bloc); without cardiopulmonary bypass	43.93	31.94	6.24	82.11	90	S
32854	00	A	Lung transplant, double (bilateral sequential or en bloc); with cardiopulmonary bypass	46.90	34.10	6.67	87.67	90	S
32900	00	A	Resection of ribs, extrapleural, all stages	18.14	8.47	1.63	28.24	90	S
32905	00	A	Thoracoplasty, Schede type or extrapleural (all stages);	19.15	12.74	2.60	34.49	90	S
32906	00	A	Thoracoplasty, Schede type or extrapleural (all stages); with closure of bronchopleural fistula	25.17	15.42	2.92	43.51	90	S
32940	00	A	Pneumonolysis, extraperiosteal, including filling or packing procedures	18.14	11.37	1.75	31.26	90	S
32960	00	A	Pneumothorax, therapeutic, intrapleural injection of air	1.84	0.93	0.13	2.90	0	N
32999	00	C	Unlisted procedure, lungs and pleura	0	0	0	0	YYY	S
33010	00	A	Pericardiocentesis; initial	2.24	1.54	0.14	3.92	0	N
33011	00	A	Pericardiocentesis; subsequent	2.24	1.11	0.12	3.47	0	N
33015	00	A	Tube pericardiostomy	5.64	4.26	0.62	10.52	90	S
33020	00	A	Pericardiotomy for removal of clot or foreign body (primary procedure)	11.08	13.26	2.52	26.86	90	S
33025	00	A	Creation of pericardial window or partial resection for drainage	10.91	13.96	2.61	27.48	90	S
33030	00	A	Pericardiectomy, subtotal or complete; without cardiopulmonary bypass	16.62	21.02	3.92	41.56	90	S
33031	00	A	Pericardiectomy, subtotal or complete; with cardiopulmonary bypass	19.64	13.25	2.50	35.39	90	S
33050	00	A	Excision of pericardial cyst or tumor	12.70	9.25	1.47	23.42	90	S
33100	00	D	Removal of heart sac	22.51*	16.37#	3.20*	42.08#	90	S
33120	00	A	Excision of intracardiac tumor, resection with cardiopulmonary bypass	22.57	28.89	5.17	56.63	90	S
33130	00	A	Resection of external cardiac tumor	19.53	13.50	2.22	35.25	90	S
33200	00	A	Insertion of permanent pacemaker with epicardial electrode(s); by thoracotomy	11.08	12.27	1.90	25.25	90	S
33201	00	A	Insertion of permanent pacemaker with epicardial electrode(s); by xiphoid approach	8.93	11.19	1.67	21.79	90	S
33206	00	A	Insertion or replacement of permanent pacemaker with transvenous electrode(s); atrial	6.04	7.73	1.34	15.11	90	S
33207	00	A	Insertion or replacement of permanent pacemaker with transvenous electrode(s); ventricular	7.28	9.01	1.33	17.62	90	S
33208	00	A	Insertion or replacement of permanent pacemaker with transvenous electrode(s); atrial and ventricular	7.28	9.50	1.54	18.32	90	N
33210	00	A	Insertion or replacement of temporary transvenous single chamber cardiac electrode or pacemaker catheter (separate procedure)	3.30	3.30	0.27	6.87	0	N
33211	00	A	Insertion or replacement of temporary transvenous dual chamber pacing electrodes (separate procedure)	3.40	3.30	0.27	6.97	0	N
33212	00	A	Insertion or replacement of pacemaker pulse generator only; single chamber, atrial or ventricular	5.21	5.38	0.88	11.47	90	S

CPT codes and descriptions only, © 1994 American Medical Association. Reimbursement information, © 1995 McGraw-Hill Inc.

Code/ CPT	Mod- ifier	Status	Description	Work value	Practice expense	Mal- practice	Total value	Global period	Up- date
33213	00	A	Insertion or replacement of pacemaker pulse generator only; dual chamber	6.15	5.38	0.88	12.41	90	N
33214	00	A	Upgrade of implanted pacemaker system, conversion of single chamber system to dual chamber system (includes removal of previously placed pulse generator, testing of existing lead, insertion of new lead, insertion of new pulse generator)	7.43	5.40	1.06	13.89	90	N
33216	00	A	Insertion, replacement or repositioning of permanent transvenous electrode(s) only (15 days or more after initial insertion); single chamber, atrial or ventricular	5.07	5.02	0.55	10.64	90	N
33217	00	A	Insertion, replacement or repositioning of permanent transvenous electrode(s) only (15 days or more after initial insertion); dual chamber	5.43	5.02	0.55	11.00	90	N
33218	00	A	Repair of pacemaker electrode(s) only; single chamber, atrial or ventricular	5.02	4.59	0.62	10.23	90	S
33220	00	A	Repair of pacemaker electrode(s) only; dual chamber	5.10	4.59	0.62	10.31	90	N
33222	00	A	Revision or relocation of skin pocket for pacemaker	4.59	5.70	1.01	11.30	90	S
33223	00	A	Revision or relocation of skin pocket for implantable cardioverter-defibrillator	6.14	5.70	1.01	12.85	90	S
33233	00	A	Removal of permanent pacemaker pulse generator;	2.97	2.64	0.05	5.66	90	N
33234	00	A	Removal of permanent pacemaker pulse generator; with transvenous electrode(s), single lead system, atrial or ventricular	8.69	4.74	0.38	13.81	90	S
33235	00	A	Removal of permanent pacemaker pulse generator; with transvenous electrode(s), dual lead system	9.93	5.21	0.55	15.69	90	N
33236	00	A	Removal of permanent epicardial pacemaker and electrodes by thoracotomy; single lead system, atrial or ventricular	11.71	3.98	0.62	16.31	90	S
33237	00	A	Removal of permanent epicardial pacemaker and electrodes by thoracotomy; dual lead system	12.69	9.60	1.13	23.42	90	S
33238	00	A	Removal of permanent transvenous electrode(s) by thoracotomy	14.15	10.29	2.01	26.45	90	S
33240	00	A	Insertion or replacement of implantable cardioverter-defibrillator pulse generator only	7.20	5.38	0.88	13.46	90	S
33241	00	A	Removal of implantable cardioverter-defibrillator pulse generator only	2.97	2.16	0.43	5.56	90	S
33242	00	A	Repair of implantable cardioverter-defibrillator pulse generator and/or leads	5.85	7.50	1.54	14.89	90	S
33243	00	A	Removal of implantable cardioverter-defibrillator pulse generator and/or lead system; by thoracotomy	21.47	9.02	1.54	32.03	90	S
33244	00	A	Removal of implantable cardioverter-defibrillator pulse generator and/or lead system; by other than thoracotomy	8.34	9.02	1.54	18.90	90	S
33245	00	A	Implantation or replacement of implantable cardioverter-defibrillator pads by thoracotomy, with or without sensing electrodes;	12.57	16.09	2.36	31.02	90	S
33246	00	A	Implantation or replacement of implantable cardioverter-defibrillator pads by thoracotomy, with or without sensing electrodes; with insertion of implantable cardioverter-defibrillator pulse generator	19.28	20.79	3.19	43.26	90	S
33247	00	A	Insertion or replacement of implantable cardioverter-defibrillator lead(s), by other than thoracotomy;	9.46	13.24	2.36	25.06	90	N
33249	00	A	Insertion or replacement of implantable cardioverter-defibrillator lead(s), by other than thoracotomy; with insertion of cardio-defibrillator pulse generator	12.83	16.81	3.19	32.83	90	S

CPT codes and descriptions only, © 1994 American Medical Association. Reimbursement information, © 1995 McGraw-Hill Inc.

Code/ CPT	Mod- ifier	Status	Description	Work value	Practice expense	Mal- practice	Total value	Global period	Up- date
33250	00	A	Operative ablation of supraventricular arrhythmogenic focus or pathway (eg, Wolff-Parkinson-White, A-V node re-entry), tract(s) and/or focus (foci); without cardiopulmonary bypass	19.54	11.56	0.86	31.96	90	S
33251	00	A	Operative ablation of supraventricular arrhythmogenic focus or pathway (eg, Wolff-Parkinson-White, A-V node re-entry), tract(s) and/or focus (foci); with cardiopulmonary bypass	22.57	16.41	3.21	42.19	90	S
33260	00	A	Operative ablation of arrhythmogenic focus or pathway; without cardiopulmonary bypass	16.19	11.77	2.29	30.25	90	S
33261	00	A	Operative ablation of arrhythmogenic focus or pathway; with cardiopulmonary bypass	22.57	13.96	2.73	39.26	90	S
33300	00	A	Repair of cardiac wound; without bypass	16.19	14.36	2.60	33.15	90	S
33305	00	A	Repair of cardiac wound; with cardiopulmonary bypass	19.22	17.40	3.07	39.69	90	S
33310	00	A	Cardiotomy, exploratory (includes removal of foreign body); without bypass	17.12	11.28	1.93	30.33	90	S
33315	00	A	Cardiotomy, exploratory (includes removal of foreign body); with cardiopulmonary bypass	20.15	14.48	2.57	37.20	90	S
33320	00	A	Suture repair of aorta or great vessels; without shunt or cardiopulmonary bypass	15.39	14.14	2.51	32.04	90	S
33321	00	A	Suture repair of aorta or great vessels; with shunt bypass	18.74	21.75	3.61	44.10	90	S
33322	00	A	Suture repair of aorta or great vessels; with cardiopulmonary bypass	18.40	21.75	3.61	43.76	90	S
33330	00	A	Insertion of graft, aorta or great vessels; without shunt, or cardiopulmonary bypass	19.15	12.67	1.93	33.75	90	S
33332	00	A	Insertion of graft, aorta or great vessels; with shunt bypass	22.50	15.07	2.39	39.96	90	S
33335	00	A	Insertion of graft, aorta or great vessels; with cardiopulmonary bypass	27.66	15.07	2.39	45.12	90	S
33350	00	C	Great vessel repair with other major procedure	0	0	0	0	90	S
33400	00	A	Valvuloplasty, aortic valve; open, with cardiopulmonary bypass	23.16	26.21	2.83	52.20	90	S
33401	00	A	Valvuloplasty, aortic valve; open, with inflow occlusion	22.45	26.21	2.83	51.49	90	S
33403	00	A	Valvuloplasty, aortic valve; using transventricular dilation, with cardiopulmonary bypass	23.43	26.21	2.83	52.47	90	S
33404	00	A	Construction of apical-aortic conduit	26.62	31.25	5.59	63.46	90	S
33405	00	A	Replacement, aortic valve, with cardiopulmonary bypass; with prosthetic valve other than homograft	28.47	30.48	5.33	64.28	90	S
33406	00	A	Replacement, aortic valve, with cardiopulmonary bypass; with homograft valve (freehand)	31.23	38.65	7.45	77.33	90	S
33411	00	A	Replacement, aortic valve; with aortic annulus enlargement, noncoronary cusp	30.37	38.65	7.45	76.47	90	S
33412	00	A	Replacement, aortic valve; with transventricular aortic annulus enlargement (Konno procedure)	32.26	38.65	7.45	78.36	90	S
33413	00	A	Replacement, aortic valve; by translocation of autologous pulmonary valve with homograft replacement of pulmonary valve (Ross procedure)	34.17	41.09	7.23	82.49	90	S
33414	00	A	Repair of left ventricular outflow tract obstruction by patch enlargement of the outflow tract	29.28	38.65	7.45	75.38	90	S
33415	00	A	Resection or incision of subvalvular tissue for discrete subvalvular aortic stenosis	25.02	30.48	5.33	60.83	90	S
33416	00	A	Ventriculomyotomy (-myectomy) for idiopathic hypertrophic subaortic stenosis (eg, asymmetric septal hypertrophy)	28.20	28.14	4.99	61.33	90	S
33417	00	A	Aortoplasty (gusset) for supravalvular stenosis	27.34	34.71	6.18	68.23	90	S
33420	00	A	Valvotomy, mitral valve; closed heart	20.69	19.82	2.45	42.96	90	S

CPT codes and descriptions only, © 1994 American Medical Association. Reimbursement information, © 1995 McGraw-Hill Inc.

Code/ CPT	Mod- ifier	Status	Description	Work value	Practice expense	Mal- practice	Total value	Global period	Up- date
33422	00	A	Valvotomy, mitral valve; open heart, with cardiopulmonary bypass	23.72	30.35	6.45	60.52	90	S
33425	00	A	Valvuloplasty, mitral valve, with cardiopulmonary bypass;	25.57	31.27	5.42	62.26	90	S
33426	00	A	Valvuloplasty, mitral valve, with cardiopulmonary bypass; with prosthetic ring	26.07	31.96	5.80	63.83	90	S
33427	00	A	Valvuloplasty, mitral valve, with cardiopulmonary bypass; radical reconstruction, with or without ring	32.07	34.71	6.30	73.08	90	S
33430	00	A	Replacement, mitral valve, with cardiopulmonary bypass	29.42	34.85	6.11	70.38	90	S
33460	00	A	Valvectomy, tricuspid valve, with cardiopulmonary bypass	21.60	26.07	4.73	52.40	90	S
33463	00	A	Valvuloplasty, tricuspid valve; without ring insertion	24.16	32.67	5.95	62.78	90	S
33464	00	A	Valvuloplasty, tricuspid valve; with ring insertion	25.87	32.67	5.95	64.49	90	S
33465	00	A	Replacement, tricuspid valve, with cardiopulmonary bypass	26.57	32.67	5.95	65.19	90	S
33468	00	A	Tricuspid valve repositioning and plication for Ebstein anomaly	28.20	34.71	6.30	69.21	90	S
33470	00	A	Valvotomy, pulmonary valve, closed heart; transventricular	19.52	19.82	2.45	41.79	90	S
33471	00	A	Valvotomy, pulmonary valve, closed heart; via pulmonary artery	21.13	26.21	2.83	50.17	90	S
33472	00	A	Valvotomy, pulmonary valve, open heart; with inflow occlusion	20.91	30.64	2.83	54.38	90	S
33474	00	A	Valvotomy, pulmonary valve, open heart; with cardiopulmonary bypass	20.91	30.64	2.83	54.38	90	S
33475	00	A	Replacement, pulmonary valve	27.34	34.85	6.11	68.30	90	S
33476	00	A	Right ventricular resection for infundibular stenosis, with or without commissurotomy	24.41	28.14	4.99	57.54	90	S
33478	00	A	Outflow tract augmentation (gusset), with or without commissurotomy or infundibular resection	25.38	31.27	5.42	62.07	90	S
33500	00	A	Repair of coronary arteriovenous or arteriocardiac chamber fistula; with cardiopulmonary bypass	23.91	29.55	5.20	58.66	90	S
33501	00	A	Repair of coronary arteriovenous or arteriocardiac chamber fistula; without cardiopulmonary bypass	16.14	14.14	2.51	32.79	90	S
33502	00	A	Repair of anomalous coronary artery; by ligation	19.80	14.14	2.51	36.45	90	S
33503	00	A	Repair of anomalous coronary artery; by graft, without cardiopulmonary bypass	20.15	29.55	5.20	54.90	90	S
33504	00	A	Repair of anomalous coronary artery; by graft, with cardiopulmonary bypass	23.16	29.55	5.20	57.91	90	S
33505	00	A	Repair of anomalous coronary artery; with construction of intrapulmonary artery tunnel (Takeuchi procedure)	25.38	34.24	6.03	65.65	90	S
33506	00	A	Repair of anomalous coronary artery; by translocation from pulmonary artery to aorta	25.38	34.24	6.03	65.65	90	S
33510	00	A	Coronary artery bypass, vein only; single coronary venous graft	23.29	29.55	5.20	58.04	90	S
33511	00	A	Coronary artery bypass, vein only; two coronary venous grafts	25.57	32.44	5.71	63.72	90	S
33512	00	A	Coronary artery bypass, vein only; three coronary venous grafts	27.84	35.33	6.22	69.39	90	S
33513	00	A	Coronary artery bypass, vein only; four coronary venous grafts	30.12	38.21	6.73	75.06	90	S
33514	00	A	Coronary artery bypass, vein only; five coronary venous grafts	32.39	41.09	7.23	80.71	90	S
33516	00	A	Coronary artery bypass, vein only; six or more coronary venous grafts	34.66	43.97	7.74	86.37	90	S
33517	00	A	Coronary artery bypass, using venous graft(s) and arterial graft(s); single vein graft (list separately in addition to code for arterial graft)	2.27	2.89	0.50	5.66	90	S

CPT codes and descriptions only, © 1994 American Medical Association. Reimbursement information, © 1995 McGraw-Hill Inc.

Code/ CPT	Mod- ifier	Status	Description	Work value	Practice expense	Mal- practice	Total value	Global period	Up- date
33518	00	A	Coronary artery bypass, using venous graft(s) and arterial graft(s); two venous grafts (list separately in addition to code for arterial graft)	4.55	5.77	1.02	11.34	90	S
33519	00	A	Coronary artery bypass, using venous graft(s) and arterial graft(s); three venous grafts (list separately in addition to code for arterial graft)	6.82	8.65	1.52	16.99	90	S
33521	00	A	Coronary artery bypass, using venous graft(s) and arterial graft(s); four venous grafts (list separately in addition to code for arterial graft)	9.10	11.54	2.03	22.67	90	S
33522	00	A	Coronary artery bypass, using venous graft(s) and arterial graft(s); five venous grafts (list separately in addition to code for arterial graft)	11.37	14.43	2.54	28.34	90	S
33523	00	A	Coronary artery bypass, using venous graft(s) and arterial graft(s); six or more venous grafts (list separately in addition to code for arterial graft)	13.65	17.32	3.05	34.02	90	S
33530	00	A	Reoperation, coronary artery bypass procedure or valve procedure, more than one month after original operation (list separately in addition to code for primary procedure)	5.86	8.87	2.18	16.91	ZZZ	S
33533	00	A	Coronary artery bypass, using arterial graft(s); single arterial graft	24.00	30.45	5.36	59.81	90	S
33534	00	A	Coronary artery bypass, using arterial graft(s); two coronary arterial grafts	26.99	34.24	6.03	67.26	90	S
33535	00	A	Coronary artery bypass, using arterial graft(s); three coronary arterial grafts	29.98	38.03	6.70	74.71	90	S
33536	00	A	Coronary artery bypass, using arterial graft(s); four or more coronary arterial grafts	32.96	41.82	7.37	82.15	90	S
33542	00	A	Myocardial resection (eg, ventricular aneurysmectomy)	26.57	30.73	5.53	62.83	90	S
33545	00	A	Repair of postinfarction ventricular septal defect, with or without myocardial resection	33.96	34.92	6.28	75.16	90	S
33570	00	D	Revise coronary circulation	21.10*	15.34#	3.00*	39.44#	90	S
33572	00	A	Coronary endarterectomy, open, any method, of left anterior descending, circumflex, or right coronary artery performed in conjunction with coronary artery bypass graft procedure, each vessel (list separately in addition to primary procedure)	4.45	3.23	0.63	8.31	ZZZ	S
33575	00	D	Revise coronary circulation	31.65*	23.01#	4.50*	59.16#	90	S
33600	00	A	Closure of atrioventricular valve (mitral or tricuspid) by suture or patch	28.31	34.85	6.11	69.27	90	S
33602	00	A	Closure of semilunar valve (aortic or pulmonary) by suture or patch	27.34	30.48	5.33	63.15	90	S
33606	00	A	Anastomosis of pulmonary artery to aorta (Damus-Kaye-Stansel procedure)	29.28	38.65	7.45	75.38	90	S
33608	00	A	Repair of complex cardiac anomaly other than pulmonary atresia with ventricular septal defect by construction or replacement of conduit from right or left ventricle to pulmonary artery	30.02	38.65	7.45	76.12	90	S
33610	00	A	Repair of complex cardiac anomalies (eg, single ventricle with subaortic obstruction) by surgical enlargement of interventricular septal defect	29.28	38.65	7.45	75.38	90	S
33611	00	A	Repair of double outlet right ventricle with intraventricular tunnel repair;	31.23	38.65	7.45	77.33	90	S
33612	00	A	Repair of double outlet right ventricle with intraventricular tunnel repair; with repair of right ventricular outflow tract obstruction	32.06	38.65	7.45	78.16	90	S

CPT codes and descriptions only, © 1994 American Medical Association. Reimbursement information, © 1995 McGraw-Hill Inc.

Code/ CPT	Mod- ifier	Status	Description	Work value	Practice expense	Mal- practice	Total value	Global period	Up- date
33615	00	A	Repair of complex cardiac anomalies (eg, tricuspid atresia) by closure of atrial septal defect and anastomosis of atria or vena cava to pulmonary artery (simple Fontan procedure)	30.50	38.65	7.45	76.60	90	S
33617	00	A	Repair of complex cardiac anomalies (eg, single ventricle) by modified Fontan procedure	32.21	38.65	7.45	78.31	90	S
33619	00	A	Repair of single ventricle with aortic outflow obstruction and aortic arch hypoplasia (hypoplastic left heart syndrome) (eg, Norwood procedure)	35.39	44.30	8.04	87.73	90	S
33641	00	A	Repair atrial septal defect, secundum, with cardiopulmonary bypass, with or without patch	19.93	25.51	4.87	50.31	90	S
33645	00	A	Direct or patch closure, sinus venosus, with or without anomalous pulmonary venous drainage	22.78	27.61	4.87	55.26	90	S
33647	00	A	Repair of atrial septal defect and ventricular septal defect, with direct or patch closure	27.44	34.92	6.28	68.64	90	S
33660	00	A	Repair of incomplete or partial atrioventricular canal (ostium primum atrial septal defect), with or without atrioventricular valve repair	24.41	31.27	5.42	61.10	90	S
33665	00	A	Repair of intermediate or transitional atrioventricular canal, with or without atrioventricular valve repair	27.34	31.27	5.42	64.03	90	S
33670	00	A	Repair of complete atrioventricular canal, with or without prosthetic valve	31.23	38.65	7.45	77.33	90	S
33681	00	A	Closure of ventricular septal defect, with or without patch	26.36	34.92	6.28	67.56	90	S
33684	00	A	Closure of ventricular septal defect, with or without patch with pulmonary valvotomy or infundibular resection (acyanotic)	28.31	34.92	6.28	69.51	90	S
33688	00	A	Closure of ventricular septal defect, with or without patch with removal of pulmonary artery band, with or without gusset	29.28	34.92	6.28	70.48	90	S
33690	00	A	Banding of pulmonary artery	18.31	22.10	4.29	44.70	90	S
33692	00	A	Complete repair tetralogy of Fallot without pulmonary atresia;	29.28	38.65	7.45	75.38	90	S
33694	00	A	Complete repair tetralogy of Fallot without pulmonary atresia; with transannular patch	30.26	38.65	7.45	76.36	90	S
33696	00	A	Complete repair tetralogy of Fallot without pulmonary atresia; with closure of previous shunt	30.12	38.65	7.45	76.22	90	S
33697	00	A	Complete repair tetralogy of Fallot with pulmonary atresia including construction of conduit from right ventricle to pulmonary artery and closure of ventricular septal defect;	32.21	38.65	7.45	78.31	90	S
33698	00	A	Complete repair tetralogy of Fallot with pulmonary atresia including construction of conduit from right ventricle to pulmonary artery and closure of ventricular septal defect; with closure of previous shunt	33.19	38.65	7.45	79.29	90	S
33702	00	A	Repair sinus of Valsalva fistula, with cardiopulmonary bypass;	25.38	30.48	5.33	61.19	90	S
33710	00	A	Repair sinus of Valsalva fistula, with cardiopulmonary bypass; with repair of ventricular septal defect	28.35	34.92	6.28	69.55	90	S
33720	00	A	Repair sinus of Valsalva aneurysm, with cardiopulmonary bypass	25.38	30.48	5.33	61.19	90	S
33722	00	A	Closure of aortico-left ventricular tunnel	27.34	30.48	5.33	63.15	90	S
33730	00	A	Complete repair of anomalous venous return (supracardiac, intracardiac, or infracardiac types)	29.89	38.65	7.45	75.99	90	S
33732	00	A	Repair of cor triatriatum or supravalvular mitral ring by resection of left atrial membrane	27.09	31.27	5.42	63.78	90	S
33735	00	A	Atrial septectomy or septostomy; closed heart (Blalock-Hanlon type operation)	19.97	25.69	4.87	50.53	90	S

CPT codes and descriptions only, © 1994 American Medical Association. Reimbursement information, © 1995 McGraw-Hill Inc.

Code/ CPT	Mod- ifier	Status	Description	Work value	Practice expense	Mal- practice	Total value	Global period	Up- date
33736	00	A	Atrial septectomy or septostomy; open heart with cardiopulmonary bypass	22.45	25.69	4.87	53.01	90	S
33737	00	A	Atrial septectomy or septostomy; open heart, with inflow occlusion	20.50	25.69	4.87	51.06	90	S
33750	00	A	Shunt; subclavian to pulmonary artery (Blalock-Taussig type operation)	20.15	22.10	4.29	46.54	90	S
33755	00	A	Shunt; ascending aorta to pulmonary artery (Waterston type operation)	20.50	22.10	4.29	46.89	90	S
33762	00	A	Shunt; descending aorta to pulmonary artery (Potts-Smith type operation)	20.50	22.10	4.29	46.89	90	S
33764	00	A	Shunt; central, with prosthetic graft	20.50	22.10	4.29	46.89	90	S
33766	00	A	Shunt; superior vena cava to pulmonary artery for flow to one lung (classical Glenn procedure)	21.47	22.10	4.29	47.86	90	S
33767	00	A	Shunt; superior vena cava to pulmonary artery for flow to both lungs (bidirectional Glenn procedure)	23.43	25.69	4.87	53.99	90	S
33770	00	A	Repair of transposition of the great arteries with ventricular septal defect and subpulmonary stenosis; without surgical enlargement of ventricular septal defect	31.96	38.65	7.45	78.06	90	S
33771	00	A	Repair of transposition of the great arteries with ventricular septal defect and subpulmonary stenosis; with surgical enlargement of ventricular septal defect	33.19	38.65	7.45	79.29	90	S
33774	00	A	Repair of transposition of the great arteries, atrial baffle procedure (eg, Mustard or Senning type) with cardiopulmonary bypass;	29.28	31.27	5.42	65.97	90	S
33775	00	A	Repair of transposition of the great arteries, atrial baffle procedure (eg, Mustard or Senning type) with cardiopulmonary bypass; with removal of pulmonary band	30.50	31.27	5.42	67.19	90	S
33776	00	A	Repair of transposition of the great arteries, atrial baffle procedure (eg, Mustard or Senning type) with cardiopulmonary bypass; with closure of ventricular septal defect	32.21	34.92	6.28	73.41	90	S
33777	00	A	Repair of transposition of the great arteries, atrial baffle procedure (eg, Mustard or Senning type) with cardiopulmonary bypass; with repair of subpulmonic obstruction	31.73	31.27	5.42	68.42	90	S
33778	00	A	Repair of transposition of the great arteries, aortic pulmonary artery reconstruction (eg, Jatene type);	34.17	41.82	7.37	83.36	90	S
33779	00	A	Repair of transposition of the great arteries, aortic pulmonary artery reconstruction (eg, Jatene type); with removal of pulmonary band	34.41	41.82	7.37	83.60	90	S
33780	00	A	Repair of transposition of the great arteries, aortic pulmonary artery reconstruction (eg, Jatene type); with closure of ventricular septal defect	35.14	41.82	7.37	84.33	90	S
33781	00	A	Repair of transposition of the great arteries, aortic pulmonary artery reconstruction (eg, Jatene type); with repair of subpulmonic obstruction	34.65	41.82	7.37	83.84	90	S
33786	00	A	Total repair, truncus arteriosus (Rastelli type operation)	33.19	38.65	7.45	79.29	90	S
33788	00	A	Reimplantation of an anomalous pulmonary artery	25.38	29.55	5.20	60.13	90	S
33800	00	A	Aortic suspension (aortopexy) for tracheal decompression (eg, for tracheomalacia) (separate procedure)	15.18	14.14	2.51	31.83	90	S
33802	00	A	Division of aberrant vessel (vascular ring);	16.60	22.10	4.29	42.99	90	S
33803	00	A	Division of aberrant vessel (vascular ring); with reanastomosis	18.54	22.10	4.29	44.93	90	S
33813	00	A	Obliteration of aortopulmonary septal defect; without cardiopulmonary bypass	19.52	22.10	4.29	45.91	90	S

CPT codes and descriptions only, © 1994 American Medical Association. Reimbursement information, © 1995 McGraw-Hill Inc.

Code/ CPT	Mod-ifier	Status	Description	Work value	Practice expense	Mal-practice	Total value	Global period	Up-date
33814	00	A	Obliteration of aortopulmonary septal defect; with cardiopulmonary bypass	24.41	30.48	5.33	60.22	90	S
33820	00	A	Repair of patent ductus arteriosus; by ligation	15.62	22.10	4.29	42.01	90	S
33822	00	A	Repair of patent ductus arteriosus; by division, under 18 years	16.60	22.10	4.29	42.99	90	S
33824	00	A	Repair of patent ductus arteriosus; by division, 18 years and older	18.54	22.10	4.29	44.93	90	S
33840	00	A	Excision of coarctation of aorta, with or without associated patent ductus arteriosus; with direct anastomosis	19.52	31.25	5.59	56.36	90	S
33845	00	A	Excision of coarctation of aorta, with or without associated patent ductus arteriosus; with graft	20.99	31.25	5.59	57.83	90	S
33851	00	A	Excision of coarctation of aorta, with or without associated patent ductus arteriosus; repair using either left subclavian artery or prosthetic material as gusset for enlargement	20.01	31.25	5.59	56.85	90	S
33852	00	A	Repair of hypoplastic or interrupted aortic arch using autogenous or prosthetic material; without cardiopulmonary bypass	22.45	31.25	5.59	59.29	90	S
33853	00	A	Repair of hypoplastic or interrupted aortic arch using autogenous or prosthetic material; with cardiopulmonary bypass	30.26	38.65	7.45	76.36	90	S
33860	00	A	Ascending aorta graft, with cardiopulmonary bypass, with or without valve suspension;	31.23	34.71	6.18	72.12	90	S
33861	00	A	Ascending aorta graft, with cardiopulmonary bypass, with or without valve suspension; with coronary reconstruction	33.19	34.71	6.18	74.08	90	S
33863	00	A	Ascending aorta graft, with cardiopulmonary bypass, with or without valve suspension; with aortic root replacement using composite prosthesis and coronary reconstruction	35.14	34.71	6.18	76.03	90	S
33870	00	A	Transverse arch graft, with cardiopulmonary bypass	37.74	44.30	8.04	90.08	90	S
33875	00	A	Descending thoracic aorta graft, with or without bypass	26.94	31.25	5.59	63.78	90	S
33877	00	A	Repair of thoracoabdominal aortic aneurysm with graft, with or without cardiopulmonary bypass	40.29	44.11	8.38	92.78	90	S
33910	00	A	Pulmonary artery embolectomy; with cardiopulmonary bypass	21.86	14.65	2.77	39.28	90	S
33915	00	A	Pulmonary artery embolectomy; without cardiopulmonary bypass	18.84	12.02	2.22	33.08	90	S
33916	00	A	Pulmonary endarterectomy, with or without embolectomy, with cardiopulmonary bypass	24.17	17.57	3.43	45.17	90	S
33917	00	A	Repair of pulmonary artery stenosis by reconstruction with patch or graft	23.43	34.71	6.30	64.44	90	S
33918	00	A	Repair of pulmonary atresia with ventricular septal defect, by unifocalization of pulmonary arteries; without cardiopulmonary bypass	25.38	29.55	5.20	60.13	90	S
33919	00	A	Repair of pulmonary atresia with ventricular septal defect, by unifocalization of pulmonary arteries; with cardiopulmonary bypass	31.11	38.65	7.45	77.21	90	S
33920	00	A	Repair of pulmonary atresia with ventricular septal defect, by construction or replacement of conduit from right or left ventricle to pulmonary artery	30.75	38.65	7.45	76.85	90	S
33922	00	A	Transection of pulmonary artery with cardiopulmonary bypass	22.45	26.21	2.83	51.49	90	S
33930	00	X	Donor cardiectomy-pneumonectomy, with preparation and maintenance of allograft	16.88*	12.27#	2.40*	31.55#	XXX	0
33935	00	R	Heart-lung transplant with recipient cardiectomy-pneumonectomy	56.87	64.80	11.05	132.72	90	S

CPT codes and descriptions only, © 1994 American Medical Association. Reimbursement information, © 1995 McGraw-Hill Inc.

Code/ CPT	Mod-ifier	Status	Description	Work value	Practice expense	Mal-practice	Total value	Global period	Up-date
33940	00	X	Donor cardiectomy, with preparation and maintenance of allograft	14.77*	10.74#	2.10*	27.61#	XXX	0
33945	00	R	Heart transplant, with or without recipient cardiectomy	39.56	64.80	11.05	115.41	90	S
33960	00	A	Prolonged extracorporeal circulation for cardiopulmonary insufficiency; initial 24 hours	19.36	7.01	0.94	27.31	XXX	S
33961	00	A	Prolonged extracorporeal circulation for cardiopulmonary insufficiency; each additional 24 hours	10.93	7.01	0.94	18.88	XXX	S
33970	00	A	Insertion of intra-aortic balloon assist device through the femoral artery, open approach	8.05	7.54	1.00	16.59	0	S
33971	00	A	Removal of intra-aortic balloon assist device including repair of femoral artery, with or without graft	4.04	5.16	0.91	10.11	90	S
33973	00	A	Insertion of intra-aortic balloon assist device through the ascending aorta	9.76	7.54	1.00	18.30	0	S
33974	00	A	Removal of intra-aortic balloon assist device from the ascending aorta, including repair of the ascending aorta, with or without graft	12.69	5.56	0.91	19.16	90	S
33975	00	A	Implantation of ventricular assist device; single ventricle support	19.52	14.19	2.77	36.48	90	S
33976	00	A	Implantation of ventricular assist device; biventricular support	26.60	19.33	3.78	49.71	90	S
33977	00	A	Removal of ventricular assist device; single ventricle support	17.08	12.41	2.43	31.92	90	S
33978	00	A	Removal of ventricular assist device; biventricular support	19.52	14.19	2.77	36.48	90	S
33999	00	C	Unlisted procedure, cardiac surgery	0	0	0	0	YYY	S
34001	00	A	Embolectomy or thrombectomy, with or without catheter; carotid, subclavian or innominate artery, by neck incision	11.69	9.58	1.87	23.14	90	S
34051	00	A	Embolectomy or thrombectomy, with or without catheter; innominate, subclavian artery, by thoracic incision	13.62	8.81	1.59	24.02	90	S
34101	00	A	Embolectomy or thrombectomy, with or without catheter; axillary, brachial, innominate, subclavian artery, by arm incision	8.73	8.34	1.71	18.78	90	S
34111	00	A	Embolectomy or thrombectomy, with or without catheter; radial or ulnar artery, by arm incision	7.18	7.59	1.59	16.36	90	S
34151	00	A	Embolectomy or thrombectomy, with or without catheter; renal, celiac, mesentery, aortoiliac artery, by abdominal incision	15.23	11.96	2.39	29.58	90	S
34201	00	A	Embolectomy or thrombectomy, with or without catheter; femoropopliteal, aortoiliac artery, by leg incision	8.04	8.90	1.78	18.72	90	S
34203	00	A	Embolectomy or thrombectomy, with or without catheter; popliteal-tibio-peroneal artery, by leg incision	11.06	8.63	1.72	21.41	90	S
34401	00	A	Thrombectomy, direct or with catheter; vena cava, iliac vein, by abdominal incision	11.64	8.07	1.39	21.10	90	S
34421	00	A	Thrombectomy, direct or with catheter; vena cava, iliac, femoropopliteal vein, by leg incision	8.89	7.45	1.51	17.85	90	S
34451	00	A	Thrombectomy, direct or with catheter; vena cava, iliac, femoropopliteal vein, by abdominal and leg incision	13.13	10.69	2.14	25.96	90	S
34471	00	A	Thrombectomy, direct or with catheter; subclavian vein, by neck incision	9.12	3.51	0.55	13.18	90	S
34490	00	A	Thrombectomy, direct or with catheter; axillary and subclavian vein, by arm incision	6.51	7.27	1.54	15.32	90	S
34501	00	A	Valvuloplasty, femoral vein	9.71	7.35	0.86	17.92	90	S
34502	00	A	Reconstruction of vena cava, any method	25.65	18.65	3.64	47.94	90	S
34510	00	A	Venous valve transposition, any vein donor	11.75	8.89	1.04	21.68	90	S
34520	00	A	Cross-over vein graft to venous system	12.33	9.33	1.09	22.75	90	S
34530	00	A	Saphenopopliteal vein anastomosis	16.33	12.35	1.44	30.12	90	S

CPT codes and descriptions only, © 1994 American Medical Association. Reimbursement information, © 1995 McGraw-Hill Inc.

Code/ CPT	Mod- ifier	Status	Description	Work value	Practice expense	Mal- practice	Total value	Global period	Up- date
35001	00	A	Direct repair of aneurysm, false aneurysm, or excision (partial or total) and graft insertion, with or without patch graft; for aneurysm and associated occlusive disease, carotid, subclavian artery, by neck incision	18.14	15.90	3.18	37.22	90	S
35002	00	A	Direct repair of aneurysm, false aneurysm, or excision (partial or total) and graft insertion, with or without patch graft; for ruptured aneurysm, carotid, subclavian artery, by neck incision	19.43	12.64	2.41	34.48	90	S
35005	00	A	Direct repair of aneurysm, false aneurysm, or excision (partial or total) and graft insertion, with or without patch graft; for aneurysm, false aneurysm, and associated occlusive disease, vertebral artery	16.62	10.28	2.19	29.09	90	S
35011	00	A	Direct repair of aneurysm, false aneurysm, or excision (partial or total) and graft insertion, with or without patch graft; for aneurysm and associated occlusive disease, axillary-brachial artery, by arm incision	10.43	13.35	2.76	26.54	90	S
35013	00	A	Direct repair of aneurysm, false aneurysm, or excision (partial or total) and graft insertion, with or without patch graft; for ruptured aneurysm, axillary-brachial artery, by arm incision	15.96	14.70	3.03	33.69	90	S
35021	00	A	Direct repair of aneurysm, false aneurysm, or excision (partial or total) and graft insertion, with or without patch graft; for aneurysm, false aneurysm, and associated occlusive disease, innominate, subclavian artery, by thoracic incision	17.62	18.13	3.06	38.81	90	S
35022	00	A	Direct repair of aneurysm, false aneurysm, or excision (partial or total) and graft insertion, with or without patch graft; for ruptured aneurysm, innominate, subclavian artery, by thoracic incision	21.15	14.78	2.80	38.73	90	S
35045	00	A	Direct repair of aneurysm, false aneurysm, or excision (partial or total) and graft insertion, with or without patch graft; for aneurysm, false aneurysm, and associated occlusive disease, radial or ulnar artery	9.98	12.35	2.50	24.83	90	S
35081	00	A	Direct repair of aneurysm, false aneurysm, or excision (partial or total) and graft insertion, with or without patch graft; for aneurysm, false aneurysm, and associated occlusive disease, abdominal aorta	22.15	21.45	4.18	47.78	90	S
35082	00	A	Direct repair of aneurysm, false aneurysm, or excision (partial or total) and graft insertion, with or without patch graft; for ruptured aneurysm, abdominal aorta	28.82	22.91	4.59	56.32	90	S
35091	00	A	Direct repair of aneurysm, false aneurysm, or excision (partial or total) and graft insertion, with or without patch graft; for aneurysm, false aneurysm, and associated occlusive disease, abdominal aorta involving visceral vessels (mesenteric, celiac, renal)	28.10	22.67	4.25	55.02	90	S
35092	00	A	Direct repair of aneurysm, false aneurysm, or excision (partial or total) and graft insertion, with or without patch graft; for ruptured aneurysm, abdominal aorta involving visceral vessels (mesenteric, celiac, renal)	36.06	26.27	5.21	67.54	90	S
35102	00	A	Direct repair of aneurysm, false aneurysm, or excision (partial or total) and graft insertion, with or without patch graft; for aneurysm, false aneurysm, and associated occlusive disease, abdominal aorta involving iliac vessels (common, hypogastric, external)	23.44	22.15	4.32	49.91	90	S
35103	00	A	Direct repair of aneurysm, false aneurysm, or excision (partial or total) and graft insertion, with or without patch graft; for ruptured aneurysm, abdominal aorta involving iliac vessels (common, hypogastric, external)	31.31	26.16	5.21	62.68	90	S

CPT codes and descriptions only, © 1994 American Medical Association. Reimbursement information, © 1995 McGraw-Hill Inc.

Code/ CPT	Mod-ifier	Status	Description	Work value	Practice expense	Mal-practice	Total value	Global period	Up-date
35111	00	A	Direct repair of aneurysm, false aneurysm, or excision (partial or total) and graft insertion, with or without patch graft; for aneurysm, false aneurysm, and associated occlusive disease, splenic artery	15.12	17.60	3.70	36.42	90	S
35112	00	A	Direct repair of aneurysm, false aneurysm, or excision (partial or total) and graft insertion, with or without patch graft; for ruptured aneurysm, splenic artery	17.38	10.45	2.22	30.05	90	S
35121	00	A	Direct repair of aneurysm, false aneurysm, or excision (partial or total) and graft insertion, with or without patch graft; for aneurysm, false aneurysm, and associated occlusive disease, hepatic, celiac, renal, or mesenteric artery	24.68	19.12	3.66	47.46	90	S
35122	00	A	Direct repair of aneurysm, false aneurysm, or excision (partial or total) and graft insertion, with or without patch graft; for ruptured aneurysm, hepatic, celiac, renal, or mesenteric artery	32.08	17.92	3.96	53.96	90	S
35131	00	A	Direct repair of aneurysm, false aneurysm, or excision (partial or total) and graft insertion, with or without patch graft; for aneurysm, false aneurysm, and associated occlusive disease, iliac artery (common, hypogastric, external)	17.00	15.88	3.15	36.03	90	S
35132	00	A	Direct repair of aneurysm, false aneurysm, or excision (partial or total) and graft insertion, with or without patch graft; for ruptured aneurysm, iliac artery (common, hypogastric, external)	20.40	18.68	3.58	42.66	90	S
35141	00	A	Direct repair of aneurysm, false aneurysm, or excision (partial or total) and graft insertion, with or without patch graft; for aneurysm, false aneurysm, and associated occlusive disease, common femoral artery (profunda femoris, superficial femoral)	13.28	14.70	2.88	30.86	90	S
35142	00	A	Direct repair of aneurysm, false aneurysm, or excision (partial or total) and graft insertion, with or without patch graft; for ruptured aneurysm, common femoral artery (profunda femoris, superficial femoral)	14.62	16.10	3.24	33.96	90	S
35151	00	A	Direct repair of aneurysm, false aneurysm, or excision (partial or total) and graft insertion, with or without patch graft; for aneurysm, false aneurysm, and associated occlusive disease, popliteal artery	15.76	15.36	2.94	34.06	90	S
35152	00	A	Direct repair of aneurysm, false aneurysm, or excision (partial or total) and graft insertion, with or without patch graft; for ruptured aneurysm, popliteal artery	15.46	9.27	1.95	26.68	90	S
35161	00	A	Direct repair of aneurysm, false aneurysm, or excision (partial or total) and graft insertion, with or without patch graft; for aneurysm, false aneurysm, and associated occlusive disease, other arteries	17.45	15.88	3.15	36.48	90	S
35162	00	A	Direct repair of aneurysm, false aneurysm, or excision (partial or total) and graft insertion, with or without patch graft; for ruptured aneurysm, other arteries	18.45	18.68	3.58	40.71	90	S
35180	00	A	Repair, congenital arteriovenous fistula; head and neck	12.16	7.37	1.48	21.01	90	S
35182	00	A	Repair, congenital arteriovenous fistula; thorax and abdomen	16.12	10.65	1.61	28.38	90	S
35184	00	A	Repair, congenital arteriovenous fistula; extremities	10.79	9.73	1.96	22.48	90	S
35188	00	A	Repair, acquired or traumatic arteriovenous fistula; head and neck	13.10	8.11	1.59	22.80	90	S
35189	00	A	Repair, acquired or traumatic arteriovenous fistula; thorax and abdomen	17.12	11.33	2.21	30.66	90	S

CPT codes and descriptions only, © 1994 American Medical Association. Reimbursement information, © 1995 McGraw-Hill Inc.

Code/ CPT	Mod-ifier	Status	Description	Work value	Practice expense	Mal-practice	Total value	Global period	Up-date
35190	00	A	Repair, acquired or traumatic arteriovenous fistula; extremities	11.79	10.34	2.14	24.27	90	S
35201	00	A	Repair blood vessel, direct; neck	8.90	10.07	1.94	20.91	90	S
35206	00	A	Repair blood vessel, direct; upper extremity	8.49	10.15	2.03	20.67	90	S
35207	00	A	Repair blood vessel, direct; hand, finger	9.06	10.80	1.93	21.79	90	S
35211	00	A	Repair blood vessel, direct; intrathoracic, with bypass	20.15	13.38	2.59	36.12	90	S
35216	00	A	Repair blood vessel, direct; intrathoracic, without bypass	17.12	10.68	2.08	29.88	90	S
35221	00	A	Repair blood vessel, direct; intra-abdominal	15.11	11.09	2.20	28.40	90	S
35226	00	A	Repair blood vessel, direct; lower extremity	8.17	10.28	1.95	20.40	90	S
35231	00	A	Repair blood vessel with vein graft; neck	10.76	13.78	2.91	27.45	90	S
35236	00	A	Repair blood vessel with vein graft; upper extremity	9.39	12.02	2.56	23.97	90	S
35241	00	A	Repair blood vessel with vein graft; intrathoracic, with bypass	21.15	13.49	2.60	37.24	90	S
35246	00	A	Repair blood vessel with vein graft; intrathoracic, without bypass	18.14	16.95	2.15	37.24	90	S
35251	00	A	Repair blood vessel with vein graft; intra-abdominal	16.12	9.59	1.88	27.59	90	S
35256	00	A	Repair blood vessel with vein graft; lower extremity	10.14	12.40	2.39	24.93	90	S
35261	00	A	Repair blood vessel with graft other than vein; neck	10.39	13.16	2.66	26.21	90	S
35266	00	A	Repair blood vessel with graft other than vein; upper extremity	9.06	11.59	2.41	23.06	90	S
35271	00	A	Repair blood vessel with graft other than vein; intrathoracic, with bypass	20.15	12.53	2.56	35.24	90	S
35276	00	A	Repair blood vessel with graft other than vein; intrathoracic, without bypass	17.12	10.85	2.26	30.23	90	S
35281	00	A	Repair blood vessel with graft other than vein; intra-abdominal	15.11	17.28	3.37	35.76	90	S
35286	00	A	Repair blood vessel with graft other than vein; lower extremity	10.78	11.71	2.33	24.82	90	S
35301	00	A	Thromboendarterectomy, with or without patch graft; carotid, vertebral, subclavian, by neck incision	15.95	14.46	2.81	33.22	90	S
35311	00	A	Thromboendarterectomy, with or without patch graft; subclavian, innominate, by thoracic incision	22.61	22.06	4.61	49.28	90	S
35321	00	A	Thromboendarterectomy, with or without patch graft; axillary-brachial	11.08	12.96	2.69	26.73	90	S
35331	00	A	Thromboendarterectomy, with or without patch graft; abdominal aorta	22.15	13.34	2.66	38.15	90	S
35341	00	A	Thromboendarterectomy, with or without patch graft; mesenteric, celiac, or renal	23.67	17.37	3.53	44.57	90	S
35351	00	A	Thromboendarterectomy, with or without patch graft; iliac	19.15	14.95	2.97	37.07	90	S
35355	00	A	Thromboendarterectomy, with or without patch graft; iliofemoral	15.11	15.42	2.99	33.52	90	S
35361	00	A	Thromboendarterectomy, with or without patch graft; combined aortoiliac	22.15	19.37	3.88	45.40	90	S
35363	00	A	Thromboendarterectomy, with or without patch graft; combined aortoiliofemoral	23.16	22.77	4.40	50.33	90	S
35371	00	A	Thromboendarterectomy, with or without patch graft; common femoral	10.49	12.51	2.50	25.50	90	S
35372	00	A	Thromboendarterectomy, with or without patch graft; deep (profunda) femoral	12.28	11.20	2.28	25.76	90	S
35381	00	A	Thromboendarterectomy, with or without patch graft; femoral and/or popliteal, and/or tibioperoneal	14.50	13.67	2.71	30.88	90	S

CPT codes and descriptions only, © 1994 American Medical Association. Reimbursement information, © 1995 McGraw-Hill Inc.

Code/ CPT	Mod- ifier	Status	Description	Work value	Practice expense	Mal- practice	Total value	Global period	Up- date
35390	00	A	Reoperation, carotid, thromboendarterectomy, more than one month after original operation (List separately in addition to code for primary procedure) (Use 35390 only with 35301)	3.19	1.67	0.39	5.25	ZZZ	S
35450	00	A	Transluminal balloon angioplasty, open; renal or other visceral artery	10.07	12.89	1.38	24.34	0	N
35452	00	A	Transluminal balloon angioplasty, open; aortic	6.91	4.35	0.61	11.87	0	S
35454	00	A	Transluminal balloon angioplasty, open; iliac	6.04	7.73	1.53	15.30	0	S
35456	00	A	Transluminal balloon angioplasty, open; femoral-popliteal	7.35	9.41	1.69	18.45	0	S
35458	00	A	Transluminal balloon angioplasty, open; brachiocephalic trunk or branches, each vessel	9.49	10.13	1.83	21.45	0	S
35459	00	A	Transluminal balloon angioplasty, open; tibioperoneal trunk and branches	8.63	10.39	1.69	20.71	0	S
35460	00	A	Transluminal balloon angioplasty, open; venous	6.04	3.16	0.74	9.94	0	S
35470	00	A	Transluminal balloon angioplasty, percutaneous; tibioperoneal trunk or branches, each vessel	8.63	10.39	1.69	20.71	0	N
35471	00	A	Transluminal balloon angioplasty, percutaneous; renal or visceral artery	10.07	12.89	1.38	24.34	0	N
35472	00	A	Transluminal balloon angioplasty, percutaneous; aortic	6.91	3.61	0.85	11.37	0	N
35473	00	A	Transluminal balloon angioplasty, percutaneous; iliac	6.04	7.73	1.53	15.30	0	N
35474	00	A	Transluminal balloon angioplasty, percutaneous; femoral-popliteal	7.36	9.42	1.69	18.47	0	N
35475	00	R	Transluminal balloon angioplasty, percutaneous; brachiocephalic trunk or branches, each vessel	9.49	10.13	1.83	21.45	0	N
35476	00	A	Transluminal balloon angioplasty, percutaneous; venous	6.04	3.16	0.74	9.94	0	N
35480	00	A	Transluminal peripheral atherectomy, open; renal or other visceral artery	11.08	13.43	1.38	25.89	0	S
35481	00	A	Transluminal peripheral atherectomy, open; aortic	7.61	4.35	0.61	12.57	0	S
35482	00	A	Transluminal peripheral atherectomy, open; iliac	6.65	8.51	1.53	16.69	0	S
35483	00	A	Transluminal peripheral atherectomy, open; femoral-popliteal	8.10	10.36	1.69	20.15	0	S
35484	00	A	Transluminal peripheral atherectomy, open; brachiocephalic trunk or branches, each vessel	10.44	10.13	1.83	22.40	0	S
35485	00	A	Transluminal peripheral atherectomy, open; tibioperoneal trunk and branches	9.49	4.52	1.06	15.07	0	S
35490	00	A	Transluminal peripheral atherectomy, percutaneous; renal or other visceral artery	11.08	13.43	1.38	25.89	0	N
35491	00	A	Transluminal peripheral atherectomy, percutaneous; aortic	7.61	4.35	0.61	12.57	0	N
35492	00	A	Transluminal peripheral atherectomy, percutaneous; iliac	6.65	8.51	1.53	16.69	0	N
35493	00	A	Transluminal peripheral atherectomy, percutaneous; femoral-popliteal	8.10	10.36	1.69	20.15	0	N
35494	00	A	Transluminal peripheral atherectomy, percutaneous; brachiocephalic trunk or branches, each vessel	10.44	10.13	1.83	22.40	0	N
35495	00	A	Transluminal peripheral atherectomy, percutaneous; tibioperoneal trunk and branches	9.49	4.52	1.06	15.07	0	N
35501	00	A	Bypass graft, with vein; carotid	18.23	19.35	3.49	41.07	90	S
35506	00	A	Bypass graft, with vein; carotid-subclavian	18.23	19.17	3.64	41.04	90	S
35507	00	A	Bypass graft, with vein; subclavian-carotid	18.23	17.92	3.61	39.76	90	S
35508	00	A	Bypass graft, with vein; carotid-vertebral	17.21	18.11	3.43	38.75	90	S
35509	00	A	Bypass graft, with vein; carotid-carotid	16.70	18.90	3.92	39.52	90	S
35511	00	A	Bypass graft, with vein; subclavian-subclavian	15.39	10.40	1.92	27.71	90	S
35515	00	A	Bypass graft, with vein; subclavian-vertebral	17.21	11.25	2.01	30.47	90	S
35516	00	A	Bypass graft, with vein; subclavian-axillary	14.88	17.37	3.54	35.79	90	S

CPT codes and descriptions only, © 1994 American Medical Association. Reimbursement information, © 1995 McGraw-Hill Inc.

Code/ CPT	Mod- ifier	Status	Description	Work value	Practice expense	Mal- practice	Total value	Global period	Up- date
35518	00	A	Bypass graft, with vein; axillary-axillary	14.05	17.47	3.38	34.90	90	S
35521	00	A	Bypass graft, with vein; axillary-femoral	14.80	17.53	3.34	35.67	90	S
35526	00	A	Bypass graft, with vein; aortosubclavian or carotid	18.63	12.95	2.44	34.02	90	S
35531	00	A	Bypass graft, with vein; aortoceliac or aortomesenteric	24.17	20.25	3.90	48.32	90	S
35533	00	A	Bypass graft, with vein; axillary-femoral-femoral	19.15	21.04	4.43	44.62	90	S
35536	00	A	Bypass graft, with vein; splenorenal	21.65	21.37	4.17	47.19	90	S
35541	00	A	Bypass graft, with vein; aortoiliac or bi-iliac	24.17	19.55	3.65	47.37	90	S
35546	00	A	Bypass graft, with vein; aortofemoral or bifemoral	24.17	21.39	4.26	49.82	90	S
35548	00	A	Bypass graft, with vein; aortoiliofemoral, unilateral	20.13	19.55	3.65	43.33	90	S
35549	00	A	Bypass graft, with vein; aortoiliofemoral, bilateral	21.91	21.39	4.26	47.56	90	S
35551	00	A	Bypass graft, with vein; aortofemoral-popliteal	25.17	19.25	3.87	48.29	90	S
35556	00	A	Bypass graft, with vein; femoral-popliteal	15.47	18.71	3.71	37.89	90	S
35558	00	A	Bypass graft, with vein; femoral-femoral	12.82	16.41	3.23	32.46	90	S
35560	00	A	Bypass graft, with vein; aortorenal	22.12	20.22	3.93	46.27	90	S
35563	00	A	Bypass graft, with vein; ilioiliac	13.83	8.32	1.70	23.85	90	S
35565	00	A	Bypass graft, with vein; iliofemoral	13.83	17.69	3.51	35.03	90	S
35566	00	A	Bypass graft, with vein; femoral-anterior tibial, posterior tibial, peroneal artery or other distal vessels	20.21	20.62	4.08	44.91	90	S
35571	00	A	Bypass graft, with vein; popliteal-tibial, -peroneal artery or other distal vessels	16.66	19.36	3.87	39.89	90	S
35582	00	A	In-situ vein bypass; aortofemoral-popliteal (only femoral-popliteal portion in-situ)	25.69	23.74	4.89	54.32	90	S
35583	00	A	In-situ vein bypass; femoral-popliteal	15.97	20.44	4.13	40.54	90	S
35585	00	A	In-situ vein bypass; femoral-anterior tibial, posterior tibial, or peroneal artery	19.05	22.95	4.63	46.63	90	S
35587	00	A	In-situ vein bypass; popliteal-tibial, peroneal	17.07	21.51	4.13	42.71	90	S
35601	00	A	Bypass graft, with other than vein; carotid	16.19	18.83	3.33	38.35	90	S
35606	00	A	Bypass graft, with other than vein; carotid-subclavian	17.40	17.55	3.51	38.46	90	S
35612	00	A	Bypass graft, with other than vein; subclavian-subclavian	14.39	16.75	3.30	34.44	90	S
35616	00	A	Bypass graft, with other than vein; subclavian-axillary	14.39	16.79	3.42	34.60	90	S
35621	00	A	Bypass graft, with other than vein; axillary-femoral	13.23	16.94	3.80	33.97	90	S
35623	00	A	Bypass graft, with other than vein; axillary-popliteal or -tibial	15.42	8.06	1.88	25.36	90	S
35626	00	A	Bypass graft, with other than vein; aortosubclavian or carotid	22.26	20.51	4.08	46.85	90	S
35631	00	A	Bypass graft, with other than vein; aortoceliac, aortomesenteric, aortorenal	23.16	17.87	3.57	44.60	90	S
35636	00	A	Bypass graft, with other than vein; splenorenal (splenic to renal arterial anastomosis)	21.15	13.50	2.45	37.10	90	S
35641	00	A	Bypass graft, with other than vein; aortoiliac or bi-iliac	22.67	20.56	4.08	47.31	90	S
35642	00	A	Bypass graft, with other than vein; carotid-vertebral	16.70	10.33	2.20	29.23	90	S
35645	00	A	Bypass graft, with other than vein; subclavian-vertebral	16.19	11.15	2.05	29.39	90	S
35646	00	A	Bypass graft, with other than vein; aortofemoral or bifemoral	24.00	23.78	4.73	52.51	90	S
35650	00	A	Bypass graft, with other than vein; axillary-axillary	13.05	16.71	3.56	33.32	90	S
35651	00	A	Bypass graft, with other than vein; aortofemoral-popliteal	23.67	24.09	4.69	52.45	90	S
35654	00	A	Bypass graft, with other than vein; axillary-femoral-femoral	17.62	22.10	4.42	44.14	90	S
35656	00	A	Bypass graft, with other than vein; femoral-popliteal	13.86	17.73	3.60	35.19	90	S
35661	00	A	Bypass graft, with other than vein; femoral-femoral	11.81	15.11	3.30	30.22	90	S
35663	00	A	Bypass graft, with other than vein; ilioiliac	12.82	16.41	3.80	33.03	90	S
35665	00	A	Bypass graft, with other than vein; iliofemoral	14.05	17.79	3.57	35.41	90	S
35666	00	A	Bypass graft, with other than vein; femoral-anterior tibial, posterior tibial, or peroneal artery	15.97	20.06	4.00	40.03	90	S

CPT codes and descriptions only, © 1994 American Medical Association. Reimbursement information, © 1995 McGraw-Hill Inc.

Code/ CPT	Mod-ifier	Status	Description	Work value	Practice expense	Mal-practice	Total value	Global period	Up-date
35671	00	A	Bypass graft, with other than vein; popliteal-tibial or -peroneal artery	12.18	16.61	4.08	32.87	90	S
35681	00	A	Bypass graft, composite	8.05	12.79	3.52	24.36	ZZZ	S
35691	00	A	Transposition and/or reimplantation; vertebral to carotid artery	16.70	19.62	3.81	40.13	90	S
35693	00	A	Transposition and/or reimplantation; vertebral to subclavian artery	14.01	9.40	1.91	25.32	90	S
35694	00	A	Transposition and/or reimplantation; subclavian to carotid artery	17.81	9.33	2.17	29.31	90	S
35695	00	A	Transposition and/or reimplantation; carotid to subclavian artery	17.81	9.33	2.17	29.31	90	S
35700	00	A	Reoperation, femoral-popliteal or femoral (popliteal) -anterior tibial, posterior tibial, peroneal artery or other distal vessels, more than one month after original operation (List separately in addition to code for primary procedure)	3.08	1.61	0.38	5.07	ZZZ	S
35701	00	A	Exploration (not followed by surgical repair), with or without lysis of artery; carotid artery	4.54	5.82	1.25	11.61	90	S
35721	00	A	Exploration (not followed by surgical repair), with or without lysis of artery; femoral artery	4.54	5.56	1.11	11.21	90	S
35741	00	A	Exploration (not followed by surgical repair), with or without lysis of artery; popliteal artery	4.54	5.73	1.15	11.42	90	S
35761	00	A	Exploration (not followed by surgical repair), with or without lysis of artery; other vessels	4.54	5.81	1.14	11.49	90	S
35800	00	A	Exploration for postoperative hemorrhage, thrombosis or infection; neck	6.04	5.28	0.97	12.29	90	S
35820	00	A	Exploration for postoperative hemorrhage, thrombosis or infection; chest	11.64	7.92	1.43	20.99	90	S
35840	00	A	Exploration for postoperative hemorrhage, thrombosis or infection; abdomen	8.63	7.23	1.44	17.30	90	S
35860	00	A	Exploration for postoperative hemorrhage, thrombosis or infection; extremity	4.54	5.81	1.15	11.50	90	S
35870	00	A	Repair of graft-enteric fistula	20.35	10.64	2.47	33.46	90	S
35875	00	A	Thrombectomy of arterial or venous graft;	9.07	8.21	1.65	18.93	90	S
35876	00	A	Thrombectomy of arterial or venous graft; with revision of arterial or venous graft	12.91	8.21	1.65	22.77	90	S
35901	00	A	Excision of infected graft; neck	7.25	7.18	1.46	15.89	90	S
35903	00	A	Excision of infected graft; extremity	8.63	7.18	1.46	17.27	90	S
35905	00	A	Excision of infected graft; thorax	16.89	7.18	1.46	25.53	90	S
35907	00	A	Excision of infected graft; abdomen	17.68	7.18	1.46	26.32	90	S
36000	00	A	Introduction of needle or intracatheter, vein	0.18	0.32	0.04	0.54	XXX	N
36005	00	A	Injection procedure for contrast venography (including introduction of needle or intracatheter)	0.95	0.47	0.04	1.46	0	N
36010	00	A	Introduction of catheter, superior or inferior vena cava	2.43	2.11	0.31	4.85	XXX	N
36011	00	A	Selective catheter placement, venous system; first order branch (eg, renal vein, jugular vein)	3.14	1.90	0.22	5.26	XXX	N
36012	00	A	Selective catheter placement, venous system; second order, or more selective, branch (eg, left adrenal vein, petrosal sinus)	3.52	2.67	0.32	6.51	XXX	N
36013	00	A	Introduction of catheter, right heart or main pulmonary artery	2.52	2.11	0.31	4.94	XXX	N
36014	00	A	Selective catheter placement, left or right pulmonary artery	3.02	2.28	0.27	5.57	XXX	N
36015	00	A	Selective catheter placement, segmental or subsegmental pulmonary artery	3.52	2.67	0.32	6.51	XXX	N

CPT codes and descriptions only, © 1994 American Medical Association. Reimbursement information, © 1995 McGraw-Hill Inc.

Code/ CPT	Mod- ifier	Status	Description	Work value	Practice expense	Mal- practice	Total value	Global period	Up- date
36100	00	A	Introduction of needle or intracatheter, carotid or vertebral artery	3.02	2.59	0.32	5.93	XXX	N
36120	00	A	Introduction of needle or intracatheter; retrograde brachial artery	2.01	2.32	0.30	4.63	XXX	N
36140	00	A	Introduction of needle or intracatheter; extremity artery	2.01	1.41	0.24	3.66	XXX	N
36145	00	A	Introduction of needle or intracatheter; arteriovenous shunt created for dialysis (cannula, fistula, or graft)	2.01	2.65	0.49	5.15	XXX	N
36160	00	A	Introduction of needle or intracatheter, aortic, translumbar	2.52	2.32	0.35	5.19	XXX	S
36200	00	A	Introduction of catheter, aorta	3.02	2.73	0.28	6.03	XXX	N
36215	00	A	Selective catheter placement, arterial system; each first order thoracic or brachiocephalic branch, within a vascular family	4.47	2.78	0.23	7.48	XXX	N
36216	00	A	Selective catheter placement, arterial system; initial second order thoracic or brachiocephalic branch, within a vascular family	5.28	3.29	0.27	8.84	XXX	N
36217	00	A	Selective catheter placement, arterial system; initial third order or more selective thoracic or brachiocephalic branch, within a vascular family	6.30	3.92	0.32	10.54	XXX	N
36218	00	A	Selective catheter placement, arterial system; additional second order, third order, and beyond, thoracic or brachiocephalic branch, within a vascular family (use in addition to 36216 or 36217 as appropriate)	1.01	0.62	0.05	1.68	XXX	N
36245	00	A	Selective catheter placement, arterial system; each first order abdominal, pelvic, or lower extremity artery branch, within a vascular family	5.07	3.15	0.26	8.48	XXX	N
36246	00	A	Selective catheter placement, arterial system; initial second order abdominal, pelvic, or lower extremity artery branch, within a vascular family	5.28	3.29	0.27	8.84	XXX	N
36247	00	A	Selective catheter placement, arterial system; initial third order or more selective abdominal, pelvic, or lower extremity artery branch, within a vascular family	6.30	3.92	0.32	10.54	XXX	N
36248	00	A	Selective catheter placement, arterial system; additional second order, third order, and beyond, abdominal, pelvic, or lower extremity artery branch, within a vascular family (use in addition to 36246 or 36247 as appropriate)	1.01	0.62	0.05	1.68	XXX	N
36260	00	A	Insertion of implantable intra-arterial infusion pump (eg, for chemotherapy of liver)	9.27	6.74	1.41	17.42	90	S
36261	00	A	Revision of implanted intra-arterial infusion pump	5.04	2.23	0.42	7.69	90	S
36262	00	A	Removal of implanted intra-arterial infusion pump	3.70	1.93	0.40	6.03	90	S
36299	00	C	Unlisted procedure, vascular injection	0	0	0	0	YYY	N
36400	00	A	Venipuncture, under age 3 years; femoral, jugular or sagittal sinus	0.18	0.09	0.01	0.28	XXX	N
36405	00	A	Venipuncture, under age 3 years; scalp vein	0.18	0.45	0.03	0.66	XXX	N
36406	00	A	Venipuncture, under age 3 years; other vein	0.18	0.16	0.01	0.35	XXX	S
36410	00	A	Venipuncture, child over age 3 years or adult, necessitating physician's skill (separate procedure), for diagnostic or therapeutic purposes. Not to be used for routine venipuncture.	0.18	0.22	0.02	0.42	XXX	N
36415	00	G	Routine venipuncture or finger/heel/ear stick for collection of specimen(s)	0.14*	0.11#	0.01*	0.26#	XXX	0
36420	00	A	Venipuncture, cutdown; under age 1 year	1.01	0.51	0.05	1.57	XXX	N
36425	00	A	Venipuncture, cutdown; age 1 or over	0.76	0.08	0.01	0.85	XXX	N
36430	00	A	Transfusion, blood or blood components	0	0.96	0.07	1.03	XXX	N
36440	00	A	Push transfusion, blood, 2 years or under	1.03	0.94	0.07	2.04	XXX	S
36450	00	A	Exchange transfusion, blood; newborn	2.23	1.88	0.18	4.29	XXX	N

CPT codes and descriptions only, © 1994 American Medical Association. Reimbursement information, © 1995 McGraw-Hill Inc.

Code/ CPT	Mod-ifier	Status	Description	Work value	Practice expense	Mal-practice	Total value	Global period	Up-date
36455	00	A	Exchange transfusion, blood; other than newborn	2.43	2.27	0.22	4.92	XXX	N
36460	00	A	Transfusion, intrauterine, fetal	6.59	4.71	1.09	12.39	XXX	N
36468	00	R	Single or multiple injections of sclerosing solutions, spider veins (telangiectasia); limb or trunk	0.63*	0.46#	0.09*	1.18#	XXX	S
36469	00	R	Single or multiple injections of sclerosing solutions, spider veins (telangiectasia); face	0.77*	0.56#	0.11*	1.44#	XXX	S
36470	00	A	Injection of sclerosing solution; single vein	1.02	0.27	0.04	1.33	10	S
36471	00	A	Injection of sclerosing solution; multiple veins, same leg	1.49	0.39	0.05	1.93	10	S
36481	00	A	Percutaneous portal vein catheterization by any method	6.99	5.30	0.61	12.90	0	S
36488	00	A	Placement of central venous catheter (subclavian, jugular, or other vein) (eg, for central venous pressure, hyperalimentation, hemodialysis, or chemotherapy); percutaneous, age 2 years or under	1.35	0.97	0.14	2.46	0	N
36489	00	A	Placement of central venous catheter (subclavian, jugular, or other vein) (eg, for central venous pressure, hyperalimentation, hemodialysis, or chemotherapy); percutaneous, over age 2	1.22	1.12	0.17	2.51	0	N
36490	00	A	Placement of central venous catheter (subclavian, jugular, or other vein) (eg, for central venous pressure, hyperalimentation, hemodialysis, or chemotherapy); cutdown, age 2 years or under	1.67	1.38	0.20	3.25	0	N
36491	00	A	Placement of central venous catheter (subclavian, jugular, or other vein) (eg, for central venous pressure, hyperalimentation, hemodialysis, or chemotherapy); cutdown, over age 2	1.43	1.71	0.32	3.46	0	N
36493	00	A	Repositioning of previously placed central venous catheter under fluoroscopic guidance	1.21	0.63	0.16	2.00	0	N
36500	00	A	Venous catheterization for selective organ blood sampling	3.52	0.08	0.01	3.61	0	N
36510	00	A	Catheterization of umbilical vein for diagnosis or therapy, newborn	1.09	0.34	0.02	1.45	0	N
36520	00	A	Therapeutic apheresis (plasma and/or cell exchange)	1.74	1.92	0.12	3.78	0	N
36522	00	A	Photopheresis, extracorporeal	1.67	3.31	0.37	5.35	ZZZ	S
36530	00	R	Insertion of implantable intravenous infusion pump	4.83	4.82	1.02	10.67	10	S
36531	00	R	Revision of implantable intravenous infusion pump	4.80	4.37	0.27	9.44	10	S
36532	00	R	Removal of implantable intravenous infusion pump	3.23	1.77	0.37	5.37	10	S
36533	00	A	Insertion of implantable venous access port, with or without subcutaneous reservoir	3.82	4.29	0.85	8.96	10	S
36534	00	A	Revision of implantable venous access port and/or subcutaneous reservoir	3.79	3.46	0.21	7.46	10	S
36535	00	A	Removal of implantable venous access port and/or subcutaneous reservoir	2.22	1.81	0.38	4.41	10	S
36600	00	A	Arterial puncture, withdrawal of blood for diagnosis	0.32	0.28	0.02	0.62	XXX	N
36620	00	A	Arterial catheterization or cannulation for sampling, monitoring or transfusion (separate procedure); percutaneous	1.15	0.66	0.14	1.95	0	N
36625	00	A	Arterial catheterization or cannulation for sampling, monitoring or transfusion (separate procedure); cutdown	2.11	0.86	0.18	3.15	0	N
36640	00	A	Arterial catheterization for prolonged infusion therapy (chemotherapy), cutdown	2.10	2.32	0.40	4.82	0	N
36660	00	A	Catheterization, umbilical artery, newborn, for diagnosis or therapy	1.40	0.49	0.04	1.93	0	N
36680	00	A	Placement of needle for intraosseous infusion	1.20	1.24	0.10	2.54	0	N
36800	00	A	Insertion of cannula for hemodialysis, other purpose (separate procedure); vein to vein	2.43	2.22	0.28	4.93	0	N

CPT codes and descriptions only, © 1994 American Medical Association. Reimbursement information, © 1995 McGraw-Hill Inc.

Code/ CPT	Mod-ifier	Status	Description	Work value	Practice expense	Mal-practice	Total value	Global period	Up-date
36810	00	A	Insertion of cannula for hemodialysis, other purpose (separate procedure); arteriovenous, external (Scribner type)	3.97	4.85	0.74	9.56	0	S
36815	00	A	Insertion of cannula for hemodialysis, other purpose (separate procedure); arteriovenous, external revision, or closure	2.62	3.35	0.70	6.67	0	S
36821	00	A	Arteriovenous anastomosis, direct, any site (eg, Cimino type) (separate procedure)	8.39	7.24	1.46	17.09	90	S
36822	00	A	Insertion of cannula(s) for prolonged extracorporeal circulation for cardiopulmonary insufficiency (ECMO) (separate procedure)	5.03	5.60	0.77	11.40	90	S
36825	00	A	Creation of arteriovenous fistula by other than direct arteriovenous anastomosis (separate procedure); autogenous graft	9.36	11.20	2.21	22.77	90	S
36830	00	A	Creation of arteriovenous fistula by other than direct arteriovenous anastomosis (separate procedure); nonautogenous graft	7.78	9.96	2.36	20.10	90	S
36832	00	A	Revision of an arteriovenous fistula, with or without thrombectomy, autogenous or non-autogenous graft (separate procedure)	5.84	8.47	2.38	16.69	90	S
36834	00	A	Plastic repair of arteriovenous aneurysm (separate procedure)	9.32	7.80	1.66	18.78	90	S
36835	00	A	Insertion of Thomas shunt (separate procedure)	6.54	3.42	0.79	10.75	90	S
36840	00	D	Insert mandril	4.57*	3.32#	0.65*	8.54#	90	S
36845	00	D	Fusion with mandril	8.44*	6.14#	1.20*	15.78#	90	S
36860	00	A	Cannula declotting (separate procedure); without balloon catheter	2.01	2.57	0.43	5.01	0	N
36861	00	A	Cannula declotting (separate procedure); with balloon catheter	2.52	3.71	1.01	7.24	0	S
37140	00	A	Venous anastomosis; portocaval	22.15	16.29	3.34	41.78	90	S
37145	00	A	Venous anastomosis; renoportal	23.16	17.13	1.72	42.01	90	S
37160	00	A	Venous anastomosis; caval-mesenteric	20.15	17.74	3.79	41.68	90	S
37180	00	A	Venous anastomosis; splenorenal, proximal	23.16	14.19	2.76	40.11	90	S
37181	00	A	Venous anastomosis; splenorenal, distal (selective decompression of esophagogastric varices, any technique)	25.17	16.41	3.52	45.10	90	S
37190	00	D	Repair of circulation defect	14.77*	10.74#	2.10*	27.61#	90	S
37200	00	A	Transcatheter biopsy	4.56	1.59	0.13	6.28	0	N
37201	00	A	Transcatheter therapy, infusion for thrombolysis other than coronary	7.25	5.50	0.64	13.39	0	N
37202	00	A	Transcatheter therapy, infusion other than for thrombolysis, any type (eg, spasmolytic, vasoconstrictive)	5.68	4.30	0.50	10.48	0	N
37203	00	A	Transcatheter retrieval, percutaneous, of intravascular foreign body (eg, fractured venous or arterial catheter)	5.03	3.82	0.45	9.30	0	N
37204	00	A	Transcatheter occlusion or embolization (eg, for tumor destruction, to achieve hemostasis, to occlude a vascular malformation), percutaneous, any method, non-central nervous system, non-head or neck	18.14	13.76	1.60	33.50	0	N
37205	00	A	Transcatheter placement of an intravascular stent(s), (non-coronary vessel), percutaneous; initial vessel	8.28	5.16	0.42	13.86	0	S
37206	00	A	Transcatheter placement of an intravascular stent(s), (non-coronary vessel), percutaneous; each additional vessel	4.13	2.58	0.21	6.92	ZZZ	S
37207	00	A	Transcatheter placement of an intravascular stent(s), (non-coronary vessel), open; initial vessel	8.28	5.16	0.42	13.86	0	S
37208	00	A	Transcatheter placement of an intravascular stent(s), (non-coronary vessel), open; each additional vessel	4.13	2.58	0.21	6.92	ZZZ	S

CPT codes and descriptions only, © 1994 American Medical Association. Reimbursement information, © 1995 McGraw-Hill Inc.

Code/ CPT	Mod- ifier	Status	Description	Work value	Practice expense	Mal- practice	Total value	Global period	Up- date
37209	00	A	Exchange of a previously placed arterial catheter during thrombolytic therapy	1.48	0.92	0.08	2.48	0	N
37565	00	A	Ligation, internal jugular vein	3.90	3.79	0.74	8.43	90	S
37600	00	A	Ligation; external carotid artery	3.90	5.10	0.80	9.80	90	S
37605	00	A	Ligation; internal or common carotid artery	4.63	5.56	1.04	11.23	90	S
37606	00	A	Ligation; internal or common carotid artery, with gradual occlusion, as with Selverstone or Crutchfield clamp	4.63	5.92	0.72	11.27	90	S
37607	00	A	Ligation or banding of angioaccess arteriovenous fistula	5.84	3.06	0.71	9.61	90	S
37609	00	A	Ligation or biopsy, temporal artery	2.27	2.22	0.38	4.87	10	S
37615	00	A	Ligation, major artery (eg, post-traumatic, rupture); neck	4.39	5.64	1.11	11.14	90	S
37616	00	A	Ligation, major artery (eg, post-traumatic, rupture); chest	14.69	4.21	0.83	19.73	90	S
37617	00	A	Ligation, major artery (eg, post-traumatic, rupture); abdomen	14.19	8.00	1.54	23.73	90	S
37618	00	A	Ligation, major artery (eg, post-traumatic, rupture); extremity	3.90	4.98	1.06	9.94	90	S
37620	00	A	Interruption, partial or complete, of inferior vena cava by suture, ligation, plication, clip, extravascular, intravascular (umbrella device)	9.24	8.81	1.48	19.53	90	S
37650	00	A	Ligation of femoral vein	4.39	4.02	0.52	8.93	90	S
37660	00	A	Ligation of common iliac vein	9.65	5.75	1.07	16.47	90	S
37700	00	A	Ligation and division of long saphenous vein at saphenofemoral junction, or distal interruptions	3.52	3.64	0.73	7.89	90	S
37720	00	A	Ligation and division and complete stripping of long or short saphenous veins	5.22	5.11	1.04	11.37	90	S
37730	00	A	Ligation and division and complete stripping of long and short saphenous veins	6.63	6.95	1.40	14.98	90	S
37735	00	A	Ligation and division and complete stripping of long or short saphenous veins with radical excision of ulcer and skin graft and/or interruption of communicating veins of lower leg, with excision of deep fascia	9.90	8.34	1.68	19.92	90	S
37760	00	A	Ligation of perforators, subfascial, radical (Linton type), with or without skin graft	9.90	7.48	1.52	18.90	90	S
37780	00	A	Ligation and division of short saphenous vein at saphenopopliteal junction (separate procedure)	3.52	1.89	0.35	5.76	90	S
37785	00	A	Ligation, division, and/or excision of recurrent or secondary varicose veins (clusters), one leg	3.56	0.98	0.18	4.72	90	S
37788	00	A	Penile revascularization, artery, with or without vein graft	21.33	15.14	1.48	37.95	90	S
37790	00	A	Penile venous occlusive procedure	8.02	5.70	0.55	14.27	90	S
37799	00	C	Unlisted procedure, vascular surgery	0	0	0	0	YYY	S
38100	00	A	Splenectomy; total (separate procedure)	11.99	8.55	1.81	22.35	90	S
38101	00	A	Splenectomy; partial (separate procedure)	12.59	6.99	1.51	21.09	90	S
38102	00	A	Splenectomy; total, en bloc for extensive disease, in conjunction with other procedure (Report in addition to code for primary procedure)	4.80	2.51	0.58	7.89	ZZZ	S
38115	00	A	Repair of ruptured spleen (splenorrhaphy) with or without partial splenectomy	12.59	7.64	1.49	21.72	90	S
38200	00	A	Injection procedure for splenoportography	2.64	1.71	0.15	4.50	0	S
38230	00	A	Bone marrow harvesting for transplantation	3.16	2.78	0.21	6.15	10	N
38240	00	A	Bone marrow transplantation; allogenic	2.24	2.08	0.14	4.46	XXX	N
38241	00	A	Bone marrow transplantation; autologous	2.24	2.04	0.13	4.41	XXX	N
38300	00	A	Drainage of lymph node abscess or lymphadenitis; simple	1.48	0.58	0.10	2.16	10	S
38305	00	A	Drainage of lymph node abscess or lymphadenitis; extensive	4.24	1.96	0.36	6.56	90	S

CPT codes and descriptions only, © 1994 American Medical Association. Reimbursement information, © 1995 McGraw-Hill Inc.

Code/ CPT	Mod- ifier	Status	Description	Work value	Practice expense	Mal- practice	Total value	Global period	Up- date
38308	00	A	Lymphangiotomy or other operations on lymphatic channels	4.55	3.37	0.45	8.37	90	S
38380	00	A	Suture and/or ligation of thoracic duct; cervical approach	6.53	4.44	0.76	11.73	90	S
38381	00	A	Suture and/or ligation of thoracic duct; thoracic approach	12.10	7.56	1.50	21.16	90	S
38382	00	A	Suture and/or ligation of thoracic duct; abdominal approach	9.24	4.84	1.13	15.21	90	S
38500	00	A	Biopsy or excision of lymph node(s); superficial (separate procedure)	2.83	1.59	0.31	4.73	10	S
38505	00	A	Biopsy or excision of lymph node(s); by needle, superficial (eg, cervical, inguinal, axillary)	1.14	1.12	0.17	2.43	0	S
38510	00	A	Biopsy or excision of lymph node(s); deep cervical node(s)	3.90	2.54	0.45	6.89	90	S
38520	00	A	Biopsy or excision of lymph node(s); deep cervical node(s) with excision scalene fat pad	4.86	2.99	0.56	8.41	90	S
38525	00	A	Biopsy or excision of lymph node(s); deep axillary node(s)	4.37	2.59	0.53	7.49	90	S
38530	00	A	Biopsy or excision of lymph node(s); internal mammary node(s) (separate procedure)	5.82	3.17	0.65	9.64	90	S
38542	00	A	Dissection, deep jugular node(s)	5.41	4.26	0.59	10.26	90	S
38550	00	A	Excision of cystic hygroma, axillary or cervical; without deep neurovascular dissection	6.42	3.23	0.63	10.28	90	S
38555	00	A	Excision of cystic hygroma, axillary or cervical; with deep neurovascular dissection	13.05	7.27	1.38	21.70	90	S
38562	00	A	Limited lymphadenectomy for staging (separate procedure); pelvic and para-aortic	9.65	6.88	1.20	17.73	90	S
38564	00	A	Limited lymphadenectomy for staging (separate procedure); retroperitoneal (aortic and/or splenic)	10.00	7.39	1.51	18.90	90	S
38700	00	A	Suprahyoid lymphadenectomy	7.56	9.64	1.31	18.51	90	S
38720	00	A	Cervical lymphadenectomy (complete)	12.29	15.73	2.04	30.06	90	S
38724	00	A	Cervical lymphadenectomy (modified radical neck dissection)	13.22	14.36	2.00	29.58	90	S
38740	00	A	Axillary lymphadenectomy; superficial	6.28	4.72	1.00	12.00	90	S
38745	00	A	Axillary lymphadenectomy; complete	8.08	8.28	1.76	18.12	90	S
38746	00	A	Thoracic lymphadenectomy, regional, including mediastinal and peritracheal nodes (Report in addition to code for primary procedure)	4.39	2.29	0.53	7.21	ZZZ	S
38747	00	A	Abdominal lymphadenectomy, regional, including celiac, para-aortic and vena caval nodes (Report in addition to code for primary procedure)	4.89	2.56	0.59	8.04	ZZZ	S
38760	00	A	Inguinofemoral lymphadenectomy, superficial, including Cloquet's node (separate procedure)	8.19	6.63	1.35	16.17	90	S
38765	00	A	Inguinofemoral lymphadenectomy, superficial, in continuity with pelvic lymphadenectomy, including external iliac, hypogastric, and obturator nodes (separate procedure)	14.98	12.67	2.42	30.07	90	S
38770	00	A	Pelvic lymphadenectomy, including external iliac, hypogastric, and obturator nodes (separate procedure)	12.10	15.40	1.73	29.23	90	S
38780	00	A	Retroperitoneal transabdominal lymphadenectomy, extensive, including pelvic, aortic, and renal nodes (separate procedure)	15.17	16.06	3.13	34.36	90	S
38790	00	A	Injection procedure for lymphangiography	1.29	1.82	0.19	3.30	0	N
38794	00	A	Cannulation, thoracic duct	4.05	2.84	0.38	7.27	90	S
38999	00	C	Unlisted procedure, hemic or lymphatic system	0	0	0	0	YYY	S
39000	00	A	Mediastinotomy with exploration, drainage, removal of foreign body, or biopsy; cervical approach	5.03	6.05	1.08	12.16	90	S

CPT codes and descriptions only, © 1994 American Medical Association. Reimbursement information, © 1995 McGraw-Hill Inc.

Code/ CPT	Mod- ifier	Status	Description	Work value	Practice expense	Mal- practice	Total value	Global period	Up- date
39010	00	A	Mediastinotomy with exploration, drainage, removal of foreign body, or biopsy; transthoracic approach, including either transthoracic or median sternotomy	10.78	11.46	2.08	24.32	90	S
39020	00	D	Exploration of chest	15.12*	10.99#	2.15*	28.26#	90	S
39200	00	A	Excision of mediastinal cyst	12.40	11.58	2.14	26.12	90	S
39220	00	A	Excision of mediastinal tumor	16.16	14.94	2.83	33.93	90	S
39400	00	A	Mediastinoscopy, with or without biopsy	5.11	5.12	0.95	11.18	10	S
39499	00	C	Unlisted procedure, mediastinum	0	0	0	0	YYY	S
39501	00	A	Repair, laceration of diaphragm, any approach	12.10	10.66	2.10	24.86	90	S
39502	00	A	Repair, paraesophageal hiatus hernia, transabdominal, with or without fundoplasty, vagotomy, and/or pyloroplasty, except neonatal	15.18	11.93	2.45	29.56	90	S
39503	00	A	Repair, neonatal diaphragmatic hernia, with or without chest tube insertion and with or without creation of ventral hernia	33.22	25.18	2.94	61.34	90	S
39520	00	A	Repair, diaphragmatic hernia (esophageal hiatal); transthoracic	15.18	12.53	2.46	30.17	90	S
39530	00	A	Repair, diaphragmatic hernia (esophageal hiatal); combined, thoracoabdominal	14.22	14.06	2.71	30.99	90	S
39531	00	A	Repair, diaphragmatic hernia (esophageal hiatal); combined, thoracoabdominal, with dilation of stricture (with or without gastroplasty)	15.23	10.00	1.80	27.03	90	S
39540	00	A	Repair, diaphragmatic hernia (other than neonatal), traumatic; acute	12.10	11.98	2.51	26.59	90	S
39541	00	A	Repair, diaphragmatic hernia (other than neonatal), traumatic; chronic	13.10	12.16	2.37	27.63	90	S
39545	00	A	Imbrication of diaphragm for eventration, transthoracic or transabdominal, paralytic or nonparalytic	12.10	7.90	1.31	21.31	90	S
39547	00	D	Revision of diaphragm	8.44*	6.14#	1.20*	15.78#	90	S
39599	00	C	Unlisted procedure, diaphragm	0	0	0	0	YYY	S
40490	00	A	Biopsy of lip	1.22	0.74	0.07	2.03	0	S
40500	00	A	Vermilionectomy (lip shave), with mucosal advancement	4.08	5.51	0.94	10.53	90	S
40510	00	A	Excision of lip; transverse wedge excision with primary closure	4.57	5.84	0.83	11.24	90	S
40520	00	A	Excision of lip; V-excision with primary direct linear closure	4.54	4.50	0.68	9.72	90	S
40525	00	A	Excision of lip; full thickness, reconstruction with local flap (eg, Estlander or fan)	7.26	9.30	1.43	17.99	90	S
40527	00	A	Excision of lip; full thickness, reconstruction with cross lip flap (Abbe-Estlander)	8.71	11.16	1.65	21.52	90	S
40530	00	A	Resection of lip, more than one-fourth, without reconstruction	5.14	5.10	0.74	10.98	90	S
40650	00	A	Repair lip, full thickness; vermilion only	3.49	4.47	0.65	8.61	90	S
40652	00	A	Repair lip, full thickness; up to half vertical height	4.08	5.23	0.79	10.10	90	S
40654	00	A	Repair lip, full thickness; over one-half vertical height, or complex	5.13	6.57	1.00	12.70	90	S
40700	00	A	Plastic repair of cleft lip/nasal deformity; primary, partial or complete, unilateral	12.04	8.46	1.28	21.78	90	S
40701	00	A	Plastic repair of cleft lip/nasal deformity; primary bilateral, one stage procedure	15.10	19.33	1.62	36.05	90	S
40702	00	A	Plastic repair of cleft lip/nasal deformity; primary bilateral, one of two stages	12.34	9.37	1.10	22.81	90	S
40720	00	A	Plastic repair of cleft lip/nasal deformity; secondary, by recreation of defect and reclosure	12.91	9.59	1.79	24.29	90	S

CPT codes and descriptions only, © 1994 American Medical Association. Reimbursement information, © 1995 McGraw-Hill Inc.

Code/ CPT	Mod- ifier	Status	Description	Work value	Practice expense	Mal- practice	Total value	Global period	Up- date
40761	00	A	Plastic repair of cleft lip/nasal deformity; with cross lip pedicle flap (Abbe-Estlander type), including sectioning and inserting of pedicle	14.00	10.84	1.74	26.58	90	S
40799	00	C	Unlisted procedure, lips	0	0	0	0	YYY	S
40800	00	A	Drainage of abscess, cyst, hematoma, vestibule of mouth; simple	1.12	0.74	0.07	1.93	10	S
40801	00	A	Drainage of abscess, cyst, hematoma, vestibule of mouth; complicated	2.48	1.70	0.16	4.34	10	S
40804	00	A	Removal of embedded foreign body, vestibule of mouth; simple	1.19	0.58	0.06	1.83	10	S
40805	00	A	Removal of embedded foreign body, vestibule of mouth; complicated	2.64	2.50	0.30	5.44	10	S
40806	00	A	Incision of labial frenum (frenotomy)	0.31	0.36	0.03	0.70	0	S
40808	00	A	Biopsy, vestibule of mouth	0.91	0.76	0.08	1.75	10	S
40810	00	A	Excision of lesion of mucosa and submucosa, vestibule of mouth; without repair	1.26	1.18	0.11	2.55	10	S
40812	00	A	Excision of lesion of mucosa and submucosa, vestibule of mouth; with simple repair	2.26	1.50	0.14	3.90	10	S
40814	00	A	Excision of lesion of mucosa and submucosa, vestibule of mouth; with complex repair	3.27	3.23	0.32	6.82	90	S
40816	00	A	Excision of lesion of mucosa and submucosa, vestibule of mouth; complex, with excision of underlying muscle	3.52	3.22	0.33	7.07	90	S
40818	00	A	Excision of mucosa of vestibule of mouth as donor graft	2.26	2.25	0.20	4.71	90	S
40819	00	A	Excision of frenum, labial or buccal (frenumectomy, frenulectomy, frenectomy)	2.26	1.23	0.14	3.63	90	S
40820	00	A	Destruction of lesion or scar of vestibule of mouth by physical methods (eg, laser, thermal, cryo, chemical)	1.23	0.53	0.06	1.82	10	S
40830	00	A	Closure of laceration, vestibule of mouth; 2.5 cm or less	1.71	0.67	0.07	2.45	10	S
40831	00	A	Closure of laceration, vestibule of mouth; over 2.5 cm or complex	2.41	1.94	0.21	4.56	10	S
40840	00	R	Vestibuloplasty; anterior	8.31	6.28	0.73	15.32	90	S
40842	00	R	Vestibuloplasty; posterior, unilateral	8.31	6.28	0.73	15.32	90	S
40843	00	R	Vestibuloplasty; posterior, bilateral	11.63	8.80	1.03	21.46	90	S
40844	00	R	Vestibuloplasty; entire arch	15.37	11.63	1.36	28.36	90	S
40845	00	R	Vestibuloplasty; complex (including ridge extension, muscle repositioning)	17.94	23.99	1.93	43.86	90	S
40899	00	C	Unlisted procedure, vestibule of mouth	0	0	0	0	YYY	S
41000	00	A	Intraoral incision and drainage of abscess, cyst, or hematoma of tongue or floor of mouth; lingual	1.25	0.76	0.08	2.09	10	S
41005	00	A	Intraoral incision and drainage of abscess, cyst, or hematoma of tongue or floor of mouth; sublingual, superficial	1.21	0.62	0.07	1.90	10	S
41006	00	A	Intraoral incision and drainage of abscess, cyst, or hematoma of tongue or floor of mouth; sublingual, deep, supramylohyoid	3.03	1.01	0.11	4.15	90	S
41007	00	A	Intraoral incision and drainage of abscess, cyst, or hematoma of tongue or floor of mouth; submental space	2.89	2.90	0.30	6.09	90	S
41008	00	A	Intraoral incision and drainage of abscess, cyst, or hematoma of tongue or floor of mouth; submandibular space	3.16	1.06	0.11	4.33	90	S
41009	00	A	Intraoral incision and drainage of abscess, cyst, or hematoma of tongue or floor of mouth; masticator space	3.35	3.31	0.34	7.00	90	S
41010	00	A	Incision of lingual frenum (frenotomy)	1.19	0.37	0.04	1.60	10	S

CPT codes and descriptions only, © 1994 American Medical Association. Reimbursement information, © 1995 McGraw-Hill Inc.

Code/ CPT	Mod-ifier	Status	Description	Work value	Practice expense	Mal-practice	Total value	Global period	Up-date
41015	00	A	Extraoral incision and drainage of abscess, cyst, or hematoma of floor of mouth; sublingual	3.72	0.87	0.10	4.69	90	S
41016	00	A	Extraoral incision and drainage of abscess, cyst, or hematoma of floor of mouth; submental	3.72	3.69	0.38	7.79	90	S
41017	00	A	Extraoral incision and drainage of abscess, cyst, or hematoma of floor of mouth; submandibular	3.72	1.40	0.14	5.26	90	S
41018	00	A	Extraoral incision and drainage of abscess, cyst, or hematoma of floor of mouth; masticator space	4.75	3.93	0.38	9.06	90	S
41100	00	A	Biopsy of tongue; anterior two-thirds	1.58	0.80	0.08	2.46	10	S
41105	00	A	Biopsy of tongue; posterior one-third	1.37	1.03	0.12	2.52	10	S
41108	00	A	Biopsy of floor of mouth	1.00	0.85	0.09	1.94	10	S
41110	00	A	Excision of lesion of tongue without closure	1.46	1.30	0.15	2.91	10	S
41112	00	A	Excision of lesion of tongue with closure; anterior two-thirds	2.63	2.39	0.23	5.25	90	S
41113	00	A	Excision of lesion of tongue with closure; posterior one-third	3.09	3.41	0.37	6.87	90	S
41114	00	A	Excision of lesion of tongue with closure; with local tongue flap	7.88	6.39	0.73	15.00	90	S
41115	00	A	Excision of lingual frenum (frenectomy)	1.69	1.78	0.17	3.64	10	S
41116	00	A	Excision, lesion of floor of mouth	2.36	2.49	0.27	5.12	90	S
41120	00	A	Glossectomy; less than one-half tongue	8.83	7.28	0.88	16.99	90	S
41130	00	A	Glossectomy; hemiglossectomy	10.27	9.06	1.14	20.47	90	S
41135	00	A	Glossectomy; partial, with unilateral radical neck dissection	14.29	18.30	2.64	35.23	90	S
41140	00	A	Glossectomy; complete or total, with or without tracheostomy, without radical neck dissection	23.46	18.89	2.45	44.80	90	S
41145	00	A	Glossectomy; complete or total, with or without tracheostomy, with unilateral radical neck dissection	27.58	22.79	2.95	53.32	90	S
41150	00	A	Glossectomy; composite procedure with resection floor of mouth and mandibular resection, without radical neck dissection	19.36	18.96	2.46	40.78	90	S
41153	00	A	Glossectomy; composite procedure with resection floor of mouth, with suprahyoid neck dissection	21.18	25.00	3.03	49.21	90	S
41155	00	A	Glossectomy; composite procedure with resection floor of mouth, mandibular resection, and radical neck dissection (Commando type)	23.40	29.95	3.75	57.10	90	S
41250	00	A	Repair of laceration 2.5 cm or less; floor of mouth and/or anterior two-thirds of tongue	1.86	1.07	0.11	3.04	10	S
41251	00	A	Repair of laceration 2.5 cm or less; posterior one-third of tongue	2.22	2.07	0.21	4.50	10	S
41252	00	A	Repair of laceration of tongue, floor of mouth, over 2.6 cm or complex	2.92	2.35	0.26	5.53	10	S
41500	00	A	Fixation of tongue, mechanical, other than suture (eg, K-wire)	3.50	3.29	0.26	7.05	90	S
41510	00	A	Suture of tongue to lip for micrognathia (Douglas type procedure)	3.32	2.53	0.45	6.30	90	S
41520	00	A	Frenoplasty (surgical revision of frenum, eg, with Z-plasty)	2.63	2.88	0.28	5.79	90	S
41599	00	C	Unlisted procedure, tongue, floor of mouth	0	0	0	0	YYY	S
41800	00	A	Drainage of abscess, cyst, hematoma from dentoalveolar structures	1.12	0.69	0.07	1.88	10	S
41805	00	A	Removal of embedded foreign body from dentoalveolar structures; soft tissues	1.19	0.84	0.08	2.11	10	S
41806	00	A	Removal of embedded foreign body from dentoalveolar structures; bone	2.64	1.64	0.15	4.43	10	S
41820	00	R	Gingivectomy, excision gingiva, each quadrant	2.81*	1.47#	0.34*	4.62#	XXX	S

CPT codes and descriptions only, © 1994 American Medical Association. Reimbursement information, © 1995 McGraw-Hill Inc.

Code/ CPT	Mod- ifier	Status	Description	Work value	Practice expense	Mal- practice	Total value	Global period	Up- date
41821	00	R	Operculectomy, excision pericoronal tissues	0.56*	0.75#	0.06*	1.37#	XXX	S
41822	00	R	Excision of fibrous tuberosities, dentoalveolar structures	2.26	3.03	0.25	5.54	10	S
41823	00	R	Excision of osseous tuberosities, dentoalveolar structures	3.15	4.20	0.34	7.69	90	S
41825	00	A	Excision of lesion or tumor (except listed above), dentoalveolar structures; without repair	1.26	1.49	0.14	2.89	10	S
41826	00	A	Excision of lesion or tumor (except listed above), dentoalveolar structures; with simple repair	2.26	2.07	0.18	4.51	10	S
41827	00	A	Excision of lesion or tumor (except listed above), dentoalveolar structures; with complex repair	3.27	3.78	0.38	7.43	90	S
41828	00	R	Excision of hyperplastic alveolar mucosa, each quadrant (specify)	1.26	1.68	0.14	3.08	10	S
41830	00	R	Alveolectomy, including curettage of osteitis or sequestrectomy	1.12	1.49	0.12	2.73	10	S
41850	00	R	Destruction of lesion (except excision), dentoalveolar structures	0.42*	0.56#	0.05*	1.03#	XXX	S
41870	00	R	Periodontal mucosal grafting	2.67*	3.57#	0.29*	6.53#	XXX	S
41872	00	R	Gingivoplasty, each quadrant (specify)	2.44	3.26	0.27	5.97	90	S
41874	00	R	Alveoloplasty, each quadrant (specify)	2.94	3.93	0.32	7.19	90	S
41899	00	C	Unlisted procedure, dentoalveolar structures	0	0	0	0	YYY	S
42000	00	A	Drainage of abscess of palate, uvula	1.18	0.62	0.06	1.86	10	S
42100	00	A	Biopsy of palate, uvula	1.26	0.79	0.08	2.13	10	S
42104	00	A	Excision, lesion of palate, uvula; without closure	1.59	1.62	0.17	3.38	10	S
42106	00	A	Excision, lesion of palate, uvula; with simple primary closure	2.63	2.22	0.21	5.06	10	S
42107	00	A	Excision, lesion of palate, uvula; with local flap closure	4.20	4.91	0.50	9.61	90	S
42120	00	A	Resection of palate or extensive resection of lesion	5.39	6.93	1.01	13.33	90	S
42140	00	A	Uvulectomy, excision of uvula	1.54	1.35	0.15	3.04	90	S
42145	00	A	Palatopharyngoplasty (eg, uvulopalatopharyngoplasty, uvulopharyngoplasty)	7.04	10.33	1.45	18.82	090[	
42160	00	A	Destruction of lesion, palate or uvula (thermal, cryo or chemical)	1.75	1.53	0.16	3.44	10	S
42180	00	A	Repair, laceration of palate; up to 2 cm	2.45	2.24	0.26	4.95	10	S
42182	00	A	Repair, laceration of palate; over 2 cm or complex	3.78	3.47	0.38	7.63	10	S
42200	00	A	Palatoplasty for cleft palate, soft and/or hard palate only	9.48	7.19	0.85	17.52	90	S
42205	00	A	Palatoplasty for cleft palate, with closure of alveolar ridge; soft tissue only	8.96	10.82	0.79	20.57	90	S
42210	00	A	Palatoplasty for cleft palate, with closure of alveolar ridge; with bone graft to alveolar ridge (includes obtaining graft)	10.02	12.51	0.95	23.48	90	S
42215	00	A	Palatoplasty for cleft palate; major revision	8.42	7.68	0.86	16.96	90	S
42220	00	A	Palatoplasty for cleft palate; secondary lengthening procedure	6.65	5.40	0.81	12.86	90	S
42225	00	A	Palatoplasty for cleft palate; attachment pharyngeal flap	9.08	6.90	1.08	17.06	90	S
42226	00	A	Lengthening of palate, and pharyngeal flap	9.42	7.89	0.86	18.17	90	S
42227	00	A	Lengthening of palate, with island flap	8.89	7.41	0.38	16.68	90	S
42235	00	A	Repair of anterior palate, including vomer flap	7.50	5.55	0.49	13.54	90	S
42260	00	A	Repair of nasolabial fistula	4.17	3.98	0.44	8.59	90	S
42280	00	A	Maxillary impression for palatal prosthesis	1.49	1.99	0.17	3.65	10	S
42281	00	A	Insertion of pin-retained palatal prosthesis	1.77	1.47	0.15	3.39	10	S
42299	00	C	Unlisted procedure, palate, uvula	0	0	0	0	YYY	S
42300	00	A	Drainage of abscess; parotid, simple	1.88	0.96	0.12	2.96	10	S
42305	00	A	Drainage of abscess; parotid, complicated	5.59	2.18	0.27	8.04	90	S
42310	00	A	Drainage of abscess; submaxillary or sublingual, intraoral	1.51	1.03	0.12	2.66	10	S
42320	00	A	Drainage of abscess; submaxillary, external	2.30	1.83	0.22	4.35	10	S

CPT codes and descriptions only, © 1994 American Medical Association. Reimbursement information, © 1995 McGraw-Hill Inc.

Code/ CPT	Mod- ifier	Status	Description	Work value	Practice expense	Mal- practice	Total value	Global period	Up- date
42325	00	A	Fistulization of sublingual salivary cyst (ranula);	2.65	2.12	0.20	4.97	90	S
42326	00	A	Fistulization of sublingual salivary cyst (ranula); with prosthesis	3.65	4.34	0.33	8.32	90	S
42330	00	A	Sialolithotomy; submandibular (submaxillary), sublingual or parotid, uncomplicated, intraoral	2.16	1.10	0.12	3.38	10	S
42335	00	A	Sialolithotomy; submandibular (submaxillary), complicated, intraoral	3.21	2.47	0.27	5.95	90	S
42340	00	A	Sialolithotomy; parotid, extraoral or complicated intraoral	4.47	4.25	0.45	9.17	90	S
42400	00	A	Biopsy of salivary gland; needle	0.78	0.79	0.10	1.67	0	S
42405	00	A	Biopsy of salivary gland; incisional	3.24	1.54	0.19	4.97	10	S
42408	00	A	Excision of sublingual salivary cyst (ranula)	4.41	3.24	0.38	8.03	90	S
42409	00	A	Marsupialization of sublingual salivary cyst (ranula)	2.71	2.81	0.30	5.82	90	S
42410	00	A	Excision of parotid tumor or parotid gland; lateral lobe, without nerve dissection	8.88	5.94	0.92	15.74	90	S
42415	00	A	Excision of parotid tumor or parotid gland; lateral lobe, with dissection and preservation of facial nerve	16.12	12.68	1.68	30.48	90	S
42420	00	A	Excision of parotid tumor or parotid gland; total, with dissection and preservation of facial nerve	18.63	14.82	1.87	35.32	90	S
42425	00	A	Excision of parotid tumor or parotid gland; total, en bloc removal with sacrifice of facial nerve	12.36	11.10	1.43	24.89	90	S
42426	00	A	Excision of parotid tumor or parotid gland; total, with unilateral radical neck dissection	19.88	24.12	3.21	47.21	90	S
42440	00	A	Excision of submandibular (submaxillary) gland	6.61	7.98	0.99	15.58	90	S
42450	00	A	Excision of sublingual gland	4.38	3.42	0.35	8.15	90	S
42500	00	A	Plastic repair of salivary duct, sialodochoplasty; primary or simple	4.06	4.61	0.50	9.17	90	S
42505	00	A	Plastic repair of salivary duct, sialodochoplasty; secondary or complicated	5.92	7.34	0.86	14.12	90	S
42507	00	A	Parotid duct diversion, bilateral (Wilke type procedure);	5.96	4.65	0.67	11.28	90	S
42508	00	A	Parotid duct diversion, bilateral (Wilke type procedure); with excision of one submandibular gland	8.64	7.61	0.94	17.19	90	S
42509	00	A	Parotid duct diversion, bilateral (Wilke type procedure); with excision of both submandibular glands	11.08	7.31	1.23	19.62	90	S
42510	00	A	Parotid duct diversion, bilateral (Wilke type procedure); with ligation of both submandibular (Wharton's) ducts	7.71	7.65	0.84	16.20	90	S
42550	00	A	Injection procedure for sialography	1.25	0.44	0.04	1.73	0	N
42600	00	A	Closure salivary fistula	4.58	3.89	0.46	8.93	90	S
42650	00	A	Dilation salivary duct	0.77	0.39	0.04	1.20	0	S
42660	00	A	Dilation and catheterization of salivary duct, with or without injection	1.13	0.50	0.06	1.69	0	S
42665	00	A	Ligation salivary duct, intraoral	2.43	2.04	0.25	4.72	90	S
42699	00	C	Unlisted procedure, salivary glands or ducts	0	0	0	0	YYY	S
42700	00	A	Incision and drainage abscess; peritonsillar	1.57	0.85	0.10	2.52	10	S
42720	00	A	Incision and drainage abscess; retropharyngeal or parapharyngeal, intraoral approach	2.61	1.89	0.22	4.72	10	S
42725	00	A	Incision and drainage abscess; retropharyngeal or parapharyngeal, external approach	7.60	4.45	0.53	12.58	90	S
42800	00	A	Biopsy; oropharynx	1.34	0.74	0.08	2.16	10	S
42802	00	A	Biopsy; hypopharynx	1.49	1.02	0.12	2.63	10	S
42804	00	A	Biopsy; nasopharynx, visible lesion, simple	1.19	1.09	0.13	2.41	10	S
42806	00	A	Biopsy; nasopharynx, survey for unknown primary lesion	1.53	1.40	0.16	3.09	10	S
42808	00	A	Excision or destruction of lesion of pharynx, any method	2.25	2.52	0.29	5.06	10	S
42809	00	A	Removal of foreign body from pharynx	1.76	0.82	0.08	2.66	10	S

CPT codes and descriptions only, © 1994 American Medical Association. Reimbursement information, © 1995 McGraw-Hill Inc.

Code/ CPT	Mod-ifier	Status	Description	Work value	Practice expense	Mal-practice	Total value	Global period	Up-date
42810	00	A	Excision branchial cleft cyst or vestige, confined to skin and subcutaneous tissues	3.20	3.14	0.47	6.81	90	S
42815	00	A	Excision branchial cleft cyst, vestige, or fistula, extending beneath subcutaneous tissues and/or into pharynx	6.75	8.47	1.12	16.34	90	S
42820	00	A	Tonsillectomy and adenoidectomy; under age 12	3.59	3.15	0.32	7.06	90	S
42821	00	A	Tonsillectomy and adenoidectomy; age 12 or over	4.10	3.93	0.46	8.49	90	S
42825	00	A	Tonsillectomy, primary or secondary; under age 12	3.21	2.64	0.33	6.18	90	S
42826	00	A	Tonsillectomy, primary or secondary; age 12 or over	3.19	3.86	0.43	7.48	90	S
42830	00	A	Adenoidectomy, primary; under age 12	2.49	1.86	0.27	4.62	90	S
42831	00	A	Adenoidectomy, primary; age 12 or over	2.61	2.36	0.25	5.22	90	S
42835	00	A	Adenoidectomy, secondary; under age 12	2.22	1.86	0.10	4.18	90	S
42836	00	A	Adenoidectomy, secondary, age 12 or over	3.10	2.79	0.31	6.20	90	S
42842	00	A	Radical resection of tonsil, tonsillar pillars, and/or retromolar trigone; without closure	8.13	6.69	0.73	15.55	90	S
42844	00	A	Radical resection of tonsil, tonsillar pillars, and/or retromolar trigone; closure with local flap (eg, tongue, buccal)	12.73	10.85	1.27	24.85	90	S
42845	00	A	Radical resection of tonsil, tonsillar pillars, and/or retromolar trigone; closure with other flap	21.88	18.62	2.22	42.72	90	S
42860	00	A	Excision of tonsil tags	2.14	1.89	0.21	4.24	90	S
42870	00	A	Excision or destruction lingual tonsil, any method (separate procedure)	5.16	2.32	0.26	7.74	90	S
42880	00	A	Excision nasopharyngeal lesion (eg, fibroma)	6.01	4.62	0.52	11.15	90	S
42890	00	A	Limited pharyngectomy	11.67	8.99	1.03	21.69	90	S
42892	00	A	Resection of lateral pharyngeal wall or pyriform sinus, direct closure by advancement of lateral and posterior pharyngeal walls	13.94	10.92	1.27	26.13	90	S
42894	00	A	Resection of pharyngeal wall requiring closure with myocutaneous flap	20.68	16.06	1.83	38.57	90	S
42900	00	A	Suture pharynx for wound or injury	4.98	4.26	0.48	9.72	10	S
42950	00	A	Pharyngoplasty (plastic or reconstructive operation on pharynx)	7.70	9.86	1.10	18.66	90	S
42953	00	A	Pharyngoesophageal repair	8.21	6.34	0.93	15.48	90	S
42955	00	A	Pharyngostomy (fistulization of pharynx, external for feeding)	6.50	3.32	0.43	10.25	90	S
42960	00	A	Control oropharyngeal hemorrhage, primary or secondary (eg, posttonsillectomy); simple	2.28	1.08	0.12	3.48	10	S
42961	00	A	Control oropharyngeal hemorrhage, primary or secondary (eg, posttonsillectomy); complicated, requiring hospitalization	5.18	1.75	0.19	7.12	90	S
42962	00	A	Control oropharyngeal hemorrhage, primary or secondary (eg, posttonsillectomy); with secondary surgical intervention	6.64	5.98	0.68	13.30	90	S
42970	00	A	Control of nasopharyngeal hemorrhage, primary or secondary (eg, postadenoidectomy); simple, with posterior nasal packs, with or without anterior packs and/or cauterization	4.78	1.03	0.10	5.91	90	N
42971	00	A	Control of nasopharyngeal hemorrhage, primary or secondary (eg, postadenoidectomy); complicated, requiring hospitalization	5.56	2.90	0.34	8.80	90	S
42972	00	A	Control of nasopharyngeal hemorrhage, primary or secondary (eg, postadenoidectomy); with secondary surgical intervention	6.55	4.55	0.73	11.83	90	S
42999	00	C	Unlisted procedure, pharynx, adenoids, or tonsils	0	0	0	0	YYY	S

CPT codes and descriptions only, © 1994 American Medical Association. Reimbursement information, © 1995 McGraw-Hill Inc.

Code/ CPT	Mod-ifier	Status	Description	Work value	Practice expense	Mal-practice	Total value	Global period	Up-date
43000	00	D	Incision of esophagus	9.29*	4.86#	1.13*	15.28#	90	S
43020	00	A	Esophagotomy, cervical approach, with removal of foreign body	7.72	6.58	0.71	15.01	90	S
43030	00	A	Cricopharyngeal myotomy	7.15	9.15	1.21	17.51	90	S
43040	00	D	Incision of esophagus	12.66*	6.62#	1.54*	20.82#	90	S
43045	00	A	Cricopharyngeal myotomy Esophagotomy, thoracic approach, with removal of foreign body	18.83	12.45	2.36	33.64	90	S
43100	00	A	Excision of lesion, esophagus, with primary repair; cervical approach	8.47	6.19	0.95	15.61	90	S
43101	00	A	Excision of lesion, esophagus, with primary repair; thoracic or abdominal approach	15.11	9.48	1.88	26.47	90	S
43105	00	D	Removal of upper esophagus	16.88*	8.83#	2.05*	27.76#	90	S
43106	00	D	Removal of upper esophagus	22.51*	11.77#	2.74*	37.02#	90	S
43107	00	A	Total or near total esophagectomy, without thoracotomy; with pharyngogastrostomy or cervical esophagogastrostomy, with or without pyloroplasty (transhiatal)	27.20	22.50	4.42	54.12	90	S
43108	00	A	Total or near total esophagectomy, without thoracotomy; with colon interposition or small bowel reconstruction, including bowel mobilization, preparation and anastomosis(es)	32.64	25.27	4.77	62.68	90	S
43110	00	D	Partial removal of esophagus	19.70*	10.30#	2.40*	32.4#	90	S
43111	00	D	Partial removal of esophagus	21.81*	11.41#	2.65*	35.87#	90	S
43112	00	A	Total or near total esophagectomy, with thoracotomy; with pharyngogastrostomy or cervical esophagogastrostomy, with or without pyloroplasty	29.67	21.65	4.22	55.54	90	S
43113	00	A	Total or near total esophagectomy, with thoracotomy; with colon interposition or small bowel reconstruction, including bowel mobilization, preparation, and anastomosis(es)	33.63	25.27	4.77	63.67	90	S
43115	00	D	Partial removal of esophagus	23.21*	12.14#	2.82*	38.17#	90	S
43116	00	A	Partial esophagectomy, cervical, with free intestinal graft, including microvascular anastomosis, obtaining the graft and intestinal reconstruction	29.67	25.27	4.77	59.71	90	S
43117	00	A	Partial esophagectomy, distal two-thirds, with thoracotomy and separate abdominal incision, with or without proximal gastrectomy; with thoracic esophagogastrostomy, with or without pyloroplasty (Ivor Lewis)	28.47	25.27	4.77	58.51	90	S
43118	00	A	Partial esophagectomy, distal two-thirds, with thoracotomy and separate abdominal incision, with or without proximal gastrectomy; with colon interposition or small bowel reconstruction, including bowel mobilization, preparation, and anastomosis(es)	31.65	25.27	4.77	61.69	90	S
43119	00	D	Removal of esophagus	24.62*	12.88#	3.00*	40.50#	90	S
43120	00	D	Remove esophagus & stomach	21.38*	11.18#	2.60*	35.16#	90	S
43121	00	A	Partial esophagectomy, distal two-thirds, with thoracotomy only, with or without proximal gastrectomy, with thoracic esophagogastrostomy, with or without pyloroplasty	27.69	21.36	4.19	53.24	90	S
43122	00	A	Partial esophagectomy, thoracoabdominal or abdominal approach, with or without proximal gastrectomy; with esophagogastrostomy, with or without pyloroplasty	27.69	21.36	4.19	53.24	90	S
43123	00	A	Partial esophagectomy, thoracoabdominal or abdominal approach, with or without proximal gastrectomy; with colon interposition or small bowel reconstruction, including bowel mobilization, preparation, and anastomosis(es)	31.65	25.27	4.77	61.69	90	S

CPT codes and descriptions only, © 1994 American Medical Association. Reimbursement information, © 1995 McGraw-Hill Inc.

Code/ CPT	Mod- ifier	Status	Description	Work value	Practice expense	Mal- practice	Total value	Global period	Up- date
43124	00	A	Total or partial esophagectomy, without reconstruction (any approach), with cervical esophagostomy	24.73	22.50	4.42	51.65	90	S
43130	00	A	Diverticulectomy of hypopharynx or esophagus, with or without myotomy; cervical approach	10.68	10.51	1.60	22.79	90	S
43135	00	A	Diverticulectomy of hypopharynx or esophagus, with or without myotomy; thoracic approach	15.11	11.72	2.17	29	90	S
43200	00	A	Esophagoscopy, rigid or flexible; diagnostic, with or without collection of specimen(s) by brushing or washing (separate procedure)	1.59	2.13	0.26	3.98	0	S
43202	00	A	Esophagoscopy, rigid or flexible; with biopsy, single or multiple	1.89	2.57	0.31	4.77	0	N
43204	00	A	Esophagoscopy, rigid or flexible; with injection sclerosis of esophageal varices	3.77	4.83	0.36	8.96	0	N
43205	00	A	Esophagoscopy, rigid or flexible; with band ligation of esophageal varices	3.79	2.70	0.18	6.67	0	N
43215	00	A	Esophagoscopy, rigid or flexible; with removal of foreign body	2.60	3.47	0.46	6.53	0	N
43216	00	A	Esophagoscopy, rigid or flexible; with removal of tumor(s), polyp(s), or other lesion(s) by hot biopsy forceps or bipolar cautery	2.40	3.64	0.37	6.41	0	N
43217	00	A	Esophagoscopy, rigid or flexible; with removal of tumor(s), polyp(s), or other lesion(s) by snare technique	2.90	3.64	0.37	6.91	0	N
43219	00	A	Esophagoscopy, rigid or flexible; with insertion of plastic tube or stent	2.80	3.58	0.34	6.72	0	N
43220	00	A	Esophagoscopy, rigid or flexible; with balloon dilation (less than 30 mm diameter)	2.10	2.68	0.27	5.05	0	N
43226	00	A	Esophagoscopy, rigid or flexible; with insertion of guide wire followed by dilation over guide wire	2.34	3.08	0.26	5.68	0	N
43227	00	A	Esophagoscopy, rigid or flexible; with control of bleeding, any method	3.60	4.61	0.34	8.55	0	N
43228	00	A	Esophagoscopy, rigid or flexible; with ablation of tumor(s), polyp(s), or other lesion(s), not amenable to removal by hot biopsy forceps, bipolar cautery or snare technique	3.77	4.79	0.38	8.94	0	N
43234	00	A	Upper gastrointestinal endoscopy, simple primary examination (eg, with small diameter flexible endoscope) (separate procedure)	2.01	2.57	0.30	4.88	0	N
43235	00	A	Upper gastrointestinal endoscopy including esophagus, stomach, and either the duodenum and/or jejunum as appropriate; diagnostic, with or without collection of specimen(s) by brushing or washing (separate procedure)	2.39	3.07	0.29	5.75	0	N
43239	00	A	Upper gastrointestinal endoscopy including esophagus, stomach, and either the duodenum and/or jejunum as appropriate; with biopsy, single or multiple	2.69	3.45	0.33	6.47	0	N
43241	00	A	Upper gastrointestinal endoscopy including esophagus, stomach, and either the duodenum and/or jejunum as appropriate; with transendoscopic tube or catheter placement	2.59	3.61	0.38	6.58	0	N
43243	00	A	Upper gastrointestinal endoscopy including esophagus, stomach, and either the duodenum and/or jejunum as appropriate; with injection sclerosis of esophageal and/or gastric varices	4.57	5.63	0.39	10.59	0	N
43244	00	A	Upper gastrointestinal endoscopy including esophagus, stomach, and either the duodenum and/or jejunum as appropriate; with band ligation of esophageal and/or gastric varices	4.59	3.47	0.41	8.47	0	N

CPT codes and descriptions only, © 1994 American Medical Association. Reimbursement information, © 1995 McGraw-Hill Inc.

Code/ CPT	Mod-ifier	Status	Description	Work value	Practice expense	Mal-practice	Total value	Global period	Up-date
43245	00	A	Upper gastrointestinal endoscopy including esophagus, stomach, and either the duodenum and/or jejunum as appropriate; with dilation of gastric outlet for obstruction, any method	3.39	4.34	0.40	8.13	0	N
43246	00	A	Upper gastrointestinal endoscopy including esophagus, stomach, and either the duodenum and/or jejunum as appropriate; with directed placement of percutaneous gastrostomy tube	4.33	5.55	0.51	10.39	0	N
43247	00	A	Upper gastrointestinal endoscopy including esophagus, stomach, and either the duodenum and/or jejunum as appropriate; with removal of foreign body	3.39	4.34	0.38	8.11	0	N
43248	00	A	Upper gastrointestinal endoscopy including esophagus, stomach, and either the duodenum and/or jejunum as appropriate; with insertion of guide wire followed by dilation of esophagus over guide wire	3.15	4.03	0.35	7.53	0	N
43249	00	A	Upper gastrointestinal endoscopy including esophagus, stomach, and either the duodenum and/or jejunum as appropriate; with balloon dilation of esophagus (less than 30 mm diameter)	2.90	3.73	0.30	6.93	0	N
43250	00	A	Upper gastrointestinal endoscopy including esophagus, stomach, and either the duodenum and/or jejunum as appropriate; with removal of tumor(s), polyp(s), or other lesion(s) by hot biopsy forceps or bipolar cautery	3.20	4.60	0.43	8.23	0	N
43251	00	A	Upper gastrointestinal endoscopy including esophagus, stomach, and either the duodenum and/or jejunum as appropriate; with removal of tumor(s), polyp(s), or other lesion(s) by snare technique	3.70	4.60	0.43	8.73	0	N
43255	00	A	Upper gastrointestinal endoscopy including esophagus, stomach, and either the duodenum and/or jejunum as appropriate; with control of bleeding, any method	4.40	5.63	0.38	10.41	0	N
43258	00	A	Upper gastrointestinal endoscopy including esophagus, stomach, and either the duodenum and/or jejunum as appropriate; with ablation of tumor(s), polyp(s), or other lesion(s) not amenable to removal by hot biopsy forceps, bipolar cautery or snare technique	4.55	5.41	0.38	10.34	0	N
43259	00	A	Upper gastrointestinal endoscopy including esophagus, stomach, and either the duodenum and/or jejunum as appropriate; with endoscopic ultrasound examination	4.89	4.02	0.35	9.26	0	N
43260	00	A	Endoscopic retrograde cholangiopancreatography (ERCP); diagnostic, with or without collection of specimen(s) by brushing or washing (separate procedure)	5.96	5.98	0.39	12.33	0	N
43261	00	A	Endoscopic retrograde cholangiopancreatography (ERCP); with biopsy, single or multiple	6.27	5.98	0.39	12.64	0	N
43262	00	A	Endoscopic retrograde cholangiopancreatography (ERCP); with sphincterotomy/papillotomy	7.39	9.00	0.58	16.97	0	N
43263	00	A	Endoscopic retrograde cholangiopancreatography (ERCP); with pressure measurement of sphincter of Oddi (pancreatic duct or common bile duct)	6.19	5.83	0.38	12.40	0	N
43264	00	A	Endoscopic retrograde cholangiopancreatography (ERCP); with endoscopic retrograde removal of stone(s) from biliary and/or pancreatic ducts	8.90	8.92	0.61	18.43	0	N
43265	00	A	Endoscopic retrograde cholangiopancreatography (ERCP); with endoscopic retrograde destruction, lithotripsy of stone(s), any method	8.90	6.82	0.49	16.21	0	N
43267	00	A	Endoscopic retrograde cholangiopancreatography (ERCP); with endoscopic retrograde insertion of nasobiliary or nasopancreatic drainage tube	7.39	7.41	0.48	15.28	0	N

CPT codes and descriptions only, © 1994 American Medical Association. Reimbursement information, © 1995 McGraw-Hill Inc.

Code/ CPT	Mod- ifier	Status	Description	Work value	Practice expense	Mal- practice	Total value	Global period	Up- date
43268	00	A	Endoscopic retrograde cholangiopancreatography (ERCP); with endoscopic retrograde insertion of tube or stent into bile or pancreatic duct	7.39	8.72	0.56	16.67	0	N
43269	00	A	Endoscopic retrograde cholangiopancreatography (ERCP); with endoscopic retrograde removal of foreign body and/or change of tube or stent	6.04	7.35	0.51	13.90	0	N
43271	00	A	Endoscopic retrograde cholangiopancreatography (ERCP); with endoscopic retrograde balloon dilation of ampulla, biliary and/or pancreatic duct(s)	7.39	7.63	0.50	15.52	0	N
43272	00	A	Endoscopic retrograde cholangiopancreatography (ERCP); with ablation of tumor(s), polyp(s), or other lesion(s) not amenable to removal by hot biopsy forceps, bipolar cautery or snare technique	7.39	5.60	0.42	13.41	0	N
43300	00	A	Esophagoplasty, (plastic repair or reconstruction), cervical approach; without repair of tracheoesophageal fistula	8.72	11.17	1.70	21.59	90	S
43305	00	A	Esophagoplasty, (plastic repair or reconstruction), cervical approach; with repair of tracheoesophageal fistula	16.14	13.71	1.78	31.63	90	S
43310	00	A	Esophagoplasty, (plastic repair or reconstruction), thoracic approach; without repair of tracheoesophageal fistula	24.20	16.99	3.23	44.42	90	S
43312	00	A	Esophagoplasty, (plastic repair or reconstruction), thoracic approach; with repair of tracheoesophageal fistula	27.26	13.72	2.30	43.28	90	S
43320	00	A	Esophagogastrostomy (cardioplasty), with or without vagotomy and pyloroplasty, transabdominal or transthoracic approach	14.49	11.68	2.05	28.22	90	S
43321	00	D	Fuse esophagus & stomach	16.53*	8.65#	2.01*	27.19#	90	S
43324	00	A	Esophagogastric fundoplasty (eg, Nissen, Belsey IV, Hill procedures)	15.18	11.88	2.53	29.59	90	S
43325	00	A	Esophagogastric fundoplasty; with fundic patch (Thal-Nissen procedure)	14.63	11.61	2.29	28.53	90	S
43326	00	A	Esophagogastric fundoplasty; with gastroplasty (eg, Collis)	14.37	7.52	1.75	23.64	90	S
43330	00	A	Esophagomyotomy (Heller type); abdominal approach	14.27	11.36	2.39	28.02	90	S
43331	00	A	Esophagomyotomy (Heller type); thoracic approach	14.73	14.33	2.64	31.70	90	S
43340	00	A	Esophagojejunostomy (without total gastrectomy); abdominal approach	14.16	12.44	2.52	29.12	90	S
43341	00	A	Esophagojejunostomy (without total gastrectomy); thoracic approach	15.26	9.90	1.56	26.72	90	S
43350	00	A	Esophagostomy, fistulization of esophagus, external; abdominal approach	11.25	7.88	1.15	20.28	90	S
43351	00	A	Esophagostomy, fistulization of esophagus, external; thoracic approach	13.42	8.77	1.53	23.72	90	S
43352	00	A	Esophagostomy, fistulization of esophagus, external; cervical approach	10.92	8.86	1.47	21.25	90	S
43360	00	A	Gastrointestinal reconstruction for previous esophagectomy, for obstructing esophageal lesion or fistula, or for previous esophageal exclusion; with stomach, with or without pyloroplasty	26.06	21.36	4.19	51.61	90	S
43361	00	A	Gastrointestinal reconstruction for previous esophagectomy, for obstructing esophageal lesion or fistula, or for previous esophageal exclusion; with colon interposition or small bowel reconstruction, including bowel mobilization, preparation, and anastomosis(es)	29.67	25.27	4.77	59.71	90	S
43400	00	A	Ligation, direct, esophageal varices	15.55	10.82	1.63	28	90	S
43401	00	A	Transection of esophagus with repair, for esophageal varices	16.26	9.59	1.93	27.78	90	S
43405	00	A	Ligation or stapling at gastroesophageal junction for pre-existing esophageal perforation	14.84	14.33	2.64	31.81	90	S

CPT codes and descriptions only, © 1994 American Medical Association. Reimbursement information, © 1995 McGraw-Hill Inc.

Code/ CPT	Mod- ifier	Status	Description	Work value	Practice expense	Mal- practice	Total value	Global period	Up- date
43410	00	A	Suture of esophageal wound or injury; cervical approach	9.61	8.90	1.54	20.05	90	S
43415	00	A	Suture of esophageal wound or injury; transthoracic or transabdominal approach	15.86	12.74	2.52	31.12	90	S
43420	00	A	Closure of esophagostomy or fistula; cervical approach	10.19	5.88	0.78	16.85	90	S
43425	00	A	Closure of esophagostomy or fistula; transthoracic or transabdominal approach	15.58	9.94	1.71	27.23	90	S
43450	00	A	Dilation of esophagus, by unguided sound or bougie, single or multiple passes	1.38	0.68	0.05	2.11	0	N
43453	00	A	Dilation of esophagus, over guide wire	1.51	1.51	0.11	3.13	0	N
43456	00	A	Dilation of esophagus, by balloon or dilator, retrograde	3.52	2.47	0.24	6.23	0	N
43458	00	A	Dilation of esophagus with balloon (30 mm diameter or larger) for achalasia	3.06	2.02	0.27	5.35	0	N
43460	00	A	Esophagogastric tamponade, with balloon (Sengstaaken type)	3.80	1.67	0.15	5.62	0	N
43499	00	C	Unlisted procedure, esophagus	0	0	0	0	YYY	N
43500	00	A	Gastrotomy; with exploration or foreign body removal	7.60	6.13	1.20	14.93	90	S
43501	00	A	Gastrotomy; with suture repair of bleeding ulcer	13.85	8.58	1.83	24.26	90	S
43502	00	A	Gastrotomy; with suture repair of pre-existing esophagogastric laceration (eg, Mallory-Weiss)	15.82	8.58	1.83	26.23	90	S
43510	00	A	Gastrotomy; with esophageal dilation and insertion of permanent intraluminal tube (eg, Celestin or Mousseaux-Barbin)	9.27	8.29	0.94	18.50	90	N
43520	00	A	Pyloromyotomy, cutting of pyloric muscle (Fredet-Ramstedt type operation)	7.00	4.48	0.87	12.35	90	S
43600	00	A	Biopsy of stomach; by capsule, tube, peroral (one or more specimens)	1.91	0.50	0.05	2.46	0	N
43605	00	A	Biopsy of stomach; by laparotomy	8.23	5.91	1.29	15.43	90	S
43610	00	A	Excision, local; ulcer or benign tumor of stomach	10.11	8.17	1.71	19.99	90	S
43611	00	A	Excision, local; malignant tumor of stomach	12.43	8.17	1.71	22.31	90	S
43620	00	A	Gastrectomy, total; with esophagoenterostomy	21.03	15.38	3.19	39.60	90	S
43621	00	A	Gastrectomy, total; with Roux-en-Y reconstruction	21.47	15.38	3.19	40.04	90	S
43622	00	A	Gastrectomy, total; with formation of intestinal pouch, any type	22.82	15.38	3.19	41.39	90	S
43631	00	A	Gastrectomy, partial, distal; with gastroduodenostomy	18.10	12.42	2.66	33.18	90	S
43632	00	A	Gastrectomy, partial, distal; with gastrojejunostomy	18.10	12.42	2.66	33.18	90	S
43633	00	A	Gastrectomy, partial, distal; with Roux-en-Y reconstruction	18.54	12.42	2.66	33.62	90	S
43634	00	A	Gastrectomy, partial, distal; with formation of intestinal pouch	19.89	20.83	4.57	45.29	90	S
43635	00	A	Vagotomy with partial distal gastrectomy (List separately in addition to code(s) for primary procedure) (Use 43635 only with 43631, 43632, 43633, 43634)	2.06	1.08	0.26	3.40	ZZZ	S
43638	00	A	Gastrectomy, partial, proximal, thoracic or abdominal approach including esophagogastrostomy, with vagotomy;	20.15	12.75	2.73	35.63	90	S
43639	00	A	Gastrectomy, partial, proximal, thoracic or abdominal approach including esophagogastrostomy, with vagotomy; with pyloroplasty or pyloromyotomy	20.64	12.75	2.73	36.12	90	S
43640	00	A	Vagotomy including pyloroplasty, with or without gastrostomy; truncal or selective	13.28	10.34	2.19	25.81	90	S
43641	00	A	Vagotomy including pyloroplasty, with or without gastrostomy; parietal cell (highly selective)	13.28	10.34	2.18	25.80	90	S
43750	00	A	Percutaneous placement of gastrostomy tube	5.71	4.35	0.56	10.62	10	N
43760	00	A	Change of gastrostomy tube	1.10	0.69	0.09	1.88	0	N
43761	00	A	Repositioning of the gastric feeding tube through the duodenum for enteric nutrition	2.01	1.06	0.25	3.32	0	N

CPT codes and descriptions only, © 1994 American Medical Association. Reimbursement information, © 1995 McGraw-Hill Inc.

Code/ CPT	Mod-ifier	Status	Description	Work value	Practice expense	Mal-practice	Total value	Global period	Up-date
43800	00	A	Pyloroplasty	9.41	6.85	1.47	17.73	90	S
43810	00	A	Gastroduodenostomy	10.08	7.64	1.53	19.25	90	S
43820	00	A	Gastrojejunostomy; without vagotomy	10.43	8.29	1.75	20.47	90	S
43825	00	A	Gastrojejunostomy; with vagotomy, any type	13.28	11.08	2.30	26.66	90	S
43830	00	A	Gastrostomy, temporary (tube, rubber or plastic) (separate procedure);	4.84	6.19	1.19	12.22	90	S
43831	00	A	Gastrostomy, temporary (tube, rubber or plastic) (separate procedure); neonatal, for feeding	6.41	5.20	0.93	12.54	90	S
43832	00	A	Gastrostomy, permanent, with construction of gastric tube	10.68	7.95	1.36	19.99	90	S
43840	00	A	Gastrorrhaphy, suture of perforated duodenal or gastric ulcer, wound, or injury	10.45	7.84	1.66	19.95	90	S
43842	00	A	Gastric restrictive procedure, without gastric bypass, for morbid obesity; vertical-banded gastroplasty	13.76	13.72	2.93	30.41	90	S
43843	00	A	Gastric restrictive procedure, without gastric bypass, for morbid obesity; other than vertical-banded gastroplasty	13.76	13.72	2.93	30.41	90	S
43844	00	D	Gastric bypass for obesity	18.29*	9.57#	2.23*	30.09#	90	S
43846	00	A	Gastric restrictive procedure, with gastric bypass for morbid obesity; with short limb (less than 100 cm) Roux-en-Y gastroenterostomy	17.84	14.80	3.30	35.94	90	S
43847	00	A	Gastric restrictive procedure, with gastric bypass for morbid obesity; with small bowel reconstruction to limit absorption	19.87	9.67	1.13	30.67	90	S
43848	00	A	Revision of gastric restrictive procedure for morbid obesity (separate procedure)	22.10	14.80	3.30	40.20	90	S
43850	00	A	Revision of gastroduodenal anastomosis (gastroduodenostomy) with reconstruction; without vagotomy	18.14	11.64	2.25	32.03	90	S
43855	00	A	Revision of gastroduodenal anastomosis (gastroduodenostomy) with reconstruction; with vagotomy	19.15	10.44	2.28	31.87	90	S
43860	00	A	Revision of gastrojejunal anastomosis (gastrojejunostomy) with reconstruction, with or without partial gastrectomy or bowel resection; without vagotomy	18.14	11.46	2.51	32.11	90	S
43865	00	A	Revision of gastrojejunal anastomosis (gastrojejunostomy) with reconstruction, with or without partial gastrectomy or bowel resection; with vagotomy	19.15	13.39	2.98	35.52	90	S
43870	00	A	Closure of gastrostomy, surgical	6.56	5.77	1.14	13.47	90	S
43880	00	A	Closure of gastrocolic fistula	18.14	8.25	1.76	28.15	90	S
43885	00	D	Revise stomach placement	9.14*	4.78#	1.11*	15.03#	90	S
43999	00	C	Unlisted procedure, stomach	0	0	0	0	YYY	N
44005	00	A	Enterolysis (freeing of intestinal adhesion) (separate procedure)	12.52	8.28	1.75	22.55	90	S
44010	00	A	Duodenotomy, for exploration, biopsy(s), or foreign body removal	9.24	6.91	1.42	17.57	90	S
44015	00	A	Tube or needle catheter jejunostomy for enteral alimentation, intraoperative, any method (List separately in addition to primary procedure)	2.62	3.22	0.45	6.29	ZZZ	S
44020	00	A	Enterotomy, small bowel, other than duodenum; for exploration, biopsy(s), or foreign body removal	10.69	7.81	1.65	20.15	90	S
44021	00	A	Enterotomy, small bowel, other than duodenum; for decompression (eg, Baker tube)	10.83	7.00	1.48	19.31	90	S
44025	00	A	Colotomy, for exploration, biopsy(s), or foreign body removal	11.07	7.74	1.61	20.42	90	S
44040	00	D	Exteriorization of bowel	12.66*	6.62#	1.54*	20.82#	90	S
44050	00	A	Reduction of volvulus, intussusception, internal hernia, by laparotomy	10.05	7.77	1.64	19.46	90	S

CPT codes and descriptions only, © 1994 American Medical Association. Reimbursement information, © 1995 McGraw-Hill Inc.

Code/ CPT	Mod- ifier	Status	Description	Work value	Practice expense	Mal- practice	Total value	Global period	Up- date
44055	00	A	Correction of malrotation by lysis of duodenal bands and/or reduction of midgut volvulus (eg, Ladd procedure)	11.92	7.66	1.60	21.18	90	S
44100	00	A	Biopsy of intestine by capsule, tube, peroral (one or more specimens)	2.01	1.38	0.13	3.52	0	N
44110	00	A	Excision of one or more lesions of small or large bowel not requiring anastomosis, exteriorization, or fistulization; single enterotomy	9.01	7.67	1.58	18.26	90	S
44111	00	A	Excision of one or more lesions of small or large bowel not requiring anastomosis, exteriorization, or fistulization; multiple enterotomies	11.05	9.67	2.14	22.86	90	S
44120	00	A	Enterectomy, resection of small intestine; single resection and anastomosis	13.15	9.46	2.02	24.63	90	S
44121	00	A	Enterectomy, resection of small intestine; each additional resection and anastomosis	4.45	2.32	0.54	7.31	ZZZ	S
44125	00	A	Enterectomy, resection of small intestine; with enterostomy	13.15	10.75	2.28	26.18	90	S
44130	00	A	Enteroenterostomy, anastomosis of intestine, with or without cutaneous enterostomy (separate procedure)	11.09	8.67	1.86	21.62	90	S
44139	00	A	Mobilization (take-down) of splenic flexure performed in conjunction with partial colectomy (List separately in addition to primary procedure)	2.23	1.17	0.27	3.67	ZZZ	S
44140	00	A	Colectomy, partial; with anastomosis	16.97	11.37	2.40	30.74	90	S
44141	00	A	Colectomy, partial; with skin level cecostomy or colostomy	17.36	11.86	2.55	31.77	90	S
44143	00	A	Colectomy, partial; with end colostomy and closure of distal segment (Hartmann type procedure)	15.00	12.26	2.62	29.88	90	S
44144	00	A	Colectomy, partial; with resection, with colostomy or ileostomy and creation of mucofistula	15.00	12.06	2.53	29.59	90	S
44145	00	A	Colectomy, partial; with coloproctostomy (low pelvic anastomosis)	21.29	13.25	2.78	37.32	90	S
44146	00	A	Colectomy, partial; with coloproctostomy (low pelvic anastomosis), with colostomy	22.22	14.98	3.14	40.34	90	S
44147	00	A	Colectomy, partial; abdominal and transanal approach	16.23	15.34	3.30	34.87	90	S
44150	00	A	Colectomy, total, abdominal, without proctectomy; with ileostomy or ileoproctostomy	19.04	14.84	3.17	37.05	90	S
44151	00	A	Colectomy, total, abdominal, without proctectomy; with continent ileostomy	17.95	10.21	2.22	30.38	90	S
44152	00	A	Colectomy, total, abdominal, without proctectomy; with rectal mucosectomy, ileoanal anastomosis, with or without loop ileostomy	22.98	15.44	3.36	41.78	90	S
44153	00	A	Colectomy, total, abdominal, without proctectomy; with rectal mucosectomy, ileoanal anastomosis, creation of ileal reservoir (S or J), with or without loop ileostomy	24.69	19.35	3.63	47.67	90	S
44155	00	A	Colectomy, total, abdominal, with proctectomy; with ileostomy	22.09	16.65	3.50	42.24	90	S
44156	00	A	Colectomy, total, abdominal, with proctectomy; with continent ileostomy	20.48	11.40	2.52	34.40	90	S
44160	00	A	Colectomy with removal of terminal ileum and ileocolostomy	14.09	12.44	2.68	29.21	90	S
44300	00	A	Enterostomy or cecostomy, tube (eg, for decompression or feeding) (separate procedure)	7.77	6.03	1.29	15.09	90	S
44310	00	A	Ileostomy or jejunostomy, non-tube (separate procedure)	10.07	7.88	1.66	19.61	90	S
44312	00	A	Revision of ileostomy; simple (release of superficial scar) (separate procedure)	5.34	3.08	0.45	8.87	90	S
44314	00	A	Revision of ileostomy; complicated (reconstruction in-depth) (separate procedure)	9.77	6.68	1.21	17.66	90	S

CPT codes and descriptions only, © 1994 American Medical Association. Reimbursement information, © 1995 McGraw-Hill Inc.

Code/ CPT	Mod-ifier	Status	Description	Work value	Practice expense	Mal-practice	Total value	Global period	Up-date
44316	00	A	Continent ileostomy (Kock procedure) (separate procedure)	13.59	9.64	1.43	24.66	90	S
44320	00	A	Colostomy or skin level cecostomy; (separate procedure)	11.39	7.46	1.57	20.42	90	S
44322	00	A	Colostomy or skin level cecostomy; with multiple biopsies (eg, for Hirschsprung disease) (separate procedure)	10.31	9.07	1.88	21.26	90	S
44340	00	A	Revision of colostomy; simple (release of superficial scar) (separate procedure)	4.92	1.68	0.35	6.95	90	S
44345	00	A	Revision of colostomy; complicated (reconstruction in-depth) (separate procedure)	10.05	4.84	1.03	15.92	90	S
44346	00	A	Revision of colostomy; with repair of paracolostomy hernia (separate procedure)	11.13	6.65	1.38	19.16	90	S
44360	00	A	Small intestinal endoscopy, enteroscopy beyond second portion of duodenum, not including ileum; diagnostic, with or without collection of specimen(s) by brushing or washing (separate procedure)	2.92	3.74	0.32	6.98	0	N
44361	00	A	Small intestinal endoscopy, enteroscopy beyond second portion of duodenum, not including ileum; with biopsy, single or multiple	3.23	4.14	0.34	7.71	0	N
44363	00	A	Small intestinal endoscopy, enteroscopy beyond second portion of duodenum, not including ileum; with removal of foreign body	3.94	2.99	0.36	7.29	0	N
44364	00	A	Small intestinal endoscopy, enteroscopy beyond second portion of duodenum, not including ileum; with removal of tumor(s), polyp(s), or other lesion(s) by snare technique	4.22	4.73	0.72	9.67	0	N
44365	00	A	Small intestinal endoscopy, enteroscopy beyond second portion of duodenum, not including ileum; with removal of tumor(s), polyp(s), or other lesion(s) by hot biopsy forceps or bipolar cautery	3.73	4.73	0.72	9.18	0	N
44366	00	A	Small intestinal endoscopy, enteroscopy beyond second portion of duodenum, not including ileum; with control of bleeding, any method	4.97	5.86	0.45	11.28	0	N
44369	00	A	Small intestinal endoscopy, enteroscopy beyond second portion of duodenum, not including ileum; with ablation of tumor(s), polyp(s), or other lesion(s) not amenable to removal by hot biopsy forceps, bipolar cautery or snare technique	5.09	6.52	0.50	12.11	0	N
44372	00	A	Small intestinal endoscopy, enteroscopy beyond second portion of duodenum, not including ileum; with placement of percutaneous jejunostomy tube	4.97	5.83	0.67	11.47	0	N
44373	00	A	Small intestinal endoscopy, enteroscopy beyond second portion of duodenum, not including ileum; with conversion of percutaneous gastrostomy tube to percutaneous jejunostomy tube	3.94	5.03	0.50	9.47	0	N
44376	00	A	Small intestinal endoscopy, enteroscopy beyond second portion of duodenum, including ileum; diagnostic, with or without collection of specimen(s) by brushing or washing (separate procedure)	5.69	4.05	0.26	10.00	0	N
44377	00	A	Small intestinal endoscopy, enteroscopy beyond second portion of duodenum, including ileum; with biopsy, single or multiple	5.98	4.26	0.28	10.52	0	N
44378	00	A	Small intestinal endoscopy, enteroscopy beyond second portion of duodenum, including ileum; with control of bleeding, any method	7.71	5.27	0.35	13.33	0	N
44380	00	A	Ileoscopy, through stoma; diagnostic, with or without collection of specimen(s) by brushing or washing (separate procedure)	1.51	1.97	0.22	3.70	0	N
44382	00	A	Ileoscopy, through stoma; with biopsy, single or multiple	1.82	2.54	0.29	4.65	0	N

CPT codes and descriptions only, © 1994 American Medical Association. Reimbursement information, © 1995 McGraw-Hill Inc.

Code/ CPT	Mod-ifier	Status	Description	Work value	Practice expense	Mal-practice	Total value	Global period	Up-date
45550	00	A	Proctopexy combined with sigmoid resection, abdominal approach	13.38	11.49	2.38	27.25	90	S
45560	00	A	Repair of rectocele (separate procedure)	7.48	4.79	0.98	13.25	90	S
45562	00	A	Exploration, repair, and presacral drainage for rectal injury;	11.13	8.09	1.58	20.80	90	S
45563	00	A	Exploration, repair, and presacral drainage for rectal injury; with colostomy	17.55	12.77	2.49	32.81	90	S
45800	00	A	Closure of rectovesical fistula;	12.75	9.82	1.45	24.02	90	S
45805	00	A	Closure of rectovesical fistula; with colostomy	15.08	12.32	2.39	29.79	90	S
45820	00	A	Closure of rectourethral fistula;	13.31	8.98	1.23	23.52	90	S
45825	00	A	Closure of rectourethral fistula; with colostomy	15.45	9.87	1.66	26.98	90	S
45900	00	A	Reduction of procidentia (separate procedure) under anesthesia	1.68	0.58	0.11	2.37	10	S
45905	00	A	Dilation of anal sphincter (separate procedure) under anesthesia other than local	1.51	0.71	0.12	2.34	10	S
45910	00	A	Dilation of rectal stricture (separate procedure) under anesthesia other than local	1.86	0.87	0.13	2.86	10	S
45915	00	A	Removal of fecal impaction or foreign body (separate procedure) under anesthesia	2.09	0.78	0.09	2.96	10	N
45999	00	C	Unlisted procedure, rectum	0	0	0	0	YYY	N
46030	00	A	Removal of anal seton, other marker	1.20	0.40	0.07	1.67	10	S
46040	00	A	Incision and drainage of ischiorectal and/or perirectal abscess (separate procedure)	4.90	1.69	0.34	6.93	90	S
46045	00	A	Incision and drainage of intramural, intramuscular or submucosal abscess, transanal, under anesthesia	3.91	1.85	0.38	6.14	90	S
46050	00	A	Incision and drainage, perianal abscess, superficial	1.14	0.60	0.11	1.85	10	S
46060	00	A	Incision and drainage of ischiorectal or intramural abscess, with fistulectomy or fistulotomy, submuscular, with or without placement of seton	5.03	5.35	1.12	11.50	90	S
46070	00	A	Incision, anal septum (infant)	2.63	1.37	0.33	4.33	90	S
46080	00	A	Sphincterotomy, anal, division of sphincter (separate procedure)	2.35	2.13	0.43	4.91	10	S
46083	00	A	Incision of thrombosed hemorrhoid, external	1.35	0.63	0.08	2.06	10	N
46200	00	A	Fissurectomy, with or without sphincterotomy	3.02	3.29	0.66	6.97	90	S
46210	00	A	Cryptectomy; single	2.52	0.77	0.14	3.43	90	S
46211	00	A	Cryptectomy; multiple (separate procedure)	4.07	1.90	0.38	6.35	90	S
46220	00	A	Papillectomy or excision of single tag, anus (separate procedure)	1.51	0.63	0.12	2.26	10	S
46221	00	A	Hemorrhoidectomy, by simple ligature (eg, rubber band)	1.38	0.66	0.14	2.18	10	S
46230	00	A	Excision of external hemorrhoid tags and/or multiple papillae	2.52	0.83	0.12	3.47	10	S
46250	00	A	Hemorrhoidectomy, external, complete	4.29	2.84	0.52	7.65	90	S
46255	00	A	Hemorrhoidectomy, internal and external, simple;	4.95	4.72	0.85	10.52	90	S
46257	00	A	Hemorrhoidectomy, internal and external, simple; with fissurectomy	5.87	5.23	1.08	12.18	90	S
46258	00	A	Hemorrhoidectomy, internal and external, simple; with fistulectomy, with or without fissurectomy	6.26	5.87	1.22	13.35	90	S
46260	00	A	Hemorrhoidectomy, internal and external, complex or extensive;	6.70	6.07	1.25	14.02	90	S
46261	00	A	Hemorrhoidectomy, internal and external, complex or extensive; with fissurectomy	6.54	6.62	1.34	14.50	90	S
46262	00	A	Hemorrhoidectomy, internal and external, complex or extensive; with fistulectomy, with or without fissurectomy	6.77	6.72	1.39	14.88	90	S

CPT codes and descriptions only, © 1994 American Medical Association. Reimbursement information, © 1995 McGraw-Hill Inc.

Code/ CPT	Mod- ifier	Status	Description	Work value	Practice expense	Mal- practice	Total value	Global period	Up- date
45309	00	A	Proctosigmoidoscopy, rigid; with removal of single tumor, polyp, or other lesion by snare technique	2.01	1.13	0.20	3.34	0	S
45315	00	A	Proctosigmoidoscopy, rigid; with removal of multiple tumors, polyps, or other lesions by hot biopsy forceps, bipolar cautery or snare technique	2.54	1.19	0.18	3.91	0	S
45317	00	A	Proctosigmoidoscopy, rigid; with control of bleeding, any method	2.73	1.26	0.19	4.18	0	S
45320	00	A	Proctosigmoidoscopy, rigid; with ablation of tumor(s), polyp(s), or other lesion(s) not amenable to removal by hot biopsy forceps, bipolar cautery or snare technique (eg, laser)	2.88	1.87	0.34	5.09	0	S
45321	00	A	Proctosigmoidoscopy, rigid; with decompression of volvulus	2.12	1.47	0.27	3.86	0	S
45330	00	A	Sigmoidoscopy, flexible; diagnostic, with or without collection of specimen(s) by brushing or washing (separate procedure)	0.96	1.23	0.12	2.31	0	N
45331	00	A	Sigmoidoscopy, flexible; with biopsy, single or multiple	1.26	1.61	0.15	3.02	0	N
45332	00	A	Sigmoidoscopy, flexible; with removal of foreign body	1.96	1.76	0.16	3.88	0	N
45333	00	A	Sigmoidoscopy, flexible; with removal of tumor(s), polyp(s), or other lesion(s) by hot biopsy forceps or bipolar cautery	1.96	2.24	0.26	4.46	0	N
45334	00	A	Sigmoidoscopy, flexible; with control of bleeding, any method	2.99	2.71	0.23	5.93	0	N
45337	00	A	Sigmoidoscopy, flexible; with decompression of volvulus, any method	2.36	3.03	0.38	5.77	0	N
45338	00	A	Sigmoidoscopy, flexible; with removal of tumor(s), polyp(s), or other lesion(s) by snare technique	2.57	2.24	0.26	5.07	0	N
45339	00	A	Sigmoidoscopy, flexible; with ablation of tumor(s), polyp(s), or other lesion(s) not amenable to removal by hot biopsy forceps, bipolar cautery or snare technique	3.14	3.24	0.31	6.69	0	N
45355	00	A	Colonoscopy, rigid or flexible, transabdominal via colotomy, single or multiple	3.52	1.17	0.10	4.79	0	N
45378	00	A	Colonoscopy, flexible, proximal to splenic flexure; diagnostic, with or without collection of specimen(s) by brushing or washing, with or without colon decompression (separate procedure)	3.70	4.13	0.39	8.22	0	N
45379	00	A	Colonoscopy, flexible, proximal to splenic flexure; with removal of foreign body	4.72	5.33	0.45	10.50	0	N
45380	00	A	Colonoscopy, flexible, proximal to splenic flexure; with biopsy, single or multiple	4.01	4.79	0.40	9.20	0	N
45382	00	A	Colonoscopy, flexible, proximal to splenic flexure; with control of bleeding, any method	5.73	5.87	0.41	12.01	0	N
45383	00	A	Colonoscopy, flexible, proximal to splenic flexure; with ablation of tumor(s), polyp(s), or other lesion(s) not amenable to removal by hot biopsy forceps, bipolar cautery or snare technique	5.87	5.92	0.50	12.29	0	N
45384	00	A	Colonoscopy, flexible, proximal to splenic flexure; with removal of tumor(s), polyp(s), or other lesion(s) by hot biopsy forceps or bipolar cautery	4.70	6.65	0.58	11.93	0	N
45385	00	A	Colonoscopy, flexible, proximal to splenic flexure; with removal of tumor(s), polyp(s), or other lesion(s) by snare technique	5.31	6.65	0.58	12.54	0	N
45500	00	A	Proctoplasty; for stenosis	6.59	5.95	1.21	13.75	90	S
45505	00	A	Proctoplasty; for prolapse of mucous membrane	5.54	6.29	1.23	13.06	90	S
45520	00	A	Perirectal injection of sclerosing solution for prolapse	0.55	0.61	0.10	1.26	0	N
45540	00	A	Proctopexy for prolapse; abdominal approach	11.98	9.89	2.10	23.97	90	S
45541	00	A	Proctopexy for prolapse; perineal approach	9.79	10.17	2.04	22.00	90	S

CPT codes and descriptions only, © 1994 American Medical Association. Reimbursement information, © 1995 McGraw-Hill Inc.

Code/ CPT	Mod- ifier	Status	Description	Work value	Practice expense	Mal- practice	Total value	Global period	Up- date
44950	00	A	Appendectomy;	6.06	4.89	1.01	11.96	90	S
44955	00	A	Appendectomy; when done for indicated purpose at time of other major procedure (not as separate procedure)	1.53	2.25	0.60	4.38	ZZZ	S
44960	00	A	Appendectomy; for ruptured appendix with abscess or generalized peritonitis	9.78	5.89	1.24	16.91	90	S
45000	00	A	Transrectal drainage of pelvic abscess	4.28	1.59	0.24	6.11	90	S
45005	00	A	Incision and drainage of submucosal abscess, rectum	1.96	1.29	0.21	3.46	10	S
45020	00	A	Incision and drainage of deep supralevator, pelvirectal, or retrorectal abscess	4.40	2.61	0.51	7.52	90	S
45100	00	A	Biopsy of anorectal wall, anal approach (eg, congenital megacolon)	3.38	1.88	0.35	5.61	90	S
45108	00	A	Anorectal myomectomy	4.28	2.66	0.53	7.47	90	S
45110	00	A	Proctectomy; complete, combined abdominoperineal, with colostomy	21.68	16.32	3.43	41.43	90	S
45111	00	A	Proctectomy; partial resection of rectum, transabdominal approach	14.97	11.77	2.49	29.23	90	S
45112	00	A	Proctectomy, combined abdominoperineal, pull-through procedure (eg, colo-anal anastomosis)	24.02	16.06	3.36	43.44	90	S
45113	00	A	Proctectomy, partial, with rectal mucosectomy, ileoanal anastomosis, creation of ileal reservoir (S or J), with or without loop ileostomy	24.69	16.06	3.36	44.11	90	S
45114	00	A	Proctectomy, partial, with anastomosis; abdominal and transsacral approach	21.20	15.39	3.24	39.83	90	S
45116	00	A	Proctectomy, partial, with anastomosis; transacral approach only (Kraske type)	19.09	10.77	2.34	32.20	90	S
45120	00	A	Proctectomy, complete (for congenital megacolon), abdominal and perineal approach; with pull-through procedure and anastomosis (eg, Swenson, Duhamel, or Soave type operation)	22.78	16.39	3.54	42.71	90	S
45121	00	A	Proctectomy, complete (for congenital megacolon), abdominal and perineal approach; with subtotal or total colectomy, with multiple biopsies	24.96	10.79	2.01	37.76	90	S
45123	00	A	Proctectomy, partial, without anastomosis, perineal approach	13.27	11.77	2.49	27.53	90	S
45130	00	A	Excision of rectal procidentia, with anastomosis; perineal approach	13.03	8.92	1.79	23.74	90	S
45135	00	A	Excision of rectal procidentia, with anastomosis; abdominal and perineal approach	15.36	15.95	3.50	34.81	90	S
45150	00	A	Division of stricture of rectum	5.26	3.38	0.63	9.27	90	S
45160	00	A	Excision of rectal tumor by proctotomy, transacral or transcoccygeal approach	12.34	7.46	1.56	21.36	90	S
45170	00	A	Excision of rectal tumor, transanal approach	9.40	4.62	0.96	14.98	90	S
45180	00	D	Removal of rectal lesion	4.22*	2.21#	0.51*	6.94#	90	S
45190	00	A	Destruction of rectal tumor, any method (eg, electrodesiccation) transanal approach	7.91	5.09	1.06	14.06	90	S
45300	00	A	Proctosigmoidoscopy, rigid; diagnostic, with or without collection of specimen(s) by brushing or washing (separate procedure)	0.70	0.55	0.07	1.32	0	S
45303	00	A	Proctosigmoidoscopy, rigid; with dilation, any method	0.50	0.65	0.12	1.27	0	S
45305	00	A	Proctosigmoidoscopy, rigid; with biopsy, single or multiple	1.01	0.84	0.14	1.99	0	S
45307	00	A	Proctosigmoidoscopy, rigid; with removal of foreign body	1.71	1.27	0.18	3.16	0	S
45308	00	A	Proctosigmoidoscopy, rigid; with removal of single tumor, polyp, or other lesion by hot biopsy forceps or bipolar cautery	1.51	1.13	0.20	2.84	0	S

CPT codes and descriptions only, © 1994 American Medical Association. Reimbursement information, © 1995 McGraw-Hill Inc.

Code/ CPT	Mod-ifier	Status	Description	Work value	Practice expense	Mal-practice	Total value	Global period	Up-date
44385	00	A	Endoscopic evaluation of small intestinal (abdominal or pelvic) pouch; diagnostic, with or without collection of specimen(s) by brushing or washing (separate procedure)	1.82	2.44	0.34	4.60	0	S
44386	00	A	Endoscopic evaluation of small intestinal (abdominal or pelvic) pouch; with biopsy, single or multiple	2.12	1.54	0.15	3.81	0	N
44388	00	A	Colonoscopy through stoma; diagnostic, with or without collection of specimen(s) by brushing or washing (separate procedure)	2.82	3.61	0.50	6.93	0	S
44389	00	A	Colonoscopy through stoma; with biopsy, single or multiple	3.13	4.00	0.45	7.58	0	N
44390	00	A	Colonoscopy through stoma; with removal of foreign body	3.83	2.63	0.28	6.74	0	N
44391	00	A	Colonoscopy through stoma; with control of bleeding, any method	4.32	5.26	0.53	10.11	0	N
44392	00	A	Colonoscopy through stoma; with removal of tumor(s), polyp(s), or other lesion(s) by hot biopsy forceps or bipolar cautery	3.82	5.16	0.70	9.68	0	N
44393	00	A	Colonoscopy through stoma; with ablation of tumor(s), polyp(s), or other lesion(s) not amenable to removal by hot biopsy forceps, bipolar cautery or snare technique	4.84	5.41	0.70	10.95	0	N
44394	00	A	Colonoscopy through stoma; with removal of tumor(s), polyp(s), or other lesion(s) by snare technique	4.43	5.16	0.70	10.29	0	N
44500	00	A	Introduction of long gastrointestinal tube (eg, Miller-Abbott) (separate procedure)	0.49	0.36	0.02	0.87	0	N
44602	00	A	Suture of small intestine (enterorrhaphy) for perforated ulcer, diverticulum, wound, injury or rupture; single perforation	9.72	7.65	1.62	18.99	90	S
44603	00	A	Suture of small intestine (enterorrhaphy) for perforated ulcer, diverticulum, wound, injury or rupture; multiple perforations	12.94	9.09	1.96	23.99	90	S
44604	00	A	Suture of large intestine (colorrhaphy) for perforated ulcer, diverticulum, wound, injury or rupture (single or multiple perforations); without colostomy	12.94	7.87	1.67	22.48	90	S
44605	00	A	Suture of large intestine (colorrhaphy) for perforated ulcer, diverticulum, wound, injury or rupture (single or multiple perforations); with colostomy	13.91	9.37	2.02	25.30	90	S
44615	00	A	Intestinal stricturoplasty (enterotomy and enterorrhaphy) with or without dilation, for intestinal obstruction	12.89	6.74	1.57	21.20	90	S
44620	00	A	Closure of enterostomy, large or small intestine;	9.65	5.97	1.26	16.88	90	S
44625	00	A	Closure of enterostomy, large or small intestine; with resection and anastomosis	12.10	9.58	2.03	23.71	90	S
44640	00	A	Closure of intestinal cutaneous fistula	13.34	6.54	1.35	21.23	90	S
44650	00	A	Closure of enteroenteric or enterocolic fistula	13.76	7.33	1.46	22.55	90	S
44660	00	A	Closure of enterovesical fistula; without intestinal or bladder resection	13.14	8.34	1.21	22.69	90	S
44661	00	A	Closure of enterovesical fistula; with bowel and/or bladder resection	15.44	13.94	2.52	31.90	90	S
44680	00	A	Intestinal plication (separate procedure)	12.41	9.71	2.14	24.26	90	S
44799	00	C	Unlisted procedure, intestine	0	0	0	0	YYY	S
44800	00	A	Excision of Meckel's diverticulum (diverticulectomy) or omphalomesenteric duct	10.12	5.24	1.08	16.44	90	S
44820	00	A	Excision of lesion of mesentery (separate procedure)	9.31	5.80	1.21	16.32	90	S
44850	00	A	Suture of mesentery (separate procedure)	8.64	5.60	1.18	15.42	90	S
44899	00	C	Unlisted procedure, Meckel's diverticulum and the mesentery	0	0	0	0	YYY	S
44900	00	A	Incision and drainage of appendiceal abscess, transabdominal	7.86	4.28	0.88	13.02	90	S

CPT codes and descriptions only, © 1994 American Medical Association. Reimbursement information, © 1995 McGraw-Hill Inc.

Code/ CPT	Mod- ifier	Status	Description	Work value	Practice expense	Mal- practice	Total value	Global period	Up- date
50135	00	A	Pyelotomy; complicated (eg, secondary operation, congenital kidney abnormality)	18.14	17.05	1.63	36.82	90	S
50200	00	A	Renal biopsy; percutaneous, by trocar or needle	2.63	2.61	0.22	5.46	0	N
50205	00	A	Renal biopsy; by surgical exposure of kidney	12.69	5.64	0.69	19.02	90	S
50220	00	A	Nephrectomy, including partial ureterectomy, any approach including rib resection;	15.98	13.31	1.43	30.72	90	S
50225	00	A	Nephrectomy, including partial ureterectomy, any approach including rib resection; complicated because of previous surgery on same kidney	18.93	16.52	1.70	37.15	90	S
50230	00	A	Nephrectomy, including partial ureterectomy, any approach including rib resection; radical, with regional lymphadenectomy and/or vena caval thrombectomy	20.56	18.40	1.84	40.80	90	S
50234	00	A	Nephrectomy with total ureterectomy and bladder cuff; through same incision	21.11	16.65	1.65	39.41	90	S
50236	00	A	Nephrectomy with total ureterectomy and bladder cuff; through separate incision	23.33	17.74	1.74	42.81	90	S
50240	00	A	Nephrectomy, partial	20.24	16.00	1.70	37.94	90	S
50280	00	A	Excision or unroofing of cyst(s) of kidney	14.63	10.86	1.16	26.65	90	S
50290	00	A	Excision of perinephric cyst	13.69	8.87	1.19	23.75	90	S
50300	00	X	Donor nephrectomy, with preparation and maintenance of allograft; from cadaver donor, unilateral or bilateral	21.10*	14.98#	1.46*	37.54#	XXX	0
50320	00	A	Donor nephrectomy, with preparation and maintenance of allograft; from living donor	21.22	16.49	2.40	40.11	90	S
50340	00	A	Recipient nephrectomy (separate procedure)	10.73	12.49	2.24	25.46	90	S
50360	00	A	Renal allotransplantation, implantation of graft; excluding donor and recipient nephrectomy	27.05	24.45	4.24	55.74	90	S
50365	00	A	Renal allotransplantation, implantation of graft; with recipient nephrectomy	32.54	30.71	3.89	67.14	90	S
50370	00	A	Removal of transplanted renal allograft	11.11	11.08	1.92	24.11	90	S
50380	00	A	Renal autotransplantation, reimplantation of kidney	16.49	10.12	1.71	28.32	90	S
50390	00	A	Aspiration and/or injection of renal cyst or pelvis by needle, percutaneous	3.24	1.69	0.15	5.08	0	N
50392	00	A	Introduction of intracatheter or catheter into renal pelvis for drainage and/or injection, percutaneous	5.59	2.36	0.20	8.15	0	N
50393	00	A	Introduction of ureteral catheter or stent into ureter through renal pelvis for drainage and/or injection, percutaneous	6.88	3.01	0.26	10.15	0	N
50394	00	A	Injection procedure for pyelography (as nephrostogram, pyelostogram, antegrade pyeloureterograms) through nephrostomy or pyelostomy tube, or indwelling ureteral catheter	0.76	0.55	0.05	1.36	0	N
50395	00	A	Introduction of guide into renal pelvis and/or ureter with dilation to establish nephrostomy tract, percutaneous	5.15	3.33	0.29	8.77	0	N
50396	00	A	Manometric studies through nephrostomy or pyelostomy tube, or indwelling ureteral catheter	2.09	0.50	0.05	2.64	0	N
50398	00	A	Change of nephrostomy or pyelostomy tube	1.46	0.53	0.05	2.04	0	S
50400	00	A	Pyeloplasty (Foley Y-pyeloplasty), plastic operation on renal pelvis, with or without plastic operation on ureter, nephropexy, nephrostomy, pyelostomy, or ureteral splinting; simple	18.07	13.66	1.36	33.09	90	S
50405	00	A	Pyeloplasty (Foley Y-pyeloplasty), plastic operation on renal pelvis, with or without plastic operation on ureter, nephropexy, nephrostomy, pyelostomy, or ureteral splinting; complicated (congenital kidney abnormality, secondary pyeloplasty, solitary kidney, calycoplasty)	22.45	17.29	1.74	41.48	90	S

CPT codes and descriptions only, © 1994 American Medical Association. Reimbursement information, © 1995 McGraw-Hill Inc.

Code/ CPT	Mod-ifier	Status	Description	Work value	Practice expense	Mal-practice	Total value	Global period	Up-date
49568	00	A	Implantation of mesh or other prosthesis for incisional hernia repair (list separately in addition to code for the incisional hernia repair)	4.89	2.56	0.59	8.04	ZZZ	S
49570	00	A	Repair epigastric hernia (eg, preperitoneal fat); reducible (separate procedure)	4.46	4.38	0.91	9.75	90	S
49572	00	A	Repair epigastric hernia (eg, preperitoneal fat); incarcerated or strangulated	5.35	5.60	1.18	12.13	90	S
49580	00	A	Repair umbilical hernia, under age 5 years; reducible	3.24	4.15	0.94	8.33	90	S
49582	00	A	Repair umbilical hernia, under age 5 years; incarcerated or strangulated	5.13	4.61	0.94	10.68	90	S
49585	00	A	Repair umbilical hernia, age 5 years or over; reducible	4.95	4.41	0.91	10.27	90	S
49587	00	A	Repair umbilical hernia, age 5 years or over; incarcerated or strangulated	5.93	4.41	0.91	11.25	90	S
49590	00	A	Repair spigelian hernia	6.55	5.63	1.22	13.40	90	S
49600	00	A	Repair of small omphalocele, with primary closure	9.48	5.26	0.77	15.51	90	S
49605	00	A	Repair of large omphalocele or gastroschisis; with or without prosthesis	21.92	8.57	1.77	32.26	90	S
49606	00	A	Repair of large omphalocele or gastroschisis; with removal of prosthesis, final reduction and closure, in operating room	17.93	8.31	0.96	27.20	90	S
49610	00	A	Repair of omphalocele (Gross type operation); first stage	9.83	5.48	1.27	16.58	90	S
49611	00	A	Repair of omphalocele (Gross type operation); second stage	8.25	9.00	0.58	17.83	90	S
49900	00	A	Suture, secondary, of abdominal wall for evisceration or dehiscence	4.54	3.66	0.75	8.95	90	S
49905	00	A	Omental flap (eg, for reconstruction of sternal and chest wall defects) (list separately in addition to code for primary procedure)	6.55	3.42	0.80	10.77	ZZZ	S
49999	00	C	Unlisted procedure, abdomen, peritoneum and omentum	0	0	0	0	YYY	S
50010	00	A	Renal exploration, not necessitating other specific procedures	10.07	9.55	1.13	20.75	90	S
50020	00	A	Drainage of perirenal or renal abscess (separate procedure)	12.41	6.80	0.85	20.06	90	S
50040	00	A	Nephrostomy, nephrotomy with drainage	13.80	7.18	0.62	21.60	90	N
50045	00	A	Nephrotomy, with exploration	14.48	9.81	0.89	25.18	90	S
50060	00	A	Nephrolithotomy; removal of calculus	18.00	12.25	1.21	31.46	90	S
50065	00	A	Nephrolithotomy; secondary surgical operation for calculus	19.62	13.93	1.35	34.90	90	S
50070	00	A	Nephrolithotomy; complicated by congenital kidney abnormality	19.15	12.87	1.35	33.37	90	S
50075	00	A	Nephrolithotomy; removal of large staghorn calculus filling renal pelvis and calyces (including anatrophic pyelolithotomy)	24.05	16.87	1.62	42.54	90	S
50080	00	A	Percutaneous nephrostolithotomy or pyelostolithotomy, with or without dilation, endoscopy, lithotripsy, stenting or basket extraction; up to 2 cm	13.98	12.20	1.15	27.33	90	S
50081	00	A	Percutaneous nephrostolithotomy or pyelostolithotomy, with or without dilation, endoscopy, lithotripsy, stenting or basket extraction; over 2 cm	20.58	14.96	1.44	36.98	90	S
50100	00	A	Transection or repositioning of aberrant renal vessels (separate procedure)	15.11	10.34	1.35	26.80	90	S
50120	00	A	Pyelotomy; with exploration	15.00	10.91	1.24	27.15	90	S
50125	00	A	Pyelotomy; with drainage, pyelostomy	15.61	10.95	1.06	27.62	90	S
50130	00	A	Pyelotomy; with removal of calculus (pyelolithotomy, pelviolithotomy, including coagulum pyelolithotomy)	16.12	12.80	1.26	30.18	90	S

CPT codes and descriptions only, © 1994 American Medical Association. Reimbursement information, © 1995 McGraw-Hill Inc.

Code/ CPT	Mod- ifier	Status	Description	Work value	Practice expense	Mal- practice	Total value	Global period	Up- date
50500	00	A	Nephrorrhaphy, suture of kidney wound or injury	18.27	12.46	1.64	32.37	90	S
50520	00	A	Closure of nephrocutaneous or pyelocutaneous fistula	15.93	10.34	1.50	27.77	90	S
50525	00	A	Closure of nephrovisceral fistula (eg, renocolic), including visceral repair; abdominal approach	20.59	12.61	1.99	35.19	90	S
50526	00	A	Closure of nephrovisceral fistula (eg, renocolic), including visceral repair; thoracic approach	22.15	7.39	2.32	31.86	90	S
50540	00	A	Symphysiotomy for horseshoe kidney with or without pyeloplasty and/or other plastic procedure, unilateral or bilateral (one operation)	19.15	13.41	1.54	34.10	90	S
50551	00	A	Renal endoscopy through established nephrostomy or pyelostomy, with or without irrigation, instillation, or ureteropyelography, exclusive of radiologic service;	5.60	2.19	0.21	8.00	0	S
50553	00	A	Renal endoscopy through established nephrostomy or pyelostomy, with or without irrigation, instillation, or ureteropyelography, exclusive of radiologic service; with ureteral catheterization, with or without dilation of ureter	5.99	1.66	0.17	7.82	0	S
50555	00	A	Renal endoscopy through established nephrostomy or pyelostomy, with or without irrigation, instillation, or ureteropyelography, exclusive of radiologic service; with biopsy	6.53	4.70	0.45	11.68	0	S
50557	00	A	Renal endoscopy through established nephrostomy or pyelostomy, with or without irrigation, instillation, or ureteropyelography, exclusive of radiologic service; with fulguration and/or incision, with or without biopsy	6.62	4.71	0.49	11.82	0	S
50559	00	A	Renal endoscopy through established nephrostomy or pyelostomy, with or without irrigation, instillation, or ureteropyelography, exclusive of radiologic service; with insertion of radioactive substance with or without biopsy and/or fulguration	6.78	1.34	0.14	8.26	0	S
50561	00	A	Renal endoscopy through established nephrostomy or pyelostomy, with or without irrigation, instillation, or ureteropyelography, exclusive of radiologic service; with removal of foreign body or calculus	7.59	5.12	0.49	13.20	0	S
50570	00	A	Renal endoscopy through nephrotomy or pyelotomy, with or without irrigation, instillation, or ureteropyelography, exclusive of radiologic service;	9.54	1.45	0.14	11.13	0	S
50572	00	A	Renal endoscopy through nephrotomy or pyelotomy, with or without irrigation, instillation, or ureteropyelography, exclusive of radiologic service; with ureteral catheterization, with or without dilation of ureter	10.35	7.25	0.75	18.35	0	S
50574	00	A	Renal endoscopy through nephrotomy or pyelotomy, with or without irrigation, instillation, or ureteropyelography, exclusive of radiologic service; with biopsy	11.02	7.08	0.64	18.74	0	S
50575	00	A	Renal endoscopy through nephrotomy or pyelotomy, with or without irrigation, instillation, or ureteropyelography, exclusive of radiologic service; with endopyelotomy (includes cystoscopy, ureteroscopy, dilation of ureter and ureteral pelvic junction, incision of ureteral pelvic junction and insertion of endopyelotomy stent)	13.98	9.93	0.97	24.88	0	S
50576	00	A	Renal endoscopy through nephrotomy or pyelotomy, with or without irrigation, instillation, or ureteropyelography, exclusive of radiologic service; with fulguration and/or incision, with or without biopsy	10.99	8.69	0.77	20.45	0	S
50578	00	A	Renal endoscopy through nephrotomy or pyelotomy, with or without irrigation, instillation, or ureteropyelography, exclusive of radiologic service; with insertion of radioactive substance, with or without biopsy and/or fulguration	11.35	3.79	1.19	16.33	0	S

CPT codes and descriptions only, © 1994 American Medical Association. Reimbursement information, © 1995 McGraw-Hill Inc.

Code/ CPT	Mod- ifier	Status	Description	Work value	Practice expense	Mal- practice	Total value	Global period	Up- date
50580	00	A	Renal endoscopy through nephrotomy or pyelotomy, with or without irrigation, instillation, or ureteropyelography, exclusive of radiologic service; with removal of foreign body or calculus	11.86	3.58	0.35	15.79	0	S
50590	00	A	Lithotripsy, extracorporeal shock wave	9.62	10.11	0.97	20.70	90	S
50600	00	A	Ureterotomy with exploration or drainage (separate procedure)	14.78	9.69	1.01	25.48	90	S
50605	00	A	Ureterotomy for insertion of indwelling stent, all types	14.40	6.11	0.60	21.11	90	S
50610	00	A	Ureterolithotomy; upper one-third of ureter	14.86	11.77	1.17	27.80	90	S
50620	00	A	Ureterolithotomy; middle one-third of ureter	14.17	11.49	1.16	26.82	90	S
50630	00	A	Ureterolithotomy; lower one-third of ureter	13.95	12.71	1.25	27.91	90	S
50650	00	A	Ureterectomy, with bladder cuff (separate procedure)	16.37	12.07	1.21	29.65	90	S
50660	00	A	Ureterectomy, total, ectopic ureter, combination abdominal, vaginal and/or perineal approach	18.44	12.49	1.53	32.46	90	S
50684	00	A	Injection procedure for ureterography or ureteropyelography through ureterostomy or indwelling ureteral catheter	0.76	0.49	0.05	1.30	0	S
50686	00	A	Manometric studies through ureterostomy or indwelling ureteral catheter	1.51	0.37	0.04	1.92	0	S
50688	00	A	Change of ureterostomy tube	1.14	0.39	0.04	1.57	10	S
50690	00	A	Injection procedure for visualization of ileal conduit and/or ureteropyelography, exclusive of radiologic service	1.16	0.32	0.03	1.51	0	S
50700	00	A	Ureteroplasty, plastic operation on ureter (eg, stricture)	14.10	12.57	1.29	27.96	90	S
50715	00	A	Ureterolysis, with or without repositioning of ureter for retroperitoneal fibrosis	17.60	11.24	1.49	30.33	90	S
50722	00	A	Ureterolysis for ovarian vein syndrome	15.11	10.32	1.97	27.40	90	S
50725	00	A	Ureterolysis for retrocaval ureter, with reanastomosis of upper urinary tract or vena cava	17.12	12.05	1.75	30.92	90	S
50727	00	A	Revision of urinary-cutaneous anastomosis (any type urostomy);	7.57	5.37	0.51	13.45	90	S
50728	00	A	Revision of urinary-cutaneous anastomosis (any type urostomy); with repair of fascial defect and hernia	11.13	7.90	0.77	19.80	90	S
50740	00	A	Ureteropyelostomy, anastomosis of ureter and renal pelvis	17.12	13.03	1.88	32.03	90	S
50750	00	A	Ureterocalycostomy, anastomosis of ureter to renal calyx	18.14	14.04	1.26	33.44	90	S
50760	00	A	Ureteroureterostomy	17.12	13.47	1.48	32.07	90	S
50770	00	A	Transureteroureterostomy, anastomosis of ureter to contralateral ureter	18.14	15.23	1.53	34.90	90	S
50780	00	A	Ureteroneocystostomy; anastomosis of single ureter to bladder	17.12	13.78	1.46	32.36	90	S
50782	00	A	Ureteroneocystostomy; anastomosis of duplicated ureter to bladder	18.23	13.78	1.46	33.47	90	S
50783	00	A	Ureteroneocystostomy; with extensive ureteral tailoring	19.17	13.78	1.46	34.41	90	S
50785	00	A	Ureteroneocystostomy; with vesico-psoas hitch or bladder flap	19.15	15.42	1.80	36.37	90	S
50800	00	A	Ureteroenterostomy, direct anastomosis of ureter to intestine	13.10	14.67	1.51	29.28	90	S
50810	00	A	Ureterosigmoidostomy, with creation of sigmoid bladder and establishment of abdominal or perineal colostomy, including bowel anastomosis	18.14	12.57	1.75	32.46	90	S
50815	00	A	Ureterocolon conduit, including bowel anastomosis	18.14	19.76	2.75	40.65	90	S
50820	00	A	Ureteroileal conduit (ileal bladder), including bowel anastomosis (Bricker operation)	20.15	18.97	2.50	41.62	90	S

CPT codes and descriptions only, © 1994 American Medical Association. Reimbursement information, © 1995 McGraw-Hill Inc.

Code/ CPT	Mod- ifier	Status	Description	Work value	Practice expense	Mal- practice	Total value	Global period	Up- date
50825	00	A	Continent diversion, including bowel anastomosis using any segment of small and/or large bowel (Kock pouch or Camey enterocystoplasty)	26.19	30.54	3.33	60.06	90	S
50830	00	A	Urinary undiversion (eg, taking down of ureteroileal conduit, ureterosigmoidostomy or ureteroenterostomy with ureteroureterostomy or ureteroneocystostomy)	29.29	20.93	2.27	52.49	90	S
50840	00	A	Replacement of all or part of ureter by bowel segment, including bowel anastomosis	18.14	13.32	1.35	32.81	90	S
50845	00	A	Cutaneous appendico-vesicostomy	19.52	13.87	1.35	34.74	90	S
50860	00	A	Ureterostomy, transplantation of ureter to skin	13.99	10.92	1.16	26.07	90	S
50900	00	A	Ureterorrhaphy, suture of ureter (separate procedure)	12.58	9.98	1.15	23.71	90	S
50920	00	A	Closure of ureterocutaneous fistula	13.22	9.52	0.99	23.73	90	S
50930	00	A	Closure of ureterovisceral fistula (including visceral repair)	17.61	12.50	1.22	31.33	90	S
50940	00	A	Deligation of ureter	13.47	9.90	0.95	24.32	90	S
50951	00	A	Ureteral endoscopy through established ureterostomy, with or without irrigation, instillation, or ureteropyelography, exclusive of radiologic service;	5.84	1.67	0.17	7.68	0	S
50953	00	A	Ureteral endoscopy through established ureterostomy, with or without irrigation, instillation, or ureteropyelography, exclusive of radiologic service; with ureteral catheterization, with or without dilation of ureter	6.24	1.66	0.16	8.06	0	S
50955	00	A	Ureteral endoscopy through established ureterostomy, with or without irrigation, instillation, or ureteropyelography, exclusive of radiologic service; with biopsy	6.75	2.55	0.25	9.55	0	S
50957	00	A	Ureteral endoscopy through established ureterostomy, with or without irrigation, instillation, or ureteropyelography, exclusive of radiologic service; with fulguration and/or incision, with or without biopsy	6.79	2.50	0.25	9.54	0	S
50959	00	A	Ureteral endoscopy through established ureterostomy, with or without irrigation, instillation, or ureteropyelography, exclusive of radiologic service; with insertion of radioactive substance, with or without biopsy and/or fulguration (not including provision of material)	4.40	3.38	0.29	8.07	0	S
50961	00	A	Ureteral endoscopy through established ureterostomy, with or without irrigation, instillation, or ureteropyelography, exclusive of radiologic service; with removal of foreign body or calculus	6.05	2.62	0.26	8.93	0	S
50970	00	A	Ureteral endoscopy through ureterotomy, with or without irrigation, instillation, or ureteropyelography, exclusive of radiologic service;	7.14	5.17	0.52	12.83	0	S
50972	00	A	Ureteral endoscopy through ureterotomy, with or without irrigation, instillation, or ureteropyelography, exclusive of radiologic service; with ureteral catheterization, with or without dilation of ureter	6.89	1.54	0.16	8.59	0	S
50974	00	A	Ureteral endoscopy through ureterotomy, with or without irrigation, instillation, or ureteropyelography, exclusive of radiologic service; with biopsy	9.17	7.01	0.65	16.83	0	S
50976	00	A	Ureteral endoscopy through ureterotomy, with or without irrigation, instillation, or ureteropyelography, exclusive of radiologic service; with fulguration and/or incision, with or without biopsy	9.04	6.41	0.62	16.07	0	S
50978	00	A	Ureteral endoscopy through ureterotomy, with or without irrigation, instillation, or ureteropyelography, exclusive of radiologic service; with insertion of radioactive substance, with or without biopsy and/or fulguration (not including provision of material)	5.10	4.05	0.48	9.63	0	S

CPT codes and descriptions only, © 1994 American Medical Association. Reimbursement information, © 1995 McGraw-Hill Inc.

Code/ CPT	Mod-ifier	Status	Description	Work value	Practice expense	Mal-practice	Total value	Global period	Up-date
50980	00	A	Ureteral endoscopy through ureterotomy, with or without irrigation, instillation, or ureteropyelography, exclusive of radiologic service; with removal of foreign body or calculus	6.85	3.13	0.30	10.28	0	S
51000	00	A	Aspiration of bladder by needle	0.78	0.48	0.05	1.31	0	S
51005	00	A	Aspiration of bladder; by trocar or intracatheter	1.02	0.46	0.04	1.52	0	S
51010	00	A	Aspiration of bladder; with insertion of suprapubic catheter	2.54	0.97	0.11	3.62	10	S
51020	00	A	Cystotomy or cystostomy; with fulguration and/or insertion of radioactive material	6.04	6.85	0.71	13.60	90	S
51030	00	A	Cystotomy or cystostomy; with cryosurgical destruction of intravesical lesion	6.04	4.53	0.43	11.00	90	S
51040	00	A	Cystostomy, cystotomy with drainage	4.08	5.70	0.75	10.53	90	S
51045	00	A	Cystotomy, with insertion of ureteral catheter or stent (separate procedure)	6.04	4.96	0.50	11.50	90	S
51050	00	A	Cystolithotomy, cystotomy with removal of calculus, without vesical neck resection	6.04	7.12	0.70	13.86	90	S
51060	00	A	Transvesical ureterolithotomy	8.05	10.31	1.19	19.55	90	S
51065	00	A	Cystotomy, with stone basket extraction and/or ultrasonic or electrohydraulic fragmentation of ureteral calculus	8.05	7.08	0.71	15.84	90	S
51080	00	A	Drainage of perivesical or prevesical space abscess	5.41	5.18	0.57	11.16	90	S
51500	00	A	Excision of urachal cyst or sinus, with or without umbilical hernia repair	9.54	6.86	1.21	17.61	90	S
51520	00	A	Cystotomy; for simple excision of vesical neck (separate procedure)	8.69	8.53	0.87	18.09	90	S
51525	00	A	Cystotomy; for excision of bladder diverticulum, single or multiple (separate procedure)	12.78	10.67	1.06	24.51	90	S
51530	00	A	Cystotomy; for excision of bladder tumor	11.32	9.25	1.02	21.59	90	S
51535	00	A	Cystotomy for excision, incision, or repair of ureterocele	11.51	7.68	1.14	20.33	90	S
51550	00	A	Cystectomy, partial; simple	14.34	10.71	1.17	26.22	90	S
51555	00	A	Cystectomy, partial; complicated (eg, postradiation, previous surgery, difficult location)	19.60	12.26	1.31	33.17	90	S
51565	00	A	Cystectomy, partial, with reimplantation of ureter(s) into bladder (ureteroneocystostomy)	20.01	15.84	1.67	37.52	90	S
51570	00	A	Cystectomy, complete; (separate procedure)	22.16	15.66	1.62	39.44	90	S
51575	00	A	Cystectomy, complete; with bilateral pelvic lymphadenectomy, including external iliac, hypogastric and obturator nodes	27.93	22.87	2.25	53.05	90	S
51580	00	A	Cystectomy, complete, with ureterosigmoidostomy or ureterocutaneous transplantations;	28.20	19.95	2.04	50.19	90	S
51585	00	A	Cystectomy, complete, with ureterosigmoidostomy or ureterocutaneous transplantations; with bilateral pelvic lymphadenectomy, including external iliac, hypogastric and obturator nodes	32.22	25.12	2.42	59.76	90	S
51590	00	A	Cystectomy, complete, with ureteroileal conduit or sigmoid bladder, including bowel anastomosis;	30.21	24.52	2.56	57.29	90	S
51595	00	A	Cystectomy, complete, with ureteroileal conduit or sigmoid bladder, including bowel anastomosis; with bilateral pelvic lymphadenectomy, including external iliac, hypogastric and obturator nodes	34.25	33.80	3.34	71.39	90	S
51596	00	A	Cystectomy, complete, with continent diversion, any technique, using any segment of small and/or large bowel to construct neobladder	36.27	34.89	3.45	74.61	90	S

CPT codes and descriptions only, © 1994 American Medical Association. Reimbursement information, © 1995 McGraw-Hill Inc.

Code/ CPT	Mod-ifier	Status	Description	Work value	Practice expense	Mal-practice	Total value	Global period	Up-date
51597	00	A	Pelvic exenteration, complete, for vesical, prostatic or urethral malignancy, with removal of bladder and ureteral transplantations, with or without hysterectomy and/or abdominoperineal resection of rectum and colon and colostomy, or any combination thereof	35.27	30.63	4.31	70.21	90	S
51600	00	A	Injection procedure for cystography or voiding urethrocystography	0.88	0.28	0.03	1.19	0	S
51605	00	A	Injection procedure and placement of chain for contrast and/or chain urethrocystography	1.13	0.30	0.03	1.46	0	S
51610	00	A	Injection procedure for retrograde urethrocystography	1.59	0.27	0.02	1.88	0	S
51700	00	A	Bladder irrigation, simple, lavage and/or instillation	0.88	0.22	0.02	1.12	0	S
51705	00	A	Change of cystostomy tube; simple	0.99	0.38	0.04	1.41	10	S
51710	00	A	Change of cystostomy tube; complicated	1.46	0.57	0.06	2.09	10	S
51715	00	A	Endoscopic injection of implant material into the submucosal tissues of the urethra and/or bladder neck	3.74	2.65	0.27	6.66	0	S
51720	00	A	Bladder instillation of anticarcinogenic agent (including detention time)	1.96	0.45	0.05	2.46	0	S
51725	00	A	Simple cystometrogram (CMG) (eg, spinal manometer)	1.51	1.01	0.11	2.63	0	S
51725	26			1.51	0.63	0.07	2.21	0	S
51725	TC			0	0.38	0.04	0.42	0	S
51726	00	A	Complex cystometrogram (eg, calibrated electronic equipment)	1.71	1.29	0.13	3.13	0	S
51726	26			1.71	0.81	0.08	2.60	0	S
51726	TC			0	0.48	0.05	0.53	0	S
51736	00	A	Simple uroflowmetry (UFR) (eg, stop-watch flow rate, mechanical uroflowmeter)	0.84	0.41	0.04	1.29	0	S
51736	26			0.84	0.26	0.03	1.13	0	S
51736	TC			0	0.15	0.01	0.16	0	S
51741	00	A	Complex uroflowmetry (eg, calibrated electronic equipment)	1.57	0.56	0.06	2.19	0	S
51741	26			1.57	0.35	0.04	1.96	0	S
51741	TC			0	0.21	0.02	0.23	0	S
51772	00	A	Urethral pressure profile studies (UPP) (urethral closure pressure profile), any technique	1.61	0.94	0.11	2.66	0	S
51772	26			1.61	0.52	0.06	2.19	0	S
51772	TC			0	0.42	0.05	0.47	0	S
51784	00	A	Electromyography studies (EMG) of anal or urethral sphincter, other than needle, any technique	1.53	1.04	0.11	2.68	0	S
51784	26			1.53	0.65	0.07	2.25	0	S
51784	TC			0	0.39	0.04	0.43	0	S
51785	00	A	Needle electromyography studies (EMG) of anal or urethral sphincter, any technique	1.53	1.04	0.11	2.68	0	S
51785	26			1.53	0.65	0.07	2.25	0	S
51785	TC			0	0.39	0.04	0.43	0	S
51792	00	A	Stimulus evoked response (eg, measurement of bulbocavernosus reflex latency time)	1.10	1.93	0.20	3.23	0	S
51792	26			1.10	0.59	0.06	1.75	0	S
51792	TC			0	1.34	0.14	1.48	0	S
51795	00	A	Voiding pressure studies (VP); bladder voiding pressure, any technique	1.53	1.44	0.16	3.13	0	S
51795	26			1.53	0.57	0.06	2.16	0	S
51795	TC			0	0.87	0.10	0.97	0	S

CPT codes and descriptions only, © 1994 American Medical Association. Reimbursement information, © 1995 McGraw-Hill Inc.

Code/ CPT	Mod- ifier	Status	Description	Work value	Practice expense	Mal- practice	Total value	Global period	Up- date
51797	00	A	Voiding pressure studies (VP); intra-abdominal voiding pressure (AP) (rectal, gastric, intraperitoneal)	1.60	0.96	0.10	2.66	0	S
51797	26			1.60	0.51	0.05	2.16	0	S
51797	TC			0	0.45	0.05	0.50	0	S
51800	00	A	Cystoplasty or cystourethroplasty, plastic operation on bladder and/or vesical neck (anterior Y-plasty, vesical fundus resection), any procedure, with or without wedge resection of posterior vesical neck	16.31	12.02	1.47	29.80	90	S
51820	00	A	Cystourethroplasty with unilateral or bilateral ureteroneocystostomy	16.67	7.39	1.32	25.38	90	S
51840	00	A	Anterior vesicourethropexy, or urethropexy (Marshall-Marchetti-Krantz type); simple	9.78	9.22	1.26	20.26	90	S
51841	00	A	Anterior vesicourethropexy, or urethropexy (Marshall-Marchetti-Krantz type); complicated (eg, secondary repair)	12.10	11.01	1.48	24.59	90	S
51845	00	A	Abdomino-vaginal vesical neck suspension, with or without endoscopic control (eg, Stamey, Raz, modified Pereyra)	9.06	10.71	1.09	20.86	90	S
51860	00	A	Cystorrhaphy, suture of bladder wound, injury or rupture; simple	11.17	7.62	0.91	19.70	90	S
51865	00	A	Cystorrhaphy, suture of bladder wound, injury or rupture; complicated	13.99	10.96	1.27	26.22	90	S
51880	00	A	Closure of cystostomy (separate procedure)	7.21	4.96	0.52	12.69	90	S
51900	00	A	Closure of vesicovaginal fistula, abdominal approach	11.67	11.65	1.41	24.73	90	S
51920	00	A	Closure of vesicouterine fistula;	10.57	7.51	0.73	18.81	90	S
51925	00	A	Closure of vesicouterine fistula; with hysterectomy	14.10	10.07	2.33	26.50	90	S
51940	00	A	Closure of bladder exstrophy	25.00	18.95	2.22	46.17	90	S
51960	00	A	Enterocystoplasty, including bowel anastomosis	21.15	21.40	2.27	44.82	90	S
51980	00	A	Cutaneous vesicostomy	10.43	7.46	0.75	18.64	90	S
52000	00	A	Cystourethroscopy (separate procedure)	2.01	1.33	0.14	3.48	0	S
52005	00	A	Cystourethroscopy, with ureteral catheterization, with or without irrigation, instillation, or ureteropyelography, exclusive of radiologic service;	2.37	2.20	0.22	4.79	0	S
52007	00	A	Cystourethroscopy, with ureteral catheterization, with or without irrigation, instillation, or ureteropyelography, exclusive of radiologic service; with brush biopsy of ureter and/or renal pelvis	3.02	2.82	0.28	6.12	0	S
52010	00	A	Cystourethroscopy, with ejaculatory duct catheterization, with or without irrigation, instillation, or duct radiography, exclusive of radiologic service	3.02	1.90	0.20	5.12	0	S
52204	00	A	Cystourethroscopy, with biopsy	2.37	2.38	0.24	4.99	0	S
52214	00	A	Cystourethroscopy, with fulguration (including cryosurgery or laser surgery) of trigone, bladder neck, prostatic fossa, urethra, or periurethral glands	3.71	2.80	0.28	6.79	0	S
52224	00	A	Cystourethroscopy, with fulguration (including cryosurgery or laser surgery) or treatment of MINOR (less than 0.5 cm) lesion(s) with or without biopsy	3.14	2.90	0.29	6.33	0	S
52234	00	A	Cystourethroscopy, with fulguration (including cryosurgery or laser surgery) and/or resection of; SMALL bladder tumor(s) (0.5 to 2.0 cm)	4.63	4.71	0.45	9.79	0	S
52235	00	A	Cystourethroscopy, with fulguration (including cryosurgery or laser surgery) and/or resection of; MEDIUM bladder tumor(s) (2.0 to 5.0 cm)	5.45	6.97	0.81	13.23	0	S
52240	00	A	Cystourethroscopy, with fulguration (including cryosurgery or laser surgery) and/or resection of; LARGE bladder tumor(s)	9.72	10.65	1.04	21.41	0	S

CPT codes and descriptions only, © 1994 American Medical Association. Reimbursement information, © 1995 McGraw-Hill Inc.

Code/ CPT	Mod- ifier	Status	Description	Work value	Practice expense	Mal- practice	Total value	Global period	Up- date
52250	00	A	Cystourethroscopy with insertion of radioactive substance, with or without biopsy or fulguration	4.50	2.86	0.29	7.65	0	S
52260	00	A	Cystourethroscopy, with dilation of bladder for interstitial cystitis; general or conduction (spinal) anesthesia	3.92	2.11	0.22	6.25	0	S
52265	00	A	Cystourethroscopy, with dilation of bladder for interstitial cystitis; local anesthesia	2.94	1.35	0.14	4.43	0	S
52270	00	A	Cystourethroscopy, with internal urethrotomy; female	3.84	3.47	0.35	7.66	0	S
52275	00	A	Cystourethroscopy, with internal urethrotomy; male	4.70	3.42	0.34	8.46	0	S
52276	00	A	Cystourethroscopy with direct vision internal urethrotomy	3.93	4.58	0.45	8.96	0	S
52277	00	A	Cystourethroscopy, with resection of external sphincter (sphincterotomy)	6.17	4.82	0.47	11.46	0	S
52281	00	A	Cystourethroscopy, with calibration and/or dilation of urethral stricture or stenosis, with or without meatotomy and injection procedure for cystography, male or female	2.80	2.31	0.23	5.34	0	S
52283	00	A	Cystourethroscopy, with steroid injection into stricture	3.74	1.51	0.15	5.40	0	S
52285	00	A	Cystourethroscopy for treatment of the female urethral syndrome with any or all of the following: urethral meatotomy, urethral dilation, internal urethrotomy, lysis of urethrovaginal septal fibrosis, lateral incisions of the bladder neck, and fulguration of polyp(s) of urethra, bladder neck, and/or trigone	3.61	2.94	0.30	6.85	0	S
52290	00	A	Cystourethroscopy; with ureteral meatotomy, unilateral or bilateral	4.59	2.34	0.24	7.17	0	S
52300	00	A	Cystourethroscopy; with resection or fulguration of ureterocele(s), unilateral or bilateral	5.35	3.47	0.36	9.18	0	S
52305	00	A	Cystourethroscopy; with incision or resection of orifice of bladder diverticulum, single or multiple	5.31	3.50	0.35	9.16	0	S
52310	00	A	Cystourethroscopy, with removal of foreign body, calculus, or ureteral stent from urethra or bladder (separate procedure); simple	2.81	2.99	0.30	6.10	0	S
52315	00	A	Cystourethroscopy, with removal of foreign body, calculus, or ureteral stent from urethra or bladder (separate procedure); complicated	5.21	4.07	0.40	9.68	0	S
52317	00	A	Litholapaxy: crushing or fragmentation of calculus by any means in bladder and removal of fragments; simple or small (less than 2.5 cm)	6.72	6.19	0.59	13.50	0	S
52318	00	A	Litholapaxy: crushing or fragmentation of calculus by any means in bladder and removal of fragments; complicated or large (over 2.5 cm)	9.19	7.88	0.77	17.84	0	S
52320	00	A	Cystourethroscopy (including ureteral catheterization); with removal of ureteral calculus	4.70	4.86	0.47	10.03	0	S
52325	00	A	Cystourethroscopy (including ureteral catheterization); with fragmentation of ureteral calculus (eg, ultrasonic or electro-hydraulic technique)	6.16	7.01	0.68	13.85	0	S
52327	00	A	Cystourethroscopy (including ureteral catheterization); with subureteric injection of implant material	5.19	3.69	0.36	9.24	0	S
52330	00	A	Cystourethroscopy (including ureteral catheterization); with manipulation, without removal of ureteral calculus	5.04	3.47	0.35	8.86	0	S
52332	00	A	Cystourethroscopy, with insertion of indwelling ureteral stent (eg, Gibbons or double-J type)	2.83	3.21	0.32	6.36	0	S
52334	00	A	Cystourethroscopy with insertion of ureteral guide wire through kidney to establish a percutaneous nephrostomy, retrograde	4.83	3.33	0.34	8.50	0	S
52335	00	A	Cystourethroscopy, with ureteroscopy and/or pyeloscopy (includes dilation of the ureter and/or pyeloureteral junction by any method);	5.86	4.69	0.45	11.00	0	S

CPT codes and descriptions only, © 1994 American Medical Association. Reimbursement information, © 1995 McGraw-Hill Inc.

Code/ CPT	Mod- ifier	Status	Description	Work value	Practice expense	Mal- practice	Total value	Global period	Up- date
52336	00	A	Cystourethroscopy, with ureteroscopy and/or pyeloscopy (includes dilation of the ureter and/or pyeloureteral junction by any method); with removal or manipulation of calculus (ureteral catheterization is included)	6.88	8.81	0.99	16.68	0	S
52337	00	A	Cystourethroscopy, with ureteroscopy and/or pyeloscopy (includes dilation of the ureter and/or pyeloureteral junction by any method); with lithotripsy (ureteral catheterization is included)	7.97	10.21	1.08	19.26	0	S
52338	00	A	Cystourethroscopy, with ureteroscopy and/or pyeloscopy (includes dilation of the ureter and/or pyeloureteral junction by any method); with biopsy and/or fulguration of lesion	7.34	5.92	0.57	13.83	0	S
52339	00	A	Cystourethroscopy, with ureteroscopy and/or pyeloscopy (includes dilation of the ureter and/or pyeloureteral junction by any method); with resection of tumor	8.82	5.92	0.57	15.31	0	S
52340	00	A	Cystourethroscopy with incision, fulguration, or resection of bladder neck and/or posterior urethra (congenital valves, obstructive hypertrophic mucosal folds)	7.76	5.15	0.50	13.41	90	S
52450	00	A	Transurethral incision of prostate	7.05	4.99	0.49	12.53	90	S
52500	00	A	Transurethral resection of bladder neck (separate procedure)	7.82	7.44	0.72	15.98	90	S
52510	00	A	Transurethral balloon dilation of the prostatic urethra, any method	6.04	7.64	0.74	14.42	90	S
52601	00	A	Transurethral electrosurgical resection of prostate, including control of postoperative bleeding, complete (vasectomy, meatotomy, cystourethroscopy, urethral calibration and/or dilation, and internal urethrotomy are included)	11.51	11.87	1.16	24.54	90	S
52606	00	A	Transurethral fulguration for postoperative bleeding occurring after the usual follow-up time	7.51	3.32	0.33	11.16	90	S
52612	00	A	Transurethral resection of prostate; first stage of two-stage resection (partial resection)	7.05	9.03	0.99	17.07	90	S
52614	00	A	Transurethral resection of prostate; second stage of two-stage resection (resection completed)	6.04	7.09	0.68	13.81	90	S
52620	00	A	Transurethral resection; of residual obstructive tissue after 90 days postoperative	6.04	5.33	0.51	11.88	90	S
52630	00	A	Transurethral resection; of regrowth of obstructive tissue longer than one year postoperative	6.55	9.01	1.13	16.69	90	S
52640	00	A	Transurethral resection; of postoperative bladder neck contracture	6.04	6.43	0.62	13.09	90	S
52647	00	A	Non-contact laser coagulation of prostate, including control of postoperative bleeding, complete (vasectomy, meatotomy, cystourethroscopy, urethral calibration and/or dilation, and internal urethrotomy are included)	7.42	11.87	1.16	20.45	90	S
52648	00	A	Contact laser vaporization with or without transurethral resection of prostate, including control of postoperative bleeding, complete (vasectomy, meatotomy, cystourethroscopy, urethral calibration and/or dilation, and internal urethrotomy are included)	8.65	11.87	1.16	21.68	90	S
52650	00	D	Prostatectomy	14.07*	9.99#	0.98*	25.04#	90	S
52700	00	A	Transurethral drainage of prostatic abscess	6.31	3.30	0.34	9.95	90	S
53000	00	A	Urethrotomy or urethrostomy, external (separate procedure); pendulous urethra	2.01	1.76	0.17	3.94	10	S
53010	00	A	Urethrotomy or urethrostomy, external (separate procedure); perineal urethra, external	3.02	3.52	0.37	6.91	90	S
53020	00	A	Meatotomy, cutting of meatus (separate procedure); except infant	1.77	0.82	0.09	2.68	0	S

CPT codes and descriptions only, © 1994 American Medical Association. Reimbursement information, © 1995 McGraw-Hill Inc.

Code/ CPT	Mod-ifier	Status	Description	Work value	Practice expense	Mal-practice	Total value	Global period	Up-date
53025	00	A	Meatotomy, cutting of meatus (separate procedure); infant	1.13	0.80	0.08	2.01	0	S
53040	00	A	Drainage of deep periurethral abscess	6.01	1.85	0.19	8.05	90	S
53060	00	A	Drainage of Skene's gland abscess or cyst	2.58	0.51	0.07	3.16	10	S
53080	00	A	Drainage of perineal urinary extravasation; uncomplicated (separate procedure)	5.87	3.98	0.45	10.30	90	S
53085	00	A	Drainage of perineal urinary extravasation; complicated	9.67	6.75	0.70	17.12	90	S
53200	00	A	Biopsy of urethra	2.59	1.10	0.12	3.81	0	S
53210	00	A	Urethrectomy, total, including cystostomy; female	11.71	6.64	0.67	19.02	90	S
53215	00	A	Urethrectomy, total, including cystostomy; male	14.59	10.00	0.96	25.55	90	S
53220	00	A	Excision or fulguration of carcinoma of urethra	6.58	4.77	0.49	11.84	90	S
53230	00	A	Excision of urethral diverticulum (separate procedure); female	9.04	7.93	0.79	17.76	90	S
53235	00	A	Excision of urethral diverticulum (separate procedure); male	9.60	5.02	0.49	15.11	90	N
53240	00	A	Marsupialization of urethral diverticulum, male or female	6.03	4.33	0.45	10.81	90	S
53250	00	A	Excision of bulbourethral gland (Cowper's gland)	5.69	4.05	0.40	10.14	90	S
53260	00	A	Excision or fulguration; urethral polyp(s), distal urethra	2.93	1.12	0.16	4.21	10	S
53265	00	A	Excision or fulguration; urethral caruncle	3.07	1.88	0.22	5.17	10	S
53270	00	A	Excision or fulguration; Skene's glands	2.93	0.84	0.18	3.95	10	S
53275	00	A	Excision or fulguration; urethral prolapse	4.37	2.37	0.25	6.99	10	S
53400	00	A	Urethroplasty; first stage, for fistula, diverticulum, or stricture (eg, Johannsen type)	11.79	7.47	0.76	20.02	90	S
53405	00	A	Urethroplasty; second stage (formation of urethra), including urinary diversion	13.70	10.38	1.21	25.29	90	S
53410	00	A	Urethroplasty, one-stage reconstruction of male anterior urethra	15.59	8.56	0.84	24.99	90	S
53415	00	A	Urethroplasty, transpubic or perineal, one stage, for reconstruction or repair of prostatic or membranous urethra	18.50	11.87	1.15	31.52	90	S
53420	00	A	Urethroplasty, two-stage reconstruction or repair of prostatic or membranous urethra; first stage	13.28	10.88	1.05	25.21	90	S
53425	00	A	Urethroplasty, two-stage reconstruction or repair of prostatic or membranous urethra; second stage	15.18	9.25	0.88	25.31	90	S
53430	00	A	Urethroplasty, reconstruction of female urethra	15.54	7.16	0.76	23.46	90	S
53440	00	A	Operation for correction of male urinary incontinence, with or without introduction of prosthesis	11.49	13.14	1.39	26.02	90	S
53442	00	A	Removal of perineal prosthesis introduced for continence	7.67	5.84	0.67	14.18	90	S
53443	00	A	Urethroplasty with tubularization of posterior urethra and/or lower bladder for incontinence (eg, Tenago, Leadbetter procedure)	18.98	10.03	1.07	30.08	90	S
53445	00	A	Operation for correction of urinary incontinence with placement of inflatable urethral or bladder neck sphincter, including placement of pump and/or reservoir	13.15	16.83	2.03	32.01	90	S
53447	00	A	Removal, repair or replacement of inflatable sphincter including pump and/or reservoir and/or cuff	12.37	9.16	0.89	22.42	90	S
53449	00	A	Surgical correction of hydraulic abnormality of inflatable sphincter device	9.16	8.41	0.82	18.39	90	S
53450	00	A	Urethromeatoplasty, with mucosal advancement	5.72	2.74	0.27	8.73	90	S
53460	00	A	Urethromeatoplasty, with partial excision of distal urethral segment (Richardson type procedure)	6.70	2.44	0.25	9.39	90	S
53502	00	A	Urethrorrhaphy, suture of urethral wound or injury, female	7.21	4.97	0.56	12.74	90	S
53505	00	A	Urethrorrhaphy, suture of urethral wound or injury; penile	7.21	5.18	0.51	12.90	90	S

CPT codes and descriptions only, © 1994 American Medical Association. Reimbursement information, © 1995 McGraw-Hill Inc.

Code/ CPT	Mod- ifier	Status	Description	Work value	Practice expense	Mal- practice	Total value	Global period	Up- date
53510	00	A	Urethrorrhaphy, suture of urethral wound or injury; perineal	9.57	6.98	0.66	17.21	90	S
53515	00	A	Urethrorrhaphy, suture of urethral wound or injury; prostatomembranous	12.71	9.03	0.88	22.62	90	S
53520	00	A	Closure of urethrostomy or urethrocutaneous fistula, male (separate procedure)	8.21	5.89	0.56	14.66	90	S
53600	00	A	Dilation of urethral stricture by passage of sound or urethral dilator, male; initial	1.21	0.33	0.03	1.57	0	S
53601	00	A	Dilation of urethral stricture by passage of sound or urethral dilator, male; subsequent	0.98	0.29	0.03	1.30	0	S
53605	00	A	Dilation of urethral stricture or vesical neck by passage of sound or urethral dilator, male, general or conduction (spinal) anesthesia	1.28	0.46	0.05	1.79	0	S
53620	00	A	Dilation of urethral stricture by passage of filiform and follower, male; initial	1.62	0.47	0.05	2.14	0	S
53621	00	A	Dilation of urethral stricture by passage of filiform and follower, male; subsequent	1.35	0.38	0.04	1.77	0	S
53640	00	A	Passage of filiform and follower for acute vesical retention, male	1.59	0.57	0.06	2.22	0	S
53660	00	A	Dilation of female urethra including suppository and/or instillation; initial	0.71	0.28	0.03	1.02	0	S
53661	00	A	Dilation of female urethra including suppository and/or instillation; subsequent	0.72	0.25	0.03	1.00	0	S
53665	00	A	Dilation of female urethra, general or conduction (spinal) anesthesia	0.76	0.36	0.04	1.16	0	S
53670	00	A	Catheterization, urethra; simple	0.50	0.22	0.02	0.74	0	S
53675	00	A	Catheterization, urethra; complicated (may include difficult removal of balloon catheter)	1.47	0.47	0.05	1.99	0	S
53800	00	D	Urinalysis; two or three glass test including examination of urine specimen(s), any method	0.14*	0.10#	0.01*	0.25#	XXX	0
53899	00	C	Unlisted procedure, urinary system	0	0	0	0	YYY	S
54000	00	A	Slitting of prepuce, dorsal or lateral (separate procedure); newborn	1.49	0.63	0.07	2.19	10	S
54001	00	A	Slitting of prepuce, dorsal or lateral (separate procedure); except newborn	2.14	0.84	0.09	3.07	10	S
54015	00	A	Incision and drainage of penis, deep	5.16	0.83	0.09	6.08	10	S
54050	00	A	Destruction of lesion(s), penis (eg, condyloma, papilloma, molluscum contagiosum, herpetic vesicle), simple; chemical	1.19	0.38	0.03	1.60	10	S
54055	00	A	Destruction of lesion(s), penis (eg, condyloma, papilloma, molluscum contagiosum, herpetic vesicle), simple; electrodesiccation	1.19	0.61	0.06	1.86	10	S
54056	00	A	Destruction of lesion(s), penis (eg, condyloma, papilloma, molluscum contagiosum, herpetic vesicle), simple; cryosurgery	1.19	0.53	0.04	1.76	10	S
54057	00	A	Destruction of lesion(s), penis (eg, condyloma, papilloma, molluscum contagiosum, herpetic vesicle), simple; laser surgery	1.19	1.61	0.21	3.01	10	S
54060	00	A	Destruction of lesion(s), penis (eg, condyloma, papilloma, molluscum contagiosum, herpetic vesicle), simple; surgical excision	1.88	1.17	0.12	3.17	10	S
54065	00	A	Destruction of lesion(s), penis (eg, condyloma, papilloma, molluscum contagiosum, herpetic vesicle), extensive, any method	2.37	2.47	0.25	5.09	10	S
54100	00	A	Biopsy of penis; cutaneous (separate procedure)	1.90	0.65	0.07	2.62	0	S
54105	00	A	Biopsy of penis; deep structures	3.45	1.01	0.11	4.57	10	S

CPT codes and descriptions only, © 1994 American Medical Association. Reimbursement information, © 1995 McGraw-Hill Inc.

Code/ CPT	Mod-ifier	Status	Description	Work value	Practice expense	Mal-practice	Total value	Global period	Up-date
54110	00	A	Excision of penile plaque (Peyronie disease);	9.66	6.03	0.61	16.30	90	S
54111	00	A	Excision of penile plaque (Peyronie disease); with graft to 5 cm in length	13.03	9.18	0.97	23.18	90	S
54112	00	A	Excision of penile plaque (Peyronie disease); with graft greater than 5 cm in length	15.14	10.84	1.14	27.12	90	S
54115	00	A	Removal foreign body from deep penile tissue (eg, plastic implant)	5.68	4.18	0.44	10.30	90	S
54120	00	A	Amputation of penis; partial	9.24	6.47	0.62	16.33	90	S
54125	00	A	Amputation of penis; complete	12.80	11.56	1.17	25.53	90	S
54130	00	A	Amputation of penis, radical; with bilateral inguinofemoral lymphadenectomy	18.92	14.66	1.32	34.90	90	S
54135	00	A	Amputation of penis, radical; in continuity with bilateral pelvic lymphadenectomy, including external iliac, hypogastric and obturator nodes	25.01	17.75	1.74	44.50	90	S
54150	00	A	Circumcision, using clamp or other device; newborn	1.78	0.54	0.05	2.37	10	S
54152	00	A	Circumcision, using clamp or other device; except newborn	2.26	1.82	0.20	4.28	10	S
54160	00	A	Circumcision, surgical excision other than clamp, device or dorsal slit; newborn	2.43	1.66	0.21	4.30	10	S
54161	00	A	Circumcision, surgical excision other than clamp, device or dorsal slit; except newborn	3.22	2.17	0.23	5.62	10	S
54200	00	A	Injection procedure for Peyronie disease;	1.01	0.32	0.03	1.36	10	S
54205	00	A	Injection procedure for Peyronie disease; with surgical exposure of plaque	7.20	5.11	0.50	12.81	90	S
54220	00	A	Irrigation of corpora cavernosa for priapism	2.42	1.58	0.17	4.17	0	S
54230	00	A	Injection procedure for corpora cavernosography	1.34	1.34	0.13	2.81	0	S
54231	00	A	Dynamic cavernosometry, including intracavernosal injection of vasoactive drugs (eg, papaverine, phentolamine)	2.04	1.44	0.14	3.62	0	S
54235	00	A	Injection of corpora cavernosa with pharmacologic agent(s) (eg, papaverine, phentolamine)	1.19	0.43	0.04	1.66	0	S
54240	00	A	Penile plethysmography	1.31	0.99	0.12	2.42	0	S
54240	26			1.31	0.51	0.06	1.88	0	S
54240	TC			0	0.48	0.06	0.54	0	S
54250	00	A	Nocturnal penile tumescence and/or rigidity test	2.22	0.80	0.08	3.10	0	S
54250	26			2.22	0.50	0.05	2.77	0	S
54250	TC			0	0.30	0.03	0.33	0	S
54300	00	A	Plastic operation of penis for straightening of chordee (eg, hypospadias), with or without mobilization of urethra	10.05	6.88	0.87	17.80	90	S
54304	00	A	Plastic operation on penis for correction of chordee or for first stage hypospadias repair with or without transplantation of prepuce and/or skin flaps	12.13	8.66	0.90	21.69	90	S
54308	00	A	Urethroplasty for second stage hypospadias repair (including urinary diversion); less than 3 cm	11.58	5.84	0.74	18.16	90	S
54312	00	A	Urethroplasty for second stage hypospadias repair (including urinary diversion); greater than 3 cm	13.16	9.37	0.91	23.44	90	S
54316	00	A	Urethroplasty for second stage hypospadias repair (including urinary diversion) with free skin graft obtained from site other than genitalia	15.97	11.34	1.12	28.43	90	S
54318	00	A	Urethroplasty for third stage hypospadias repair to release penis from scrotum (eg, third stage Cecil repair)	10.47	7.53	1.11	19.11	90	S
54322	00	A	One stage distal hypospadias repair (with or without chordee or circumcision); with simple meatal advancement (eg, Magpi, V-flap)	12.34	7.61	0.74	20.69	90	S

CPT codes and descriptions only, © 1994 American Medical Association. Reimbursement information, © 1995 McGraw-Hill Inc.

Code/ CPT	Mod- ifier	Status	Description	Work value	Practice expense	Mal- practice	Total value	Global period	Up- date
54324	00	A	One stage distal hypospadias repair (with or without chordee or circumcision); with urethroplasty by local skin flaps (eg, flip-flap, prepucial flap)	15.46	10.98	1.08	27.52	90	S
54326	00	A	One stage distal hypospadias repair (with or without chordee or circumcision); with urethroplasty by local skin flaps and mobilization of urethra	14.81	10.51	1.03	26.35	90	S
54328	00	A	One stage distal hypospadias repair (with or without chordee or circumcision); with extensive dissection to correct chordee and urethroplasty with local skin flaps, skin graft patch, and/or island flap	14.80	10.72	1.24	26.76	90	S
54332	00	A	One stage proximal penile or penoscrotal hypospadias repair requiring extensive dissection to correct chordee and urethroplasty by use of skin graft tube and/or island flap	16.17	12.52	1.13	29.82	90	S
54336	00	A	One stage perineal hypospadias repair requiring extensive dissection to correct chordee and urethroplasty by use of skin graft tube and/or island flap	18.95	18.79	1.40	39.14	90	S
54340	00	A	Repair of hypospadias complications (ie, fistula, stricture, diverticula); by closure, incision, or excision, simple	8.55	6.07	0.59	15.21	90	S
54344	00	A	Repair of hypospadias complications (ie, fistula, stricture, diverticula); requiring mobilization of skin flaps and urethroplasty with flap or patch graft	15.22	16.61	1.10	32.93	90	S
54348	00	A	Repair of hypospadias complications (ie, fistula, stricture, diverticula); requiring extensive dissection and urethroplasty with flap, patch or tubed graft (includes urinary diversion)	16.37	11.62	1.14	29.13	90	S
54352	00	A	Repair of hypospadias cripple requiring extensive dissection and excision of previously constructed structures including re-release of chordee and reconstruction of urethra and penis by use of local skin as grafts and island flaps and skin brought in as flaps or grafts	23.84	16.18	1.49	41.51	90	S
54360	00	A	Plastic operation on penis to correct angulation	11.39	7.02	0.73	19.14	90	S
54380	00	A	Plastic operation on penis for epispadias distal to external sphincter;	12.59	9.42	0.75	22.76	90	S
54385	00	A	Plastic operation on penis for epispadias distal to external sphincter; with incontinence	14.75	10.46	0.89	26.10	90	S
54390	00	A	Plastic operation on penis for epispadias distal to external sphincter; with exstrophy of bladder	20.97	13.57	1.58	36.12	90	S
54400	00	A	Insertion of penile prosthesis; non-inflatable (semi-rigid)	8.58	10.99	1.27	20.84	90	S
54401	00	A	Insertion of penile prosthesis; inflatable (self-contained)	9.67	13.76	1.73	25.16	90	S
54402	00	A	Removal or replacement of non-inflatable (semi-rigid) or inflatable (self-contained) penile prosthesis	8.67	6.00	0.58	15.25	90	S
54405	00	A	Insertion of inflatable (multi-component) penile prosthesis, including placement of pump, cylinders, and/or reservoir	12.63	17.10	2.10	31.83	90	S
54407	00	A	Removal, repair, or replacement of inflatable (multi-component) penile prosthesis, including pump and/or reservoir and/or cylinders	12.61	11.22	1.10	24.93	90	S
54409	00	A	Surgical correction of hydraulic abnormality of inflatable (multi-component) prosthesis including pump and/or reservoir and/or cylinders	11.53	8.97	0.87	21.37	90	S
54420	00	A	Corpora cavernosa-saphenous vein shunt (priapism operation), unilateral or bilateral	10.75	7.74	0.87	19.36	90	S
54430	00	A	Corpora cavernosa-corpus spongiosum shunt (priapism operation), unilateral or bilateral	9.55	6.99	0.69	17.23	90	S
54435	00	A	Corpora cavernosa-glans penis fistulization (eg, biopsy needle, Winter procedure, rongeur, or punch) for priapism	5.63	4.15	0.39	10.17	90	S

CPT codes and descriptions only, © 1994 American Medical Association. Reimbursement information, © 1995 McGraw-Hill Inc.

Code/ CPT	Mod- ifier	Status	Description	Work value	Practice expense	Mal- practice	Total value	Global period	Up- date
57105	00	A	Biopsy of vaginal mucosa; extensive, requiring suture (including cysts)	1.64	1.57	0.33	3.54	10	S
57108	00	A	Colpectomy, obliteration of vagina; partial	5.69	5.28	1.10	12.07	90	S
57110	00	A	Colpectomy, obliteration of vagina; complete	13.48	7.88	1.76	23.12	90	S
57120	00	A	Colpocleisis (Le Fort type)	6.73	6.99	1.51	15.23	90	S
57130	00	A	Excision of vaginal septum	2.40	2.62	0.55	5.57	10	S
57135	00	A	Excision of vaginal cyst or tumor	2.64	1.93	0.38	4.95	10	S
57150	00	A	Irrigation of vagina and/or application of medicament for treatment of bacterial, parasitic, or fungoid disease	0.94	0.19	0.04	1.17	0	S
57160	00	A	Insertion of pessary	0.89	0.25	0.05	1.19	0	S
57170	00	A	Diaphragm or cervical cap fitting with instructions	0.91	0.32	0.06	1.29	0	S
57180	00	A	Introduction of any hemostatic agent or pack for spontaneous or traumatic nonobstetrical vaginal hemorrhage (separate procedure)	1.53	0.55	0.11	2.19	10	S
57200	00	A	Colporrhaphy, suture of injury of vagina (nonobstetrical)	3.68	2.71	0.60	6.99	90	S
57210	00	A	Colpoperineorrhaphy, suture of injury of vagina and/or perineum (nonobstetrical)	4.73	3.27	0.65	8.65	90	S
57220	00	A	Plastic operation on urethral sphincter, vaginal approach (eg, Kelly urethral plication)	3.87	4.44	0.80	9.11	90	S
57230	00	A	Plastic repair of urethrocele	5.07	3.84	0.64	9.55	90	S
57240	00	A	Anterior colporrhaphy, repair of cystocele with or without repair of urethrocele	5.39	6.90	1.60	13.89	90	S
57250	00	A	Posterior colporrhaphy, repair of rectocele with or without perineorrhaphy	4.96	6.40	1.69	13.05	90	S
57260	00	A	Combined anteroposterior colporrhaphy;	7.59	8.65	1.88	18.12	90	S
57265	00	A	Combined anteroposterior colporrhaphy; with enterocele repair	7.36	9.42	2.11	18.89	90	S
57268	00	A	Repair of enterocele, vaginal approach (separate procedure)	6.14	7.02	1.50	14.66	90	S
57270	00	A	Repair of enterocele, abdominal approach (separate procedure)	7.36	6.83	1.44	15.63	90	S
57280	00	A	Colpopexy, abdominal approach	8.35	8.53	1.85	18.73	90	S
57282	00	A	Sacrospinous ligament fixation for prolapse of vagina	8.06	8.72	1.89	18.67	90	S
57288	00	A	Sling operation for stress incontinence (eg, fascia or synthetic)	12.34	10.72	1.36	24.42	90	S
57289	00	A	Pereyra procedure, including anterior colporrhaphy	6.40	8.19	1.13	15.72	90	S
57291	00	A	Construction of artificial vagina; without graft	7.46	5.35	1.19	14.00	90	S
57292	00	A	Construction of artificial vagina; with graft	12.34	6.55	1.38	20.27	90	S
57300	00	A	Closure of rectovaginal fistula; vaginal or transanal approach	6.81	7.91	1.66	16.38	90	S
57305	00	A	Closure of rectovaginal fistula; abdominal approach	8.69	7.55	1.56	17.80	90	S
57307	00	A	Closure of rectovaginal fistula; abdominal approach, with concomitant colostomy	10.05	6.11	1.28	17.44	90	S
57310	00	A	Closure of urethrovaginal fistula;	6.10	4.32	0.48	10.90	90	S
57311	00	A	Closure of urethrovaginal fistula; with bulbocavernosus transplant	7.23	5.58	0.41	13.22	90	S
57320	00	A	Closure of vesicovaginal fistula; vaginal approach	7.33	9.38	1.35	18.06	90	S
57330	00	A	Closure of vesicovaginal fistula; transvesical and vaginal approach	11.67	8.29	0.81	20.77	90	S
57335	00	A	Vaginoplasty for intersex state	9.11	6.91	0.81	16.83	90	S
57400	00	A	Dilation of vagina under anesthesia	0.83	0.33	0.06	1.22	0	S
57410	00	A	Pelvic examination under anesthesia	0.59	0.36	0.05	1.00	0	S

CPT codes and descriptions only, © 1994 American Medical Association. Reimbursement information, © 1995 McGraw-Hill Inc.

Code/ CPT	Mod- ifier	Status	Description	Work value	Practice expense	Mal- practice	Total value	Global period	Up- date
57415	00	A	Removal of impacted vaginal foreign body (separate procedure) under anesthesia	0.91	0.36	0.05	1.32	10	S
57452	00	A	Colposcopy (vaginoscopy); (separate procedure)	0.99	0.65	0.14	1.78	0	S
57454	00	A	Colposcopy (vaginoscopy); with biopsy(s) of the cervix and/or endocervical curettage	1.27	1.21	0.26	2.74	0	S
57460	00	A	Colposcopy (vaginoscopy); with loop electrode excision procedure of the cervix	2.83	2.02	0.46	5.31	0	S
57500	00	A	Biopsy, single or multiple, or local excision of lesion, with or without fulguration (separate procedure)	0.97	0.57	0.12	1.66	0	S
57505	00	A	Endocervical curettage (not done as part of a dilation and curettage)	1.09	0.63	0.13	1.85	10	S
57510	00	A	Cauterization of cervix; electro or thermal	1.85	0.52	0.09	2.46	10	S
57511	00	A	Cauterization of cervix; cryocautery, initial or repeat	1.85	0.85	0.17	2.87	10	S
57513	00	A	Cauterization of cervix; laser ablation	1.85	2.47	0.67	4.99	10	S
57520	00	A	Conization of cervix, with or without fulguration, with or without dilation and curettage, with or without repair; cold knife or laser	3.96	3.45	0.73	8.14	90	S
57522	00	A	Conization of cervix, with or without fulguration, with or without dilation and curettage, with or without repair; loop electrode excision	3.26	3.45	0.73	7.44	90	S
57530	00	A	Trachelectomy (cervicectomy), amputation of cervix (separate procedure)	4.42	3.61	0.78	8.81	90	S
57540	00	A	Excision of cervical stump, abdominal approach;	6.01	6.74	1.51	14.26	90	S
57545	00	A	Excision of cervical stump, abdominal approach; with pelvic floor repair	6.63	4.58	1.03	12.24	90	S
57550	00	A	Excision of cervical stump, vaginal approach;	4.91	6.28	1.54	12.73	90	S
57555	00	A	Excision of cervical stump, vaginal approach; with anterior and/or posterior repair	8.14	10.10	2.17	20.41	90	S
57556	00	A	Excision of cervical stump, vaginal approach; with repair of enterocele	7.56	9.44	1.92	18.92	90	S
57700	00	A	Cerclage of uterine cervix, nonobstetrical	3.30	2.39	0.34	6.03	90	S
57720	00	A	Trachelorrhaphy, plastic repair of uterine cervix, vaginal approach	3.87	2.76	0.50	7.13	90	S
57800	00	A	Dilation of cervical canal, instrumental (separate procedure)	0.77	0.48	0.10	1.35	0	S
57820	00	A	Dilation and curettage of cervical stump	1.62	2.08	0.46	4.16	10	S
58100	00	A	Endometrial and/or endocervical sampling (biopsy), without cervical dilation, any method (separate procedure)	0.71	0.66	0.14	1.51	0	S
58120	00	A	Dilation and curettage, diagnostic and/or therapeutic (nonobstetrical)	2.45	2.70	0.56	5.71	10	S
58140	00	A	Myomectomy, excision of fibroid tumor of uterus, single or multiple (separate procedure); abdominal approach	7.61	8.33	1.71	17.65	90	S
58145	00	A	Myomectomy, excision of fibroid tumor of uterus, single or multiple (separate procedure); vaginal approach	7.36	8.24	1.54	17.14	90	S
58150	00	A	Total abdominal hysterectomy (corpus and cervix), with or without removal of tube(s), with or without removal of ovary(s);	13.00	9.57	2.08	24.65	90	S
58152	00	A	Total abdominal hysterectomy (corpus and cervix), with or without removal of tube(s), with or without removal of ovary(s); with colpo-urethrocystopexy (Marshall-Marchetti-Krantz type)	14.10	11.99	2.59	28.68	90	S
58180	00	A	Supracervical abdominal hysterectomy (subtotal hysterectomy), with or without removal of tube(s), with or without removal of ovary(s)	9.06	9.76	2.11	20.93	90	S

CPT codes and descriptions only, © 1994 American Medical Association. Reimbursement information, © 1995 McGraw-Hill Inc.

Code/ CPT	Mod- ifier	Status	Description	Work value	Practice expense	Mal- practice	Total value	Global period	Up- date
58200	00	A	Total abdominal hysterectomy, including partial vaginectomy, with para-aortic and pelvic lymph node sampling, with or without removal of tube(s), with or without removal of ovary(s)	20.34	12.98	2.80	36.12	90	S
58210	00	A	Radical abdominal hysterectomy, with bilateral total pelvic lymphadenectomy and para-aortic lymph node sampling (biopsy), with or without removal of tube(s), with or without removal of ovary(s)	23.97	17.77	3.87	45.61	90	S
58240	00	A	Pelvic exenteration for gynecologic malignancy, with total abdominal hysterectomy or cervicectomy, with or without removal of tube(s), with or without removal of ovary(s), with removal of bladder and ureteral transplantations, and/or abdominoperineal resection of rectum and colon and colostomy, or any combination thereof	28.79	28.73	6.15	63.67	90	S
58260	00	A	Vaginal hysterectomy;	11.39	9.39	2.07	22.85	90	S
58262	00	A	Vaginal hysterectomy; with removal of tube(s), and/or ovary(s)	13.06	9.39	2.07	24.52	90	S
58263	00	A	Vaginal hysterectomy; with removal of tube(s), and/or ovary(s), with repair of enterocele	14.27	10.32	2.22	26.81	90	S
58267	00	A	Vaginal hysterectomy; with colpo-urethrocystopexy (Marshall-Marchetti-Krantz type, Pereyra type, with or without endoscopic control)	13.94	11.53	2.46	27.93	90	S
58270	00	A	Vaginal hysterectomy; with repair of enterocele	12.60	10.32	2.22	25.14	90	S
58275	00	A	Vaginal hysterectomy, with total or partial colpectomy;	13.99	11.02	2.32	27.33	90	S
58280	00	A	Vaginal hysterectomy, with total or partial colpectomy; with repair of enterocele	14.35	10.50	2.30	27.15	90	S
58285	00	A	Vaginal hysterectomy, radical (Schauta type operation)	17.45	11.60	2.70	31.75	90	S
58300	00	N	Insertion of intrauterine device (IUD)	1.01	0.77	0.13	1.91	XXX	0
58301	00	A	Removal of intrauterine device (IUD)	0.73	0.45	0.08	1.26	0	S
58321	00	A	Artificial insemination; intra-cervical	0.92	0.71	0.15	1.78	0	S
58322	00	A	Artificial insemination; intra-uterine	1.10	0.71	0.15	1.96	0	S
58323	00	A	Sperm washing for artificial insemination	0.23	0.16	0.04	0.43	0	S
58340	00	A	Injection procedure for hysterosalpingography	0.88	0.57	0.08	1.53	0	S
58345	00	A	Transcervical introduction of fallopian tube catheter for diagnosis and/or re-establishing patency (any method), with or without hysterosalpingography	4.61	3.49	0.41	8.51	10	S
58350	00	A	Chromotubation of oviduct, including materials	0.96	0.69	0.16	1.81	10	S
58400	00	A	Uterine suspension, with or without shortening of round ligaments, with or without shortening of sacrouterine ligaments; (separate procedure)	5.66	5.64	1.16	12.46	90	S
58410	00	A	Uterine suspension, with or without shortening of round ligaments, with or without shortening of sacrouterine ligaments; with presacral sympathectomy	6.78	5.53	0.84	13.15	90	S
58520	00	A	Hysterorrhaphy, repair of ruptured uterus (nonobstetrical)	6.35	4.24	0.99	11.58	90	S
58540	00	A	Hysteroplasty, repair of uterine anomaly (Strassman type)	8.58	6.13	1.42	16.13	90	S
58600	00	A	Ligation or transection of fallopian tube(s), abdominal or vaginal approach, unilateral or bilateral	3.74	5.36	1.38	10.48	90	S
58605	00	A	Ligation or transection of fallopian tube(s), abdominal or vaginal approach, postpartum, unilateral or bilateral, during same hospitalization (separate procedure)	3.29	4.21	1.01	8.51	90	S
58611	00	A	Ligation or transection of fallopian tube(s) when done at the time of cesarean section or intra-abdominal surgery (not a separate procedure)	0.63	0.47	0.10	1.20	ZZZ	S
58615	00	A	Occlusion of fallopian tube(s) by device (eg, band, clip, Falope ring) vaginal or suprapubic approach	3.85	2.91	0.35	7.11	10	S

CPT codes and descriptions only, © 1994 American Medical Association. Reimbursement information, © 1995 McGraw-Hill Inc.

Code/ CPT	Mod-ifier	Status	Description	Work value	Practice expense	Mal-practice	Total value	Global period	Up-date
58700	00	A	Salpingectomy, complete or partial, unilateral or bilateral (separate procedure)	5.92	6.33	1.31	13.56	90	S
58720	00	A	Salpingo-oophorectomy, complete or partial, unilateral or bilateral (separate procedure)	6.20	7.50	1.63	15.33	90	S
58740	00	A	Lysis of adhesions (salpingolysis, ovariolysis)	5.28	6.94	1.88	14.10	90	S
58750	00	A	Tubotubal anastomosis	8.82	6.31	1.46	16.59	90	S
58752	00	A	Tubouterine implantation	7.94	6.74	0.93	15.61	90	S
58760	00	A	Fimbrioplasty	7.16	5.11	1.19	13.46	90	S
58770	00	A	Salpingostomy (salpingoneostomy)	6.96	5.28	1.11	13.35	90	S
58800	00	A	Drainage of ovarian cyst(s), unilateral or bilateral, (separate procedure); vaginal approach	3.77	2.68	0.53	6.98	90	S
58805	00	A	Drainage of ovarian cyst(s), unilateral or bilateral, (separate procedure); abdominal approach	5.44	6.38	1.36	13.18	90	S
58820	00	A	Drainage of ovarian abscess; vaginal approach	3.96	2.76	0.49	7.21	90	S
58822	00	A	Drainage of ovarian abscess; abdominal approach	6.18	3.55	0.81	10.54	90	S
58825	00	A	Transposition, ovary(s)	5.63	4.03	0.93	10.59	90	S
58900	00	A	Biopsy of ovary, unilateral or bilateral (separate procedure)	5.49	5.19	1.07	11.75	90	S
58920	00	A	Wedge resection or bisection of ovary, unilateral or bilateral	6.28	6.78	1.41	14.47	90	S
58925	00	A	Ovarian cystectomy, unilateral or bilateral	6.40	6.56	1.38	14.34	90	S
58940	00	A	Oophorectomy, partial or total, unilateral or bilateral;	6.54	6.49	1.33	14.36	90	S
58943	00	A	Oophorectomy, partial or total, unilateral or bilateral; for ovarian malignancy, with para-aortic and pelvic lymph node biopsies, peritoneal washings, peritoneal biopsies, diaphragmatic assessments, with or without salpingectomy(s), with or without omentectomy	17.49	12.11	2.63	32.23	90	S
58950	00	A	Resection of ovarian malignancy with bilateral salpingo-oophorectomy and omentectomy;	14.10	11.24	2.38	27.72	90	S
58951	00	A	Resection of ovarian malignancy with bilateral salpingo-oophorectomy and omentectomy; with total abdominal hysterectomy, pelvic and limited para-aortic lymphadenectomy	20.34	18.34	3.93	42.61	90	S
58952	00	A	Resection of ovarian malignancy with bilateral salpingo-oophorectomy and omentectomy; with radical dissection for debulking	21.35	18.11	3.92	43.38	90	S
58960	00	A	Laparotomy, for staging or restaging of ovarian malignancy ("second look"), with or without omentectomy, peritoneal washing, biopsy of abdominal and pelvic peritoneum, diaphragmatic assessment with pelvic and limited para-aortic lymphadenectomy	10.14	12.98	2.95	26.07	90	S
58970	00	A	Follicle puncture for oocyte retrieval, any method	3.53	2.52	0.58	6.63	0	N
58972	00	C	Culture and fertilization of oocyte(s)	4.92*	3.52#	0.81*	9.25#	0	N
58974	00	C	Embryo transfer, any method (separate procedure)	6.33*	4.52#	1.05*	11.90#	0	N
58976	00	A	Gamete or zygote intrafallopian transfer, any method	3.83	2.73	0.63	7.19	0	N
58999	00	C	Unlisted procedure, female genital system (nonobstetrical)	0	0	0	0	YYY	S
59000	00	A	Amniocentesis, any method	1.30	0.97	0.18	2.45	0	S
59012	00	A	Cordocentesis (intrauterine), any method	3.45	2.62	0.31	6.38	0	S
59015	00	A	Chorionic villus sampling, any method	2.20	1.20	0.10	3.50	0	S
59020	00	A	Fetal contraction stress test	0.66	1.35	0.29	2.30	0	S
59020	26			0.66	0.85	0.19	1.70	0	S
59020	TC			0	0.50	0.10	0.60	0	S
59025	00	A	Fetal non-stress test	0.53	0.61	0.12	1.26	0	S
59025	26			0.53	0.39	0.08	1.00	0	S

CPT codes and descriptions only, © 1994 American Medical Association. Reimbursement information, © 1995 McGraw-Hill Inc.

Code/ CPT	Mod-ifier	Status	Description	Work value	Practice expense	Mal-practice	Total value	Global period	Up-date
59025	TC			0	0.22	0.04	0.26	0	S
59030	00	A	Fetal scalp blood sampling	1.99	1.58	0.21	3.78	0	S
59050	00	A	Fetal monitoring during labor by consulting physician (ie, non-attending physician) with written report (separate procedure); supervision and interpretation	0.89	0.81	0.15	1.85	XXX	S
59051	00	A	Fetal monitoring during labor by consulting physician (ie, non-attending physician) with written report (separate procedure); interpretation only	0.74	0.81	0.15	1.70	XXX	N
59100	00	A	Hysterotomy, abdominal (eg, for hydatidiform mole, abortion)	5.96	4.14	0.96	11.06	90	S
59120	00	A	Surgical treatment of ectopic pregnancy; tubal or ovarian, requiring salpingectomy and/or oophorectomy, abdominal or vaginal approach	7.11	7.86	1.50	16.47	90	S
59121	00	A	Surgical treatment of ectopic pregnancy; tubal or ovarian, without salpingectomy and/or oophorectomy	6.99	5.38	1.07	13.44	90	S
59130	00	A	Surgical treatment of ectopic pregnancy; abdominal pregnancy	7.88	5.96	0.70	14.54	90	S
59135	00	A	Surgical treatment of ectopic pregnancy; interstitial, uterine pregnancy requiring total hysterectomy	13.00	9.85	1.15	24.00	90	S
59136	00	A	Surgical treatment of ectopic pregnancy; interstitial, uterine pregnancy with partial resection of uterus	8.69	6.22	1.44	16.35	90	S
59140	00	A	Surgical treatment of ectopic pregnancy; cervical, with evacuation	5.09	4.66	0.29	10.04	90	S
59150	00	A	Laparoscopic treatment of ectopic pregnancy; without salpingectomy and/or oophorectomy	6.34	4.53	1.05	11.92	90	S
59151	00	A	Laparoscopic treatment of ectopic pregnancy; with salpingectomy and/or oophorectomy	7.24	8.61	0.64	16.49	90	S
59160	00	A	Curettage, postpartum (separate procedure)	2.66	2.93	0.52	6.11	10	S
59200	00	A	Insertion of cervical dilator (eg, laminaria, prostaglandin) (separate procedure)	0.79	0.54	0.11	1.44	0	S
59300	00	A	Episiotomy or vaginal repair, by other than attending physician	2.41	0.99	0.10	3.50	0	S
59320	00	A	Cerclage of cervix, during pregnancy; vaginal	2.48	1.78	0.41	4.67	0	S
59325	00	A	Cerclage of cervix, during pregnancy; abdominal	4.07	2.89	0.29	7.25	0	S
59350	00	A	Hysterorrhaphy of ruptured uterus	4.95	3.54	0.82	9.31	0	S
59400	00	A	Routine obstetric care including antepartum care, vaginal delivery (with or without episiotomy, and/or forceps) and postpartum care	20.99	14.99	3.47	39.45	MMM	S
59409	00	A	Vaginal delivery only (with or without episiotomy and/or forceps);	13.28	9.48	2.20	24.96	MMM	S
59410	00	A	Vaginal delivery only (with or without episiotomy and/or forceps); including postpartum care	14.44	10.31	2.39	27.14	MMM	S
59412	00	A	External cephalic version, with or without tocolysis (list in addition to code(s) for delivery)	1.71	1.22	0.29	3.22	MMM	S
59414	00	A	Delivery of placenta (separate procedure)	1.61	1.15	0.27	3.03	MMM	S
59425	00	A	Antepartum care only; 4-6 visits	4.04	2.88	0.66	7.58	MMM	S
59426	00	A	Antepartum care only; 7 or more visits	6.91	4.94	1.14	12.99	MMM	S
59430	00	A	Postpartum care only (separate procedure)	2.01	0.38	0.07	2.46	MMM	S
59510	00	A	Routine obstetric care including antepartum care, cesarean delivery, and postpartum care	23.67	16.90	3.92	44.49	MMM	S
59514	00	A	Cesarean delivery only;	15.39	10.99	2.55	28.93	MMM	S
59515	00	A	Cesarean delivery only; including postpartum care	16.55	11.82	2.73	31.10	MMM	S
59525	00	A	Subtotal or total hysterectomy after cesarean delivery (list in addition to 59510 or 59515)	8.54	3.81	0.88	13.23	MMM	S

CPT codes and descriptions only, © 1994 American Medical Association. Reimbursement information, © 1995 McGraw-Hill Inc.

Code/ CPT	Mod- ifier	Status	Description	Work value	Practice expense	Mal- practice	Total value	Global period	Up- date
59812	00	A	Treatment of incomplete abortion, any trimester, completed surgically	3.10	3.61	0.77	7.48	90	S
59820	00	A	Treatment of missed abortion, completed surgically; first trimester	3.73	3.75	0.77	8.25	90	S
59821	00	A	Treatment of missed abortion, completed surgically; second trimester	4.26	2.72	0.62	7.60	90	S
59830	00	A	Treatment of septic abortion, completed surgically	5.96	4.53	0.52	11.01	90	S
59840	00	A	Induced abortion, by dilation and curettage	2.91	3.22	0.69	6.82	10	S
59841	00	A	Induced abortion, by dilation and evacuation	3.24	3.75	0.76	7.75	10	S
59850	00	A	Induced abortion, by one or more intra-amniotic injections (amniocentesis-injections), including hospital admission and visits, deliver of fetus and secundines;	5.46	4.00	0.85	10.31	90	S
59851	00	A	Induced abortion, by one or more intra-amniotic injections (amniocentesis-injections), including hospital admission and visits, deliver of fetus and secundines; with dilation and curettage and/or evacuation	5.62	4.28	0.88	10.78	90	S
59852	00	A	Induced abortion, by one or more intra-amniotic injections (amniocentesis-injections), including hospital admission and visits, deliver of fetus and secundines; with hysterotomy (failed intra-amniotic injection)	7.70	5.51	1.27	14.48	90	S
59855	00	A	Induced abortion, by one or more vaginal suppositories (eg, prostaglandin) with or without cervical dilation (eg, laminaria), including hospital admission and visits, delivery of fetus and secundines;	4.75	3.39	0.78	8.92	90	S
59856	00	A	Induced abortion, by one or more vaginal suppositories (eg, prostaglandin) with or without cervical dilation (eg, laminaria), including hospital admission and visits, delivery of fetus and secundines; with dilation and curettage and/or evacuation	7.16	5.11	1.19	13.46	90	S
59857	00	A	Induced abortion, by one or more vaginal suppositories (eg, prostaglandin) with or without cervical dilation (eg, laminaria), including hospital admission and visits, delivery of fetus and secundines; with hysterotomy (failed medical evaluation)	8.71	6.22	1.44	16.37	90	S
59870	00	A	Uterine evacuation and curettage for hydatidiform mole	4.08	2.91	0.67	7.66	90	S
59899	00	C	Unlisted procedure, maternity care and delivery	0	0	0	0	YYY	S
60000	00	A	Incision and drainage of thyroglossal cyst, infected	1.71	0.60	0.09	2.40	10	N
60001	00	A	Aspiration and/or injection, thyroid cyst	0.97	1.05	0.12	2.14	0	N
60100	00	A	Biopsy thyroid, percutaneous core needle	0.97	1.05	0.12	2.14	0	N
60200	00	A	Excision of cyst or adenoma of thyroid, or transection of isthmus	8.83	6.02	1.04	15.89	90	S
60210	00	A	Partial thyroid lobectomy, unilateral; with or without isthmusectomy	10.51	8.68	1.65	20.84	90	S
60212	00	A	Partial thyroid lobectomy, unilateral; with contralateral subtotal lobectomy, including isthmusectomy	15.48	9.04	1.74	26.26	90	S
60220	00	A	Total thyroid lobectomy, unilateral; with or without isthmusectomy	9.86	8.54	1.61	20.01	90	S
60225	00	A	Total thyroid lobectomy, unilateral; with contralateral subtotal lobectomy, including isthmusectomy	11.65	10.49	1.92	24.06	90	S
60240	00	A	Thyroidectomy, total or complete	15.66	10.58	1.96	28.20	90	S
60245	00	D	Partial removal of thyroid	11.96*	10.83#	1.17*	23.96#	90	S
60246	00	D	Partial removal of thyroid	15.48*	14.02#	1.52*	31.02#	90	S
60252	00	A	Thyroidectomy, total or subtotal for malignancy; with limited neck dissection	15.40	13.65	2.55	31.60	90	S

CPT codes and descriptions only, © 1994 American Medical Association. Reimbursement information, © 1995 McGraw-Hill Inc.

Code/ CPT	Mod- ifier	Status	Description	Work value	Practice expense	Mal- practice	Total value	Global period	Up- date
60254	00	A	Thyroidectomy, total or subtotal for malignancy; with radical neck dissection	16.68	19.21	3.08	38.97	90	S
60260	00	A	Thyroidectomy, removal of all remaining thyroid tissue following previous removal of a portion of thyroid	14.49	3.14	0.34	17.97	90	S
60270	00	A	Thyroidectomy, including substernal thyroid gland; sternal split or transthoracic approach	16.44	13.97	2.54	32.95	90	S
60271	00	A	Thyroidectomy, including substernal thyroid gland; cervical approach	14.16	12.14	2.25	28.55	90	S
60280	00	A	Excision of thyroglossal duct cyst or sinus;	5.55	7.10	1.11	13.76	90	S
60281	00	A	Excision of thyroglossal duct cyst or sinus; recurrent	8.00	5.04	0.95	13.99	90	S
60500	00	A	Parathyroidectomy or exploration of parathyroid(s);	15.40	11.36	2.31	29.07	90	S
60502	00	A	Parathyroidectomy or exploration of parathyroid(s); re-exploration	19.25	11.39	2.33	32.97	90	S
60505	00	A	Parathyroidectomy or exploration of parathyroid(s); with mediastinal exploration, sternal split or transthoracic approach	19.93	13.14	2.56	35.63	90	S
60512	00	A	Parathyroid autotransplantation	4.45	2.32	0.54	7.31	ZZZ	S
60520	00	A	Thymectomy, partial or total; transcervical approach (separate procedure)	15.82	13.54	2.46	31.82	90	S
60521	00	A	Thymectomy, partial or total; sternal split or transthoracic approach, without radical mediastinal dissection (separate procedure)	17.80	13.54	2.46	33.80	90	S
60522	00	A	Thymectomy, partial or total; sternal split or transthoracic approach, with radical mediastinal dissection (separate procedure)	21.76	13.54	2.46	37.76	90	S
60540	00	A	Adrenalectomy, partial or complete, or exploration of adrenal gland with or without biopsy, transabdominal, lumbar or dorsal (separate procedure);	15.72	12.05	2.08	29.85	90	S
60545	00	A	Adrenalectomy, partial or complete, or exploration of adrenal gland with or without biopsy, transabdominal, lumbar or dorsal (separate procedure); with excision of adjacent retroperitoneal tumor	18.51	14.27	2.34	35.12	90	S
60600	00	A	Excision of carotid body tumor; without excision of carotid artery	16.13	11.46	1.88	29.47	90	S
60605	00	A	Excision of carotid body tumor; with excision of carotid artery	18.20	10.71	2.21	31.12	90	S
60699	00	C	Unlisted procedure, endocrine system	0	0	0	0	YYY	S
61000	00	A	Subdural tap through fontanelle, or suture, infant, unilateral or bilateral; initial	1.58	1.07	0.17	2.82	0	S
61001	00	A	Subdural tap through fontanelle, or suture, infant, unilateral or bilateral; subsequent taps	1.49	0.88	0.17	2.54	0	S
61020	00	A	Ventricular puncture through previous burr hole, fontanelle, suture, or implanted ventricular catheter/reservoir; without injection	1.51	1.26	0.20	2.97	0	S
61026	00	A	Ventricular puncture through previous burr hole, fontanelle, suture, or implanted ventricular catheter/reservoir; with injection of drug or other substance for diagnosis or treatment	1.69	2.03	0.22	3.94	0	N
61050	00	A	Cisternal or lateral cervical (C1-C2) puncture; without injection (separate procedure)	1.51	1.23	0.15	2.89	0	N
61055	00	A	Cisternal or lateral cervical (C1-C2) puncture; with injection of drug or other substance for diagnosis or treatment (eg, C1-C2)	2.10	1.88	0.19	4.17	0	N
61070	00	A	Puncture of shunt tubing or reservoir for aspiration or injection procedure	0.89	0.49	0.03	1.41	0	N

CPT codes and descriptions only, © 1994 American Medical Association. Reimbursement information, © 1995 McGraw-Hill Inc.

Code/ CPT	Mod- ifier	Status	Description	Work value	Practice expense	Mal- practice	Total value	Global period	Up- date
61105	00	A	Twist drill hole for subdural or ventricular puncture; not followed by other surgery	8.19	6.89	1.24	16.32	90	S
61106	00	A	Twist drill hole for subdural or ventricular puncture; followed by other surgery	7.35	6.15	1.15	14.65	ZZZ	S
61107	00	A	Twist drill hole for subdural or ventricular puncture; for implanting ventricular catheter or pressure recording device	4.35	5.68	1.26	11.29	0	S
61108	00	A	Twist drill hole for subdural or ventricular puncture; for evacuation and/or drainage of subdural hematoma	10.80	12.05	2.22	25.07	90	S
61120	00	A	Burr hole(s) for ventricular puncture (including injection of gas, contrast media, dye, or radioactive material); not followed by other surgery	9.31	5.95	1.08	16.34	90	S
61130	00	A	Burr hole(s) for ventricular puncture (including injection of gas, contrast media, dye, or radioactive material); followed by other surgery	6.37	4.95	0.96	12.28	ZZZ	S
61140	00	A	Burr hole(s) or trephine; with biopsy of brain or intracranial lesion	14.84	14.13	2.56	31.53	90	S
61150	00	A	Burr hole(s) or trephine; with drainage of brain abscess or cyst	16.37	14.65	2.63	33.65	90	S
61151	00	A	Burr hole(s) or trephine; with subsequent tapping (aspiration) of intracranial abscess or cyst	11.40	2.13	0.37	13.90	90	S
61154	00	A	Burr hole(s) with evacuation and/or drainage of hematoma, extradural or subdural	13.67	17.50	3.27	34.44	90	S
61156	00	A	Burr hole(s); with aspiration of hematoma or cyst, intracerebral	15.23	16.19	3.05	34.47	90	S
61210	00	A	Burr hole(s); for implanting ventricular catheter, reservoir, EEG electrode(s) or pressure recording device (separate procedure)	4.72	6.54	1.53	12.79	0	S
61215	00	A	Insertion of subcutaneous reservoir, pump or continuous infusion system for connection to ventricular catheter	10.05	9.00	1.63	20.68	90	S
61250	00	A	Burr hole(s) or trephine, supratentorial, exploratory, not followed by other surgery	11.03	8.03	1.44	20.50	90	S
61253	00	A	Burr hole(s) or trephine, infratentorial, unilateral or bilateral	13.00	9.62	1.69	24.31	90	S
61304	00	A	Craniectomy or craniotomy, exploratory; supratentorial	20.63	26.03	4.78	51.44	90	S
61305	00	A	Craniectomy or craniotomy, exploratory; infratentorial (posterior fossa)	24.77	29.11	5.05	58.93	90	S
61312	00	A	Craniectomy or craniotomy for evacuation of hematoma, supratentorial; extradural or subdural	20.54	24.13	4.46	49.13	90	S
61313	00	A	Craniectomy or craniotomy for evacuation of hematoma, supratentorial; intracerebral	20.54	24.04	4.38	48.96	90	S
61314	00	A	Craniectomy or craniotomy for evacuation of hematoma, infratentorial; extradural or subdural	22.78	25.62	4.68	53.08	90	S
61315	00	A	Craniectomy or craniotomy for evacuation of hematoma, infratentorial; intracerebellar	25.91	24.41	4.47	54.79	90	S
61320	00	A	Craniectomy or craniotomy, drainage of intracranial abscess; supratentorial	23.90	18.70	3.41	46.01	90	S
61321	00	A	Craniectomy or craniotomy, drainage of intracranial abscess; infratentorial	26.66	19.83	3.54	50.03	90	S
61330	00	A	Decompression of orbit only, transcranial approach	15.65	12.97	1.22	29.84	90	S
61332	00	A	Exploration of orbit (transcranial approach); with biopsy	26.08	20.72	2.76	49.56	90	S
61333	00	A	Exploration of orbit (transcranial approach); with removal of lesion	26.75	20.46	3.26	50.47	90	S
61334	00	A	Exploration of orbit (transcranial approach); with removal of foreign body	17.07	14.65	1.82	33.54	90	S
61340	00	A	Other cranial decompression (eg, subtemporal), supratentorial	11.56	14.80	2.54	28.90	90	S

CPT codes and descriptions only, © 1994 American Medical Association. Reimbursement information, © 1995 McGraw-Hill Inc.

Code/ CPT	Mod-ifier	Status	Description	Work value	Practice expense	Mal-practice	Total value	Global period	Up-date
61343	00	A	Craniectomy, suboccipital with cervical laminectomy for decompression of medulla and spinal cord, with or without dural graft (eg, Arnold-Chiari malformation)	27.87	30.05	5.28	63.20	90	S
61345	00	A	Other cranial decompression, posterior fossa	25.36	19.18	3.45	47.99	90	S
61440	00	A	Craniotomy for section of tentorium cerebelli (separate procedure)	24.79	20.75	3.00	48.54	90	S
61450	00	A	Craniectomy, subtemporal, for section, compression, or decompression of sensory root of gasserian ganglion	24.29	20.43	3.43	48.15	90	S
61458	00	A	Craniectomy, suboccipital; for exploration or decompression of cranial nerves	25.97	27.28	4.87	58.12	90	S
61460	00	A	Craniectomy, suboccipital; for section of one or more cranial nerves	26.75	25.05	3.98	55.78	90	S
61470	00	A	Craniectomy, suboccipital; for medullary tractotomy	20.79	13.86	2.53	37.18	90	S
61480	00	A	Craniectomy, suboccipital; for mesencephalic tractotomy or pedunculotomy	16.77	15.07	1.78	33.62	90	S
61490	00	A	Craniotomy for lobotomy, including cingulotomy	15.63	11.72	2.16	29.51	90	S
61500	00	A	Craniectomy; with excision of tumor or other bone lesion of skull	16.93	20.07	3.58	40.58	90	S
61501	00	A	Craniectomy; for osteomyelitis	13.59	17.40	3.33	34.32	90	S
61510	00	A	Craniectomy, trephination, bone flap craniotomy; for excision of brain tumor, supratentorial, except meningioma	23.39	27.04	4.90	55.33	90	S
61512	00	A	Craniectomy, trephination, bone flap craniotomy; for excision of meningioma, supratentorial	24.26	29.02	5.28	58.56	90	S
61514	00	A	Craniectomy, trephination, bone flap craniotomy; for excision of brain abscess, supratentorial	23.49	25.52	4.74	53.75	90	S
61516	00	A	Craniectomy, trephination, bone flap craniotomy; for excision or fenestration of cyst, supratentorial	22.84	26.48	4.57	53.89	90	S
61518	00	A	Craniectomy for excision of brain tumor, infratentorial or posterior fossa; except meningioma, cerebellopontine angle tumor, or midline tumor at base of skull	32.27	30.02	5.46	67.75	90	S
61519	00	A	Craniectomy for excision of brain tumor, infratentorial or posterior fossa; meningioma	33.84	31.22	5.77	70.83	90	S
61520	00	A	Craniectomy for excision of brain tumor, infratentorial or posterior fossa; cerebellopontine angle tumor	38.35	33.85	5.89	78.09	90	S
61521	00	A	Craniectomy for excision of brain tumor, infratentorial or posterior fossa; midline tumor at base of skull	39.48	32.97	5.85	78.30	90	S
61522	00	A	Craniectomy, infratentorial or posterior fossa; for excision of brain abscess	27.55	19.96	3.79	51.30	90	S
61524	00	A	Craniectomy, infratentorial or posterior fossa; for excision or fenestration of cyst	26.02	27.45	5.15	58.62	90	S
61526	00	A	Craniectomy, bone flap craniotomy, transtemporal (mastoid) for excision of cerebellopontine angle tumor;	29.71	34.01	4.79	68.51	90	S
61530	00	A	Craniectomy, bone flap craniotomy, transtemporal (mastoid) for excision of cerebellopontine angle tumor; combined with middle/posterior fossa craniotomy/craniectomy	42.35	34.01	4.79	81.15	90	S
61531	00	A	Subdural implantation of strip electrodes through one or more burr or trephine hole(s) for long term seizure monitoring	20.50	14.98	1.75	37.23	90	S
61533	00	A	Craniotomy with elevation of bone flap; for subdural implantation of an electrode array, for long term seizure monitoring	23.41	17.02	3.33	43.76	90	S
61534	00	A	Craniotomy with elevation of bone flap; for excision of epileptogenic focus without electrocorticography during surgery	19.13	6.38	2.01	27.52	90	S

CPT codes and descriptions only, © 1994 American Medical Association. Reimbursement information, © 1995 McGraw-Hill Inc.

Code/ CPT	Mod-ifier	Status	Description	Work value	Practice expense	Mal-practice	Total value	Global period	Up-date
61535	00	A	Craniotomy with elevation of bone flap; for removal of epidural or subdural electrode array, without excision of cerebral tissue (separate procedure)	10.23	7.66	1.25	19.14	90	S
61536	00	A	Craniotomy with elevation of bone flap; for excision of cerebral epileptogenic focus, with electrocorticography during surgery (includes removal of electrode array)	29.43	21.96	3.99	55.38	90	S
61538	00	A	Craniotomy with elevation of bone flap; for lobectomy with electrocorticography during surgery, temporal lobe	28.05	29.08	4.97	62.10	90	S
61539	00	A	Craniotomy with elevation of bone flap; for lobectomy with electrocorticography during surgery, other than temporal lobe, partial or total	30.05	22.96	4.07	57.08	90	S
61541	00	A	Craniotomy with elevation of bone flap; for transection of corpus callosum	26.95	19.80	3.78	50.53	90	S
61542	00	A	Craniotomy with elevation of bone flap; for total hemispherectomy	27.39	19.91	3.90	51.20	90	S
61543	00	A	Craniotomy with elevation of bone flap; for partial or subtotal hemispherectomy	20.62	17.24	2.49	40.35	90	S
61544	00	A	Craniotomy with elevation of bone flap; for excision or coagulation of choroid plexus	23.71	28.19	2.11	54.01	90	S
61545	00	A	Craniotomy with elevation of bone flap; for excision of craniopharyngioma	34.50	25.66	4.80	64.96	90	S
61546	00	A	Craniotomy for hypophysectomy or excision of pituitary tumor, intracranial approach	29.33	27.01	4.78	61.12	90	S
61548	00	A	Hypophysectomy or excision of pituitary tumor, transnasal or transseptal approach, nonstereotactic	20.15	24.78	4.03	48.96	90	S
61550	00	A	Craniectomy for craniosynostosis; single cranial suture	14.24	11.81	1.11	27.16	90	S
61552	00	A	Craniectomy for craniosynostosis; multiple cranial sutures	19.02	13.83	2.70	35.55	90	S
61556	00	A	Craniotomy for craniosynostosis; frontal or parietal bone flap	21.35	15.53	3.04	39.92	90	S
61557	00	A	Craniotomy for craniosynostosis; bifrontal bone flap	21.47	15.62	3.05	40.14	90	S
61558	00	A	Extensive craniectomy for multiple cranial suture craniosynostosis (eg, cloverleaf skull); not requiring bone grafts	24.41	17.74	3.47	45.62	90	S
61559	00	A	Extensive craniectomy for multiple cranial suture craniosynostosis (eg, cloverleaf skull); recontouring with multiple osteotomies and bone autografts (eg, barrel-stave procedure) (includes obtaining grafts)	31.65	23.01	4.50	59.16	90	S
61563	00	A	Excision, intra and extracranial, benign tumor of cranial bone (eg, fibrous dysplasia); without optic nerve decompression	25.87	18.81	3.68	48.36	90	S
61564	00	A	Excision, intra and extracranial, benign tumor of cranial bone (eg, fibrous dysplasia); with optic nerve decompression	32.64	23.73	4.64	61.01	90	S
61570	00	A	Craniectomy or craniotomy; with excision of foreign body from brain	22.89	16.49	3.06	42.44	90	S
61571	00	A	Craniectomy or craniotomy; with treatment of penetrating wound of brain	24.55	18.32	3.21	46.08	90	S
61575	00	A	Transoral approach to skull base, brain stem or upper spinal cord for biopsy, decompression or excision of lesion;	32.33	32.99	5.05	70.37	90	S
61576	00	A	Transoral approach to skull base, brain stem or upper spinal cord for biopsy, decompression or excision of lesion; requiring splitting of tongue and/or mandible (including tracheostomy)	33.82	28.23	3.91	65.96	90	S

CPT codes and descriptions only, © 1994 American Medical Association. Reimbursement information, © 1995 McGraw-Hill Inc.

Code/ CPT	Mod- ifier	Status	Description	Work value	Practice expense	Mal- practice	Total value	Global period	Up- date
61580	00	A	Craniofacial approach to anterior cranial fossa; extradural, including lateral rhinotomy, ethmoidectomy, sphenoidectomy, without maxillectomy or orbital exenteration	28.90	21.01	4.10	54.01	90	S
61581	00	A	Craniofacial approach to anterior cranial fossa; extradural, including lateral rhinotomy, orbital exenteration, ethmoidectomy, sphenoidectomy and/or maxillectomy	32.80	23.84	4.66	61.30	90	S
61582	00	A	Craniofacial approach to anterior cranial fossa; extradural, including unilateral or bifrontal craniotomy, elevation of frontal lobe(s), osteotomy of base of anterior cranial fossa	29.77	21.65	4.22	55.64	90	S
61583	00	A	Craniofacial approach to anterior cranial fossa; intradural, including unilateral or bifrontal craniotomy, elevation or resection of frontal lobe, osteotomy of base of anterior cranial fossa	33.97	24.70	4.83	63.50	90	S
61584	00	A	Orbitocranial approach to anterior cranial fossa, extradural, including supraorbital ridge osteotomy and elevation of frontal and/or temporal lobe(s); without orbital exenteration	32.89	23.91	4.68	61.48	90	S
61585	00	A	Orbitocranial approach to anterior cranial fossa, extradural, including supraorbital ridge osteotomy and elevation of frontal and/or temporal lobe(s); with orbital exenteration	36.80	26.75	5.23	68.78	90	S
61590	00	A	Infratemporal pre-auricular approach to middle cranial fossa (parapharyngeal space, infratemporal and midline skull base, nasopharynx), with or without disarticulation of the mandible, including parotidectomy, craniotomy, decompression and/or mobilization of the facial nerve and/or petrous carotid artery	40.02	29.10	5.68	74.80	90	S
61591	00	A	Infratemporal post-auricular approach to middle cranial fossa (internal auditory meatus, petrous apex, tentorium, cavernous sinus, parasellar area, infratemporal fossa) including mastoidectomy, resection of sigmoid sinus, with or without decompression and/or mobilization of contents of auditory canal or petrous carotid artery	41.97	30.52	5.96	78.45	90	S
61592	00	A	Orbitocranial zygomatic approach to middle cranial fossa (cavernous sinus and carotid artery, clivus, basilar artery or petrous apex) including osteotomy of zygoma, craniotomy, extra- or intradural elevation of temporal lobe	38.07	27.68	5.41	71.16	90	S
61595	00	A	Transtemporal approach to posterior cranial fossa, jugular foramen or midline skull base, including mastoidectomy, decompression of sigmoid sinus and/or facial nerve, with or without mobilization	28.12	20.44	4.00	52.56	90	S
61596	00	A	Transcochlear approach to posterior cranial fossa, jugular foramen or midline skull base, including labyrinthectomy, decompression, with or without mobilization of facial nerve and/or petrous carotid artery	34.17	24.84	4.86	63.87	90	S
61597	00	A	Transcondylar (far lateral) approach to posterior cranial fossa, jugular foramen or midline skull base, including occipital condylectomy, mastoidectomy, resection of C1-C3 vertebral body(s), decompression of vertebral artery, with or without mobilization	36.12	26.26	5.13	67.51	90	S
61598	00	A	Transpetrosal approach to posterior cranial fossa, clivus or foramen magnum, including ligation of superior petrosal sinus and/or sigmoid sinus	31.83	23.13	4.52	59.48	90	S
61600	00	A	Resection or excision of neoplastic, vascular or infectious lesion of base of anterior cranial fossa; extradural	24.41	17.74	3.46	45.61	90	S

CPT codes and descriptions only, © 1994 American Medical Association. Reimbursement information, © 1995 McGraw-Hill Inc.

Code/ CPT	Mod-ifier	Status	Description	Work value	Practice expense	Mal-practice	Total value	Global period	Up-date
61601	00	A	Resection or excision of neoplastic, vascular or infectious lesion of base of anterior cranial fossa; intradural, including dural repair, with or without graft	26.16	19.03	3.72	48.91	90	S
61605	00	A	Resection or excision of neoplastic, vascular or infectious lesion of infratemporal fossa, parapharyngeal space, petrous apex; extradural	27.62	20.09	3.93	51.64	90	S
61606	00	A	Resection or excision of neoplastic, vascular or infectious lesion of infratemporal fossa, parapharyngeal space, petrous apex; intradural, including dural repair, with or without graft	37	26.90	5.25	69.15	90	S
61607	00	A	Resection or excision of neoplastic, vascular or infectious lesion of parasellar area, cavernous sinus, clivus or midline skull base; extradural	34.56	25.13	4.91	64.60	90	S
61608	00	A	Resection or excision of neoplastic, vascular or infectious lesion of parasellar area, cavernous sinus, clivus or midline skull base; intradural, including dural repair, with or without graft	40.21	29.24	5.71	75.16	90	S
61609	00	A	Transection or ligation, carotid artery in cavernous sinus; without repair	9.89	7.19	1.40	18.48	ZZZ	S
61610	00	A	Transection or ligation, carotid artery in cavernous sinus; with repair by anastomosis or graft	29.67	21.57	4.21	55.45	ZZZ	S
61611	00	A	Transection or ligation, carotid artery in petrous canal; without repair	7.42	5.39	1.06	13.87	ZZZ	S
61612	00	A	Transection or ligation, carotid artery in petrous canal; with repair by anastomosis or graft	27.88	20.27	3.96	52.11	ZZZ	S
61613	00	A	Obliteration of carotid aneurysm, arteriovenous malformation, or carotid-cavernous fistula by dissection within cavernous sinus	39.43	28.67	5.61	73.71	90	S
61615	00	A	Resection or excision of neoplastic, vascular or infectious lesion of base of posterior cranial fossa, jugular foramen, foramen magnum, or C1-C3 vertebral bodies; extradural	30.36	22.07	4.31	56.74	90	S
61616	00	A	Resection or excision of neoplastic, vascular or infectious lesion of base of posterior cranial fossa, jugular foramen, foramen magnum, or C1-C3 vertebral bodies; intradural, including dural repair, with or without graft	41.29	30.03	5.86	77.18	90	S
61618	00	A	Secondary repair of dura for CSF leak, anterior, middle or posterior cranial fossa following surgery of the skull base; by free tissue graft (eg, pericranium, fascia, tensor fascia lata, adipose tissue, homologous or synthetic grafts)	15.62	11.35	2.22	29.19	90	S
61619	00	A	Secondary repair of dura for CSF leak, anterior, middle or posterior cranial fossa following surgery of the skull base; by local or regionalized vascularized pedicle flap or myocutaneous flap (including galea, temporalis, frontalis or occipitalis muscle)	19.52	14.19	2.77	36.48	90	S
61624	00	A	Transcatheter occlusion or embolization (eg, for tumor destruction, to achieve hemostasis, to occlude a vascular malformation), percutaneous, any method; central nervous system (intracranial, spinal cord)	20.15	15.28	1.79	37.22	0	N
61626	00	A	Transcatheter occlusion or embolization (eg, for tumor destruction, to achieve hemostasis, to occlude a vascular malformation), percutaneous, any method; non-central nervous system, head or neck (extracranial, brachiocephalic branch)	16.62	12.60	1.47	30.69	0	N
61680	00	A	Surgery of intracranial arteriovenous malformation; supratentorial, simple	36.45	31.06	5.79	73.30	90	S
61682	00	A	Surgery of intracranial arteriovenous malformation; supratentorial, complex	42.21	35.31	6.36	83.88	90	S

CPT codes and descriptions only, © 1994 American Medical Association. Reimbursement information, © 1995 McGraw-Hill Inc.

Code/ CPT	Mod- ifier	Status	Description	Work value	Practice expense	Mal- practice	Total value	Global period	Up- date
63266	00	A	Laminectomy for excision or evacuation of intraspinal lesion other than neoplasm, extradural; thoracic	20.65	24.76	4.43	49.84	90	S
63267	00	A	Laminectomy for excision or evacuation of intraspinal lesion other than neoplasm, extradural; lumbar	16.70	21.38	4.20	42.28	90	S
63268	00	A	Laminectomy for excision or evacuation of intraspinal lesion other than neoplasm, extradural; sacral	17.27	12.56	2.46	32.29	90	S
63270	00	A	Laminectomy for excision of intraspinal lesion other than neoplasm, intradural; cervical	24.84	18.14	3.42	46.40	90	S
63271	00	A	Laminectomy for excision of intraspinal lesion other than neoplasm, intradural; thoracic	24.96	26.60	4.79	56.35	90	S
63272	00	A	Laminectomy for excision of intraspinal lesion other than neoplasm, intradural; lumbar	23.69	23.15	4.26	51.10	90	S
63273	00	A	Laminectomy for excision of intraspinal lesion other than neoplasm, intradural; sacral	22.66	17.56	3.12	43.34	90	S
63275	00	A	Laminectomy for biopsy/excision of intraspinal neoplasm; extradural, cervical	22.05	27.82	5.09	54.96	90	S
63276	00	A	Laminectomy for biopsy/excision of intraspinal neoplasm; extradural, thoracic	21.76	25.31	4.62	51.69	90	S
63277	00	A	Laminectomy for biopsy/excision of intraspinal neoplasm; extradural, lumbar	19.51	23.75	4.25	47.51	90	S
63278	00	A	Laminectomy for biopsy/excision of intraspinal neoplasm; extradural, sacral	19.24	23.34	4.32	46.90	90	S
63280	00	A	Laminectomy for biopsy/excision of intraspinal neoplasm; intradural, extramedullary, cervical	26.72	28.08	4.99	59.79	90	S
63281	00	A	Laminectomy for biopsy/excision of intraspinal neoplasm; intradural, extramedullary, thoracic	26.42	27.67	4.96	59.05	90	S
63282	00	A	Laminectomy for biopsy/excision of intraspinal neoplasm; intradural, extramedullary, lumbar	24.96	24.11	4.44	53.51	90	S
63283	00	A	Laminectomy for biopsy/excision of intraspinal neoplasm; intradural, sacral	23.57	18.77	3.44	45.78	90	S
63285	00	A	Laminectomy for biopsy/excision of intraspinal neoplasm; intradural, intramedullary, cervical	34.24	24.49	4.49	63.22	90	S
63286	00	A	Laminectomy for biopsy/excision of intraspinal neoplasm; intradural, intramedullary, thoracic	33.94	28.76	4.92	67.62	90	S
63287	00	A	Laminectomy for biopsy/excision of intraspinal neoplasm; intradural, intramedullary, thoracolumbar	34.43	25.72	4.53	64.68	90	S
63290	00	A	Laminectomy for biopsy/excision of intraspinal neoplasm; combined extradural-intradural lesion, any level	35.04	27.16	4.65	66.85	90	S
63300	00	A	Vertebral corpectomy (vertebral body resection), partial or complete, for excision of intraspinal lesion, single segment; extradural, cervical	22.78	17.27	2.02	42.07	90	S
63301	00	A	Vertebral corpectomy (vertebral body resection), partial or complete, for excision of intraspinal lesion, single segment; extradural, thoracic by transthoracic approach	25.08	18.45	3.58	47.11	90	S
63302	00	A	Vertebral corpectomy (vertebral body resection), partial or complete, for excision of intraspinal lesion, single segment; extradural, thoracic by thoracolumbar approach	25.60	21.36	3.02	49.98	90	S
63303	00	A	Vertebral corpectomy (vertebral body resection), partial or complete, for excision of intraspinal lesion, single segment; extradural, lumbar or sacral by transperitoneal or retroperitoneal approach	28.47	18.50	3.39	50.36	90	S
63304	00	A	Vertebral corpectomy (vertebral body resection), partial or complete, for excision of intraspinal lesion, single segment; intradural, cervical	28.10	21.31	2.49	51.90	90	S

CPT codes and descriptions only, © 1994 American Medical Association. Reimbursement information, © 1995 McGraw-Hill Inc.

Code/ CPT	Mod- ifier	Status	Description	Work value	Practice expense	Mal- practice	Total value	Global period	Up- date
63305	00	A	Vertebral corpectomy (vertebral body resection), partial or complete, for excision of intraspinal lesion, single segment; intradural, thoracic by transthoracic approach	29.42	22.49	3.75	55.66	90	S
63306	00	A	Vertebral corpectomy (vertebral body resection), partial or complete, for excision of intraspinal lesion, single segment; intradural, thoracic by thoracolumbar approach	30.01	22.76	2.65	55.42	90	S
63307	00	A	Vertebral corpectomy (vertebral body resection), partial or complete, for excision of intraspinal lesion, single segment; intradural, lumbar or sacral by transperitoneal or retroperitoneal approach	29.42	24.42	2.98	56.82	90	S
63308	00	A	Vertebral corpectomy (vertebral body resection), partial or complete, for excision of intraspinal lesion, single segment; each additional segment (list separately in addition to codes for single segment 63300-63307)	5.25	4.05	0.73	10.03	ZZZ	S
63600	00	A	Creation of lesion of spinal cord by stereotactic method, percutaneous, any modality (including stimulation and/or recording)	13.08	10.70	2.63	26.41	90	N
63610	00	A	Stereotactic stimulation of spinal cord, percutaneous, separate procedure not followed by other surgery	8.73	6.73	2.06	17.52	0	N
63615	00	A	Stereotactic biopsy, aspiration, or excision of lesion, spinal cord	15.40	11.55	2.03	28.98	90	S
63650	00	A	Percutaneous implantation of neurostimulator electrodes; epidural	5.99	8.05	2.13	16.17	90	S
63655	00	A	Laminectomy for implantation of neurostimulator electrodes; epidural	8.95	14.90	3.64	27.49	90	S
63660	00	A	Revision or removal of spinal neurostimulator electrodes	5.54	7.09	1.56	14.19	90	S
63685	00	A	Incision and subcutaneous placement of spinal neurostimulator pulse generator or receiver, direct or inductive coupling	6.29	7.40	1.46	15.15	90	S
63688	00	A	Revision or removal of implanted spinal neurostimulator pulse generator or receiver	4.77	6.10	1.26	12.13	90	S
63690	00	A	Electronic analysis of implanted neurostimulator pulse generator system (may include rate, pulse amplitude and duration, configuration of wave form, battery status, electrode selectability, output modulation, cycling, impedance and patient compliance measurements); without reprogramming of pulse generator	0.45	0.65	0.12	1.22	XXX	N
63691	00	A	Electronic analysis of implanted neurostimulator pulse generator system (may include rate, pulse amplitude and duration, configuration of wave form, battery status, electrode selectability, output modulation, cycling, impedance and patient compliance measurements); with reprogramming of pulse generator	0.65	0.41	0.11	1.17	XXX	N
63700	00	A	Repair of meningocele; less than 5 cm diameter	15.62	11.35	2.22	29.19	90	S
63702	00	A	Repair of meningocele; larger than 5 cm diameter	17.57	12.78	2.49	32.84	90	S
63704	00	A	Repair of myelomeningocele; less than 5 cm diameter	19.52	14.19	2.77	36.48	90	S
63706	00	A	Repair of myelomeningocele; larger than 5 cm diameter	22.45	16.33	3.18	41.96	90	S
63707	00	A	Repair of dural/CSF leak, not requiring laminectomy	10.14	12.98	2.56	25.68	90	S
63709	00	A	Repair of dural/CSF leak or pseudomeningocele, with laminectomy	13.26	16.97	3.30	33.53	90	S
63710	00	A	Dural graft, spinal	13.01	9.75	1.58	24.34	90	S
63740	00	A	Creation of shunt, lumbar, subarachnoid-peritoneal, -pleural, or other; including laminectomy	10.43	13.35	2.99	26.77	90	S
63741	00	A	Creation of shunt, lumbar, subarachnoid-peritoneal, -pleural, or other; percutaneous, not requiring laminectomy	7.13	9.92	2.39	19.44	90	S

CPT codes and descriptions only, © 1994 American Medical Association. Reimbursement information, © 1995 McGraw-Hill Inc.

Code/ CPT	Mod- ifier	Status	Description	Work value	Practice expense	Mal- practice	Total value	Global period	Up- date
63744	00	A	Replacement, irrigation or revision of lumbosubarachnoid shunt	6.83	8.15	1.68	16.66	90	S
63746	00	A	Removal of entire lumbosubarachnoid shunt system without replacement	5.60	5.52	1.08	12.20	90	S
63750	00	A	Insertion, subarachnoid catheter with reservoir and/or pump for intermittent or continuous infusion of drug, including laminectomy	7.23	11.24	3.03	21.50	90	S
63780	00	A	Insertion or replacement, subarachnoid or epidural catheter, with reservoir and/or pump for drug infusion, without laminectomy	6.22	1.93	0.55	8.70	90	N
64400	00	A	Injection, anesthetic agent; trigeminal nerve, any division or branch	1.11	0.48	0.05	1.64	0	N
64402	00	A	Injection, anesthetic agent; facial nerve	1.25	0.62	0.09	1.96	0	S
64405	00	A	Injection, anesthetic agent; greater occipital nerve	1.32	0.64	0.07	2.03	0	N
64408	00	A	Injection, anesthetic agent; vagus nerve	1.41	1.04	0.11	2.56	0	N
64410	00	A	Injection, anesthetic agent; phrenic nerve	1.43	0.71	0.15	2.29	0	N
64412	00	A	Injection, anesthetic agent; spinal accessory nerve	1.18	0.62	0.08	1.88	0	N
64413	00	A	Injection, anesthetic agent; cervical plexus	1.40	0.74	0.08	2.22	0	N
64415	00	A	Injection, anesthetic agent; brachial plexus	1.48	0.26	0.07	1.81	0	N
64417	00	A	Injection, anesthetic agent; axillary nerve	1.44	0.63	0.15	2.22	0	N
64418	00	A	Injection, anesthetic agent; suprascapular nerve	1.32	0.85	0.10	2.27	0	N
64420	00	A	Injection, anesthetic agent; intercostal nerve, single	1.18	0.64	0.07	1.89	0	N
64421	00	A	Injection, anesthetic agent; intercostal nerves, multiple, regional block	1.68	0.83	0.17	2.68	0	N
64425	00	A	Injection, anesthetic agent; ilioinguinal, iliohypogastric nerves	1.75	0.57	0.10	2.42	0	N
64430	00	A	Injection, anesthetic agent; pudendal nerve	1.46	0.70	0.12	2.28	0	S
64435	00	A	Injection, anesthetic agent; paracervical (uterine) nerve	1.45	0.47	0.09	2.01	0	S
64440	00	A	Injection, anesthetic agent; paravertebral nerve (thoracic, lumbar, sacral, coccygeal), single vertebral level	1.34	0.79	0.09	2.22	0	N
64441	00	A	Injection, anesthetic agent; paravertebral nerves, multiple levels (eg, regional block)	1.79	1.01	0.12	2.92	0	N
64442	00	A	Injection, anesthetic agent; paravertebral facet joint nerve, lumbar, single level	1.41	1.19	0.16	2.76	0	N
64443	00	A	Injection, anesthetic agent; paravertebral facet joint nerve, lumbar, each additional level	1.35	0.63	0.12	2.10	ZZZ	N
64445	00	A	Injection, anesthetic agent; sciatic nerve	1.48	2.03	0.49	0.06	0	N
64450	00	A	Injection, anesthetic agent; other peripheral nerve or branch	1.27	0.53	0.05	1.85	0	S
64505	00	A	Injection, anesthetic agent; sphenopalatine ganglion	1.36	0.62	0.06	2.04	0	N
64508	00	A	Injection, anesthetic agent; carotid sinus (separate procedure)	1.12	1.04	0.08	2.24	0	N
64510	00	A	Injection, anesthetic agent; stellate ganglion (cervical sympathetic)	1.22	0.71	0.18	2.11	0	N
64520	00	A	Injection, anesthetic agent; lumbar or thoracic (paravertebral sympathetic)	1.35	0.72	0.17	2.24	0	N
64530	00	A	Injection, anesthetic agent; celiac plexus, with or without radiologic monitoring	1.58	1.17	0.28	3.03	0	N
64550	00	A	Application of surface (transcutaneous) neurostimulator	0.18	0.44	0.04	0.66	0	N
64553	00	A	Percutaneous implantation of neurostimulator electrodes; cranial nerve	2.26	1.02	0.10	3.38	10	N
64555	00	A	Percutaneous implantation of neurostimulator electrodes; peripheral nerve	2.22	0.42	0.10	2.74	10	N

CPT codes and descriptions only, © 1994 American Medical Association. Reimbursement information, © 1995 McGraw-Hill Inc.

Code/ CPT	Mod-ifier	Status	Description	Work value	Practice expense	Mal-practice	Total value	Global period	Up-date
64560	00	A	Percutaneous implantation of neurostimulator electrodes; autonomic nerve	2.31	1.45	0.24	4.00	10	S
64565	00	A	Percutaneous implantation of neurostimulator electrodes; neuromuscular	1.71	0.76	0.08	2.55	10	N
64573	00	A	Incision for implantation of neurostimulator electrodes; cranial nerve	4.35	3.16	0.61	8.12	90	S
64575	00	A	Incision for implantation of neurostimulator electrodes; peripheral nerve	4.27	3.07	0.40	7.74	90	S
64577	00	A	Incision for implantation of neurostimulator electrodes; autonomic nerve	4.54	2.76	0.45	7.75	90	S
64580	00	A	Incision for implantation of neurostimulator electrodes; neuromuscular	4.04	2.91	0.20	7.15	90	S
64585	00	A	Revision or removal of peripheral neurostimulator electrodes	2.01	0.97	0.09	3.07	10	S
64590	00	A	Incision and subcutaneous placement of peripheral neurostimulator pulse generator or receiver, direct or inductive coupling	2.35	1.84	0.35	4.54	10	S
64595	00	A	Revision or removal of peripheral neurostimulator pulse generator or receiver	1.68	1.12	0.21	3.01	10	S
64600	00	A	Destruction by neurolytic agent, trigeminal nerve; supraorbital, infraorbital, mental, or inferior alveolar branch	3.40	1.69	0.17	5.26	10	N
64605	00	A	Destruction by neurolytic agent, trigeminal nerve; second and third division branches at foramen ovale	5.56	1.56	0.33	7.45	10	N
64610	00	A	Destruction by neurolytic agent, trigeminal nerve; second and third division branches at foramen ovale under radiologic monitoring	7.11	7.26	1.35	15.72	10	N
64612	00	A	Destruction by neurolytic agent (chemodenervation of muscle endplate); muscles enervated by facial nerve (eg, for blepharospasm, hemifacial spasm)	1.91	1.45	0.17	3.53	10	S
64613	00	A	Destruction by neurolytic agent (chemodenervation of muscle endplate); cervical spinal muscles (eg, for spasmodic torticollis)	1.91	1.45	0.17	3.53	10	S
64620	00	A	Destruction by neurolytic agent; intercostal nerve	2.79	1.00	0.19	3.98	10	N
64622	00	A	Destruction by neurolytic agent; paravertebral facet joint nerve, lumbar, single level	2.95	1.82	0.35	5.12	10	N
64623	00	A	Destruction by neurolytic agent; paravertebral facet joint nerve, lumbar, each additional level	0.99	0.85	0.17	2.01	ZZZ	N
64630	00	A	Destruction by neurolytic agent; pudendal nerve	2.95	1.74	0.38	5.07	10	N
64640	00	A	Destruction by neurolytic agent; other peripheral nerve or branch	2.49	0.92	0.09	3.50	10	N
64680	00	A	Destruction by neurolytic agent, celiac plexus, with or without radiologic monitoring	2.57	1.55	0.41	4.53	10	N
64702	00	A	Neuroplasty; digital, one or both, same digit	4.02	4.22	0.70	8.94	90	S
64704	00	A	Neuroplasty; nerve of hand or foot	4.44	5.38	0.74	10.56	90	S
64708	00	A	Neuroplasty, major peripheral nerve, arm or leg; other than specified	5.71	7.31	1.26	14.28	90	S
64712	00	A	Neuroplasty, major peripheral nerve, arm or leg; sciatic nerve	7.18	9.19	1.68	18.05	90	S
64713	00	A	Neuroplasty, major peripheral nerve, arm or leg; brachial plexus	10.34	9.40	1.72	21.46	90	S
64714	00	A	Neuroplasty, major peripheral nerve, arm or leg; lumbar plexus	9.87	6.13	1.41	17.41	90	S
64716	00	A	Neuroplasty and/or transposition; cranial nerve (specify)	5.80	4.83	0.67	11.30	90	S
64718	00	A	Neuroplasty and/or transposition; ulnar nerve at elbow	5.48	6.72	1.13	13.33	90	S
64719	00	A	Neuroplasty and/or transposition; ulnar nerve at wrist	4.72	4.95	0.85	10.52	90	S

CPT codes and descriptions only, © 1994 American Medical Association. Reimbursement information, © 1995 McGraw-Hill Inc.

Code/ CPT	Mod- ifier	Status	Description	Work value	Practice expense	Mal- practice	Total value	Global period	Up- date
64721	00	A	Neuroplasty and/or transposition; median nerve at carpal tunnel	3.99	4.90	0.83	9.72	90	S
64722	00	A	Decompression; unspecified nerve(s) (specify)	4.46	5.71	1.11	11.28	90	S
64726	00	A	Decompression; plantar digital nerve	3.97	0.72	0.07	4.76	90	S
64727	00	A	Internal neurolysis, requiring use of operating microscope (list separately in addition to code for neuroplasty) (Neuroplasty includes external neurolysis)	3.10	3.24	0.55	6.89	ZZZ	S
64732	00	A	Transection or avulsion of; supraorbital nerve	4.15	4.31	0.72	9.18	90	S
64734	00	A	Transection or avulsion of; infraorbital nerve	4.62	4.61	0.67	9.90	90	S
64736	00	A	Transection or avulsion of; mental nerve	4.40	4.46	0.42	9.28	90	S
64738	00	A	Transection or avulsion of; inferior alveolar nerve by osteotomy	5.42	5.07	0.61	11.10	90	S
64740	00	A	Transection or avulsion of; lingual nerve	5.28	5.18	0.62	11.08	90	S
64742	00	A	Transection or avulsion of; facial nerve, differential or complete	5.91	5.00	0.44	11.35	90	S
64744	00	A	Transection or avulsion of; greater occipital nerve	4.87	6.10	1.10	12.07	90	S
64746	00	A	Transection or avulsion of; phrenic nerve	5.62	3.77	0.77	10.16	90	S
64752	00	A	Transection or avulsion of; vagus nerve (vagotomy), transthoracic	6.64	3.93	0.85	11.42	90	S
64755	00	A	Transection or avulsion of; vagi limited to proximal stomach (selective proximal vagotomy, proximal gastric vagotomy, parietal cell vagotomy, supra- or highly selective vagotomy)	13.10	10.47	2.27	25.84	90	S
64760	00	A	Transection or avulsion of; vagus nerve (vagotomy), abdominal	6.54	6.65	1.50	14.69	90	S
64761	00	A	Transection or avulsion of; pudendal nerve	6.10	4.66	0.50	11.26	90	S
64763	00	A	Transection or avulsion of obturator nerve, extrapelvic, with or without adductor tenotomy	6.72	4.80	0.92	12.44	90	S
64766	00	A	Transection or avulsion of obturator nerve, intrapelvic, with or without adductor tenotomy	8.31	6.67	1.20	16.18	90	S
64771	00	A	Transection or avulsion of other cranial nerve, extradural	6.99	6.42	0.73	14.14	90	S
64772	00	A	Transection or avulsion of other spinal nerve, extradural	6.79	6.77	1.30	14.86	90	S
64774	00	A	Excision of neuroma; cutaneous nerve, surgically identifiable	4.86	2.74	0.45	8.05	90	S
64776	00	A	Excision of neuroma; digital nerve, one or both, same digit	4.86	2.78	0.41	8.05	90	S
64778	00	A	Excision of neuroma; digital nerve, each additional digit (list separately by this number)	3.11	2.73	0.43	6.27	ZZZ	S
64782	00	A	Excision of neuroma; hand or foot, except digital nerve	5.81	4.70	0.46	10.97	90	S
64783	00	A	Excision of neuroma; hand or foot, each additional nerve, except same digit (list separately by this number)	3.72	3.26	0.47	7.45	ZZZ	S
64784	00	A	Excision of neuroma; major peripheral nerve, except sciatic	9.46	5.64	0.96	16.06	90	S
64786	00	A	Excision of neuroma; sciatic nerve	15.10	12.66	2.14	29.90	90	S
64787	00	A	Implantation of nerve end into bone or muscle (list separately in addition to neuroma excision)	4.30	3.47	0.60	8.37	ZZZ	S
64788	00	A	Excision of neurofibroma or neurolemmoma; cutaneous nerve	4.30	3.63	0.50	8.43	90	S
64790	00	A	Excision of neurofibroma or neurolemmoma; major peripheral nerve	10.95	7.11	1.22	19.28	90	S
64792	00	A	Excision of neurofibroma or neurolemmoma; extensive (including malignant type)	14.40	8.99	1.66	25.05	90	S
64795	00	A	Biopsy of nerve	3.01	2.38	0.39	5.78	0	S
64802	00	A	Sympathectomy, cervical	8.22	5.40	1.10	14.72	90	S
64804	00	A	Sympathectomy, cervicothoracic	13.65	12.77	2.44	28.86	90	S

CPT codes and descriptions only, © 1994 American Medical Association. Reimbursement information, © 1995 McGraw-Hill Inc.

Code/ CPT	Mod- ifier	Status	Description	Work value	Practice expense	Mal- practice	Total value	Global period	Up- date
64809	00	A	Sympathectomy, thoracolumbar	12.79	10.55	2.04	25.38	90	S
64818	00	A	Sympathectomy, lumbar	9.42	8.57	1.72	19.71	90	S
64820	00	A	Sympathectomy, digital arteries, with magnification, each digit	9.10	6.62	1.30	17.02	90	S
64830	00	A	Microdissection and/or microrepair of nerve (list separately in addition to code for nerve repair)	3.10	2.01	0.38	5.49	ZZZ	S
64831	00	A	Suture of digital nerve, hand or foot; one nerve	8.84	3.38	0.56	12.78	90	S
64832	00	A	Suture of digital nerve, hand or foot; each additional digital nerve	5.66	1.40	0.24	7.30	ZZZ	S
64834	00	A	Suture of one nerve, hand or foot; common sensory nerve	9.77	3.50	0.56	13.83	90	S
64835	00	A	Suture of one nerve, hand or foot; median motor thenar	10.47	5.96	1.03	17.46	90	S
64836	00	A	Suture of one nerve, hand or foot; ulnar motor	10.47	6.70	1.22	18.39	90	S
64837	00	A	Suture of each additional nerve, hand or foot	6.26	4.45	0.85	11.56	ZZZ	S
64840	00	A	Suture of posterior tibial nerve	12.43	10.35	0.53	23.31	90	S
64856	00	A	Suture of major peripheral nerve, arm or leg, except sciatic; including transposition	12.81	8.21	1.46	22.48	90	S
64857	00	A	Suture of major peripheral nerve, arm or leg, except sciatic; without transposition	13.43	9.53	1.54	24.50	90	S
64858	00	A	Suture of sciatic nerve	15.43	10.98	2.11	28.52	90	S
64859	00	A	Suture of each additional major peripheral nerve	4.26	3.50	0.58	8.34	ZZZ	S
64861	00	A	Suture of; brachial plexus	17.94	13.42	1.38	32.74	90	S
64862	00	A	Suture of; lumbar plexus	18.14	21.56	1.61	41.31	90	S
64864	00	A	Suture of facial nerve; extracranial	11.87	7.86	1.16	20.89	90	S
64865	00	A	Suture of facial nerve; infratemporal, with or without grafting	14.70	12.34	1.50	28.54	90	S
64866	00	A	Anastomosis; facial-spinal accessory	14.94	11.19	1.84	27.97	90	S
64868	00	A	Anastomosis; facial-hypoglossal	13.36	11.19	1.47	26.02	90	S
64870	00	A	Anastomosis; facial-phrenic	15.19	13.91	1.70	30.80	90	S
64872	00	A	Suture of nerve; requiring secondary or delayed suture (list separately in addition to code for primary neurorrhaphy)	1.99	1.44	0.29	3.72	ZZZ	S
64874	00	A	Suture of nerve; requiring extensive mobilization, or transposition of nerve (list separately in addition to code for nerve suture)	2.98	2.17	0.43	5.58	ZZZ	S
64876	00	A	Suture of nerve; requiring shortening of bone of extremity (list separately in addition to code for nerve suture)	3.38	2.46	0.48	6.32	ZZZ	N
64885	00	A	Nerve graft (includes obtaining graft), head or neck; up to 4 cm in length	16.73	12.69	1.48	30.90	90	S
64886	00	A	Nerve graft (includes obtaining graft), head or neck; more than 4 cm in length	19.95	15.13	1.77	36.85	90	S
64890	00	A	Nerve graft (includes obtaining graft), single strand, hand or foot; up to 4 cm length	14.35	12.26	2.12	28.73	90	S
64891	00	A	Nerve graft (includes obtaining graft), single strand, hand or foot; more than 4 cm length	15.21	10.42	1.73	27.36	90	S
64892	00	A	Nerve graft (includes obtaining graft), single strand, arm or leg; up to 4 cm length	13.85	11.04	1.69	26.58	90	S
64893	00	A	Nerve graft (includes obtaining graft), single strand, arm or leg; more than 4 cm length	14.61	13.93	2.27	30.81	90	S
64895	00	A	Nerve graft (includes obtaining graft), multiple strands (cable), hand or foot; up to 4 cm length	18.39	13.16	2.55	34.10	90	S
64896	00	A	Nerve graft (includes obtaining graft), multiple strands (cable), hand or foot; more than 4 cm length	19.38	17.53	1.90	38.81	90	S
64897	00	A	Nerve graft (includes obtaining graft), multiple strands (cable), arm or leg; up to 4 cm length	17.38	12.63	2.47	32.48	90	S

CPT codes and descriptions only, © 1994 American Medical Association. Reimbursement information, © 1995 McGraw-Hill Inc.

Code/ CPT	Mod- ifier	Status	Description	Work value	Practice expense	Mal- practice	Total value	Global period	Up- date
64898	00	A	Nerve graft (includes obtaining graft), multiple strands (cable), arm or leg; more than 4 cm length	18.39	14.40	2.35	35.14	90	S
64901	00	A	Nerve graft, each additional nerve; single strand	10.22	10.16	0.87	21.25	ZZZ	S
64902	00	A	Nerve graft, each additional nerve; multiple strands (cable)	11.83	11.92	0.99	24.74	ZZZ	S
64905	00	A	Nerve pedicle transfer; first stage	13.22	9.40	0.70	23.32	90	S
64907	00	A	Nerve pedicle transfer; second stage	17.90	13.02	2.55	33.47	90	S
64999	00	C	Unlisted procedure, nervous system	0	0	0	0	YYY	N
65091	00	A	Evisceration of ocular contents; without implant	6.10	7.81	0.45	14.36	90	S
65093	00	A	Evisceration of ocular contents; with implant	6.47	8.28	0.52	15.27	90	S
65101	00	A	Enucleation of eye; without implant	6.52	8.35	0.47	15.34	90	S
65103	00	A	Enucleation of eye; with implant, muscles not attached to implant	7.06	9.04	0.50	16.60	90	S
65105	00	A	Enucleation of eye; with implant, muscles attached to implant	7.82	10.01	0.55	18.38	90	S
65110	00	A	Exenteration of orbit (does not include skin graft), removal of orbital contents; only	13.18	15.99	1.14	30.31	90	S
65112	00	A	Exenteration of orbit (does not include skin graft), removal of orbital contents; with therapeutic removal of bone	15.44	12.16	1.09	28.69	90	S
65114	00	A	Exenteration of orbit (does not include skin graft), removal of orbital contents; with muscle or myocutaneous flap	16.59	13.07	1.65	31.31	90	S
65125	00	A	Modification of ocular implant with placement or replacement of pegs (eg, drilling receptacle for prosthesis appendage) (separate procedure)	2.97	2.47	0.13	5.57	90	S
65130	00	A	Insertion of ocular implant secondary; after evisceration, in scleral shell	6.75	8.64	0.50	15.89	90	S
65135	00	A	Insertion of ocular implant secondary; after enucleation, muscles not attached to implant	6.93	5.42	0.35	12.70	90	S
65140	00	A	Insertion of ocular implant secondary; after enucleation, muscles attached to implant	7.46	6.22	0.33	14.01	90	S
65150	00	A	Reinsertion of ocular implant; with or without conjunctival graft	5.97	8.44	0.56	14.97	90	S
65155	00	A	Reinsertion of ocular implant; with use of foreign material for reinforcement and/or attachment of muscles to implant	8.21	11.11	0.90	20.22	90	S
65175	00	A	Removal of ocular implant	5.93	7.49	0.40	13.82	90	S
65205	00	A	Removal of foreign body, external eye; conjunctival superficial	0.78	0.37	0.02	1.17	0	S
65210	00	A	Removal of foreign body, external eye; conjunctival embedded (includes concretions), subconjunctival, or scleral nonperforating	0.84	0.46	0.03	1.33	0	S
65220	00	A	Removal of foreign body, external eye; corneal, without slit lamp	0.71	0.52	0.04	1.27	0	N
65222	00	A	Removal of foreign body, external eye; corneal, with slit lamp	0.93	0.57	0.03	1.53	0	S
65235	00	A	Removal of foreign body, intraocular; from anterior chamber or lens	7.12	5.61	0.30	13.03	90	S
65260	00	A	Removal of foreign body, intraocular; from posterior segment, magnetic extraction, anterior or posterior route	10.35	8.63	0.45	19.43	90	S
65265	00	A	Removal of foreign body, intraocular; from posterior segment, nonmagnetic extraction	12.04	10.04	0.51	22.59	90	S
65270	00	A	Repair of laceration; conjunctiva, with or without nonperforating laceration sclera, direct closure	1.85	1.17	0.07	3.09	10	S
65272	00	A	Repair of laceration; conjunctiva, by mobilization and rearrangement, without hospitalization	3.57	1.64	0.10	5.31	90	S

CPT codes and descriptions only, © 1994 American Medical Association. Reimbursement information, © 1995 McGraw-Hill Inc.

Code/ CPT	Mod- ifier	Status	Description	Work value	Practice expense	Mal- practice	Total value	Global period	Up- date
65273	00	A	Repair of laceration; conjunctiva, by mobilization and rearrangement, with hospitalization	3.89	3.22	0.21	7.32	90	S
65275	00	A	Repair of laceration; cornea, nonperforating, with or without removal foreign body	5.04	0.66	0.04	5.74	90	S
65280	00	A	Repair of laceration; cornea and/or sclera, perforating, not involving uveal tissue	7.10	9.09	0.49	16.68	90	S
65285	00	A	Repair of laceration; cornea and/or sclera, perforating, with reposition or resection of uveal tissue	12.06	12.26	0.64	24.96	90	S
65286	00	A	Repair of laceration; application of tissue glue, wounds of cornea and/or sclera	5.16	4.79	0.25	10.20	90	S
65290	00	A	Repair of wound, extraocular muscle, tendon and/or Tenon's capsule	5.06	6.20	0.37	11.63	90	S
65400	00	A	Excision of lesion, cornea (keratectomy, lamellar, partial), except pterygium	5.61	6.46	0.35	12.42	90	S
65410	00	A	Biopsy of cornea	1.47	1.59	0.11	3.17	0	S
65420	00	A	Excision or transposition of pterygium; without graft	3.97	4.28	0.23	8.48	90	S
65426	00	A	Excision or transposition of pterygium; with graft	5.05	6.47	0.38	11.90	90	S
65430	00	A	Scraping of cornea, diagnostic, for smear and/or culture	0.87	0.54	0.03	1.44	0	S
65435	00	A	Removal of corneal epithelium; with or without chemocauterization (abrasion, curettage)	0.92	0.77	0.04	1.73	0	S
65436	00	A	Removal of corneal epithelium; with application of chelating agent (eg, EDTA)	3.99	1.53	0.08	5.60	90	S
65450	00	A	Destruction of lesion of cornea by cryotherapy, photocoagulation or thermocauterization	3.07	3.28	0.17	6.52	90	S
65600	00	A	Multiple punctures of anterior cornea (eg, for corneal erosion, tattoo)	3.15	2.62	0.14	5.91	90	S
65710	00	A	Keratoplasty (corneal transplant); lamellar	9.52	15.38	1.13	26.03	90	S
65730	00	A	Keratoplasty (corneal transplant); penetrating (except in aphakia)	11.83	18.27	1.29	31.39	90	S
65750	00	A	Keratoplasty (corneal transplant); penetrating (in aphakia)	12.58	19.00	1.33	32.91	90	S
65755	00	A	Keratoplasty (corneal transplant); penetrating (in pseudophakia)	12.58	19.52	1.39	33.49	90	S
65760	00	N	Keratomileusis	22.51*	18.75#	0.97*	42.23#	XXX	0
65765	00	N	Keratophakia	24.62*	20.51#	1.06*	46.19#	XXX	0
65767	00	N	Epikeratoplasty	19.70*	16.41#	0.85*	36.96#	XXX	0
65770	00	A	Keratoprosthesis	16.56	13.81	0.71	31.08	90	S
65771	00	N	Radial keratotomy	9.85*	8.21#	0.43*	18.49#	XXX	0
65772	00	A	Corneal relaxing incision for correction of surgically induced astigmatism	4.04	5.16	0.31	9.51	90	S
65775	00	A	Corneal wedge resection for correction of surgically induced astigmatism	5.44	7.62	0.50	13.56	90	S
65800	00	A	Paracentesis of anterior chamber of eye (separate procedure); with diagnostic aspiration of aqueous	1.91	1.72	0.10	3.73	0	S
65805	00	A	Paracentesis of anterior chamber of eye (separate procedure); with therapeutic release of aqueous	1.91	1.81	0.10	3.82	0	S
65810	00	A	Paracentesis of anterior chamber of eye (separate procedure); with removal of vitreous and/or discission of anterior hyaloid membrane, with or without air injection	4.57	5.45	0.30	10.32	90	S
65815	00	A	Paracentesis of anterior chamber of eye (separate procedure); with removal of blood, with or without irrigation and/or air injection	4.75	4.49	0.24	9.48	90	S
65820	00	A	Goniotomy	7.60	9.54	0.51	17.65	90	S
65850	00	A	Trabeculotomy ab externo	10.18	13.03	0.69	23.90	90	S

CPT codes and descriptions only, © 1994 American Medical Association. Reimbursement information, © 1995 McGraw-Hill Inc.

Code/ CPT	Mod-ifier	Status	Description	Work value	Practice expense	Mal-practice	Total value	Global period	Up-date
65855	00	A	Trabeculoplasty by laser surgery, one or more sessions (defined treatment series)	4.65	7.38	0.52	12.55	90	S
65860	00	A	Severing adhesions of anterior segment, laser technique (separate procedure)	3.37	5.12	0.37	8.86	90	S
65865	00	A	Severing adhesions of anterior segment of eye, incisional technique (with or without injection of air or liquid) (separate procedure); goniosynechiae	5.42	6.93	0.41	12.76	90	S
65870	00	A	Severing adhesions of anterior segment of eye, incisional technique (with or without injection of air or liquid) (separate procedure); anterior synechiae, except goniosynechiae	5.92	5.86	0.31	12.09	90	S
65875	00	A	Severing adhesions of anterior segment of eye, incisional technique (with or without injection of air or liquid) (separate procedure); posterior synechiae	6.14	6.28	0.34	12.76	90	S
65880	00	A	Severing adhesions of anterior segment of eye, incisional technique (with or without injection of air or liquid) (separate procedure); corneovitreal adhesions	6.69	6.85	0.37	13.91	90	S
65900	00	A	Removal of epithelial downgrowth, anterior chamber eye	10.43	7.91	0.92	19.26	90	S
65920	00	A	Removal of implanted material, anterior segment eye	7.90	8.36	0.44	16.70	90	S
65930	00	A	Removal of blood clot, anterior segment eye	7.03	7.68	0.41	15.12	90	S
66020	00	A	Injection, anterior chamber (separate procedure); air or liquid	1.54	2.02	0.14	3.70	10	S
66030	00	A	Injection, anterior chamber (separate procedure); medication	1.20	0.54	0.03	1.77	10	S
66130	00	A	Excision of lesion, sclera	7.54	5.28	0.28	13.10	90	S
66150	00	A	Fistulization of sclera for glaucoma; trephination with iridectomy	7.60	9.72	0.59	17.91	90	S
66155	00	A	Fistulization of sclera for glaucoma; thermocauterization with iridectomy	7.48	9.57	0.50	17.55	90	S
66160	00	A	Fistulization of sclera for glaucoma; sclerectomy with punch or scissors, with iridectomy	9.47	10.77	0.55	20.79	90	S
66165	00	A	Fistulization of sclera for glaucoma; iridencleisis or iridotasis	7.31	9.36	0.57	17.24	90	S
66170	00	A	Fistulization of sclera for glaucoma; trabeculectomy ab externo in absence of previous surgery	11.31	12.15	0.63	24.09	90	S
66172	00	A	Fistulization of sclera for glaucoma; trabeculectomy ab externo with scarring from previous ocular surgery or trauma (includes injection of antifibrotic agents)	13.67	12.15	0.63	26.45	90	S
66180	00	A	Aqueous shunt to extraocular reservoir (eg, Molteno, Schocket, Denver-Krupin)	12.63	16.17	1.03	29.83	90	S
66185	00	A	Revision of aqueous shunt to extraocular reservoir	7.69	9.85	0.58	18.12	90	S
66220	00	A	Repair of scleral staphyloma; without graft	7.32	5.95	0.34	13.61	90	S
66225	00	A	Repair of scleral staphyloma; with graft	10.55	13.64	0.86	25.05	90	S
66250	00	A	Revision or repair of operative wound of anterior segment, any type, early or late, major or minor procedure	5.63	7.20	0.38	13.21	90	S
66500	00	A	Iridotomy by stab incision (separate procedure); except transfixion	3.58	4.58	0.27	8.43	90	S
66505	00	A	Iridotomy by stab incision (separate procedure); with transfixion as for iris bombe	3.93	3.27	0.17	7.37	90	S
66600	00	A	Iridectomy, with corneoscleral or corneal section; for removal of lesion	8.23	9.36	0.51	18.10	90	S
66605	00	A	Iridectomy, with corneoscleral or corneal section; with cyclectomy	12.34	11.87	0.67	24.88	90	S
66625	00	A	Iridotomy by stab incision (separate procedure); peripheral for glaucoma (separate procedure)	4.95	7.10	0.48	12.53	90	S

CPT codes and descriptions only, © 1994 American Medical Association. Reimbursement information, © 1995 McGraw-Hill Inc.

Code/ CPT	Mod-ifier	Status	Description	Work value	Practice expense	Mal-practice	Total value	Global period	Up-date
66630	00	A	Iridotomy by stab incision (separate procedure); sector for glaucoma (separate procedure)	5.81	7.43	0.45	13.69	90	S
66635	00	A	Iridotomy by stab incision (separate procedure); "optical" (separate procedure)	5.90	7.72	0.49	14.11	90	S
66680	00	A	Repair of iris, ciliary body (as for iridodialysis)	5.14	6.42	0.35	11.91	90	S
66682	00	A	Suture of iris, ciliary body (separate procedure) with retrieval of suture through small incision (eg, McCannel suture)	5.86	7.33	0.38	13.57	90	S
66700	00	A	Ciliary body destruction; diathermy	4.55	5.83	0.35	10.73	90	S
66710	00	A	Ciliary body destruction; cyclophotocoagulation	4.55	6.08	0.41	11.04	90	S
66720	00	A	Ciliary body destruction; cryotherapy	4.55	5.83	0.38	10.76	90	S
66740	00	A	Ciliary body destruction; cyclodialysis	4.55	6.01	0.39	10.95	90	S
66761	00	A	Iridotomy/iridectomy by laser surgery (eg, for glaucoma) (one or more sessions)	3.77	6.46	0.47	10.70	90	S
66762	00	A	Iridoplasty by photocoagulation (one or more sessions) (eg, for improvement of vision, for widening of anterior chamber angle)	4.33	7.53	0.55	12.41	90	S
66770	00	A	Destruction of cyst or lesion iris or ciliary body (nonexcisional procedure)	4.88	6.79	0.45	12.12	90	S
66820	00	A	Discission of secondary membranous cataract (opacified posterior lens capsule and/or anterior hyaloid); stab incision technique (Ziegler or Wheeler knife)	3.76	4.81	0.29	8.86	90	S
66821	00	A	Discission of secondary membranous cataract (opacified posterior lens capsule and/or anterior hyaloid); laser surgery (eg, YAG laser) (one or more stages)	2.78	4.83	0.37	7.98	90	S
66825	00	A	Repositioning of intraocular lens prosthesis, requiring an incision (separate procedure)	7.73	7.33	0.38	15.44	90	S
66830	00	A	Removal of secondary membranous cataract (opacified posterior lens capsule and/or anterior hyaloid) with corneo-scleral section, with or without iridectomy (iridocapsulotomy, iridocapsulectomy)	7.80	7.67	0.40	15.87	90	S
66840	00	A	Removal of lens material; aspiration technique, one or more stages	7.51	9.61	0.54	17.66	90	S
66850	00	A	Removal of lens material; phacofragmentation technique (mechanical or ultrasonic) (eg, phacoemulsification), with aspiration	8.66	11.09	0.70	20.45	90	S
66852	00	A	Removal of lens material; pars plana approach, with or without vitrectomy	9.52	13.23	0.90	23.65	90	S
66920	00	A	Removal of lens material; intracapsular	8.46	10.82	0.60	19.88	90	S
66930	00	A	Removal of lens material; intracapsular, for dislocated lens	9.73	10.49	0.57	20.79	90	S
66940	00	A	Removal of lens material; extracapsular (other than 66840, 66850, 66852)	8.48	10.85	0.62	19.95	90	S
66983	00	A	Intracapsular cataract extraction with insertion of intraocular lens prosthesis (one stage procedure)	8.54	13.20	0.95	22.69	90	S
66984	00	A	Extracapsular cataract removal with insertion of intraocular lens prosthesis (one stage procedure), manual or mechanical technique (eg, irrigation and aspiration or phacoemulsification)	9.89	13.93	0.94	24.76	90	S
66985	00	A	Insertion of intraocular lens prosthesis (secondary implant), not associated with concurrent cataract removal	7.89	10.10	0.63	18.62	90	S
66986	00	A	Exchange of intraocular lens	11.78	12.20	0.63	24.61	90	S
66999	00	C	Unlisted procedure, anterior segment of eye	0	0	0	0	YYY	S
67005	00	A	Removal of vitreous, anterior approach (open sky technique or limbal incision); partial removal	6.63	13.93	1.13	21.69	90	S

CPT codes and descriptions only, © 1994 American Medical Association. Reimbursement information, © 1995 McGraw-Hill Inc.

Code/ CPT	Mod- ifier	Status	Description	Work value	Practice expense	Mal- practice	Total value	Global period	Up- date
67010	00	A	Removal of vitreous, anterior approach (open sky technique or limbal incision); subtotal removal with mechanical vitrectomy	6.67	13.28	1.04	20.99	90	S
67015	00	A	Aspiration or release of vitreous, subretinal or choroidal fluid, pars plana approach (posterior sclerotomy)	6.69	6.45	0.35	13.49	90	S
67025	00	A	Injection of vitreous substitute, pars plana or limbal approach, (fluid-gas exchange), with or without aspiration (separate procedure)	6.44	6.75	0.36	13.55	90	S
67028	00	A	Intravitreal injection of a pharmacologic agent (separate procedure)	2.52	3.22	0.18	5.92	0	S
67030	00	A	Discission of vitreous strands (without removal), pars plana approach	4.44	7.06	0.50	12.00	90	S
67031	00	A	Severing of vitreous strands, vitreous face adhesions, sheets, membranes or opacities, laser surgery (one or more stages)	3.42	8.88	0.75	13.05	90	S
67036	00	A	Vitrectomy, mechanical, pars plana approach;	11.33	19.99	1.49	32.81	90	S
67038	00	A	Vitrectomy, mechanical, pars plana approach; with epiretinal membrane stripping	20.20	27.25	1.80	49.25	90	S
67039	00	A	Vitrectomy, mechanical, pars plana approach; with focal endolaser photocoagulation	13.60	22.84	1.68	38.12	90	S
67040	00	A	Vitrectomy, mechanical, pars plana approach; with endolaser panretinal photocoagulation	16.26	24.86	1.75	42.87	90	S
67101	00	A	Repair of retinal detachment, one or more sessions; cryotherapy or diathermy, with or without drainage of subretinal fluid	7.02	9.83	0.66	17.51	90	S
67105	00	A	Repair of retinal detachment, one or more sessions; photocoagulation (laser or xenon arc, one or more sessions), with or without drainage of subretinal fluid	7.06	11.22	0.80	19.08	90	S
67107	00	A	Repair of retinal detachment, one or more sessions; scleral buckling (such as lamellar excision, imbrication or encircling procedure), with or without implant, may include procedures 67101, 67105	13.99	17.91	1.10	33	90	S
67108	00	A	Repair of retinal detachment, one or more sessions; with vitrectomy, any method, with or without air or gas tamponade, with or without focal endolaser photocoagulation, may include procedures 67101-67107 and/or removal of lens by same technique	19.90	26.71	1.76	48.37	90	S
67109	00	A	Repair of retinal detachment, one or more sessions; by technique other than 67101-67108 and 67110	11.51	16.40	1.12	29.03	90	S
67110	00	A	Repair of retinal detachment, one or more sessions; by injection of air or other gas (eg, pneumatic retinopexy)	8.14	13.06	0.97	22.17	90	S
67112	00	A	Repair of retinal detachment, one or more sessions; previously operated upon, any technique	16.15	16.51	0.86	33.52	90	S
67115	00	A	Release of encircling material (posterior segment)	4.64	6.36	0.44	11.44	90	S
67120	00	A	Removal of implanted material, posterior segment; extraocular	5.63	7.15	0.38	13.16	90	S
67121	00	A	Removal of implanted material, posterior segment; intraocular	10.17	9.42	0.49	20.08	90	S
67141	00	A	Prophylaxis of retinal detachment (eg, retinal break, lattice degeneration) without drainage, one or more sessions; cryotherapy, diathermy	4.90	7.09	0.48	12.47	90	S
67145	00	A	Prophylaxis of retinal detachment (eg, retinal break, lattice degeneration) without drainage, one or more sessions; photocoagulation (laser or xenon arc)	5.07	7.23	0.49	12.79	90	S

CPT codes and descriptions only, © 1994 American Medical Association. Reimbursement information, © 1995 McGraw-Hill Inc.

Code/ CPT	Mod- ifier	Status	Description	Work value	Practice expense	Mal- practice	Total value	Global period	Up- date
67208	00	A	Destruction of localized lesion of retina (eg, maculopathy, choroidopathy, small tumors), one or more sessions; cryotherapy, diathermy	6.40	8.28	0.52	15.20	90	S
67210	00	A	Destruction of localized lesion of retina (eg, maculopathy, choroidopathy, small tumors), one or more sessions; photocoagulation (laser or xenon arc)	9.48	9.02	0.47	18.97	90	S
67218	00	A	Destruction of localized lesion of retina (eg, maculopathy, choroidopathy, small tumors), one or more sessions; radiation by implantation of source (includes removal of source)	12.73	13.31	0.70	26.74	90	S
67227	00	A	Destruction of extensive or progressive retinopathy (eg, diabetic retinopathy), one or more sessions; cryotherapy, diathermy	6.28	8.11	0.51	14.90	90	S
67228	00	A	Destruction of extensive or progressive retinopathy (eg, diabetic retinopathy), one or more sessions; photocoagulation (laser or xenon arc)	12.39	9.39	0.48	22.26	90	S
67250	00	A	Scleral reinforcement (separate procedure); without graft	8.36	6.99	0.40	15.75	90	S
67255	00	A	Scleral reinforcement (separate procedure); with graft	8.39	12.60	0.87	21.86	90	S
67299	00	C	Unlisted procedure, posterior segment	0	0	0	0	YYY	S
67311	00	A	Strabismus surgery, recession or resection procedure (patient not previously operated on); one horizontal muscle	6.30	8.06	0.47	14.83	90	S
67312	00	A	Strabismus surgery, recession or resection procedure (patient not previously operated on); two horizontal muscles	7.55	9.66	0.53	17.74	90	S
67314	00	A	Strabismus surgery, recession or resection procedure (patient not previously operated on); one vertical muscle (excluding superior oblique)	7.12	9.18	0.58	16.88	90	S
67316	00	A	Strabismus surgery, recession or resection procedure (patient not previously operated on); two or more vertical muscles (excluding superior oblique)	8.02	10.34	0.67	19.03	90	S
67318	00	A	Strabismus surgery, any procedure (patient not previously operated on), superior oblique muscle	7.45	6.21	0.33	13.99	90	S
67320	00	A	Transposition procedure (eg, for paretic extraocular muscle), any extraocular muscle (specify)	8.26	10.57	0.69	19.52	90	S
67331	00	A	Strabismus surgery on patient with previous eye surgery or injury that did not involve the extraocular muscles	7.72	9.89	0.54	18.15	90	S
67332	00	A	Strabismus surgery on patient with scarring of extraocular muscles (eg, prior ocular injury, strabismus or retinal detachment surgery) or restrictive myopathy (eg, dysthyroid ophthalmopathy)	8.59	11.00	0.58	20.17	90	S
67334	00	A	Strabismus surgery by posterior fixation suture technique, with or without muscle recession	7.56	6.30	0.33	14.19	90	S
67335	00	A	Placement of adjustable suture(s) during strabismus surgery, including postoperative adjustment(s) of suture(s) (Report in addition to code for specific strabismus surgery)	2.49	5.28	0.43	8.20	ZZZ	S
67340	00	A	Strabismus surgery involving exploration and/or repair of detached extraocular muscle(s)	9.45	7.88	0.41	17.74	90	S
67343	00	A	Release of extensive scar tissue without detaching extraocular muscle (separate procedure)	7.00	5.83	0.31	13.14	90	S
67345	00	A	Chemodenervation of extraocular muscle	2.91	2.22	0.26	5.39	10	S
67350	00	A	Biopsy of extraocular muscle	2.87	2.39	0.13	5.39	0	S
67399	00	C	Unlisted procedure, ocular muscle	0	0	0	0	YYY	S
67400	00	A	Orbitotomy without bone flap (frontal or transconjunctival approach); for exploration, with or without biopsy	9.20	10.91	0.62	20.73	90	S
67405	00	A	Orbitotomy without bone flap (frontal or transconjunctival approach); with drainage only	7.42	9.49	0.67	17.58	90	S

CPT codes and descriptions only, © 1994 American Medical Association. Reimbursement information, © 1995 McGraw-Hill Inc.

Code/ CPT	Mod- ifier	Status	Description	Work value	Practice expense	Mal- practice	Total value	Global period	Up- date
67412	00	A	Orbitotomy without bone flap (frontal or transconjunctival approach); with removal of lesion	9.14	11.70	0.67	21.51	90	S
67413	00	A	Orbitotomy without bone flap (frontal or transconjunctival approach); with removal of foreign body	9.75	8.09	0.57	18.41	90	S
67414	00	A	Orbitotomy without bone flap (frontal or transconjunctival approach); with removal of bone for decompression	10.07	8.39	0.44	18.90	90	S
67415	00	A	Fine needle aspiration of orbital contents	1.76	2.02	0.12	3.90	0	S
67420	00	A	Orbitotomy with bone flap or window, lateral approach (eg, Kroenlein); with removal of lesion	13.36	16.78	1.11	31.25	90	S
67430	00	A	Orbitotomy with bone flap or window, lateral approach (eg, Kroenlein); with removal of foreign body	12.79	10.65	0.54	23.98	90	S
67440	00	A	Orbitotomy with bone flap or window, lateral approach (eg, Kroenlein); with drainage	12.43	15.91	0.97	29.31	90	S
67445	00	A	Orbitotomy with bone flap or window, lateral approach (eg, Kroenlein); with removal of bone for decompression	13.36	11.13	0.57	25.06	90	S
67450	00	A	Orbitotomy with bone flap or window, lateral approach (eg, Kroenlein); for exploration, with or without biopsy	12.80	15.29	0.87	28.96	90	S
67500	00	A	Retrobulbar injection; medication (separate procedure, does not include supply of medication)	0.79	0.73	0.06	1.58	0	S
67505	00	A	Retrobulbar injection; alcohol	0.82	1.04	0.06	1.92	0	S
67515	00	A	Injection of therapeutic agent into Tenon's capsule	0.61	0.56	0.03	1.20	0	S
67550	00	A	Orbital implant (implant outside muscle cone); insertion	9.69	9.62	0.70	20.01	90	S
67560	00	A	Orbital implant (implant outside muscle cone); removal or revision	10.10	8.30	0.48	18.88	90	S
67570	00	A	Optic nerve decompression (eg, incision or fenestration of optic nerve sheath)	12.52	7.56	0.39	20.47	90	S
67599	00	C	Unlisted procedure, orbit	0	0	0	0	YYY	S
67700	00	A	Blepharotomy, drainage of abscess, eyelid	1.30	0.49	0.03	1.82	10	S
67710	00	A	Severing of tarsorrhaphy	0.97	1.01	0.06	2.04	10	S
67715	00	A	Canthotomy (separate procedure)	1.17	1.49	0.09	2.75	10	S
67800	00	A	Excision of chalazion; single	1.35	0.94	0.05	2.34	10	S
67801	00	A	Excision of chalazion; multiple, same lid	1.85	1.39	0.08	3.32	10	S
67805	00	A	Excision of chalazion; multiple, different lids	2.17	1.38	0.08	3.63	10	S
67808	00	A	Excision of chalazion; under general anesthesia and/or requiring hospitalization, single or multiple	3.55	2.13	0.13	5.81	90	S
67810	00	A	Biopsy of eyelid	1.48	0.81	0.05	2.34	0	S
67820	00	A	Correction of trichiasis; epilation, by forceps only	0.89	0.38	0.02	1.29	0	S
67825	00	A	Correction of trichiasis; epilation, (eg, by electrosurgery or cryotherapy)	1.33	0.90	0.05	2.28	10	S
67830	00	A	Correction of trichiasis; incision of lid margin	1.65	2.36	0.17	4.18	10	S
67835	00	A	Correction of trichiasis; incision of lid margin, with free mucous membrane graft	5.41	6.95	0.45	12.81	90	S
67840	00	A	Excision of lesion of eyelid (except chalazion) without closure or with simple direct closure	1.99	1.22	0.07	3.28	10	S
67850	00	A	Destruction of lesion of lid margin (up to 1 cm)	1.64	0.82	0.05	2.51	10	S
67875	00	A	Temporary closure of eyelids by suture (eg, Frost suture)	1.35	1.72	0.13	3.20	0	S
67880	00	A	Construction of intermarginal adhesions, median tarsorrhaphy, or canthorrhaphy;	3.55	3.94	0.23	7.72	90	S
67882	00	A	Construction of intermarginal adhesions, median tarsorrhaphy, or canthorrhaphy; with transposition of tarsal plate	4.77	6.10	0.37	11.24	90	S
67900	00	A	Repair of brow ptosis (supraciliary, mid-forehead or coronal approach)	4.54	3.78	0.20	8.52	90	S

CPT codes and descriptions only, © 1994 American Medical Association. Reimbursement information, © 1995 McGraw-Hill Inc.

Code/ CPT	Mod- ifier	Status	Description	Work value	Practice expense	Mal- practice	Total value	Global period	Up- date
67901	00	A	Repair of blepharoptosis; frontalis muscle technique with suture or other material	6.82	8.73	0.64	16.19	90	S
67902	00	A	Repair of blepharoptosis; frontalis muscle technique with fascial sling (includes obtaining fascia)	6.88	8.81	0.72	16.41	90	S
67903	00	A	Repair of blepharoptosis; (tarso)levator resection or advancement, internal approach	6.22	9.25	0.73	16.20	90	S
67904	00	A	Repair of blepharoptosis; (tarso)levator resection or advancement, external approach	5.96	8.98	0.71	15.65	90	S
67906	00	A	Repair of blepharoptosis; superior rectus technique with fascial sling (includes obtaining fascia)	6.64	5.46	0.36	12.46	90	S
67908	00	A	Repair of blepharoptosis; conjunctivo-tarso-Muller's muscle-levator resection (eg, Fasanella-Servat type)	4.95	7.52	0.54	13.01	90	S
67909	00	A	Reduction of overcorrection of ptosis	5.22	6.69	0.48	12.39	90	S
67911	00	A	Correction of lid retraction	5.09	8.06	0.79	13.94	90	S
67914	00	A	Repair of ectropion; suture	3.60	5.17	0.39	9.16	90	S
67915	00	A	Repair of ectropion; thermocauterization	3.10	1.25	0.07	4.42	90	S
67916	00	A	Repair of ectropion; blepharoplasty, excision tarsal wedge	5.13	6.50	0.38	12.01	90	S
67917	00	A	Repair of ectropion; blepharoplasty, extensive (eg, Kuhnt-Szymanowski or tarsal strip operations)	5.84	7.48	0.47	13.79	90	S
67921	00	A	Repair of entropion; suture	3.32	3.82	0.20	7.34	90	S
67922	00	A	Repair of entropion; thermocauterization	2.98	1.19	0.07	4.24	90	S
67923	00	A	Repair of entropion; blepharoplasty, excision tarsal wedge	5.70	6.88	0.38	12.96	90	S
67924	00	A	Repair of entropion; blepharoplasty, extensive (eg, Wheeler operation)	5.64	7.22	0.43	13.29	90	S
67930	00	A	Suture of recent wound, eyelid, involving lid margin, tarsus, and/or palpebral conjunctiva direct closure; partial thickness	3.56	1.27	0.08	4.91	10	S
67935	00	A	Suture of recent wound, eyelid, involving lid margin, tarsus, and/or palpebral conjunctiva direct closure; full thickness	6.07	3.79	0.24	10.10	90	S
67938	00	A	Removal of embedded foreign body, eyelid	1.28	0.52	0.03	1.83	10	S
67950	00	A	Canthoplasty (reconstruction of canthus)	5.64	7.22	0.45	13.31	90	S
67961	00	A	Excision and repair of eyelid, involving lid margin, tarsus, conjunctiva, canthus, or full thickness, may include preparation for skin graft or pedicle flap with adjacent tissue transfer or rearrangement; up to one-fourth of lid margin	5.51	7.05	0.50	13.06	90	S
67966	00	A	Excision and repair of eyelid, involving lid margin, tarsus, conjunctiva, canthus, or full thickness, may include preparation for skin graft or pedicle flap with adjacent tissue transfer or rearrangement; over one-fourth of lid margin	6.39	8.37	0.66	15.42	90	S
67971	00	A	Reconstruction of eyelid, full thickness by transfer of tarsoconjunctival flap from opposing eyelid; up to two-thirds of eyelid, one stage or first stage	9.56	10.68	0.64	20.88	90	S
67973	00	A	Reconstruction of eyelid, full thickness by transfer of tarsoconjunctival flap from opposing eyelid; total eyelid, lower, one stage or first stage	12.59	13.54	0.91	27.04	90	S
67974	00	A	Reconstruction of eyelid, full thickness by transfer of tarsoconjunctival flap from opposing eyelid; total eyelid, upper, one stage or first stage	12.56	14.07	0.87	27.50	90	S
67975	00	A	Reconstruction of eyelid, full thickness by transfer of tarsoconjunctival flap from opposing eyelid; second stage	8.90	4.15	0.24	13.29	90	S
67999	00	C	Unlisted procedure, eyelids	0	0	0	0	YYY	S
68020	00	A	Incision of conjunctiva, drainage of cyst	1.32	0.51	0.03	1.86	10	S
68040	00	A	Expression of conjunctival follicles, eg, for trachoma	0.85	0.45	0.02	1.32	0	S

CPT codes and descriptions only, © 1994 American Medical Association. Reimbursement information, © 1995 McGraw-Hill Inc.

Code/ CPT	Mod- ifier	Status	Description	Work value	Practice expense	Mal- practice	Total value	Global period	Up- date
68100	00	A	Biopsy of conjunctiva	1.35	0.99	0.06	2.40	0	S
68110	00	A	Excision of lesion, conjunctiva; up to 1 cm	1.72	1.24	0.07	3.03	10	S
68115	00	A	Excision of lesion, conjunctiva; over 1 cm	2.31	1.93	0.11	4.35	10	S
68130	00	A	Excision of lesion, conjunctiva; with adjacent sclera	4.75	4.09	0.22	9.06	90	S
68135	00	A	Destruction of lesion, conjunctiva	1.79	0.74	0.04	2.57	10	S
68200	00	A	Subconjunctival injection	0.49	0.52	0.03	1.04	0	S
68320	00	A	Conjunctivoplasty; with conjunctival graft or extensive rearrangement	4.97	6.37	0.42	11.76	90	S
68325	00	A	Conjunctivoplasty; with buccal mucous membrane graft (includes obtaining graft)	6.96	8.91	0.62	16.49	90	S
68326	00	A	Conjunctivoplasty, reconstruction cul-de-sac; with conjunctival graft or extensive rearrangement	6.75	8.62	0.49	15.86	90	S
68328	00	A	Conjunctivoplasty, reconstruction cul-de-sac; with buccal mucous membrane graft (includes obtaining graft)	7.78	9.96	0.82	18.56	90	S
68330	00	A	Repair of symblepharon; conjunctivoplasty, without graft	4.53	5.80	0.35	10.68	90	S
68335	00	A	Repair of symblepharon; with free graft conjunctiva or buccal mucous membrane (includes obtaining graft)	6.79	9.14	0.68	16.61	90	S
68340	00	A	Repair of symblepharon; division of symblepharon, with or without insertion of conformer or contact lens	3.92	3.14	0.17	7.23	90	S
68360	00	A	Conjunctival flap; bridge or partial (separate procedure)	4.12	5.28	0.33	9.73	90	S
68362	00	A	Conjunctival flap; total (such as Gunderson thin flap or purse string flap)	6.94	8.01	0.42	15.37	90	S
68399	00	C	Unlisted procedure, conjunctiva	0	0	0	0	YYY	S
68400	00	A	Incision, drainage of lacrimal gland	1.64	1.00	0.06	2.70	10	S
68420	00	A	Incision, drainage of lacrimal sac (dacryocystotomy or dacryocystostomy)	2.25	1.02	0.06	3.33	10	S
68440	00	A	Snip incision of lacrimal punctum	0.89	0.76	0.04	1.69	10	S
68500	00	A	Excision of lacrimal gland (dacryoadenectomy), except for tumor; total	10.47	7.61	0.75	18.83	90	S
68505	00	A	Excision of lacrimal gland (dacryoadenectomy), except for tumor; partial	10.39	8.69	0.49	19.57	90	S
68510	00	A	Biopsy of lacrimal gland	4.61	3.69	0.28	8.58	0	S
68520	00	A	Excision of lacrimal sac (dacryocystectomy)	7.11	9.10	0.51	16.72	90	S
68525	00	A	Biopsy of lacrimal sac	4.43	3.68	0.23	8.34	0	S
68530	00	A	Removal of foreign body or dacryolith, lacrimal passages	3.61	2.85	0.17	6.63	10	S
68540	00	A	Excision of lacrimal gland tumor; frontal approach	10.10	8.31	0.50	18.91	90	S
68550	00	A	Excision of lacrimal gland tumor; involving osteotomy	12.66	11.34	0.74	24.74	90	S
68700	00	A	Plastic repair of canaliculi	6.20	2.69	0.15	9.04	90	S
68705	00	A	Correction of everted punctum, cautery	2.01	1.02	0.05	3.08	10	S
68720	00	A	Dacryocystorhinostomy (fistulization of lacrimal sac to nasal cavity)	7.68	10.20	0.74	18.62	90	S
68745	00	A	Conjunctivorhinostomy (fistulization of conjunctiva to nasal cavity); without tube	8.23	6.56	0.45	15.24	90	S
68750	00	A	Conjunctivorhinostomy (fistulization of conjunctiva to nasal cavity); with insertion of tube or stent	8.21	11.49	0.83	20.53	90	S
68760	00	A	Closure of the lacrimal punctum; by thermocauterization, ligation, or laser surgery	1.68	0.92	0.04	2.64	10	S
68761	00	A	Closure of the lacrimal punctum; by plug, each	1.31	0.92	0.04	2.27	10	S
68770	00	A	Closure of lacrimal fistula (separate procedure)	6.62	4.24	0.23	11.09	90	S
68800	00	A	Dilation of lacrimal punctum, with or without irrigation, unilateral or bilateral	1.11	0.42	0.02	1.55	10	S
68820	00	A	Probing of nasolacrimal duct, with or without irrigation, unilateral or bilateral;	1.47	0.55	0.03	2.05	10	S

CPT codes and descriptions only, © 1994 American Medical Association. Reimbursement information, © 1995 McGraw-Hill Inc.

Code/ CPT	Mod- ifier	Status	Description	Work value	Practice expense	Mal- practice	Total value	Global period	Up- date
68825	00	A	Probing of nasolacrimal duct, with or without irrigation, unilateral or bilateral; requiring general anesthesia	1.53	1.49	0.09	3.11	10	S
68830	00	A	Probing of nasolacrimal duct, with or without irrigation, unilateral or bilateral; with insertion of tube or stent	2.12	1.93	0.10	4.15	10	S
68840	00	A	Probing of lacrimal canaliculi, with or without irrigation	1.22	0.49	0.03	1.74	10	S
68850	00	A	Injection of contrast medium for dacryocystography	0.80	0.51	0.04	1.35	0	S
68899	00	C	Unlisted procedure, lacrimal system	0	0	0	0	YYY	S
69000	00	A	Drainage external ear, abscess or hematoma; simple	1.40	0.35	0.03	1.78	10	S
69005	00	A	Drainage external ear, abscess or hematoma; complicated	2.06	1.16	0.13	3.35	10	S
69020	00	A	Drainage external auditory canal, abscess	1.43	0.45	0.04	1.92	10	S
69090	00	N	Ear piercing	0.56*	0.51#	0.05*	1.12#	XXX	0
69100	00	A	Biopsy external ear	0.76	0.66	0.07	1.49	0	S
69105	00	A	Biopsy external auditory canal	0.85	0.80	0.09	1.74	0	S
69110	00	A	Excision external ear; partial, simple repair	3.34	2.63	0.37	6.34	90	S
69120	00	A	Excision external ear; complete amputation	3.95	0.78	0.07	4.80	90	S
69140	00	A	Excision exostosis(es), external auditory canal	7.68	8.00	0.88	16.56	90	S
69145	00	A	Excision soft tissue lesion, external auditory canal	2.54	2.51	0.28	5.33	90	S
69150	00	A	Radical excision external auditory canal lesion; without neck dissection	13.01	10.46	1.25	24.72	90	S
69155	00	A	Radical excision external auditory canal lesion; with neck dissection	17.03	15.92	1.61	34.56	90	S
69200	00	A	Removal foreign body from external auditory canal; without general anesthesia	0.77	0.42	0.04	1.23	0	N
69205	00	A	Removal foreign body from external auditory canal; with general anesthesia	1.15	1.07	0.11	2.33	10	S
69210	00	A	Removal impacted cerumen (separate procedure), one or both ears	0.61	0.23	0.02	0.86	0	N
69220	00	A	Debridement, mastoidectomy cavity, simple (eg, routine cleaning)	0.83	0.50	0.05	1.38	0	S
69222	00	A	Debridement, mastoidectomy cavity, complex (eg, with anesthesia or more than routine cleaning)	1.35	0.74	0.08	2.17	10	S
69300	00	R	Otoplasty, protruding ear, with or without size reduction	6.36	5.30	0.28	11.94	YYY	S
69310	00	A	Reconstruction of external auditory canal (meatoplasty) (eg, for stenosis due to trauma, infection) (separate procedure)	10.59	9.84	1.08	21.51	90	S
69320	00	A	Reconstruction external auditory canal for congenital atresia, single stage	16.60	14.65	1.66	32.91	90	S
69399	00	C	Unlisted procedure, external ear	0	0	0	0	YYY	S
69400	00	A	Eustachian tube inflation, transnasal; with catheterization	0.83	0.45	0.05	1.33	0	S
69401	00	A	Eustachian tube inflation, transnasal; without catheterization	0.63	0.25	0.03	0.91	0	S
69405	00	A	Eustachian tube catheterization, transtympanic	2.58	0.48	0.04	3.10	10	S
69410	00	A	Focal application of phase control substance, middle ear (baffle technique)	0.33	0.60	0.07	1.00	0	S
69420	00	A	Myringotomy including aspiration and/or eustachian tube inflation	1.28	0.69	0.08	2.05	10	S
69421	00	A	Myringotomy including aspiration and/or eustachian tube inflation requiring general anesthesia	1.68	1.14	0.13	2.95	10	S
69424	00	A	Ventilating tube removal when originally inserted by another physician	0.85	0.60	0.06	1.51	0	S
69433	00	A	Tympanostomy (requiring insertion of ventilating tube), local or topical anesthesia	1.47	1.33	0.15	2.95	10	S
69436	00	A	Tympanostomy (requiring insertion of ventilating tube), general anesthesia	1.91	2.13	0.23	4.27	10	S

CPT codes and descriptions only, © 1994 American Medical Association. Reimbursement information, © 1995 McGraw-Hill Inc.

Code/ CPT	Mod- ifier	Status	Description	Work value	Practice expense	Mal- practice	Total value	Global period	Up- date
69440	00	A	Middle ear exploration through postauricular or ear canal incision	7.31	8.69	0.93	16.93	90	S
69450	00	A	Tympanolysis, transcanal	5.44	8.08	1.15	14.67	90	S
69501	00	A	Transmastoid antrotomy ("simple" mastoidectomy)	8.81	10.90	1.17	20.88	90	S
69502	00	A	Mastoidectomy; complete	11.96	13.36	1.45	26.77	90	S
69505	00	A	Mastoidectomy; modified radical	12.57	16.09	1.79	30.45	90	S
69511	00	A	Mastoidectomy; radical	13.10	16.77	1.84	31.71	90	S
69530	00	A	Petrous apicectomy including radical mastoidectomy	18.04	16.71	1.72	36.47	90	S
69535	00	A	Resection temporal bone, external approach	34.50	25.27	2.85	62.62	90	S
69540	00	A	Excision aural polyp	1.15	1.27	0.14	2.56	10	S
69550	00	A	Excision aural glomus tumor; transcanal	10.70	14.51	2.00	27.21	90	S
69552	00	A	Excision aural glomus tumor; transmastoid	18.84	16.73	1.86	37.43	90	S
69554	00	A	Excision aural glomus tumor; extended (extratemporal)	25.78	22.87	2.63	51.28	90	S
69601	00	A	Revision mastoidectomy; resulting in complete mastoidectomy	12.79	14.02	1.55	28.36	90	S
69602	00	A	Revision mastoidectomy; resulting in modified radical mastoidectomy	13.16	16.27	1.75	31.18	90	S
69603	00	A	Revision mastoidectomy; resulting in radical mastoidectomy	13.60	17.34	1.88	32.82	90	S
69604	00	A	Revision mastoidectomy; resulting in tympanoplasty	13.60	19.70	2.70	36	90	S
69605	00	A	Revision mastoidectomy; with apicectomy	18.04	14.95	1.86	34.85	90	S
69610	00	A	Tympanic membrane repair, with or without site preparation or perforation for closure, with or without patch	4.38	0.93	0.10	5.41	10	S
69620	00	A	Myringoplasty (surgery confined to drumhead and donor area)	5.74	8.33	1.16	15.23	90	S
69631	00	A	Tympanoplasty without mastoidectomy (including canalplasty, atticotomy and/or middle ear surgery), initial or revision; without ossicular chain reconstruction	9.55	12.32	1.61	23.48	90	S
69632	00	A	Tympanoplasty without mastoidectomy (including canalplasty, atticotomy and/or middle ear surgery), initial or revision; with ossicular chain reconstruction (eg, postfenestration)	12.41	15.88	1.73	30.02	90	S
69633	00	A	Tympanoplasty without mastoidectomy (including canalplasty, atticotomy and/or middle ear surgery), initial or revision; with ossicular chain reconstruction and synthetic prosthesis (eg, partial ossicular replacement prosthesis, (PORP), total ossicular replacement prosthesis (TORP))	11.76	15.05	1.78	28.59	90	S
69635	00	A	Tympanoplasty with antrotomy or mastoidotomy (including canalplasty, atticotomy, middle ear surgery, and/or tympanic membrane repair); without ossicular chain reconstruction	13.02	16.65	1.91	31.58	90	S
69636	00	A	Tympanoplasty with antrotomy or mastoidotomy (including canalplasty, atticotomy, middle ear surgery, and/or tympanic membrane repair); with ossicular chain reconstruction	14.88	19.05	2.11	36.04	90	S
69637	00	A	Tympanoplasty with antrotomy or mastoidotomy (including canalplasty, atticotomy, middle ear surgery, and/or tympanic membrane repair); with ossicular chain reconstruction and synthetic prosthesis (eg, partial ossicular replacement prosthesis, (PORP), total ossicular replacement prosthesis (TORP))	14.77	18.90	2.22	35.89	90	S
69641	00	A	Tympanoplasty with mastoidectomy (including canalplasty, middle ear surgery, tympanic membrane repair); without ossicular chain reconstruction	12.29	15.73	1.87	29.89	90	S

CPT codes and descriptions only, © 1994 American Medical Association. Reimbursement information, © 1995 McGraw-Hill Inc.

Code/ CPT	Mod-ifier	Status	Description	Work value	Practice expense	Mal-practice	Total value	Global period	Up-date
69642	00	A	Tympanoplasty with mastoidectomy (including canalplasty, middle ear surgery, tympanic membrane repair); with ossicular chain reconstruction	16.37	20.62	2.21	39.20	90	S
69643	00	A	Tympanoplasty with mastoidectomy (including canalplasty, middle ear surgery, tympanic membrane repair); with intact or reconstructed wall, without ossicular chain reconstruction	14.81	18.95	2.51	36.27	90	S
69644	00	A	Tympanoplasty with mastoidectomy (including canalplasty, middle ear surgery, tympanic membrane repair); with intact or reconstructed canal wall, with ossicular chain reconstruction	16.46	21.07	2.70	40.23	90	S
69645	00	A	Tympanoplasty with mastoidectomy (including canalplasty, middle ear surgery, tympanic membrane repair); radical or complete, without ossicular chain reconstruction	15.80	20.23	2.51	38.54	90	S
69646	00	A	Tympanoplasty with mastoidectomy (including canalplasty, middle ear surgery, tympanic membrane repair); radical or complete, with ossicular chain reconstruction	17.35	21.97	2.40	41.72	90	S
69650	00	A	Stapes mobilization	9.40	12.03	1.33	22.76	90	S
69660	00	A	Stapedectomy or stapedotomy with reestablishment of ossicular continuity, with or without use of foreign material;	11.64	14.90	1.82	28.36	90	S
69661	00	A	Stapedectomy or stapedotomy with reestablishment of ossicular continuity, with or without use of foreign material; with footplate drill out	15.32	18.44	1.93	35.69	90	S
69662	00	A	Revision of stapedectomy or stapedotomy	15.04	18.02	1.94	35	90	S
69666	00	A	Repair oval window fistula	9.38	12.71	1.77	23.86	90	S
69667	00	A	Repair round window fistula	9.39	12.55	1.66	23.60	90	S
69670	00	A	Mastoid obliteration (separate procedure)	11.05	10.18	1.08	22.31	90	S
69676	00	A	Tympanic neurectomy	9.23	8.53	0.86	18.62	90	S
69700	00	A	Closure postauricular fistula, mastoid (separate procedure)	7.97	7.86	0.84	16.67	90	S
69710	00	N	Implantation or replacement of electromagnetic bone conduction hearing device in temporal bone	7.03*	6.37#	0.69*	14.09#	XXX	0
69711	00	A	Removal or repair of electromagnetic bone conduction hearing device in temporal bone	10.13	8.44	0.44	19.01	90	S
69720	00	A	Decompression facial nerve, intratemporal; lateral to geniculate ganglion	13.80	17.66	2.27	33.73	90	S
69725	00	A	Decompression facial nerve, intratemporal; including medial to geniculate ganglion	18.98	14.65	1.51	35.14	90	S
69740	00	A	Suture facial nerve, intratemporal, with or without graft or decompression; lateral to geniculate ganglion	15.39	11.83	1.69	28.91	90	S
69745	00	A	Suture facial nerve, intratemporal, with or without graft or decompression; including medial to geniculate ganglion	16.10	15.95	1.53	33.58	90	S
69799	00	C	Unlisted procedure, middle ear	0	0	0	0	YYY	S
69801	00	A	Labyrinthotomy, with or without cryosurgery or other nonexcisional destructive procedures or tack procedure; transcanal	8.19	12.38	1.84	22.41	90	S
69802	00	A	Labyrinthotomy, with or without cryosurgery or other nonexcisional destructive procedures or tack procedure; with mastoidectomy	12.44	11.24	1.22	24.90	90	S
69805	00	A	Endolymphatic sac operation; without shunt	10.27	14.53	2.00	26.80	90	S
69806	00	A	Endolymphatic sac operation; with shunt	11.82	17.45	2.54	31.81	90	S
69820	00	A	Fenestration semicircular canal	10.14	8.85	1.00	19.99	90	S
69840	00	A	Revision fenestration operation	10.06	8.49	0.51	19.06	90	S
69905	00	A	Labyrinthectomy; transcanal	10.70	14.55	2.07	27.32	90	S
69910	00	A	Labyrinthectomy; with mastoidectomy	13.10	18.00	2.34	33.44	90	S
69915	00	A	Vestibular nerve section, translabyrinthine approach	19.89	17.71	2.02	39.62	90	S

CPT codes and descriptions only, © 1994 American Medical Association. Reimbursement information, © 1995 McGraw-Hill Inc.

Code/ CPT	Mod- ifier	Status	Description	Work value	Practice expense	Mal- practice	Total value	Global period	Up- date
69930	00	A	Cochlear device implantation, with or without mastoidectomy	14.00	23.12	3.34	40.46	90	S
69949	00	C	Unlisted procedure, inner ear	0	0	0	0	YYY	S
69950	00	A	Vestibular nerve section, transcranial approach	21.15	17.99	2.31	41.45	90	S
69955	00	A	Total facial nerve decompression and/or repair (may include graft)	22.12	20.28	2.25	44.65	90	S
69960	00	A	Decompression internal auditory canal	19.75	17.85	1.93	39.53	90	S
69970	00	A	Removal of tumor, temporal bone	22.30	19.69	2.26	44.25	90	S
69979	00	C	Unlisted procedure, temporal bone, middle fossa approach	0	0	0	0	YYY	S

CPT codes and descriptions only, © 1994 American Medical Association. Reimbursement information, © 1995 McGraw-Hill Inc.

CHAPTER 3

Radiology

The editors have elected to indicate that a relative value is not available for procedures with a "0" in the individual units column.

I. **General:** Listed values for radiology procedures apply only when these services are performed by or under the supervision of a physician.

A. **Total:** The unit value listed next to the modifier column (modifier 00) represents the global value of the procedure. The five digit code is used to represent this service including the professional services and technical value of providing that service. The following sections, professional and technical, provide additional definitions for each component.

B. **Professional:** The unit value listed next to the modifier column (modifier -26) is used to designate professional services. Modifier -26 is added to the procedure code to indicate the use of this value. The professional component includes examination of the patient, when indicated, performance and/or supervision of the procedure, interpretation and written report of the examination, and consultation with referring physicians.

C. **Technical:** The unit value listed next to the modifier column (modifier TC) is used to designate the technical value of providing the service. Modifier TC may be used to designate this component. (Note: Modifier TC is not CPT compatible and may not be accepted by all payers. Check with the specific payer prior to use of this modifier. TC is accepted by Medicare.) The technical component includes personnel, materials, space, equipment, and other allocated facility overhead normally included in providing the service.

II. **Supervision and Interpretation Only:** A code designated as Supervision and Interpretation Only is used to indicate radiological services provided by a radiologist and staff, in conjunction with services provided by another physician (i.e., injection, insertion of catheter). In this instance, a physician other than the radiologist should list separately the appropriate procedure code, and the radiologist should bill using the appropriate Supervision and Interpretation code. If the Radiologist and Staff provide both portions of the service, current CPT requires reporting with the Supervision and Interpretation code and the appropriate procedure code.

III. **Unlisted Services or Procedure:** A service or procedure that is not identified by a particular code should be listed under the appropriate "Unlisted Procedure." These procedures often have 99 as the final two digits. Values should be substantiated by report. (See BY REPORT.)

CPT codes and descriptions only, © 1994 American Medical Association. Reimbursement information, © 1995 McGraw-Hill Inc.

IV. Procedures without Values: Procedures which have a BR or RNE in the units column require a report (see BY REPORT) to substantiate value.

V. Unusual Service or Procedure: When a procedure of unusual nature is performed, modifier -22 should be added and value substantiated by report. (See BY REPORT.)

VI. By Report: Value of a procedure should be established for any by report circumstance by identifying a similar service and justifying value difference. Procedures which require a report should include the following:

1. Accurate definition;
2. Clinical history;
3. Related procedure values; and
4. Reason for value adjustment.

VII. Portable X-ray: Use code Q0092 to indicate set-up of portable x-ray. Medicare should increase payment by 32%.

VIII. Separate or Multiple Procedures: Multiple procedures performed on the same date should be listed separately. Medicare allows 100% for each code between 70000–79999 billed on the same date. Codes falling in the 10000–69979 series are subject to the surgical guidelines, regardless of physician specialty.

IX. Reduced Value: If a physician elects to reduce the value of a procedure, modifier -52 should be added to the procedure code. Modifier -52 and the appropriate code may be used to indicate a limited or follow-up CT scan.

X. Services or Procedures Listed in Other Sections: Services or procedures provided by a radiologist may be listed in an alternate section of the book (i.e., consultations listed in MEDICINE). The radiologist should use these procedure codes following the guidelines appropriate to that section.

XI. Modifiers: A comprehensive listing of modifiers is provided in the introduction. Value adjustments significant to radiology and modifiers for those adjustments are listed above.

CPT codes and descriptions only, © 1994 American Medical Association. Reimbursement information, © 1995 McGraw-Hill Inc.

RADIOLOGY VALUES

Code/ CPT	Mod-ifier	Status	Description	Work value	Practice expense	Mal-practice	Total value	Global period	Up-date
70010	00	A	Myelography, posterior fossa, radiological supervision and interpretation	1.19	4.65	0.34	6.18	XXX	N
70010	26			1.19	0.52	0.08	1.79	XXX	N
70010	TC			0	4.13	0.26	4.39	XXX	N
70015	00	A	Cisternography, positive contrast, radiological supervision and interpretation	1.19	1.81	0.17	3.17	XXX	N
70015	26			1.19	0.52	0.08	1.79	XXX	N
70015	TC			0	1.29	0.09	1.38	XXX	N
70030	00	A	Radiologic examination, eye, for detection of foreign body	0.17	0.48	0.04	0.69	XXX	N
70030	26			0.17	0.08	0.01	0.26	XXX	N
70030	TC			0	0.40	0.03	0.43	XXX	N
70100	00	A	Radiologic examination, mandible; partial, less than four views	0.18	0.59	0.04	0.81	XXX	N
70100	26			0.18	0.09	0.01	0.28	XXX	N
70100	TC			0	0.50	0.03	0.53	XXX	N
70110	00	A	Radiologic examination, mandible; complete, minimum of four views	0.25	0.71	0.06	1.02	XXX	N
70110	26			0.25	0.12	0.02	0.39	XXX	N
70110	TC			0	0.59	0.04	0.63	XXX	N
70120	00	A	Radiologic examination, mastoids; less than three views per side	0.18	0.68	0.05	0.91	XXX	N
70120	26			0.18	0.09	0.01	0.28	XXX	N
70120	TC			0	0.59	0.04	0.63	XXX	N
70130	00	A	Radiologic examination, mastoids; complete, minimum of three views per side	0.34	0.91	0.07	1.32	XXX	N
70130	26			0.34	0.16	0.02	0.52	XXX	N
70130	TC			0	0.75	0.05	0.80	XXX	N
70134	00	A	Radiologic examination, internal auditory meati, complete	0.34	0.86	0.07	1.27	XXX	N
70134	26			0.34	0.16	0.02	0.52	XXX	N
70134	TC			0	0.70	0.05	0.75	XXX	N
70140	00	A	Radiologic examination, facial bones; less than three views	0.19	0.68	0.05	0.92	XXX	N
70140	26			0.19	0.09	0.01	0.29	XXX	N
70140	TC			0	0.59	0.04	0.63	XXX	N
70150	00	A	Radiologic examination, facial bones; complete, minimum of three views	0.26	0.87	0.07	1.20	XXX	N
70150	26			0.26	0.12	0.02	0.40	XXX	N
70150	TC			0	0.75	0.05	0.80	XXX	N
70160	00	A	Radiologic examination, nasal bones, complete, minimum of three views	0.17	0.58	0.04	0.79	XXX	N
70160	26			0.17	0.08	0.01	0.26	XXX	N

CPT codes and descriptions only, © 1994 American Medical Association. Reimbursement information, © 1995 McGraw-Hill Inc.

Code/ CPT	Mod- ifier	Status	Description	Work value	Practice expense	Mal- practice	Total value	Global period	Up- date
70160	TC			0	0.50	0.03	0.53	XXX	N
70170	00	A	Dacryocystography, nasolacrimal duct, radiological supervision and interpretation	0.30	1.04	0.08	1.42	XXX	N
70170	26			0.30	0.14	0.02	0.46	XXX	N
70170	TC			0	0.90	0.06	0.96	XXX	N
70190	00	A	Radiologic examination; optic foramina	0.21	0.69	0.05	0.95	XXX	N
70190	26			0.21	0.10	0.01	0.32	XXX	N
70190	TC			0	0.59	0.04	0.63	XXX	N
70200	00	A	Radiologic examination; orbits, complete, minimum of four views	0.28	0.88	0.07	1.23	XXX	N
70200	26			0.28	0.13	0.02	0.43	XXX	N
70200	TC			0	0.75	0.05	0.80	XXX	N
70210	00	A	Radiologic examination, sinuses, paranasal, less than three views	0.17	0.67	0.05	0.89	XXX	N
70210	26			0.17	0.08	0.01	0.26	XXX	N
70210	TC			0	0.59	0.04	0.63	XXX	N
70220	00	A	Radiologic examination, sinuses, paranasal, complete, minimum of three views	0.25	0.87	0.07	1.19	XXX	N
70220	26			0.25	0.12	0.02	0.39	XXX	N
70220	TC			0	0.75	0.05	0.80	XXX	N
70240	00	A	Radiologic examination, sella turcica	0.19	0.49	0.04	0.72	XXX	N
70240	26			0.19	0.09	0.01	0.29	XXX	N
70240	TC			0	0.40	0.03	0.43	XXX	N
70250	00	A	Radiologic examination, skull; less than four views, with or without stereo	0.24	0.70	0.06	1.00	XXX	N
70250	26			0.24	0.11	0.02	0.37	XXX	N
70250	TC			0	0.59	0.04	0.63	XXX	N
70260	00	A	Radiologic examination, skull; complete, minimum of four views, with or without stereo	0.34	1.01	0.08	1.43	XXX	N
70260	26			0.34	0.16	0.02	0.52	XXX	N
70260	TC			0	0.85	0.06	0.91	XXX	N
70300	00	A	Radiologic examination, teeth; single view	0.10	0.30	0.03	0.43	XXX	N
70300	26			0.10	0.05	0.01	0.16	XXX	N
70300	TC			0	0.25	0.02	0.27	XXX	N
70310	00	A	Radiologic examination, teeth; partial examination, less than full mouth	0.16	0.47	0.04	0.67	XXX	N
70310	26			0.16	0.07	0.01	0.24	XXX	N
70310	TC			0	0.40	0.03	0.43	XXX	N
70320	00	A	Radiologic examination, teeth; complete, full mouth	0.22	0.85	0.07	1.14	XXX	N
70320	26			0.22	0.10	0.02	0.34	XXX	N
70320	TC			0	0.75	0.05	0.80	XXX	N
70328	00	A	Radiologic examination, temporomandibular joint, open and closed mouth; unilateral	0.18	0.56	0.04	0.78	XXX	N
70328	26			0.18	0.09	0.01	0.28	XXX	N
70328	TC			0	0.47	0.03	0.50	XXX	N
70330	00	A	Radiologic examination, temporomandibular joint, open and closed mouth; bilateral	0.24	0.91	0.07	1.22	XXX	N
70330	26			0.24	0.11	0.02	0.37	XXX	N
70330	TC			0	0.80	0.05	0.85	XXX	N
70332	00	A	Temporomandibular joint arthrography, radiological supervision and interpretation	0.54	2.25	0.17	2.96	XXX	N
70332	26			0.54	0.25	0.04	0.83	XXX	N

CPT codes and descriptions only, © 1994 American Medical Association. Reimbursement information, © 1995 McGraw-Hill Inc.

Code/ CPT	Mod- ifier	Status	Description	Work value	Practice expense	Mal- practice	Total value	Global period	Up- date
70332	TC			0	2.00	0.13	2.13	XXX	N
70336	00	A	Magnetic resonance (eg, proton) imaging, temporomandibular joint	0.95	11.11	0.73	12.79	XXX	N
70336	26			0.95	0.43	0.06	1.44	XXX	N
70336	TC			0	10.68	0.67	11.35	XXX	N
70350	00	A	Cephalogram, orthodontic	0.17	0.44	0.03	0.64	XXX	N
70350	26			0.17	0.08	0.01	0.26	XXX	N
70350	TC			0	0.36	0.02	0.38	XXX	N
70355	00	A	Orthopantogram	0.20	0.63	0.05	0.88	XXX	N
70355	26			0.20	0.09	0.01	0.30	XXX	N
70355	TC			0	0.54	0.04	0.58	XXX	N
70360	00	A	Radiologic examination; neck, soft tissue	0.17	0.48	0.04	0.69	XXX	N
70360	26			0.17	0.08	0.01	0.26	XXX	N
70360	TC			0	0.40	0.03	0.43	XXX	N
70370	00	A	Radiologic examination; pharynx or larynx, including fluoroscopy and/or magnification technique	0.32	1.39	0.10	1.81	XXX	N
70370	26			0.32	0.15	0.02	0.49	XXX	N
70370	TC			0	1.24	0.08	1.32	XXX	N
70371	00	A	Complex dynamic pharyngeal and speech evaluation by cine or video recording	0.84	2.38	0.19	3.41	XXX	N
70371	26			0.84	0.38	0.06	1.28	XXX	N
70371	TC			0	2.00	0.13	2.13	XXX	N
70373	00	A	Laryngography, contrast, radiological supervision and interpretation	0.44	1.90	0.14	2.48	XXX	N
70373	26			0.44	0.20	0.03	0.67	XXX	N
70373	TC			0	1.70	0.11	1.81	XXX	N
70380	00	A	Radiologic examination, salivary gland for calculus	0.17	0.72	0.05	0.94	XXX	N
70380	26			0.17	0.08	0.01	0.26	XXX	N
70380	TC			0	0.64	0.04	0.68	XXX	N
70390	00	A	Sialography, radiological supervision and interpretation	0.38	1.87	0.14	2.39	XXX	N
70390	26			0.38	0.17	0.03	0.58	XXX	N
70390	TC			0	1.70	0.11	1.81	XXX	N
70450	00	A	Computerized axial tomography, head or brain; without contrast material	0.85	4.88	0.35	6.08	XXX	N
70450	26			0.85	0.38	0.06	1.29	XXX	N
70450	TC			0	4.50	0.29	4.79	XXX	N
70460	00	A	Computerized axial tomography, head or brain; with contrast material(s)	1.13	5.89	0.43	7.45	XXX	N
70460	26			1.13	0.50	0.08	1.71	XXX	N
70460	TC			0	5.39	0.35	5.74	XXX	N
70470	00	A	Computerized axial tomography, head or brain; without contrast material, followed by contrast material(s) and further sections	1.27	7.30	0.52	9.09	XXX	N
70470	26			1.27	0.56	0.09	1.92	XXX	N
70470	TC			0	6.74	0.43	7.17	XXX	N
70480	00	A	Computerized axial tomography, orbit, sella, or posterior fossa or outer, middle, or inner ear; without contrast material	1.28	5.07	0.38	6.73	XXX	N
70480	26			1.28	0.57	0.09	1.94	XXX	N
70480	TC			0	4.50	0.29	4.79	XXX	N

CPT codes and descriptions only, © 1994 American Medical Association. Reimbursement information, © 1995 McGraw-Hill Inc.

Code/ CPT	Mod- ifier	Status	Description	Work value	Practice expense	Mal- practice	Total value	Global period	Up- date
70481	00	A	Computerized axial tomography, orbit, sella, or posterior fossa or outer, middle, or inner ear; with contrast material(s)	1.38	6.00	0.44	7.82	XXX	N
70481	26			1.38	0.61	0.09	2.08	XXX	N
70481	TC			0	5.39	0.35	5.74	XXX	N
70482	00	A	Computerized axial tomography, orbit, sella, or posterior fossa or outer, middle, or inner ear; without contrast material, followed by contrast material(s) and further sections	1.45	7.38	0.53	9.36	XXX	N
70482	26			1.45	0.64	0.10	2.19	XXX	N
70482	TC			0	6.74	0.43	7.17	XXX	N
70486	00	A	Computerized axial tomography, maxillofacial area; without contrast material	1.14	5.00	0.37	6.51	XXX	N
70486	26			1.14	0.50	0.08	1.72	XXX	N
70486	TC			0	4.50	0.29	4.79	XXX	N
70487	00	A	Computerized axial tomography, maxillofacial area; with contrast material(s)	1.30	5.96	0.44	7.70	XXX	N
70487	26			1.30	0.57	0.09	1.96	XXX	N
70487	TC			0	5.39	0.35	5.74	XXX	N
70488	00	A	Computerized axial tomography, maxillofacial area; without contrast material, followed by contrast material(s) and further sections	1.42	7.37	0.53	9.32	XXX	N
70488	26			1.42	0.63	0.10	2.15	XXX	N
70488	TC			0	6.74	0.43	7.17	XXX	N
70490	00	A	Computerized axial tomography, soft tissue neck; without contrast material	1.28	5.07	0.38	6.73	XXX	N
70490	26			1.28	0.57	0.09	1.94	XXX	N
70490	TC			0	4.50	0.29	4.79	XXX	N
70491	00	A	Computerized axial tomography, soft tissue neck; with contrast material(s)	1.38	6.00	0.44	7.82	XXX	N
70491	26			1.38	0.61	0.09	2.08	XXX	N
70491	TC			0	5.39	0.35	5.74	XXX	N
70492	00	A	Computerized axial tomography, soft tissue neck; without contrast material followed by contrast material(s) and further sections	1.45	7.38	0.53	9.36	XXX	N
70492	26			1.45	0.64	0.10	2.19	XXX	N
70492	TC			0	6.74	0.43	7.17	XXX	N
70540	00	A	Magnetic resonance (eg, proton) imaging, orbit, face, and neck	1.48	11.34	0.77	13.59	XXX	N
70540	26			1.48	0.66	0.10	2.24	XXX	N
70540	TC			0	10.68	0.67	11.35	XXX	N
70541	00	A	Magnetic resonance angiography, head and/or neck, with or without contrast material(s)	1.81	11.34	0.77	13.92	XXX	N
70541	26			1.81	0.66	0.10	2.57	XXX	N
70541	TC			0	10.68	0.67	11.35	XXX	N
70551	00	A	Magnetic resonance (eg, proton) imaging, brain (including brain stem); without contrast material	1.48	11.34	0.77	13.59	XXX	N
70551	26			1.48	0.66	0.10	2.24	XXX	N
70551	TC			0	10.68	0.67	11.35	XXX	N
70552	00	A	Magnetic resonance (eg, proton) imaging, brain (including brain stem); with contrast material(s)	1.78	13.61	0.93	16.32	XXX	N
70552	26			1.78	0.80	0.12	2.70	XXX	N
70552	TC			0	12.81	0.81	13.62	XXX	N

CPT codes and descriptions only, © 1994 American Medical Association. Reimbursement information, © 1995 McGraw-Hill Inc.

Code/ CPT	Mod- ifier	Status	Description	Work value	Practice expense	Mal- practice	Total value	Global period	Up- date
70553	00	A	Magnetic resonance (eg, proton) imaging, brain (including brain stem); without contrast material, followed by contrast material(s) and further sequences	2.36	24.79	1.65	28.80	XXX	N
70553	26			2.36	1.07	0.16	3.59	XXX	N
70553	TC			0	23.72	1.49	25.21	XXX	N
71010	00	A	Radiologic examination, chest; single view, frontal	0.18	0.53	0.04	0.75	XXX	N
71010	26			0.18	0.08	0.01	0.27	XXX	N
71010	TC			0	0.45	0.03	0.48	XXX	N
71015	00	A	Radiologic examination, chest; stereo, frontal	0.21	0.60	0.04	0.85	XXX	N
71015	26			0.21	0.10	0.01	0.32	XXX	N
71015	TC			0	0.50	0.03	0.53	XXX	N
71020	00	A	Radiologic examination, chest, two views, frontal and lateral;	0.22	0.69	0.05	0.96	XXX	N
71020	26			0.22	0.10	0.01	0.33	XXX	N
71020	TC			0	0.59	0.04	0.63	XXX	N
71021	00	A	Radiologic examination, chest, two views, frontal and lateral; with apical lordotic procedure	0.27	0.82	0.07	1.16	XXX	N
71021	26			0.27	0.12	0.02	0.41	XXX	N
71021	TC			0	0.70	0.05	0.75	XXX	N
71022	00	A	Radiologic examination, chest, two views, frontal and lateral; with oblique projections	0.31	0.84	0.07	1.22	XXX	N
71022	26			0.31	0.14	0.02	0.47	XXX	N
71022	TC			0	0.70	0.05	0.75	XXX	N
71023	00	A	Radiologic examination, chest, two views, frontal and lateral; with fluoroscopy	0.38	0.92	0.08	1.38	XXX	N
71023	26			0.38	0.17	0.03	0.58	XXX	N
71023	TC			0	0.75	0.05	0.80	XXX	N
71030	00	A	Radiologic examination, chest, complete, minimum of four views;	0.31	0.89	0.07	1.27	XXX	N
71030	26			0.31	0.14	0.02	0.47	XXX	N
71030	TC			0	0.75	0.05	0.80	XXX	N
71034	00	A	Radiologic examination, chest, complete, minimum of four views; with fluoroscopy	0.46	1.58	0.12	2.16	XXX	N
71034	26			0.46	0.21	0.03	0.70	XXX	N
71034	TC			0	1.37	0.09	1.46	XXX	N
71035	00	A	Radiologic examination, chest, special views (eg, lateral decubitus, Bucky studies)	0.18	0.58	0.04	0.80	XXX	N
71035	26			0.18	0.08	0.01	0.27	XXX	N
71035	TC			0	0.50	0.03	0.53	XXX	N
71036	00	A	Needle biopsy of intrathoracic lesion, including follow-up films, fluoroscopic localization only, radiological supervision and interpretation	0.54	1.75	0.14	2.43	XXX	N
71036	26			0.54	0.25	0.04	0.83	XXX	N
71036	TC			0	1.50	0.10	1.60	XXX	N
71038	00	A	Fluoroscopic localization for transbronchial biopsy or brushing	0.54	1.85	0.15	2.54	XXX	N
71038	26			0.54	0.25	0.04	0.83	XXX	N
71038	TC			0	1.60	0.11	1.71	XXX	N
71040	00	A	Bronchography, unilateral, radiological supervision and interpretation	0.58	1.66	0.13	2.37	XXX	N
71040	26			0.58	0.27	0.04	0.89	XXX	N
71040	TC			0	1.39	0.09	1.48	XXX	N

CPT codes and descriptions only, © 1994 American Medical Association. Reimbursement information, © 1995 McGraw-Hill Inc.

Code/ CPT	Mod- ifier	Status	Description	Work value	Practice expense	Mal- practice	Total value	Global period	Up- date
71060	00	A	Bronchography, bilateral, radiological supervision and interpretation	0.74	2.44	0.19	3.37	XXX	N
71060	26			0.74	0.34	0.05	1.13	XXX	N
71060	TC			0	2.10	0.14	2.24	XXX	N
71090	00	A	Insertion pacemaker, fluoroscopy and radiography, radiological supervision and interpretation	0.54	1.85	0.15	2.54	XXX	N
71090	26			0.54	0.25	0.04	0.83	XXX	N
71090	TC			0	1.60	0.11	1.71	XXX	N
71100	00	A	Radiologic examination, ribs, unilateral; two views	0.22	0.64	0.06	0.92	XXX	N
71100	26			0.22	0.10	0.02	0.34	XXX	N
71100	TC			0	0.54	0.04	0.58	XXX	N
71101	00	A	Radiologic examination, ribs, unilateral; including posteroanterior chest, minimum of three views	0.27	0.77	0.06	1.10	XXX	N
71101	26			0.27	0.13	0.02	0.42	XXX	N
71101	TC			0	0.64	0.04	0.68	XXX	N
71110	00	A	Radiologic examination, ribs, bilateral; three views	0.27	0.88	0.07	1.22	XXX	N
71110	26			0.27	0.13	0.02	0.42	XXX	N
71110	TC			0	0.75	0.05	0.80	XXX	N
71111	00	A	Radiologic examination, ribs, bilateral; including posteroanterior chest, minimum of four views	0.32	1.00	0.08	1.40	XXX	N
71111	26			0.32	0.15	0.02	0.49	XXX	N
71111	TC			0	0.85	0.06	0.91	XXX	N
71120	00	A	Radiologic examination; sternum, minimum of two views	0.20	0.71	0.05	0.96	XXX	N
71120	26			0.20	0.09	0.01	0.30	XXX	N
71120	TC			0	0.62	0.04	0.66	XXX	N
71130	00	A	Radiologic examination; sternoclavicular joint or joints, minimum of three views	0.22	0.77	0.05	1.04	XXX	N
71130	26			0.22	0.10	0.01	0.33	XXX	N
71130	TC			0	0.67	0.04	0.71	XXX	N
71250	00	A	Computerized axial tomography, thorax; without contrast material	1.16	6.14	0.44	7.74	XXX	N
71250	26			1.16	0.51	0.08	1.75	XXX	N
71250	TC			0	5.63	0.36	5.99	XXX	N
71260	00	A	Computerized axial tomography, thorax; with contrast material(s)	1.24	7.29	0.51	9.04	XXX	N
71260	26			1.24	0.55	0.08	1.87	XXX	N
71260	TC			0	6.74	0.43	7.17	XXX	N
71270	00	A	Computerized axial tomography, thorax; without contrast material, followed by contrast material(s) and further sections	1.38	9.04	0.61	11.03	XXX	N
71270	26			1.38	0.61	0.09	2.08	XXX	N
71270	TC			0	8.43	0.52	8.95	XXX	N
71550	00	A	Magnetic resonance (eg, proton) imaging, chest (eg, for evaluation of hilar and mediastinal lymphadenopathy)	1.60	11.40	0.78	13.78	XXX	N
71550	26			1.60	0.72	0.11	2.43	XXX	N
71550	TC			0	10.68	0.67	11.35	XXX	N
71555	00	A	Magnetic resonance angiography, chest (excluding myocardium), with or without contrast material(s)	1.81	11.40	0.78	13.99	XXX	N
71555	26			1.81	0.72	0.11	2.64	XXX	N
71555	TC			0	10.68	0.67	11.35	XXX	N
72010	00	A	Radiologic examination, spine, entire, survey study, anteroposterior and lateral	0.45	1.18	0.09	1.72	XXX	N

CPT codes and descriptions only, © 1994 American Medical Association. Reimbursement information, © 1995 McGraw-Hill Inc.

Code/ CPT	Mod- ifier	Status	Description	Work value	Practice expense	Mal- practice	Total value	Global period	Up- date
72010	26			0.45	0.20	0.03	0.68	XXX	N
72010	TC			0	0.98	0.06	1.04	XXX	N
72020	00	A	Radiologic examination, spine, single view, specify level	0.15	0.47	0.04	0.66	XXX	N
72020	26			0.15	0.07	0.01	0.23	XXX	N
72020	TC			0	0.40	0.03	0.43	XXX	N
72040	00	A	Radiologic examination, spine, cervical; anteroposterior and lateral	0.22	0.67	0.05	0.94	XXX	N
72040	26			0.22	0.10	0.01	0.33	XXX	N
72040	TC			0	0.57	0.04	0.61	XXX	N
72050	00	A	Radiologic examination, spine, cervical; minimum of four views	0.31	0.99	0.08	1.38	XXX	N
72050	26			0.31	0.14	0.02	0.47	XXX	N
72050	TC			0	0.85	0.06	0.91	XXX	N
72052	00	A	Radiologic examination, spine, cervical; complete, including oblique and flexion and/or extension studies	0.36	1.25	0.09	1.70	XXX	N
72052	26			0.36	0.17	0.02	0.55	XXX	N
72052	TC			0	1.08	0.07	1.15	XXX	N
72069	00	A	Radiologic examination, spine, thoracolumbar, standing (scoliosis)	0.22	0.57	0.04	0.83	XXX	N
72069	26			0.22	0.10	0.01	0.33	XXX	N
72069	TC			0	0.47	0.03	0.50	XXX	N
72070	00	A	Radiologic examination, spine; thoracic, anteroposterior and lateral	0.22	0.72	0.05	0.99	XXX	N
72070	26			0.22	0.10	0.01	0.33	XXX	N
72070	TC			0	0.62	0.04	0.66	XXX	N
72072	00	A	Radiologic examination, spine; thoracic, anteroposterior and lateral, including swimmer's view of the cervicothoracic junction	0.22	0.80	0.06	1.08	XXX	N
72072	26			0.22	0.10	0.01	0.33	XXX	N
72072	TC			0	0.70	0.05	0.75	XXX	N
72074	00	A	Radiologic examination, spine; thoracic, complete, including obliques, minimum of four views	0.22	0.97	0.07	1.26	XXX	N
72074	26			0.22	0.10	0.01	0.33	XXX	N
72074	TC			0	0.87	0.06	0.93	XXX	N
72080	00	A	Radiologic examination, spine; thoracolumbar, anteroposterior and lateral	0.22	0.74	0.05	1.01	XXX	N
72080	26			0.22	0.10	0.01	0.33	XXX	N
72080	TC			0	0.64	0.04	0.68	XXX	N
72090	00	A	Radiologic examination, spine; scoliosis study, including supine and erect studies	0.28	0.77	0.06	1.11	XXX	N
72090	26			0.28	0.13	0.02	0.43	XXX	N
72090	TC			0	0.64	0.04	0.68	XXX	N
72100	00	A	Radiologic examination, spine, lumbosacral; anteroposterior and lateral	0.22	0.74	0.05	1.01	XXX	N
72100	26			0.22	0.10	0.01	0.33	XXX	N
72100	TC			0	0.64	0.04	0.68	XXX	N
72110	00	A	Radiologic examination, spine, lumbosacral; complete, with oblique views	0.31	1.01	0.08	1.40	XXX	N
72110	26			0.31	0.14	0.02	0.47	XXX	N
72110	TC			0	0.87	0.06	0.93	XXX	N
72114	00	A	Radiologic examination, spine, lumbosacral; complete, including bending views	0.36	1.30	0.09	1.75	XXX	N

CPT codes and descriptions only, © 1994 American Medical Association. Reimbursement information, © 1995 McGraw-Hill Inc.

Code/ CPT	Mod-ifier	Status	Description	Work value	Practice expense	Mal-practice	Total value	Global period	Up-date
72114	26			0.36	0.17	0.02	0.55	XXX	N
72114	TC			0	1.13	0.07	1.20	XXX	N
72120	00	A	Radiologic examination, spine, lumbosacral, bending views only, minimum of four views	0.22	0.95	0.07	1.24	XXX	N
72120	26			0.22	0.10	0.01	0.33	XXX	N
72120	TC			0	0.85	0.06	0.91	XXX	N
72125	00	A	Computerized axial tomography, cervical spine; without contrast material	1.16	6.14	0.44	7.74	XXX	N
72125	26			1.16	0.51	0.08	1.75	XXX	N
72125	TC			0	5.63	0.36	5.99	XXX	N
72126	00	A	Computerized axial tomography, cervical spine; with contrast material	1.22	7.27	0.51	9.00	XXX	N
72126	26			1.22	0.53	0.08	1.83	XXX	N
72126	TC			0	6.74	0.43	7.17	XXX	N
72127	00	A	Computerized axial tomography, cervical spine; without contrast material, followed by contrast material(s) and further sections	1.27	8.99	0.61	10.87	XXX	N
72127	26			1.27	0.56	0.09	1.92	XXX	N
72127	TC			0	8.43	0.52	8.95	XXX	N
72128	00	A	Computerized axial tomography, thoracic spine; without contrast material	1.16	6.14	0.44	7.74	XXX	N
72128	26			1.16	0.51	0.08	1.75	XXX	N
72128	TC			0	5.63	0.36	5.99	XXX	N
72129	00	A	Computerized axial tomography, thoracic spine; with contrast material	1.22	7.27	0.51	9.00	XXX	N
72129	26			1.22	0.53	0.08	1.83	XXX	N
72129	TC			0	6.74	0.43	7.17	XXX	N
72130	00	A	Computerized axial tomography, thoracic spine; without contrast material, followed by contrast material(s) and further sections	1.27	8.99	0.61	10.87	XXX	N
72130	26			1.27	0.56	0.09	1.92	XXX	N
72130	TC			0	8.43	0.52	8.95	XXX	N
72131	00	A	Computerized axial tomography, lumbar spine; without contrast material	1.16	6.14	0.44	7.74	XXX	N
72131	26			1.16	0.51	0.08	1.75	XXX	N
72131	TC			0	5.63	0.36	5.99	XXX	N
72132	00	A	Computerized axial tomography, lumbar spine; with contrast material	1.22	7.27	0.51	9.00	XXX	N
72132	26			1.22	0.53	0.08	1.83	XXX	N
72132	TC			0	6.74	0.43	7.17	XXX	N
72133	00	A	Computerized axial tomography, lumbar spine; without contrast material, followed by contrast material(s) and further sections	1.27	8.99	0.61	10.87	XXX	N
72133	26			1.27	0.56	0.09	1.92	XXX	N
72133	TC			0	8.43	0.52	8.95	XXX	N
72141	00	A	Magnetic resonance (eg, proton) imaging, spinal canal and contents, cervical; without contrast material	1.60	11.40	0.78	13.78	XXX	N
72141	26			1.60	0.72	0.11	2.43	XXX	N
72141	TC			0	10.68	0.67	11.35	XXX	N
72142	00	A	Magnetic resonance (eg, proton) imaging, spinal canal and contents, cervical; with contrast material(s)	1.92	13.67	0.94	16.53	XXX	N
72142	26			1.92	0.86	0.13	2.91	XXX	N
72142	TC			0	12.81	0.81	13.62	XXX	N

CPT codes and descriptions only, © 1994 American Medical Association. Reimbursement information, © 1995 McGraw-Hill Inc.

Code/ CPT	Mod- ifier	Status	Description	Work value	Practice expense	Mal- practice	Total value	Global period	Up- date
72146	00	A	Magnetic resonance (eg, proton) imaging, spinal canal and contents, thoracic; without contrast material	1.60	12.58	0.85	15.03	XXX	N
72146	26			1.60	0.72	0.11	2.43	XXX	N
72146	TC			0	11.86	0.74	12.60	XXX	N
72147	00	A	Magnetic resonance (eg, proton) imaging, spinal canal and contents, thoracic; with contrast material(s)	1.92	13.67	0.94	16.53	XXX	N
72147	26			1.92	0.86	0.13	2.91	XXX	N
72147	TC			0	12.81	0.81	13.62	XXX	N
72148	00	A	Magnetic resonance (eg, proton) imaging, spinal canal and contents, lumbar; without contrast material	1.48	12.52	0.84	14.84	XXX	N
72148	26			1.48	0.66	0.10	2.24	XXX	N
72148	TC			0	11.86	0.74	12.60	XXX	N
72149	00	A	Magnetic resonance (eg, proton) imaging, spinal canal and contents, lumbar; with contrast material(s)	1.78	13.61	0.93	16.32	XXX	N
72149	26			1.78	0.80	0.12	2.70	XXX	N
72149	TC			0	12.81	0.81	13.62	XXX	N
72156	00	A	Magnetic resonance (eg, proton) imaging, spinal canal and contents, without contrast material, followed by contrast material(s) and further sequences; cervical	2.57	24.87	1.66	29.10	XXX	N
72156	26			2.57	1.15	0.17	3.89	XXX	N
72156	TC			0	23.72	1.49	25.21	XXX	N
72157	00	A	Magnetic resonance (eg, proton) imaging, spinal canal and contents, without contrast material, followed by contrast material(s) and further sequences; thoracic	2.57	24.87	1.66	29.10	XXX	N
72157	26			2.57	1.15	0.17	3.89	XXX	N
72157	TC			0	23.72	1.49	25.21	XXX	N
72158	00	A	Magnetic resonance (eg, proton) imaging, spinal canal and contents, without contrast material, followed by contrast material(s) and further sequences; lumbar	2.36	24.79	1.65	28.80	XXX	N
72158	26			2.36	1.07	0.16	3.59	XXX	N
72158	TC			0	23.72	1.49	25.21	XXX	N
72159	00	A	Magnetic resonance angiography, spinal canal and contents, with or without contrast material(s)	1.80	12.52	0.84	15.16	XXX	N
72159	26			1.80	0.66	0.10	2.56	XXX	N
72159	TC			0	11.86	0.74	12.60	XXX	N
72170	00	A	Radiologic examination, pelvis; anteroposterior only	0.17	0.57	0.04	0.78	XXX	N
72170	26			0.17	0.07	0.01	0.25	XXX	N
72170	TC			0	0.50	0.03	0.53	XXX	N
72190	00	A	Radiologic examination, pelvis; complete, minimum of three views	0.21	0.74	0.05	1.00	XXX	N
72190	26			0.21	0.10	0.01	0.32	XXX	N
72190	TC			0	0.64	0.04	0.68	XXX	N
72192	00	A	Computerized axial tomography, pelvis; without contrast material	1.09	6.11	0.43	7.63	XXX	N
72192	26			1.09	0.48	0.07	1.64	XXX	N
72192	TC			0	5.63	0.36	5.99	XXX	N
72193	00	A	Computerized axial tomography, pelvis; with contrast material(s)	1.16	7.03	0.49	8.68	XXX	N
72193	26			1.16	0.51	0.08	1.75	XXX	N
72193	TC			0	6.52	0.41	6.93	XXX	N
72194	00	A	Computerized axial tomography, pelvis; without contrast material, followed by contrast material(s) and further sections	1.22	8.62	0.58	10.42	XXX	N

CPT codes and descriptions only, © 1994 American Medical Association. Reimbursement information, © 1995 McGraw-Hill Inc.

Code/ CPT	Mod- ifier	Status	Description	Work value	Practice expense	Mal- practice	Total value	Global period	Up- date
72194	26			1.22	0.53	0.08	1.83	XXX	N
72194	TC			0	8.09	0.50	8.59	XXX	N
72196	00	A	Magnetic resonance (eg, proton) imaging, pelvis	1.60	11.40	0.78	13.78	XXX	N
72196	26			1.60	0.72	0.11	2.43	XXX	N
72196	TC			0	10.68	0.67	11.35	XXX	N
72198	00	A	Magnetic resonance angiography, pelvis, with or without contrast material(s)	1.80	11.40	0.78	13.98	XXX	N
72198	26			1.80	0.72	0.11	2.63	XXX	N
72198	TC			0	10.68	0.67	11.35	XXX	N
72200	00	A	Radiologic examination, sacroiliac joints; less than three views	0.17	0.58	0.04	0.79	XXX	N
72200	26			0.17	0.08	0.01	0.26	XXX	N
72200	TC			0	0.50	0.03	0.53	XXX	N
72202	00	A	Radiologic examination, sacroiliac joints; three or more views	0.19	0.68	0.05	0.92	XXX	N
72202	26			0.19	0.09	0.01	0.29	XXX	N
72202	TC			0	0.59	0.04	0.63	XXX	N
72220	00	A	Radiologic examination, sacrum and coccyx, minimum of two views	0.17	0.62	0.05	0.84	XXX	N
72220	26			0.17	0.08	0.01	0.26	XXX	N
72220	TC			0	0.54	0.04	0.58	XXX	N
72240	00	A	Myelography, cervical, radiological supervision and interpretation	0.91	4.93	0.35	6.19	XXX	N
72240	26			0.91	0.41	0.06	1.38	XXX	N
72240	TC			0	4.52	0.29	4.81	XXX	N
72255	00	A	Myelography, thoracic, radiological supervision and interpretation	0.91	4.54	0.32	5.77	XXX	N
72255	26			0.91	0.41	0.06	1.38	XXX	N
72255	TC			0	4.13	0.26	4.39	XXX	N
72265	00	A	Myelography, lumbosacral, radiological supervision and interpretation	0.83	4.26	0.31	5.40	XXX	N
72265	26			0.83	0.38	0.06	1.27	XXX	N
72265	TC			0	3.88	0.25	4.13	XXX	N
72270	00	A	Myelography, entire spinal canal, radiological supervision and interpretation	1.33	6.40	0.46	8.19	XXX	N
72270	26			1.33	0.59	0.09	2.01	XXX	N
72270	TC			0	5.81	0.37	6.18	XXX	N
72285	00	A	Diskography, cervical, radiological supervision and interpretation	0.83	8.37	0.56	9.76	XXX	N
72285	26			0.83	0.38	0.06	1.27	XXX	N
72285	TC			0	7.99	0.50	8.49	XXX	N
72295	00	A	Diskography, lumbar, radiological supervision and interpretation	0.83	7.87	0.52	9.22	XXX	N
72295	26			0.83	0.38	0.06	1.27	XXX	N
72295	TC			0	7.49	0.46	7.95	XXX	N
73000	00	A	Radiologic examination; clavicle, complete	0.16	0.57	0.04	0.77	XXX	N
73000	26			0.16	0.07	0.01	0.24	XXX	N
73000	TC			0	0.50	0.03	0.53	XXX	N
73010	00	A	Radiologic examination; scapula, complete	0.17	0.58	0.04	0.79	XXX	N
73010	26			0.17	0.08	0.01	0.26	XXX	N
73010	TC			0	0.50	0.03	0.53	XXX	N
73020	00	A	Radiologic examination, shoulder; one view	0.15	0.52	0.04	0.71	XXX	N

CPT codes and descriptions only, © 1994 American Medical Association. Reimbursement information, © 1995 McGraw-Hill Inc.

Code/ CPT	Mod- ifier	Status	Description	Work value	Practice expense	Mal- practice	Total value	Global period	Up- date
73020	26			0.15	0.07	0.01	0.23	XXX	N
73020	TC			0	0.45	0.03	0.48	XXX	N
73030	00	A	Radiologic examination, shoulder; complete, minimum of two views	0.18	0.62	0.05	0.85	XXX	N
73030	26			0.18	0.08	0.01	0.27	XXX	N
73030	TC			0	0.54	0.04	0.58	XXX	N
73040	00	A	Radiologic examination, shoulder, arthrography, radiological supervision and interpretation	0.54	2.25	0.17	2.96	XXX	N
73040	26			0.54	0.25	0.04	0.83	XXX	N
73040	TC			0	2.00	0.13	2.13	XXX	N
73050	00	A	Radiologic examination; acromioclavicular joints, bilateral, with or without weighted distraction	0.20	0.73	0.05	0.98	XXX	N
73050	26			0.20	0.09	0.01	0.30	XXX	N
73050	TC			0	0.64	0.04	0.68	XXX	N
73060	00	A	Radiologic examination; humerus, minimum of two views	0.17	0.62	0.05	0.84	XXX	N
73060	26			0.17	0.08	0.01	0.26	XXX	N
73060	TC			0	0.54	0.04	0.58	XXX	N
73070	00	A	Radiologic examination, elbow; anteroposterior and lateral views	0.15	0.57	0.04	0.76	XXX	N
73070	26			0.15	0.07	0.01	0.23	XXX	N
73070	TC			0	0.50	0.03	0.53	XXX	N
73080	00	A	Radiologic examination, elbow; complete, minimum of three views	0.17	0.62	0.05	0.84	XXX	N
73080	26			0.17	0.08	0.01	0.26	XXX	N
73080	TC			0	0.54	0.04	0.58	XXX	N
73085	00	A	Radiologic examination, elbow, arthrography, radiological supervision and interpretation	0.54	2.25	0.17	2.96	XXX	N
73085	26			0.54	0.25	0.04	0.83	XXX	N
73085	TC			0	2.00	0.13	2.13	XXX	N
73090	00	A	Radiologic examination; forearm, anteroposterior and lateral views	0.16	0.57	0.04	0.77	XXX	N
73090	26			0.16	0.07	0.01	0.24	XXX	N
73090	TC			0	0.50	0.03	0.53	XXX	N
73092	00	A	Radiologic examination; upper extremity, infant, minimum of two views	0.16	0.54	0.04	0.74	XXX	N
73092	26			0.16	0.07	0.01	0.24	XXX	N
73092	TC			0	0.47	0.03	0.50	XXX	N
73100	00	A	Radiologic examination, wrist; anteroposterior and lateral views	0.16	0.54	0.04	0.74	XXX	N
73100	26			0.16	0.07	0.01	0.24	XXX	N
73100	TC			0	0.47	0.03	0.50	XXX	N
73110	00	A	Radiologic examination, wrist; complete, minimum of three views	0.17	0.59	0.04	0.80	XXX	N
73110	26			0.17	0.08	0.01	0.26	XXX	N
73110	TC			0	0.51	0.03	0.54	XXX	N
73115	00	A	Radiologic examination, wrist, arthrography, radiological supervision and interpretation	0.54	1.75	0.14	2.43	XXX	N
73115	26			0.54	0.25	0.04	0.83	XXX	N
73115	TC			0	1.50	0.10	1.60	XXX	N
73120	00	A	Radiologic examination, hand; two views	0.16	0.54	0.04	0.74	XXX	N
73120	26			0.16	0.07	0.01	0.24	XXX	N
73120	TC			0	0.47	0.03	0.50	XXX	N

CPT codes and descriptions only, © 1994 American Medical Association. Reimbursement information, © 1995 McGraw-Hill Inc.

Code/ CPT	Mod- ifier	Status	Description	Work value	Practice expense	Mal- practice	Total value	Global period	Up- date
73130	00	A	Radiologic examination, hand; minimum of three views	0.17	0.59	0.04	0.80	XXX	N
73130	26			0.17	0.08	0.01	0.26	XXX	N
73130	TC			0	0.51	0.03	0.54	XXX	N
73140	00	A	Radiologic examination, finger(s), minimum of two views	0.13	0.46	0.04	0.63	XXX	N
73140	26			0.13	0.06	0.01	0.20	XXX	N
73140	TC			0	0.40	0.03	0.43	XXX	N
73200	00	A	Computerized axial tomography, upper extremity; without contrast material	1.09	5.21	0.37	6.67	XXX	N
73200	26			1.09	0.48	0.07	1.64	XXX	N
73200	TC			0	4.73	0.30	5.03	XXX	N
73201	00	A	Computerized axial tomography, upper extremity; with contrast material(s)	1.16	6.14	0.44	7.74	XXX	N
73201	26			1.16	0.51	0.08	1.75	XXX	N
73201	TC			0	5.63	0.36	5.99	XXX	N
73202	00	A	Computerized axial tomography, upper extremity; without contrast material, followed by contrast material(s) and further sections	1.22	7.61	0.53	9.36	XXX	N
73202	26			1.22	0.53	0.08	1.83	XXX	N
73202	TC			0	7.08	0.45	7.53	XXX	N
73220	00	A	Magnetic resonance (eg, proton) imaging, upper extremity, other than joint	1.48	11.34	0.77	13.59	XXX	N
73220	26			1.48	0.66	0.10	2.24	XXX	N
73220	TC			0	10.68	0.67	11.35	XXX	N
73221	00	A	Magnetic resonance (eg, proton) imaging, any joint of upper extremity	0.95	11.11	0.73	12.79	XXX	N
73221	26			0.95	0.43	0.06	1.44	XXX	N
73221	TC			0	10.68	0.67	11.35	XXX	N
73225	00	A	Magnetic resonance angiography, upper extremity, with or without contrast material(s)	1.73	11.34	0.77	13.84	XXX	N
73225	26			1.73	0.66	0.10	2.49	XXX	N
73225	TC			0	10.68	0.67	11.35	XXX	N
73500	00	A	Radiologic examination, hip unilateral; one view	0.17	0.53	0.04	0.74	XXX	N
73500	26			0.17	0.08	0.01	0.26	XXX	N
73500	TC			0	0.45	0.03	0.48	XXX	N
73510	00	A	Radiologic examination, hip unilateral; complete, minimum of two views	0.21	0.64	0.05	0.90	XXX	N
73510	26			0.21	0.10	0.01	0.32	XXX	N
73510	TC			0	0.54	0.04	0.58	XXX	N
73520	00	A	Radiologic examination, hips, bilateral, minimum of two views of each hip, including anteroposterior view of pelvis	0.26	0.76	0.06	1.08	XXX	N
73520	26			0.26	0.12	0.02	0.40	XXX	N
73520	TC			0	0.64	0.04	0.68	XXX	N
73525	00	A	Radiologic examination, hip, arthrography, radiological supervision and interpretation	0.54	2.25	0.17	2.96	XXX	N
73525	26			0.54	0.25	0.04	0.83	XXX	N
73525	TC			0	2.00	0.13	2.13	XXX	N
73530	00	A	Radiologic examination, hip, during operative procedure	0.29	0.63	0.05	0.97	XXX	N
73530	26			0.29	0.13	0.02	0.44	XXX	N
73530	TC			0	0.50	0.03	0.53	XXX	N
73540	00	A	Radiologic examination, pelvis and hips, infant or child, minimum of two views	0.20	0.64	0.05	0.89	XXX	N
73540	26			0.20	0.10	0.01	0.31	XXX	N

CPT codes and descriptions only, © 1994 American Medical Association. Reimbursement information, © 1995 McGraw-Hill Inc.

Code/ CPT	Mod-ifier	Status	Description	Work value	Practice expense	Mal-practice	Total value	Global period	Up-date
73540	TC			0	0.54	0.04	0.58	XXX	N
73550	00	A	Radiologic examination, femur, anteroposterior and lateral views	0.17	0.62	0.05	0.84	XXX	N
73550	26			0.17	0.08	0.01	0.26	XXX	N
73550	TC			0	0.54	0.04	0.58	XXX	N
73560	00	A	Radiologic examination, knee; anteroposterior and lateral views	0.17	0.57	0.04	0.78	XXX	N
73560	26			0.17	0.07	0.01	0.25	XXX	N
73560	TC			0	0.50	0.03	0.53	XXX	N
73562	00	A	Radiologic examination, knee; anteroposterior and lateral, with oblique(s), minimum of three views	0.18	0.63	0.05	0.86	XXX	N
73562	26			0.18	0.09	0.01	0.28	XXX	N
73562	TC			0	0.54	0.04	0.58	XXX	N
73564	00	A	Radiologic examination, knee; complete, including oblique(s), and tunnel, and/or patellar and/or standing views	0.22	0.69	0.06	0.97	XXX	N
73564	26			0.22	0.10	0.02	0.34	XXX	N
73564	TC			0	0.59	0.04	0.63	XXX	N
73565	00	A	Radiologic examination, knee; both knees, standing, anteroposterior	0.17	0.54	0.04	0.75	XXX	N
73565	26			0.17	0.07	0.01	0.25	XXX	N
73565	TC			0	0.47	0.03	0.50	XXX	N
73580	00	A	Radiologic examination, knee, arthrography, radiological supervision and interpretation	0.54	2.75	0.21	3.50	XXX	N
73580	26			0.54	0.25	0.04	0.83	XXX	N
73580	TC			0	2.50	0.17	2.67	XXX	N
73590	00	A	Radiologic examination; tibia and fibula, anteroposterior and lateral views	0.17	0.57	0.04	0.78	XXX	N
73590	26			0.17	0.07	0.01	0.25	XXX	N
73590	TC			0	0.50	0.03	0.53	XXX	N
73592	00	A	Radiologic examination; lower extremity, infant, minimum of two views	0.16	0.54	0.04	0.74	XXX	N
73592	26			0.16	0.07	0.01	0.24	XXX	N
73592	TC			0	0.47	0.03	0.50	XXX	N
73600	00	A	Radiologic examination, ankle; anteroposterior and lateral views	0.16	0.54	0.04	0.74	XXX	N
73600	26			0.16	0.07	0.01	0.24	XXX	N
73600	TC			0	0.47	0.03	0.50	XXX	N
73610	00	A	Radiologic examination, ankle; complete, minimum of three views	0.17	0.59	0.04	0.80	XXX	N
73610	26			0.17	0.08	0.01	0.26	XXX	N
73610	TC			0	0.51	0.03	0.54	XXX	N
73615	00	A	Radiologic examination, ankle, arthrography, radiological supervision and interpretation	0.54	2.25	0.17	2.96	XXX	N
73615	26			0.54	0.25	0.04	0.83	XXX	N
73615	TC			0	2.00	0.13	2.13	XXX	N
73620	00	A	Radiologic examination, foot; anteroposterior and lateral views	0.16	0.54	0.04	0.74	XXX	N
73620	26			0.16	0.07	0.01	0.24	XXX	N
73620	TC			0	0.47	0.03	0.50	XXX	N
73630	00	A	Radiologic examination, foot; complete, minimum of three views	0.17	0.59	0.04	0.80	XXX	N

CPT codes and descriptions only, © 1994 American Medical Association. Reimbursement information, © 1995 McGraw-Hill Inc.

Code/ CPT	Mod-ifier	Status	Description	Work value	Practice expense	Mal-practice	Total value	Global period	Up-date
73630	26			0.17	0.08	0.01	0.26	XXX	N
73630	TC			0	0.51	0.03	0.54	XXX	N
73650	00	A	Radiologic examination; calcaneus, minimum of two views	0.16	0.52	0.04	0.72	XXX	N
73650	26			0.16	0.07	0.01	0.24	XXX	N
73650	TC			0	0.45	0.03	0.48	XXX	N
73660	00	A	Radiologic examination; toe(s), minimum of two views	0.13	0.46	0.04	0.63	XXX	N
73660	26			0.13	0.06	0.01	0.20	XXX	N
73660	TC			0	0.40	0.03	0.43	XXX	N
73700	00	A	Computerized axial tomography, lower extremity; without contrast material	1.09	5.21	0.37	6.67	XXX	N
73700	26			1.09	0.48	0.07	1.64	XXX	N
73700	TC			0	4.73	0.30	5.03	XXX	N
73701	00	A	Computerized axial tomography, lower extremity; with contrast material(s)	1.16	6.14	0.44	7.74	XXX	N
73701	26			1.16	0.51	0.08	1.75	XXX	N
73701	TC			0	5.63	0.36	5.99	XXX	N
73702	00	A	Computerized axial tomography, lower extremity; without contrast material, followed by contrast material(s) and further sections	1.22	7.61	0.53	9.36	XXX	N
73702	26			1.22	0.53	0.08	1.83	XXX	N
73702	TC			0	7.08	0.45	7.53	XXX	N
73720	00	A	Magnetic resonance (eg, proton) imaging, lower extremity, other than joint	1.48	11.34	0.77	13.59	XXX	N
73720	26			1.48	0.66	0.10	2.24	XXX	N
73720	TC			0	10.68	0.67	11.35	XXX	N
73721	00	A	Magnetic resonance (eg, proton) imaging, any joint of lower extremity	0.95	11.11	0.73	12.79	XXX	N
73721	26			0.95	0.43	0.06	1.44	XXX	N
73721	TC			0	10.68	0.67	11.35	XXX	N
73725	00	A	Magnetic resonance angiography, lower extremity, with or without contrast material(s)	1.82	11.34	0.77	13.93	XXX	N
73725	26			1.82	0.66	0.10	2.58	XXX	N
73725	TC			0	10.68	0.67	11.35	XXX	N
74000	00	A	Radiologic examination, abdomen; single anteroposterior view	0.18	0.58	0.04	0.80	XXX	N
74000	26			0.18	0.08	0.01	0.27	XXX	N
74000	TC			0	0.50	0.03	0.53	XXX	N
74010	00	A	Radiologic examination, abdomen; anteroposterior and additional oblique and cone views	0.23	0.65	0.06	0.94	XXX	N
74010	26			0.23	0.11	0.02	0.36	XXX	N
74010	TC			0	0.54	0.04	0.58	XXX	N
74020	00	A	Radiologic examination, abdomen; complete, including decubitus and/or erect views	0.27	0.72	0.06	1.05	XXX	N
74020	26			0.27	0.13	0.02	0.42	XXX	N
74020	TC			0	0.59	0.04	0.63	XXX	N
74022	00	A	Radiologic examination, abdomen; complete acute abdomen series, including supine, erect, and/or decubitus views, upright PA chest	0.32	0.85	0.07	1.24	XXX	N
74022	26			0.32	0.15	0.02	0.49	XXX	N
74022	TC			0	0.70	0.05	0.75	XXX	N
74150	00	A	Computerized axial tomography, abdomen; without contrast material	1.19	5.91	0.43	7.53	XXX	N

CPT codes and descriptions only, © 1994 American Medical Association. Reimbursement information, © 1995 McGraw-Hill Inc.

Code/ CPT	Mod- ifier	Status	Description	Work value	Practice expense	Mal- practice	Total value	Global period	Up- date
74150	26			1.19	0.52	0.08	1.79	XXX	N
74150	TC			0	5.39	0.35	5.74	XXX	N
74160	00	A	Computerized axial tomography, abdomen; with contrast material(s)	1.27	7.08	0.50	8.85	XXX	N
74160	26			1.27	0.56	0.09	1.92	XXX	N
74160	TC			0	6.52	0.41	6.93	XXX	N
74170	00	A	Computerized axial tomography, abdomen; without contrast material, followed by contrast material(s) and further sections	1.40	8.71	0.60	10.71	XXX	N
74170	26			1.40	0.62	0.10	2.12	XXX	N
74170	TC			0	8.09	0.50	8.59	XXX	N
74181	00	A	Magnetic resonance (eg, proton) imaging, abdomen	1.60	11.40	0.78	13.78	XXX	N
74181	26			1.60	0.72	0.11	2.43	XXX	N
74181	TC			0	10.68	0.67	11.35	XXX	N
74185	00	A	Magnetic resonance angiography, abdomen, with or without contrast material(s)	1.80	11.40	0.78	13.98	XXX	N
74185	26			1.80	0.72	0.11	2.63	XXX	N
74185	TC			0	10.68	0.67	11.35	XXX	N
74190	00	A	Peritoneogram (eg, after injection of air or contrast), radiological supervision and interpretation	0.48	1.37	0.10	1.95	XXX	N
74190	26			0.48	0.13	0.02	0.63	XXX	N
74190	TC			0	1.24	0.08	1.32	XXX	N
74210	00	A	Radiologic examination; pharynx and/or cervical esophagus	0.36	1.29	0.09	1.74	XXX	N
74210	26			0.36	0.16	0.02	0.54	XXX	N
74210	TC			0	1.13	0.07	1.20	XXX	N
74220	00	A	Radiologic examination; esophagus	0.46	1.34	0.10	1.90	XXX	N
74220	26			0.46	0.21	0.03	0.70	XXX	N
74220	TC			0	1.13	0.07	1.20	XXX	N
74230	00	A	Swallowing function, pharynx and/or esophagus, with cineradiography and/or video	0.53	1.49	0.12	2.14	XXX	N
74230	26			0.53	0.25	0.04	0.82	XXX	N
74230	TC			0	1.24	0.08	1.32	XXX	N
74235	00	A	Removal of foreign body(s), esophageal, with use of balloon catheter, radiological supervision and interpretation	1.19	3.02	0.25	4.46	XXX	N
74235	26			1.19	0.52	0.08	1.79	XXX	N
74235	TC			0	2.50	0.17	2.67	XXX	N
74240	00	A	Radiologic examination, gastrointestinal tract, upper; with or without delayed films, without KUB	0.69	1.71	0.14	2.54	XXX	N
74240	26			0.69	0.32	0.05	1.06	XXX	N
74240	TC			0	1.39	0.09	1.48	XXX	N
74241	00	A	Radiologic examination, gastrointestinal tract, upper; with or without delayed films, with KUB	0.69	1.74	0.14	2.57	XXX	N
74241	26			0.69	0.32	0.05	1.06	XXX	N
74241	TC			0	1.42	0.09	1.51	XXX	N
74245	00	A	Radiologic examination, gastrointestinal tract, upper; with small bowel, includes multiple serial films	0.91	2.68	0.21	3.80	XXX	N
74245	26			0.91	0.41	0.06	1.38	XXX	N
74245	TC			0	2.27	0.15	2.42	XXX	N
74246	00	A	Radiological examination, gastrointestinal tract, upper, air contrast, with specific high density barium, effervescent agent, with or without glucagon; with or without delayed films, without KUB	0.69	1.89	0.15	2.73	XXX	N

CPT codes and descriptions only, © 1994 American Medical Association. Reimbursement information, © 1995 McGraw-Hill Inc.

Code/ CPT	Mod- ifier	Status	Description	Work value	Practice expense	Mal- practice	Total value	Global period	Up- date
74246	26			0.69	0.32	0.05	1.06	XXX	N
74246	TC			0	1.57	0.10	1.67	XXX	N
74247	00	A	Radiological examination, gastrointestinal tract, upper, air contrast, with specific high density barium, effervescent agent, with or without glucagon; with or without delayed films, with KUB	0.69	1.92	0.16	2.77	XXX	N
74247	26			0.69	0.32	0.05	1.06	XXX	N
74247	TC			0	1.60	0.11	1.71	XXX	N
74249	00	A	Radiological examination, gastrointestinal tract, upper, air contrast, with specific high density barium, effervescent agent, with or without glucagon; with small bowel follow-through	0.91	2.86	0.22	3.99	XXX	N
74249	26			0.91	0.41	0.06	1.38	XXX	N
74249	TC			0	2.45	0.16	2.61	XXX	N
74250	00	A	Radiologic examination, small bowel, includes multiple serial films;	0.47	1.45	0.11	2.03	XXX	N
74250	26			0.47	0.21	0.03	0.71	XXX	N
74250	TC			0	1.24	0.08	1.32	XXX	N
74251	00	A	Radiologic examination, small bowel, includes multiple serial films; via enteroclysis tube	0.69	1.45	0.11	2.25	XXX	N
74251	26			0.69	0.21	0.03	0.93	XXX	N
74251	TC			0	1.24	0.08	1.32	XXX	N
74260	00	A	Duodenography, hypotonic	0.50	1.65	0.12	2.27	XXX	N
74260	26			0.50	0.23	0.03	0.76	XXX	N
74260	TC			0	1.42	0.09	1.51	XXX	N
74270	00	A	Radiologic examination, colon; barium enema, with or without KUB	0.69	1.94	0.16	2.79	XXX	N
74270	26			0.69	0.32	0.05	1.06	XXX	N
74270	TC			0	1.62	0.11	1.73	XXX	N
74280	00	A	Radiologic examination, colon; air contrast with specific high density barium, with or without glucagon	0.99	2.58	0.21	3.78	XXX	N
74280	26			0.99	0.45	0.07	1.51	XXX	N
74280	TC			0	2.13	0.14	2.27	XXX	N
74283	00	A	Barium enema, therapeutic, for reduction of intussusception	2.02	3.34	0.30	5.66	XXX	N
74283	26			2.02	0.90	0.14	3.06	XXX	N
74283	TC			0	2.44	0.16	2.60	XXX	N
74290	00	A	Cholecystography, oral contrast;	0.32	0.85	0.07	1.24	XXX	N
74290	26			0.32	0.15	0.02	0.49	XXX	N
74290	TC			0	0.70	0.05	0.75	XXX	N
74291	00	A	Cholecystography, oral contrast; additional or repeat examination or multiple day examination	0.20	0.49	0.04	0.73	XXX	N
74291	26			0.20	0.09	0.01	0.30	XXX	N
74291	TC			0	0.40	0.03	0.43	XXX	N
74300	00	C	Cholangiography and/or pancreatography; intraoperative, radiological supervision and interpretation	0.36*	0.53#	0.03*	0.92#	XXX	N
74300	26			0.36	0.17	0.02	0.55	XXX	N
74300	TC			0	0.36#	0.01*	0.37#	XXX	N
74301	00	C	Cholangiography and/or pancreatography; additional set intraoperative, radiological supervision and interpretation	0.21*	0.25#	0.01*	0.47#	XXX	N
74301	26			0.21	0.10	0.01	0.32	XXX	N
74301	TC			0	0.15#	0	0.15#	XXX	N

CPT codes and descriptions only, © 1994 American Medical Association. Reimbursement information, © 1995 McGraw-Hill Inc.

Code/ CPT	Mod- ifier	Status	Description	Work value	Practice expense	Mal- practice	Total value	Global period	Up- date
74305	00	A	Cholangiography and/or pancreatography; postoperative, radiological supervision and interpretation	0.42	0.94	0.08	1.44	XXX	N
74305	26			0.42	0.19	0.03	0.64	XXX	N
74305	TC			0	0.75	0.05	0.80	XXX	N
74320	00	A	Cholangiography, percutaneous, transhepatic, radiological supervision and interpretation	0.54	3.25	0.23	4.02	XXX	N
74320	26			0.54	0.25	0.04	0.83	XXX	N
74320	TC			0	3.00	0.19	3.19	XXX	N
74327	00	A	Postoperative biliary duct stone removal, percutaneous via T-tube tract, basket or snare (eg, Burhenne technique), radiological supervision and interpretation	0.70	2.00	0.16	2.86	XXX	N
74327	26			0.70	0.32	0.05	1.07	XXX	N
74327	TC			0	1.68	0.11	1.79	XXX	N
74328	00	A	Endoscopic catheterization of the biliary ductal system, radiological supervision and interpretation	0.70	3.32	0.24	4.26	XXX	N
74328	26			0.70	0.32	0.05	1.07	XXX	N
74328	TC			0	3.00	0.19	3.19	XXX	N
74329	00	A	Endoscopic catheterization of the pancreatic ductal system, radiological supervision and interpretation	0.70	3.32	0.24	4.26	XXX	N
74329	26			0.70	0.32	0.05	1.07	XXX	N
74329	TC			0	3.00	0.19	3.19	XXX	N
74330	00	A	Combined endoscopic catheterization of the biliary and pancreatic ductal systems, radiological supervision and interpretation	0.70	3.32	0.24	4.26	XXX	N
74330	26			0.70	0.32	0.05	1.07	XXX	N
74330	TC			0	3.00	0.19	3.19	XXX	N
74340	00	A	Introduction of long gastrointestinal tube (eg, Miller-Abbott), including multiple fluoroscopies and films, radiological supervision and interpretation	0.54	2.75	0.21	3.50	XXX	N
74340	26			0.54	0.25	0.04	0.83	XXX	N
74340	TC			0	2.50	0.17	2.67	XXX	N
74350	00	A	Percutaneous placement of gastrostomy tube, radiological supervision and interpretation	0.76	3.35	0.24	4.35	XXX	N
74350	26			0.76	0.35	0.05	1.16	XXX	N
74350	TC			0	3.00	0.19	3.19	XXX	N
74355	00	A	Percutaneous placement of enteroclysis tube, radiological supervision and interpretation	0.76	2.85	0.22	3.83	XXX	N
74355	26			0.76	0.35	0.05	1.16	XXX	N
74355	TC			0	2.50	0.17	2.67	XXX	N
74360	00	A	Intraluminal dilation of strictures and/or obstructions (eg, esophagus), radiological supervision and interpretation	0.54	3.25	0.23	4.02	XXX	N
74360	26			0.54	0.25	0.04	0.83	XXX	N
74360	TC			0	3.00	0.19	3.19	XXX	N
74363	00	A	Percutaneous transhepatic dilatation of biliary duct stricture with or without placement of stent, radiological supervision and interpretation	0.88	6.21	0.43	7.52	XXX	N
74363	26			0.88	0.40	0.06	1.34	XXX	N
74363	TC			0	5.81	0.37	6.18	XXX	N
74400	00	A	Urography (pyelography), intravenous, with or without KUB, with or without tomography;	0.49	1.82	0.14	2.45	XXX	N
74400	26			0.49	0.22	0.03	0.74	XXX	N
74400	TC			0	1.60	0.11	1.71	XXX	N

CPT codes and descriptions only, © 1994 American Medical Association. Reimbursement information, © 1995 McGraw-Hill Inc.

Code/ CPT	Mod- ifier	Status	Description	Work value	Practice expense	Mal- practice	Total value	Global period	Up- date
74405	00	A	Urography (pyelography), intravenous, with or without KUB, with or without tomography; with special hypertensive contrast concentration and/or clearance studies	0.49	2.11	0.16	2.76	XXX	N
74405	26			0.49	0.22	0.03	0.74	XXX	N
74405	TC			0	1.89	0.13	2.02	XXX	N
74410	00	A	Urography, infusion, drip technique and/or bolus technique;	0.49	2.08	0.15	2.72	XXX	N
74410	26			0.49	0.22	0.03	0.74	XXX	N
74410	TC			0	1.86	0.12	1.98	XXX	N
74415	00	A	Urography, infusion, drip technique and/or bolus technique; with nephrotomography	0.49	2.24	0.16	2.89	XXX	N
74415	26			0.49	0.22	0.03	0.74	XXX	N
74415	TC			0	2.02	0.13	2.15	XXX	N
74420	00	A	Urography, retrograde, with or without KUB	0.36	2.66	0.19	3.21	XXX	N
74420	26			0.36	0.16	0.02	0.54	XXX	N
74420	TC			0	2.50	0.17	2.67	XXX	N
74425	00	A	Urography, antegrade, (pyelostogram, nephrostogram, loopogram), radiological supervision and interpretation	0.36	1.40	0.10	1.86	XXX	N
74425	26			0.36	0.16	0.02	0.54	XXX	N
74425	TC			0	1.24	0.08	1.32	XXX	N
74430	00	A	Cystography, minimum of three views, radiological supervision and interpretation	0.32	1.15	0.09	1.56	XXX	N
74430	26			0.32	0.15	0.02	0.49	XXX	N
74430	TC			0	1.00	0.07	1.07	XXX	N
74440	00	A	Vasography, vesiculography, or epididymography, radiological supervision and interpretation	0.38	1.25	0.10	1.73	XXX	N
74440	26			0.38	0.17	0.03	0.58	XXX	N
74440	TC			0	1.08	0.07	1.15	XXX	N
74445	00	A	Corpora cavernosography, radiological supervision and interpretation	1.14	1.58	0.15	2.87	XXX	N
74445	26			1.14	0.50	0.08	1.72	XXX	N
74445	TC			0	1.08	0.07	1.15	XXX	N
74450	00	A	Urethrocystography, retrograde, radiological supervision and interpretation	0.33	1.54	0.11	1.98	XXX	N
74450	26			0.33	0.15	0.02	0.50	XXX	N
74450	TC			0	1.39	0.09	1.48	XXX	N
74455	00	A	Urethrocystography, voiding, radiological supervision and interpretation	0.33	1.65	0.12	2.10	XXX	N
74455	26			0.33	0.15	0.02	0.50	XXX	N
74455	TC			0	1.50	0.10	1.60	XXX	N
74470	00	A	Radiologic examination, renal cyst study, translumbar, contrast visualization, radiological supervision and interpretation	0.54	1.44	0.12	2.10	XXX	N
74470	26			0.54	0.25	0.04	0.83	XXX	N
74470	TC			0	1.19	0.08	1.27	XXX	N
74475	00	A	Introduction of intracatheter or catheter into renal pelvis for drainage and/or injection, percutaneous, radiological supervision and interpretation	0.54	4.13	0.29	4.96	XXX	N
74475	26			0.54	0.25	0.04	0.83	XXX	N
74475	TC			0	3.88	0.25	4.13	XXX	N

CPT codes and descriptions only, © 1994 American Medical Association. Reimbursement information, © 1995 McGraw-Hill Inc.

Code/ CPT	Mod- ifier	Status	Description	Work value	Practice expense	Mal- practice	Total value	Global period	Up- date
74480	00	A	Introduction of ureteral catheter or stent into ureter through renal pelvis for drainage and/or injection, percutaneous, radiological supervision and interpretation	0.54	4.13	0.29	4.96	XXX	N
74480	26			0.54	0.25	0.04	0.83	XXX	N
74480	TC			0	3.88	0.25	4.13	XXX	N
74485	00	A	Dilation of nephrostomy, ureters, or urethra, radiological supervision and interpretation	0.54	3.25	0.23	4.02	XXX	N
74485	26			0.54	0.25	0.04	0.83	XXX	N
74485	TC			0	3.00	0.19	3.19	XXX	N
74710	00	A	Pelvimetry, with or without placental localization	0.34	1.16	0.09	1.59	XXX	N
74710	26			0.34	0.16	0.02	0.52	XXX	N
74710	TC			0	1.00	0.07	1.07	XXX	N
74740	00	A	Hysterosalpingography, radiological supervision and interpretation	0.38	1.41	0.11	1.90	XXX	N
74740	26			0.38	0.17	0.03	0.58	XXX	N
74740	TC			0	1.24	0.08	1.32	XXX	N
74742	00	A	Transcervical catheterization of fallopian tube, radiological supervision and interpretation	0.61	3.25	0.23	4.09	XXX	N
74742	26			0.61	0.25	0.04	0.90	XXX	N
74742	TC			0	3.00	0.19	3.19	XXX	N
74775	00	A	Perineogram (eg, vaginogram, for sex determination or extent of anomalies)	0.62	1.68	0.13	2.43	XXX	N
74775	26			0.62	0.29	0.04	0.95	XXX	N
74775	TC			0	1.39	0.09	1.48	XXX	N
75552	00	A	Cardiac magnetic resonance imaging for morphology; without contrast material	1.60	11.40	0.78	13.78	XXX	N
75552	26			1.60	0.72	0.11	2.43	XXX	N
75552	TC			0	10.68	0.67	11.35	XXX	N
75553	00	A	Cardiac magnetic resonance imaging for morphology; with contrast material	2.00	11.40	0.78	14.18	XXX	N
75553	26			2.00	0.72	0.11	2.83	XXX	N
75553	TC			0	10.68	0.67	11.35	XXX	N
75554	00	A	Cardiac magnetic resonance imaging for function, with or without morphology; complete study (eg, multiple chambers)	1.83	11.40	0.78	14.01	XXX	N
75554	26			1.83	0.72	0.11	2.66	XXX	N
75554	TC			0	10.68	0.67	11.35	XXX	N
75555	00	A	Cardiac magnetic resonance imaging for function, with or without morphology; limited study (eg, single chamber)	1.74	11.40	0.78	13.92	XXX	N
75555	26			1.74	0.72	0.11	2.57	XXX	N
75555	TC			0	10.68	0.67	11.35	XXX	N
75556	00	N	Cardiac magnetic resonance imaging for velocity flow mapping	1.77*	7.98#	0.34*	10.09#	XXX	0
75556	26			1.77*	0.65#	0.07*	2.49#		
75556	TC			1.77*	7.33#	0.28*	9.38#		
75600	00	A	Aortography, thoracic, without serialography, radiological supervision and interpretation	0.49	12.23	0.78	13.50	XXX	N
75600	26			0.49	0.22	0.03	0.74	XXX	N
75600	TC			0	12.01	0.75	12.76	XXX	N
75605	00	A	Aortography, thoracic, by serialography, radiological supervision and interpretation	1.14	12.51	0.83	14.48	XXX	N
75605	26			1.14	0.50	0.08	1.72	XXX	N

CPT codes and descriptions only, © 1994 American Medical Association. Reimbursement information, © 1995 McGraw-Hill Inc.

Code/ CPT	Mod- ifier	Status	Description	Work value	Practice expense	Mal- practice	Total value	Global period	Up- date
75605	TC			0	12.01	0.75	12.76	XXX	N
75625	00	A	Aortography, abdominal, by serialography, radiological supervision and interpretation	1.14	12.51	0.83	14.48	XXX	N
75625	26			1.14	0.50	0.08	1.72	XXX	N
75625	TC			0	12.01	0.75	12.76	XXX	N
75630	00	A	Aortography, abdominal plus bilateral iliofemoral lower extremity, catheter, by serialography, radiological supervision and interpretation	1.31	13.09	0.88	15.28	XXX	N
75630	26			1.31	0.58	0.09	1.98	XXX	N
75630	TC			0	12.51	0.79	13.30	XXX	N
75650	00	A	Angiography, cervicocerebral, catheter, including vessel origin, radiological supervision and interpretation	1.49	12.67	0.85	15.01	XXX	N
75650	26			1.49	0.66	0.10	2.25	XXX	N
75650	TC			0	12.01	0.75	12.76	XXX	N
75658	00	A	Angiography, brachial, retrograde, radiological supervision and interpretation	1.31	12.59	0.84	14.74	XXX	N
75658	26			1.31	0.58	0.09	1.98	XXX	N
75658	TC			0	12.01	0.75	12.76	XXX	N
75660	00	A	Angiography, external carotid, unilateral, selective, radiological supervision and interpretation	1.31	12.59	0.84	14.74	XXX	N
75660	26			1.31	0.58	0.09	1.98	XXX	N
75660	TC			0	12.01	0.75	12.76	XXX	N
75662	00	A	Angiography, external carotid, bilateral, selective, radiological supervision and interpretation	1.66	12.75	0.86	15.27	XXX	N
75662	26			1.66	0.74	0.11	2.51	XXX	N
75662	TC			0	12.01	0.75	12.76	XXX	N
75665	00	A	Angiography, carotid, cerebral, unilateral, radiological supervision and interpretation	1.31	12.59	0.84	14.74	XXX	N
75665	26			1.31	0.58	0.09	1.98	XXX	N
75665	TC			0	12.01	0.75	12.76	XXX	N
75671	00	A	Angiography, carotid, cerebral, bilateral, radiological supervision and interpretation	1.66	12.75	0.86	15.27	XXX	N
75671	26			1.66	0.74	0.11	2.51	XXX	N
75671	TC			0	12.01	0.75	12.76	XXX	N
75676	00	A	Angiography, carotid, cervical, unilateral, radiological supervision and interpretation	1.31	12.59	0.84	14.74	XXX	N
75676	26			1.31	0.58	0.09	1.98	XXX	N
75676	TC			0	12.01	0.75	12.76	XXX	N
75680	00	A	Angiography, carotid, cervical, bilateral, radiological supervision and interpretation	1.66	12.75	0.86	15.27	XXX	N
75680	26			1.66	0.74	0.11	2.51	XXX	N
75680	TC			0	12.01	0.75	12.76	XXX	N
75685	00	A	Angiography, vertebral, cervical, and/or intracranial, radiological supervision and interpretation	1.31	12.59	0.84	14.74	XXX	N
75685	26			1.31	0.58	0.09	1.98	XXX	N
75685	TC			0	12.01	0.75	12.76	XXX	N
75705	00	A	Angiography, spinal, selective, radiological supervision and interpretation	2.18	12.99	0.90	16.07	XXX	N
75705	26			2.18	0.98	0.15	3.31	XXX	N
75705	TC			0	12.01	0.75	12.76	XXX	N
75710	00	A	Angiography, extremity, unilateral, radiological supervision and interpretation	1.14	12.51	0.83	14.48	XXX	N

CPT codes and descriptions only, © 1994 American Medical Association. Reimbursement information, © 1995 McGraw-Hill Inc.

Code/ CPT	Mod- ifier	Status	Description	Work value	Practice expense	Mal- practice	Total value	Global period	Up- date
75710	26			1.14	0.50	0.08	1.72	XXX	N
75710	TC			0	12.01	0.75	12.76	XXX	N
75716	00	A	Angiography, extremity, bilateral, radiological supervision and interpretation	1.31	12.59	0.84	14.74	XXX	N
75716	26			1.31	0.58	0.09	1.98	XXX	N
75716	TC			0	12.01	0.75	12.76	XXX	N
75722	00	A	Angiography, renal, unilateral, selective (including flush aortogram), radiological supervision and interpretation	1.14	12.51	0.83	14.48	XXX	N
75722	26			1.14	0.50	0.08	1.72	XXX	N
75722	TC			0	12.01	0.75	12.76	XXX	N
75724	00	A	Angiography, renal, bilateral, selective (including flush aortogram), radiological supervision and interpretation	1.49	12.67	0.85	15.01	XXX	N
75724	26			1.49	0.66	0.10	2.25	XXX	N
75724	TC			0	12.01	0.75	12.76	XXX	N
75726	00	A	Angiography, visceral, selective or supraselective, (with or without flush aortogram), radiological supervision and interpretation	1.14	12.51	0.83	14.48	XXX	N
75726	26			1.14	0.50	0.08	1.72	XXX	N
75726	TC			0	12.01	0.75	12.76	XXX	N
75731	00	A	Angiography, adrenal, unilateral, selective, radiological supervision and interpretation	1.14	12.51	0.83	14.48	XXX	N
75731	26			1.14	0.50	0.08	1.72	XXX	N
75731	TC			0	12.01	0.75	12.76	XXX	N
75733	00	A	Angiography, adrenal, bilateral, selective, radiological supervision and interpretation	1.31	12.59	0.84	14.74	XXX	N
75733	26			1.31	0.58	0.09	1.98	XXX	N
75733	TC			0	12.01	0.75	12.76	XXX	N
75736	00	A	Angiography, pelvic, selective or supraselective, radiological supervision and interpretation	1.14	12.51	0.83	14.48	XXX	N
75736	26			1.14	0.50	0.08	1.72	XXX	N
75736	TC			0	12.01	0.75	12.76	XXX	N
75741	00	A	Angiography, pulmonary, unilateral, selective, radiological supervision and interpretation	1.31	12.59	0.84	14.74	XXX	N
75741	26			1.31	0.58	0.09	1.98	XXX	N
75741	TC			0	12.01	0.75	12.76	XXX	N
75743	00	A	Angiography, pulmonary, bilateral, selective, radiological supervision and interpretation	1.66	12.75	0.86	15.27	XXX	N
75743	26			1.66	0.74	0.11	2.51	XXX	N
75743	TC			0	12.01	0.75	12.76	XXX	N
75746	00	A	Angiography, pulmonary, by nonselective catheter or venous injection, radiological supervision and interpretation	1.14	12.51	0.83	14.48	XXX	N
75746	26			1.14	0.50	0.08	1.72	XXX	N
75746	TC			0	12.01	0.75	12.76	XXX	N
75756	00	A	Angiography, internal mammary, radiological supervision and interpretation	1.14	12.51	0.83	14.48	XXX	N
75756	26			1.14	0.50	0.08	1.72	XXX	N
75756	TC			0	12.01	0.75	12.76	XXX	N
75774	00	A	Angiography, selective, each additional vessel studied after basic examination, radiological supervision and interpretation	0.36	12.17	0.77	13.30	XXX	N
75774	26			0.36	0.16	0.02	0.54	XXX	N
75774	TC			0	12.01	0.75	12.76	XXX	N

CPT codes and descriptions only, © 1994 American Medical Association. Reimbursement information, © 1995 McGraw-Hill Inc.

Code/ CPT	Mod-ifier	Status	Description	Work value	Practice expense	Mal-practice	Total value	Global period	Up-date
75896	00	A	Transcatheter therapy, infusion, any method (eg, thrombolysis other than coronary), radiological supervision and interpretation	1.31	20.58	1.34	23.23	XXX	N
75896	26			1.31	0.58	0.09	1.98	XXX	N
75896	TC			0	20	1.25	21.25	XXX	N
75898	00	A	Angiogram through existing catheter for follow-up study for transcatheter therapy, embolization or infusion	1.65	1.74	0.18	3.57	XXX	N
75898	26			1.65	0.74	0.11	2.50	XXX	N
75898	TC			0	1.00	0.07	1.07	XXX	N
75900	00	A	Exchange of a previously placed arterial catheter during thrombolytic therapy with contrast monitoring, radiological supervision and interpretation	0.49	20.22	1.29	22	XXX	N
75900	26			0.49	0.23	0.03	0.75	XXX	N
75900	TC			0	19.99	1.26	21.25	XXX	N
75940	00	A	Percutaneous placement of IVC filter, radiological supervision and interpretation	0.54	12.26	0.79	13.59	XXX	N
75940	26			0.54	0.25	0.04	0.83	XXX	N
75940	TC			0	12.01	0.75	12.76	XXX	N
75960	00	A	Transcatheter introduction of intravascular stent(s), (non-coronary vessel), percutaneous and/or open, radiological supervision and interpretation, each vessel	0.82	14.57	0.94	16.33	XXX	N
75960	26			0.82	0.37	0.06	1.25	XXX	N
75960	TC			0	14.20	0.88	15.08	XXX	N
75961	00	A	Transcatheter retrieval, percutaneous, of intravascular foreign body (eg, fractured venous or arterial catheter), radiological supervision and interpretation	4.25	11.91	0.90	17.06	XXX	N
75961	26			4.25	1.90	0.28	6.43	XXX	N
75961	TC			0	10.01	0.62	10.63	XXX	N
75962	00	A	Transluminal balloon angioplasty, peripheral artery, radiological supervision and interpretation	0.54	15.25	0.98	16.77	XXX	N
75962	26			0.54	0.25	0.04	0.83	XXX	N
75962	TC			0	15	0.94	15.94	XXX	N
75964	00	A	Transluminal balloon angioplasty, each additional peripheral artery, radiological supervision and interpretation	0.36	8.16	0.52	9.04	XXX	N
75964	26			0.36	0.16	0.02	0.54	XXX	N
75964	TC			0	8.00	0.50	8.50	XXX	N
75966	00	A	Transluminal balloon angioplasty, renal or other visceral artery, radiological supervision and interpretation	1.31	15.58	1.03	17.92	XXX	N
75966	26			1.31	0.58	0.09	1.98	XXX	N
75966	TC			0	15	0.94	15.94	XXX	N
75968	00	A	Transluminal balloon angioplasty, each additional visceral artery, radiological supervision and interpretation	0.36	8.16	0.52	9.04	XXX	N
75968	26			0.36	0.16	0.02	0.54	XXX	N
75968	TC			0	8.00	0.50	8.50	XXX	N
75970	00	A	Transcatheter biopsy, radiological supervision and interpretation	0.83	11.38	0.75	12.96	XXX	N
75970	26			0.83	0.38	0.06	1.27	XXX	N
75970	TC			0	11	0.69	11.69	XXX	N
75978	00	A	Transluminal balloon angioplasty, venous (eg, subclavian stenosis), radiological supervision and interpretation	0.54	15.48	0.98	17	XXX	N
75978	26			0.54	0.48	0.04	1.06	XXX	N
75978	TC			0	15	0.94	15.94	XXX	N

CPT codes and descriptions only, © 1994 American Medical Association. Reimbursement information, © 1995 McGraw-Hill Inc.

Code/ CPT	Mod-ifier	Status	Description	Work value	Practice expense	Mal-practice	Total value	Global period	Up-date
75980	00	A	Percutaneous transhepatic biliary drainage with contrast monitoring, radiological supervision and interpretation	1.44	5.80	0.43	7.67	XXX	N
75980	26			1.44	0.64	0.10	2.18	XXX	N
75980	TC			0	5.16	0.33	5.49	XXX	N
75982	00	A	Percutaneous placement of drainage catheter for combined internal and external biliary drainage or of a drainage stent for internal biliary drainage in patients with an inoperable mechanical biliary obstruction, radiological supervision and interpretation	1.44	6.45	0.47	8.36	XXX	N
75982	26			1.44	0.64	0.10	2.18	XXX	N
75982	TC			0	5.81	0.37	6.18	XXX	N
75984	00	A	Change of percutaneous tube or drainage catheter with contrast monitoring (eg, gastrointestinal system, genitourinary system, abscess), radiological supervision and interpretation	0.72	2.19	0.17	3.08	XXX	N
75984	26			0.72	0.33	0.05	1.10	XXX	N
75984	TC			0	1.86	0.12	1.98	XXX	N
75989	00	A	Radiological guidance for percutaneous drainage of abscess, or specimen collection (ie, fluoroscopy, ultrasound, or computed tomography), with or without placement of indwelling catheter, radiological supervision and interpretation	1.19	3.52	0.27	4.98	XXX	N
75989	26			1.19	0.52	0.08	1.79	XXX	N
75989	TC			0	3.00	0.19	3.19	XXX	N
75992	00	A	Transluminal atherectomy, peripheral artery, radiological supervision and interpretation	0.54	15.25	0.98	16.77	XXX	N
75992	26			0.54	0.25	0.04	0.83	XXX	N
75992	TC			0	15	0.94	15.94	XXX	N
75993	00	A	Transluminal atherectomy, each additional peripheral artery, radiological supervision and interpretation	0.36	8.16	0.52	9.04	XXX	N
75993	26			0.36	0.16	0.02	0.54	XXX	N
75993	TC			0	8.00	0.50	8.50	XXX	N
75994	00	A	Transluminal atherectomy, renal, radiological supervision and interpretation	1.31	15.58	1.03	17.92	XXX	N
75994	26			1.31	0.58	0.09	1.98	XXX	N
75994	TC			0	15	0.94	15.94	XXX	N
75995	00	A	Transluminal atherectomy, visceral, radiological supervision and interpretation	1.31	15.58	1.03	17.92	XXX	N
75995	26			1.31	0.58	0.09	1.98	XXX	N
75995	TC			0	15	0.94	15.94	XXX	N
75996	00	A	Transluminal atherectomy, each additional visceral artery, radiological supervision and interpretation	0.36	8.16	0.52	9.04	XXX	N
75996	26			0.36	0.16	0.02	0.54	XXX	N
75996	TC			0	8.00	0.50	8.50	XXX	N
76000	00	A	Fluoroscopy (separate procedure), up to one hour physician time, other than 71023 or 71034 (eg, cardiac fluoroscopy)	0.17	1.31	0.09	1.57	XXX	N
76000	26			0.17	0.07	0.01	0.25	XXX	N
76000	TC			0	1.24	0.08	1.32	XXX	N
76001	00	A	Fluoroscopy, physician time more than one hour, assisting a non-radiologic physician (eg, nephrostolithotomy, ERCP, bronchoscopy, transbronchial biopsy)	0.67	2.81	0.22	3.70	XXX	N
76001	26			0.67	0.31	0.05	1.03	XXX	N
76001	TC			0	2.50	0.17	2.67	XXX	N

CPT codes and descriptions only, © 1994 American Medical Association. Reimbursement information, © 1995 McGraw-Hill Inc.

Code/ CPT	Mod- ifier	Status	Description	Work value	Practice expense	Mal- practice	Total value	Global period	Up- date
76003	00	A	Fluoroscopic localization for needle biopsy or fine needle aspiration	0.54	1.49	0.12	2.15	XXX	N
76003	26			0.54	0.25	0.04	0.83	XXX	N
76003	TC			0	1.24	0.08	1.32	XXX	N
76010	00	A	Radiologic examination from nose to rectum for foreign body, single film, child	0.18	0.58	0.04	0.80	XXX	N
76010	26			0.18	0.08	0.01	0.27	XXX	N
76010	TC			0	0.50	0.03	0.53	XXX	N
76020	00	A	Bone age studies	0.19	0.59	0.04	0.82	XXX	N
76020	26			0.19	0.09	0.01	0.29	XXX	N
76020	TC			0	0.50	0.03	0.53	XXX	N
76040	00	A	Bone length studies (orthoroentgenogram, scanogram)	0.27	0.88	0.07	1.22	XXX	N
76040	26			0.27	0.13	0.02	0.42	XXX	N
76040	TC			0	0.75	0.05	0.80	XXX	N
76061	00	A	Radiologic examination, osseous survey; limited (eg, for metastases)	0.45	1.15	0.09	1.69	XXX	N
76061	26			0.45	0.20	0.03	0.68	XXX	N
76061	TC			0	0.95	0.06	1.01	XXX	N
76062	00	A	Radiologic examination, osseous survey; complete (axial and appendicular skeleton)	0.54	1.62	0.13	2.29	XXX	N
76062	26			0.54	0.25	0.04	0.83	XXX	N
76062	TC			0	1.37	0.09	1.46	XXX	N
76065	00	A	Radiologic examination, osseous survey, infant	0.28	0.83	0.07	1.18	XXX	N
76065	26			0.28	0.13	0.02	0.43	XXX	N
76065	TC			0	0.70	0.05	0.75	XXX	N
76066	00	A	Joint survey, single view, one or more joints (specify)	0.31	1.20	0.09	1.60	XXX	N
76066	26			0.31	0.14	0.02	0.47	XXX	N
76066	TC			0	1.06	0.07	1.13	XXX	N
76070	00	A	Computerized tomography, bone density study	0.25	2.93	0.20	3.38	XXX	N
76070	26			0.25	0.12	0.02	0.39	XXX	N
76070	TC			0	2.81	0.18	2.99	XXX	N
76075	00	A	Dual energy x-ray absorptiometry (DEXA), bone density study	0.30	3.07	0.21	3.58	XXX	N
76075	26			0.30	0.12	0.02	0.44	XXX	N
76075	TC			0	2.95	0.19	3.14	XXX	N
76080	00	A	Radiologic examination, fistula or sinus tract study, radiological supervision and interpretation	0.54	1.25	0.11	1.90	XXX	N
76080	26			0.54	0.25	0.04	0.83	XXX	N
76080	TC			0	1.00	0.07	1.07	XXX	N
76086	00	A	Mammary ductogram or galactogram, single duct, radiological supervision and interpretation	0.36	2.67	0.19	3.22	XXX	N
76086	26			0.36	0.17	0.02	0.55	XXX	N
76086	TC			0	2.50	0.17	2.67	XXX	N
76088	00	A	Mammary ductogram or galactogram, multiple ducts, radiological supervision and interpretation	0.45	3.69	0.25	4.39	XXX	N
76088	26			0.45	0.20	0.03	0.68	XXX	N
76088	TC			0	3.49	0.22	3.71	XXX	N
76090	00	A	Mammography; unilateral	0.25	1.12	0.09	1.46	XXX	N
76090	26			0.25	0.12	0.02	0.39	XXX	N
76090	TC			0	1.00	0.07	1.07	XXX	N
76091	00	A	Mammography; bilateral	0.41	1.42	0.11	1.94	XXX	N

CPT codes and descriptions only, © 1994 American Medical Association. Reimbursement information, © 1995 McGraw-Hill Inc.

Code/ CPT	Mod- ifier	Status	Description	Work value	Practice expense	Mal- practice	Total value	Global period	Up- date
76091	26			0.41	0.18	0.03	0.62	XXX	N
76091	TC			0	1.24	0.08	1.32	XXX	N
76092	00	X	Screening mammography, bilateral (two view film study of each breast)	0.25*	0.55#	0.03*	0.83#	XXX	0
76092	26			0.25*	0.05#	0	0.30#		
76092	TC			0.25*	0.50#	0.03*	0.78#		
76093	00	A	Magnetic resonance imaging, breast, without and/or with contrast material(s); unilateral	1.63	17.52	1.16	20.31	XXX	N
76093	26			1.63	0.72	0.11	2.46	XXX	N
76093	TC			0	16.80	1.05	17.85	XXX	N
76094	00	A	Magnetic resonance imaging, breast, without and/or with contrast material(s); bilateral	1.63	23.51	1.53	26.67	XXX	N
76094	26			1.63	0.72	0.11	2.46	XXX	N
76094	TC			0	22.79	1.42	24.21	XXX	N
76095	00	A	Stereotactic localization for breast biopsy, each lesion, radiological supervision and interpretation	1.59	7.54	0.54	9.67	XXX	N
76095	26			1.59	0.71	0.11	2.41	XXX	N
76095	TC			0	6.83	0.43	7.26	XXX	N
76096	00	A	Preoperative placement of needle localization wire, breast, radiological supervision and interpretation	0.56	1.50	0.12	2.18	XXX	N
76096	26			0.56	0.26	0.04	0.86	XXX	N
76096	TC			0	1.24	0.08	1.32	XXX	N
76098	00	A	Radiological examination, surgical specimen	0.16	0.47	0.04	0.67	XXX	N
76098	26			0.16	0.07	0.01	0.24	XXX	N
76098	TC			0	0.40	0.03	0.43	XXX	N
76100	00	A	Radiologic examination, single plane body section (eg, tomography), other than with urography	0.58	1.46	0.12	2.16	XXX	N
76100	26			0.58	0.27	0.04	0.89	XXX	N
76100	TC			0	1.19	0.08	1.27	XXX	N
76101	00	A	Radiologic examination, complex motion (ie, hypercycloidal) body section (eg, mastoid polytomography), other than with urography; unilateral	0.58	1.62	0.13	2.33	XXX	N
76101	26			0.58	0.27	0.04	0.89	XXX	N
76101	TC			0	1.35	0.09	1.44	XXX	N
76102	00	A	Radiologic examination, complex motion (ie, hypercycloidal) body section (eg, mastoid polytomography), other than with urography; bilateral	0.58	1.92	0.15	2.65	XXX	N
76102	26			0.58	0.27	0.04	0.89	XXX	N
76102	TC			0	1.65	0.11	1.76	XXX	N
76120	00	A	Cineradiography, except where specifically included	0.38	1.17	0.10	1.65	XXX	N
76120	26			0.38	0.17	0.03	0.58	XXX	N
76120	TC			0	1.00	0.07	1.07	XXX	N
76125	00	A	Cineradiography to complement routine examination	0.27	0.87	0.07	1.21	XXX	N
76125	26			0.27	0.12	0.02	0.41	XXX	N
76125	TC			0	0.75	0.05	0.80	XXX	N
76140	00	G	Consultation on x-ray examination made elsewhere, written report	0.44*	0	0.02*	0.46#	XXX	0
76140	26			0.32*	0	0.01*	0.33#		
76140	TC			0	0	0	0		
76150	00	A	Xeroradiography	0	0.40	0.03	0.43	XXX	N
76350	00	C	Subtraction in conjunction with contrast studies	0.32*	0	0.01*	0.33#	XXX	N
76350	26			0.32*	0	0.01*	0.33#		

CPT codes and descriptions only, © 1994 American Medical Association. Reimbursement information, © 1995 McGraw-Hill Inc.

Code/ CPT	Mod- ifier	Status	Description	Work value	Practice expense	Mal- practice	Total value	Global period	Up- date
76350	TC			0	0	0	0		
76355	00	A	Computerized tomography guidance for stereotactic localization	1.21	8.40	0.57	10.18	XXX	N
76355	26			1.21	0.53	0.08	1.82	XXX	N
76355	TC			0	7.87	0.49	8.36	XXX	N
76360	00	A	Computerized tomography guidance for needle biopsy, radiological supervision and interpretation	1.16	8.37	0.57	10.10	XXX	N
76360	26			1.16	0.50	0.08	1.74	XXX	N
76360	TC			0	7.87	0.49	8.36	XXX	N
76365	00	A	Computerized tomography guidance for cyst aspiration, radiological supervision and interpretation	1.16	8.37	0.57	10.10	XXX	N
76365	26			1.16	0.50	0.08	1.74	XXX	N
76365	TC			0	7.87	0.49	8.36	XXX	N
76370	00	A	Computerized tomography guidance for placement of radiation therapy fields	0.85	3.19	0.24	4.28	XXX	N
76370	26			0.85	0.38	0.06	1.29	XXX	N
76370	TC			0	2.81	0.18	2.99	XXX	N
76375	00	A	Computerized tomography, coronal, sagittal, multiplanar, oblique and/or 3-dimensional reconstruction	0.16	3.44	0.22	3.82	XXX	N
76375	26			0.16	0.07	0.01	0.24	XXX	N
76375	TC			0	3.37	0.21	3.58	XXX	N
76380	00	A	Computerized tomography, limited or localized follow-up study	0.98	3.78	0.28	5.04	XXX	N
76380	26			0.98	0.44	0.07	1.49	XXX	N
76380	TC			0	3.34	0.21	3.55	XXX	N
76400	00	A	Magnetic resonance (eg, proton) imaging, bone marrow blood supply	1.60	11.40	0.78	13.78	XXX	N
76400	26			1.60	0.72	0.11	2.43	XXX	N
76400	TC			0	10.68	0.67	11.35	XXX	N
76499	00	C	Unlisted diagnostic radiologic procedure	0	0	0	0	XXX	N
76499	26			0	0	0	0	XXX	N
76499	TC			0	0	0	0	XXX	N
76506	00	A	Echoencephalography, B-scan and/or real time with image documentation (gray scale) (for determination of ventricular size, delineation of cerebral contents and detection of fluid masses or other intracranial abnormalities), including A-mode encephalography as secondary component where indicated	0.63	1.64	0.13	2.40	XXX	N
76506	26			0.63	0.29	0.04	0.96	XXX	N
76506	TC			0	1.35	0.09	1.44	XXX	N
76511	00	A	Ophthalmic ultrasound, echography, diagnostic; A-scan only, with amplitude quantification	0.94	1.44	0.12	2.50	XXX	N
76511	26			0.94	0.25	0.04	1.23	XXX	N
76511	TC			0	1.19	0.08	1.27	XXX	N
76512	00	A	Ophthalmic ultrasound, echography, diagnostic; contact B-scan (with or without simultaneous A-scan)	0.66	1.75	0.15	2.56	XXX	N
76512	26			0.66	0.30	0.05	1.01	XXX	N
76512	TC			0	1.45	0.10	1.55	XXX	N
76513	00	A	Ophthalmic ultrasound, echography, diagnostic; immersion (water bath) B-scan	0.66	1.75	0.15	2.56	XXX	N
76513	26			0.66	0.30	0.05	1.01	XXX	N
76513	TC			0	1.45	0.10	1.55	XXX	N
76516	00	A	Ophthalmic biometry by ultrasound echography, A-scan;	0.54	1.44	0.12	2.10	XXX	N

CPT codes and descriptions only, © 1994 American Medical Association. Reimbursement information, © 1995 McGraw-Hill Inc.

Code/ CPT	Mod-ifier	Status	Description	Work value	Practice expense	Mal-practice	Total value	Global period	Up-date
76516	26			0.54	0.25	0.04	0.83	XXX	N
76516	TC			0	1.19	0.08	1.27	XXX	N
76519	00	A	Ophthalmic biometry by ultrasound echography, A-scan; with intraocular lens power calculation	0.54	1.44	0.12	2.10	XXX	N
76519	26			0.54	0.25	0.04	0.83	XXX	N
76519	TC			0	1.19	0.08	1.27	XXX	N
76529	00	A	Ophthalmic ultrasonic foreign body localization	0.57	1.56	0.13	2.26	XXX	N
76529	26			0.57	0.26	0.04	0.87	XXX	N
76529	TC			0	1.30	0.09	1.39	XXX	N
76536	00	A	Echography, soft tissues of head and neck (eg, thyroid, parathyroid, parotid), B-scan and/or real time with image documentation	0.56	1.61	0.13	2.30	XXX	N
76536	26			0.56	0.26	0.04	0.86	XXX	N
76536	TC			0	1.35	0.09	1.44	XXX	N
76604	00	A	Echography, chest, B-scan (includes mediastinum) and/or real time with image documentation	0.55	1.50	0.12	2.17	XXX	N
76604	26			0.55	0.26	0.04	0.85	XXX	N
76604	TC			0	1.24	0.08	1.32	XXX	N
76645	00	A	Echography, breast(s) (unilateral or bilateral), B-scan and/or real time with image documentation	0.54	1.25	0.11	1.90	XXX	N
76645	26			0.54	0.25	0.04	0.83	XXX	N
76645	TC			0	1.00	0.07	1.07	XXX	N
76700	00	A	Echography, abdominal, B-scan and/or real time with image documentation; complete	0.81	2.25	0.17	3.23	XXX	N
76700	26			0.81	0.37	0.05	1.23	XXX	N
76700	TC			0	1.88	0.12	2.00	XXX	N
76705	00	A	Echography, abdominal, B-scan and/or real time with image documentation; limited (eg, single organ, quadrant, follow-up)	0.59	1.62	0.13	2.34	XXX	N
76705	26			0.59	0.27	0.04	0.90	XXX	N
76705	TC			0	1.35	0.09	1.44	XXX	N
76770	00	A	Echography, retroperitoneal (eg, renal, aorta, nodes), B-scan and/or real time with image documentation; complete	0.74	2.22	0.17	3.13	XXX	N
76770	26			0.74	0.34	0.05	1.13	XXX	N
76770	TC			0	1.88	0.12	2.00	XXX	N
76775	00	A	Echography, retroperitoneal (eg, renal, aorta, nodes), B-scan and/or real time with image documentation; limited	0.58	1.62	0.13	2.33	XXX	N
76775	26			0.58	0.27	0.04	0.89	XXX	N
76775	TC			0	1.35	0.09	1.44	XXX	N
76778	00	A	Echography of transplanted kidney, B-scan and/or real time with image documentation, with or without duplex Doppler studies	0.74	2.22	0.17	3.13	XXX	N
76778	26			0.74	0.34	0.05	1.13	XXX	N
76778	TC			0	1.88	0.12	2.00	XXX	N
76800	00	A	Echography, spinal canal and contents	1.13	1.85	0.17	3.15	XXX	N
76800	26			1.13	0.50	0.08	1.71	XXX	N
76800	TC			0	1.35	0.09	1.44	XXX	N
76805	00	A	Echography, pregnant uterus, B-scan and/or real time with image documentation; complete (complete fetal and maternal evaluation)	0.99	2.45	0.20	3.64	XXX	N
76805	26			0.99	0.45	0.07	1.51	XXX	N
76805	TC			0	2.00	0.13	2.13	XXX	N

CPT codes and descriptions only, © 1994 American Medical Association. Reimbursement information, © 1995 McGraw-Hill Inc.

Code/ CPT	Mod-ifier	Status	Description	Work value	Practice expense	Mal-practice	Total value	Global period	Up-date
76810	00	A	Echography, pregnant uterus, B-scan and/or real time with image documentation; complete (complete fetal and maternal evaluation), multiple gestation, after the first trimester	1.97	4.88	0.38	7.23	XXX	N
76810	26			1.97	0.88	0.13	2.98	XXX	N
76810	TC			0	4.00	0.25	4.25	XXX	N
76815	00	A	Echography, pregnant uterus, B-scan and/or real time with image documentation; limited (gestational age, heart beat, placental location, fetal position, or emergency in the delivery room)	0.65	1.65	0.13	2.43	XXX	N
76815	26			0.65	0.30	0.04	0.99	XXX	N
76815	TC			0	1.35	0.09	1.44	XXX	N
76816	00	A	Echography, pregnant uterus, B-scan and/or real time with image documentation; follow-up or repeat	0.57	1.32	0.11	2.00	XXX	N
76816	26			0.57	0.26	0.04	0.87	XXX	N
76816	TC			0	1.06	0.07	1.13	XXX	N
76818	00	A	Fetal biophysical profile	0.77	1.89	0.15	2.81	XXX	N
76818	26			0.77	0.35	0.05	1.17	XXX	N
76818	TC			0	1.54	0.10	1.64	XXX	N
76825	00	A	Echocardiography, fetal, cardiovascular system, real time with image documentation (2D) with or without M-mode recording;	0.98	2.23	0.17	3.38	XXX	N
76825	26			0.98	0.35	0.05	1.38	XXX	N
76825	TC			0	1.88	0.12	2.00	XXX	N
76826	00	A	Echocardiography, fetal, cardiovascular system, real time with image documentation (2D) with or without M-mode recording; follow-up or repeat study	0.83	1.35	0.10	2.28	XXX	N
76826	26			0.83	0.68	0.05	1.56	XXX	N
76826	TC			0	0.67	0.05	0.72	XXX	N
76827	00	A	Doppler echocardiography, fetal, cardiovascular system, pulsed wave and/or continuous wave with spectral display; complete	0.58	2.33	0.18	3.09	XXX	N
76827	26			0.58	0.69	0.05	1.32	XXX	N
76827	TC			0	1.64	0.13	1.77	XXX	N
76828	00	A	Doppler echocardiography, fetal, cardiovascular system, pulsed wave and/or continuous wave with spectral display; follow-up or repeat study	0.56	1.34	0.11	2.01	XXX	N
76828	26			0.56	0.28	0.02	0.86	XXX	N
76828	TC			0	1.06	0.09	1.15	XXX	N
76830	00	A	Echography, transvaginal	0.69	1.77	0.15	2.61	XXX	N
76830	26			0.69	0.32	0.05	1.06	XXX	N
76830	TC			0	1.45	0.10	1.55	XXX	N
76856	00	A	Echography, pelvic (nonobstetric), B-scan and/or real time with image documentation; complete	0.69	1.77	0.15	2.61	XXX	N
76856	26			0.69	0.32	0.05	1.06	XXX	N
76856	TC			0	1.45	0.10	1.55	XXX	N
76857	00	A	Echography, pelvic (nonobstetric), B-scan and/or real time with image documentation; limited or follow-up (eg, for follicles)	0.38	1.17	0.10	1.65	XXX	N
76857	26			0.38	0.17	0.03	0.58	XXX	N
76857	TC			0	1.00	0.07	1.07	XXX	N
76870	00	A	Echography, scrotum and contents	0.64	1.74	0.14	2.52	XXX	N
76870	26			0.64	0.29	0.04	0.97	XXX	N

CPT codes and descriptions only, © 1994 American Medical Association. Reimbursement information, © 1995 McGraw-Hill Inc.

Code/ CPT	Mod-ifier	Status	Description	Work value	Practice expense	Mal-practice	Total value	Global period	Up-date
76870	TC			0	1.45	0.10	1.55	XXX	N
76872	00	A	Echography, transrectal	0.69	1.77	0.15	2.61	XXX	N
76872	26			0.69	0.32	0.05	1.06	XXX	N
76872	TC			0	1.45	0.10	1.55	XXX	N
76880	00	A	Echography, extremity, non-vascular, B-scan and/or real time with image documentation	0.59	1.62	0.13	2.34	XXX	N
76880	26			0.59	0.27	0.04	0.90	XXX	N
76880	TC			0	1.35	0.09	1.44	XXX	N
76930	00	A	Ultrasonic guidance for pericardiocentesis, radiological supervision and interpretation	0.67	1.76	0.15	2.58	XXX	N
76930	26			0.67	0.31	0.05	1.03	XXX	N
76930	TC			0	1.45	0.10	1.55	XXX	N
76932	00	A	Ultrasonic guidance for endomyocardial biopsy, radiological supervision and interpretation	0.67	1.76	0.15	2.58	XXX	N
76932	26			0.67	0.31	0.05	1.03	XXX	N
76932	TC			0	1.45	0.10	1.55	XXX	N
76934	00	A	Ultrasonic guidance for thoracentesis or abdominal paracentesis, radiological supervision and interpretation	0.67	1.76	0.15	2.58	XXX	N
76934	26			0.67	0.31	0.05	1.03	XXX	N
76934	TC			0	1.45	0.10	1.55	XXX	N
76936	00	A	Ultrasound guided compression repair of arterial pseudo-aneurysm or arteriovenous fistulae (includes diagnostic ultrasound evaluation, compression of lesion and imaging)	1.31	6.81	0.45	8.57	XXX	N
76936	26			1.31	0.81	0.07	2.19	XXX	N
76936	TC			0	6.00	0.38	6.38	XXX	N
76938	00	A	Ultrasonic guidance for cyst (any location), or renal pelvis aspiration, radiological supervision and interpretation	0.67	1.76	0.15	2.58	XXX	N
76938	26			0.67	0.31	0.05	1.03	XXX	N
76938	TC			0	1.45	0.10	1.55	XXX	N
76941	00	A	Ultrasonic guidance for intrauterine fetal transfusion or cordocentesis, radiological supervision and interpretation	1.34	2.07	0.19	3.60	XXX	N
76941	26			1.34	0.61	0.10	2.05	XXX	N
76941	TC			0	1.46	0.09	1.55	XXX	N
76942	00	A	Ultrasonic guidance for needle biopsy, radiological supervision and interpretation	0.67	1.76	0.15	2.58	XXX	N
76942	26			0.67	0.31	0.05	1.03	XXX	N
76942	TC			0	1.45	0.10	1.55	XXX	N
76945	00	A	Ultrasonic guidance for chorionic villus sampling, radiological supervision and interpretation	0.67	2.07	0.19	2.93	XXX	N
76945	26			0.67	0.61	0.10	1.38	XXX	N
76945	TC			0	1.46	0.09	1.55	XXX	N
76946	00	A	Ultrasonic guidance for amniocentesis, radiological supervision and interpretation	0.38	1.62	0.13	2.13	XXX	N
76946	26			0.38	0.17	0.03	0.58	XXX	N
76946	TC			0	1.45	0.10	1.55	XXX	N
76948	00	A	Ultrasonic guidance for aspiration of ova, radiological supervision and interpretation	0.38	1.62	0.13	2.13	XXX	N
76948	26			0.38	0.17	0.03	0.58	XXX	N
76948	TC			0	1.45	0.10	1.55	XXX	N
76950	00	A	Echography for placement of radiation therapy fields, B-scan	0.58	1.51	0.12	2.21	XXX	N

CPT codes and descriptions only, © 1994 American Medical Association. Reimbursement information, © 1995 McGraw-Hill Inc.

Code/ CPT	Mod-ifier	Status	Description	Work value	Practice expense	Mal-practice	Total value	Global period	Up-date
76950	26			0.58	0.27	0.04	0.89	XXX	N
76950	TC			0	1.24	0.08	1.32	XXX	N
76960	00	A	Ultrasonic guidance for placement of radiation therapy fields, except for B-scan echography	0.58	1.51	0.12	2.21	XXX	N
76960	26			0.58	0.27	0.04	0.89	XXX	N
76960	TC			0	1.24	0.08	1.32	XXX	N
76970	00	A	Ultrasound study follow-up (specify)	0.40	1.18	0.10	1.68	XXX	N
76970	26			0.40	0.18	0.03	0.61	XXX	N
76970	TC			0	1.00	0.07	1.07	XXX	N
76975	00	A	Gastrointestinal endoscopic ultrasound, radiological supervision and interpretation	0.81	1.79	0.15	2.75	XXX	N
76975	26			0.81	0.34	0.05	1.20	XXX	N
76975	TC			0	1.45	0.10	1.55	XXX	N
76986	00	A	Echography, intraoperative	1.20	3.03	0.25	4.48	XXX	N
76986	26			1.20	0.53	0.08	1.81	XXX	N
76986	TC			0	2.50	0.17	2.67	XXX	N
76999	00	C	Unlisted ultrasound procedure	0	0	0	0	XXX	N
76999	26			0	0	0	0	XXX	N
76999	TC			0	0	0	0	XXX	N
77261	00	A	Therapeutic radiology treatment planning; simple	1.39	0.62	0.09	2.10	XXX	N
77262	00	A	Therapeutic radiology treatment planning; intermediate	2.11	0.94	0.14	3.19	XXX	N
77263	00	A	Therapeutic radiology treatment planning; complex	3.14	1.40	0.20	4.74	XXX	N
77280	00	A	Therapeutic radiology simulation-aided field setting; simple	0.70	3.63	0.26	4.59	XXX	N
77280	26			0.70	0.32	0.05	1.07	XXX	N
77280	TC			0	3.31	0.21	3.52	XXX	N
77285	00	A	Therapeutic radiology simulation-aided field setting; intermediate	1.05	5.77	0.41	7.23	XXX	N
77285	26			1.05	0.46	0.07	1.58	XXX	N
77285	TC			0	5.31	0.34	5.65	XXX	N
77290	00	A	Therapeutic radiology simulation-aided field setting; complex	1.56	6.90	0.50	8.96	XXX	N
77290	26			1.56	0.70	0.11	2.37	XXX	N
77290	TC			0	6.20	0.39	6.59	XXX	N
77295	00	A	Therapeutic radiology simulation-aided field setting; by three-dimensional reconstruction of tumor volume	4.57	28.68	1.93	35.18	XXX	N
77295	26			4.57	2.06	0.23	6.86	XXX	N
77295	TC			0	26.62	1.70	28.32	XXX	N
77299	00	C	Unlisted procedure, therapeutic radiology clinical treatment planning	0	0	0	0	XXX	N
77299	26			0	0	0	0	XXX	N
77299	TC			0	0	0	0	XXX	N
77300	00	A	Basic radiation dosimetry calculation, central axis depth dose, TDF, NSD, gap calculation, off axis factor, tissue inhomogeneity factors, as required during course of treatment, only when prescribed by the treating physician	0.62	1.56	0.12	2.30	XXX	N
77300	26			0.62	0.28	0.04	0.94	XXX	N
77300	TC			0	1.28	0.08	1.36	XXX	N
77305	00	A	Teletherapy, isodose plan (whether hand or computer calculated); simple (one or two parallel opposed unmodified ports directed to a single area of interest)	0.70	2.09	0.17	2.96	XXX	N
77305	26			0.70	0.32	0.05	1.07	XXX	N
77305	TC			0	1.77	0.12	1.89	XXX	N

CPT codes and descriptions only, © 1994 American Medical Association. Reimbursement information, © 1995 McGraw-Hill Inc.

Code/ CPT	Mod-ifier	Status	Description	Work value	Practice expense	Mal-practice	Total value	Global period	Up-date
77310	00	A	Teletherapy, isodose plan (whether hand or computer calculated); intermediate (three or more treatment ports directed to a single area of interest)	1.05	2.68	0.22	3.95	XXX	N
77310	26			1.05	0.46	0.07	1.58	XXX	N
77310	TC			0	2.22	0.15	2.37	XXX	N
77315	00	A	Teletherapy, isodose plan (whether hand or computer calculated); complex (mantle or inverted Y, tangential ports, the use of wedges, compensators, complex blocking, rotational beam, or special beam considerations)	1.56	3.23	0.28	5.07	XXX	N
77315	26			1.56	0.70	0.11	2.37	XXX	N
77315	TC			0	2.53	0.17	2.70	XXX	N
77321	00	A	Special teletherapy port plan, particles, hemi-body, total body	0.95	4.28	0.30	5.53	XXX	N
77321	26			0.95	0.43	0.06	1.44	XXX	N
77321	TC			0	3.85	0.24	4.09	XXX	N
77326	00	A	Brachytherapy isodose calculation; simple (calculation made from single plane, one to four sources/ribbon application, remote afterloading brachytherapy, 1 to 8 sources)	0.93	2.67	0.21	3.81	XXX	N
77326	26			0.93	0.42	0.06	1.41	XXX	N
77326	TC			0	2.25	0.15	2.40	XXX	N
77327	00	A	Brachytherapy isodose calculation; intermediate (multiplane dosage calculations, application involving five to ten sources/ribbons, remote afterloading brachytherapy, 9 to 12 sources)	1.39	3.93	0.30	5.62	XXX	N
77327	26			1.39	0.62	0.09	2.10	XXX	N
77327	TC			0	3.31	0.21	3.52	XXX	N
77328	00	A	Brachytherapy isodose calculation; complex (multiplane isodose plan, volume implant calculations, over ten sources/ribbons used, special spatial reconstruction, remote afterloading brachytherapy, over 12 sources)	2.09	5.66	0.44	8.19	XXX	N
77328	26			2.09	0.93	0.14	3.16	XXX	N
77328	TC			0	4.73	0.30	5.03	XXX	N
77331	00	A	Special dosimetry (eg, TLD, microdosimetry) (specify), only when prescribed by the treating physician	0.87	0.87	0.09	1.83	XXX	N
77331	26			0.87	0.39	0.06	1.32	XXX	N
77331	TC			0	0.48	0.03	0.51	XXX	N
77332	00	A	Treatment devices, design and construction; simple (simple block, simple bolus)	0.54	1.53	0.12	2.19	XXX	N
77332	26			0.54	0.25	0.04	0.83	XXX	N
77332	TC			0	1.28	0.08	1.36	XXX	N
77333	00	A	Treatment devices, design and construction; intermediate (multiple blocks, stents, bite blocks, special bolus)	0.84	2.19	0.18	3.21	XXX	N
77333	26			0.84	0.38	0.06	1.28	XXX	N
77333	TC			0	1.81	0.12	1.93	XXX	N
77334	00	A	Treatment devices, design and construction; complex (irregular blocks, special shields, compensators, wedges, molds or casts)	1.24	3.64	0.27	5.15	XXX	N
77334	26			1.24	0.54	0.08	1.86	XXX	N
77334	TC			0	3.10	0.19	3.29	XXX	N
77336	00	A	Continuing medical radiation physics consultation in support of therapeutic radiologist including continuing quality assurance reported per week of therapy	0	2.84	0.18	3.02	XXX	N
77370	00	A	Special medical radiation physics consultation	0	3.33	0.21	3.54	XXX	N

CPT codes and descriptions only, © 1994 American Medical Association. Reimbursement information, © 1995 McGraw-Hill Inc.

Code/ CPT	Mod- ifier	Status	Description	Work value	Practice expense	Mal- practice	Total value	Global period	Up- date
77399	00	C	Unlisted procedure, medical radiation physics, dosimetry and treatment devices	0	0	0	0	XXX	N
77399	26			0	0	0	0	XXX	N
77399	TC			0	0	0	0	XXX	N
77401	00	A	Radiation treatment delivery, superficial and/or ortho voltage	0	1.69	0.11	1.80	XXX	N
77402	00	A	Radiation treatment delivery, single treatment area, single port or parallel opposed ports, simple blocks or no blocks; up to 5 MeV	0	1.69	0.11	1.80	XXX	N
77403	00	A	Radiation treatment delivery, single treatment area, single port or parallel opposed ports, simple blocks or no blocks; 6-10 MeV	0	1.69	0.11	1.80	XXX	N
77404	00	A	Radiation treatment delivery, single treatment area, single port or parallel opposed ports, simple blocks or no blocks; 11-19 MeV	0	1.69	0.11	1.80	XXX	N
77406	00	A	Radiation treatment delivery, single treatment area, single port or parallel opposed ports, simple blocks or no blocks; 20 MeV or greater	0	1.69	0.11	1.80	XXX	N
77407	00	A	Radiation treatment delivery, two separate treatment areas, three or more ports on a single treatment area, use of multiple blocks; up to 5 MeV	0	1.99	0.13	2.12	XXX	N
77408	00	A	Radiation treatment delivery, two separate treatment areas, three or more ports on a single treatment area, use of multiple blocks; 6-10 MeV	0	1.99	0.13	2.12	XXX	N
77409	00	A	Radiation treatment delivery, two separate treatment areas, three or more ports on a single treatment area, use of multiple blocks; 11-19 MeV	0	1.99	0.13	2.12	XXX	N
77411	00	A	Radiation treatment delivery, two separate treatment areas, three or more ports on a single treatment area, use of multiple blocks; 20 MeV or greater	0	1.99	0.13	2.12	XXX	N
77412	00	A	Radiation treatment delivery, three or more separate treatment areas, custom blocking, tangential ports, wedges, rotational beam, compensators, special particle beam (eg, electron or neutrons); up to 5 MeV	0	2.22	0.15	2.37	XXX	N
77413	00	A	Radiation treatment delivery, three or more separate treatment areas, custom blocking, tangential ports, wedges, rotational beam, compensators, special particle beam (eg, electron or neutrons); 6-10 MeV	0	2.22	0.15	2.37	XXX	N
77414	00	A	Radiation treatment delivery, three or more separate treatment areas, custom blocking, tangential ports, wedges, rotational beam, compensators, special particle beam (eg, electron or neutrons); 11-19 MeV	0	2.22	0.15	2.37	XXX	N
77416	00	A	Radiation treatment delivery, three or more separate treatment areas, custom blocking, tangential ports, wedges, rotational beam, compensators, special particle beam (eg, electron or neutrons); 20 MeV or greater	0	2.22	0.15	2.37	XXX	N
77417	00	A	Therapeutic radiology port film(s)	0	0.56	0.04	0.60	XXX	N
77417	26			0	0	0	0		
77417	TC			0	0	0	0		
77419	00	A	Weekly radiation therapy management; conformal	3.60	1.61	0.23	5.44	XXX	N
77419	26			0	0	0	0		
77419	TC			0	0	0	0		
77420	00	A	Weekly radiation therapy management; simple	1.61	0.72	0.11	2.44	XXX	N
77425	00	A	Weekly radiation therapy management; intermediate	2.44	1.10	0.17	3.71	XXX	N
77430	00	A	Weekly radiation therapy management; complex	3.60	1.61	0.23	5.44	XXX	N

CPT codes and descriptions only, © 1994 American Medical Association. Reimbursement information, © 1995 McGraw-Hill Inc.

Code/ CPT	Mod- ifier	Status	Description	Work value	Practice expense	Mal- practice	Total value	Global period	Up- date
77431	00	A	Radiation therapy management with complete course of therapy consisting of one or two fractions only	1.81	0.81	0.12	2.74	XXX	N
77431	26			0	0	0	0		
77431	TC			0	0	0	0		
77432	00	A	Stereotactic radiation treatment management of cerebral lesion(s) (complete course of treatment consisting of one session)	7.93	4.94	0.40	13.27	XXX	N
77432	26			0	0	0	0		
77432	TC			0	0	0	0		
77470	00	A	Special treatment procedure (eg, total body irradiation, hemibody irradiation, per oral, vaginal cone irradiation)	2.09	11.55	0.80	14.44	XXX	N
77470	26			2.09	0.93	0.14	3.16	XXX	N
77470	TC			0	10.62	0.66	11.28	XXX	N
77499	00	C	Unlisted procedure, therapeutic radiology clinical treatment management	0	0	0	0	XXX	N
77499	26			0	0	0	0	XXX	N
77499	TC			0	0	0	0	XXX	N
77600	00	A	Hyperthermia, externally generated; superficial (ie, heating to a depth of 4 cm or less)	1.56	3.60	0.29	5.45	ZZZ	N
77600	26			1.56	0.70	0.11	2.37	ZZZ	N
77600	TC			0	2.90	0.18	3.08	ZZZ	N
77605	00	A	Hyperthermia, externally generated; deep (ie, heating to depths greater than 4 cm)	2.09	4.80	0.39	7.28	ZZZ	N
77605	26			2.09	0.93	0.14	3.16	ZZZ	N
77605	TC			0	3.87	0.25	4.12	ZZZ	N
77610	00	A	Hyperthermia generated by interstitial probe(s); 5 or fewer interstitial applicators	1.56	3.60	0.29	5.45	ZZZ	N
77610	26			1.56	0.70	0.11	2.37	ZZZ	N
77610	TC			0	2.90	0.18	3.08	ZZZ	N
77615	00	A	Hyperthermia generated by interstitial probe(s); more than 5 interstitial applicators	2.09	4.80	0.39	7.28	ZZZ	N
77615	26			2.09	0.93	0.14	3.16	ZZZ	N
77615	TC			0	3.87	0.25	4.12	ZZZ	N
77620	00	A	Hyperthermia generated by intracavitary probe(s)	1.56	3.60	0.29	5.45	ZZZ	N
77620	26			1.56	0.70	0.11	2.37	ZZZ	N
77620	TC			0	2.90	0.18	3.08	ZZZ	N
77750	00	A	Infusion or instillation of radioelement solution	4.59	3.32	0.38	8.29	90	N
77750	26			4.59	2.05	0.30	6.94	90	N
77750	TC			0	1.27	0.08	1.35	90	N
77761	00	A	Intracavitary radioelement application; simple	3.56	3.98	0.39	7.93	90	N
77761	26			3.56	1.59	0.23	5.38	90	N
77761	TC			0	2.39	0.16	2.55	90	N
77762	00	A	Intracavitary radioelement application; intermediate	5.35	5.83	0.57	11.75	90	N
77762	26			5.35	2.39	0.35	8.09	90	N
77762	TC			0	3.44	0.22	3.66	90	N
77763	00	A	Intracavitary radioelement application; complex	8.01	7.86	0.77	16.64	90	N
77763	26			8.01	3.58	0.50	12.09	90	N
77763	TC			0	4.28	0.27	4.55	90	N
77776	00	A	Interstitial radioelement application; simple	4.66	4.16	0.45	9.27	XXX	N
77776	26			4.66	2.09	0.31	7.06	XXX	N
77776	TC			0	2.07	0.14	2.21	XXX	N
77777	00	A	Interstitial radioelement application; intermediate	6.99	7.17	0.71	14.87	90	N

CPT codes and descriptions only, © 1994 American Medical Association. Reimbursement information, © 1995 McGraw-Hill Inc.

Code/ CPT	Mod- ifier	Status	Description	Work value	Practice expense	Mal- practice	Total value	Global period	Up- date
77777	26			6.99	3.13	0.45	10.57	90	N
77777	TC			0	4.04	0.26	4.30	90	N
77778	00	A	Interstitial radioelement application; complex	10.46	9.58	0.98	21.02	90	N
77778	26			10.46	4.69	0.67	15.82	90	N
77778	TC			0	4.89	0.31	5.20	90	N
77781	00	A	Remote afterloading high intensity brachytherapy; 1-4 source positions or catheters	1.55	20.04	1.32	22.91	90	N
77781	26			1.55	0.69	0.11	2.35	90	N
77781	TC			0	19.35	1.21	20.56	90	N
77782	00	A	Remote afterloading high intensity brachytherapy; 5-8 source positions or catheters	2.33	20.40	1.37	24.10	90	N
77782	26			2.33	1.05	0.16	3.54	90	N
77782	TC			0	19.35	1.21	20.56	90	N
77783	00	A	Remote afterloading high intensity brachytherapy; 9-12 source positions or catheters	3.49	20.90	1.44	25.83	90	N
77783	26			3.49	1.55	0.23	5.27	90	N
77783	TC			0	19.35	1.21	20.56	90	N
77784	00	A	Remote afterloading high intensity brachytherapy; over 12 source positions or catheters	5.24	21.69	1.56	28.49	90	N
77784	26			5.24	2.34	0.35	7.93	90	N
77784	TC			0	19.35	1.21	20.56	90	N
77789	00	A	Surface application of radioelement	1.05	0.89	0.10	2.04	90	N
77789	26			1.05	0.46	0.07	1.58	90	N
77789	TC			0	0.43	0.03	0.46	90	N
77790	00	A	Supervision, handling, loading of radioelement	1.05	0.94	0.10	2.09	XXX	N
77790	26			1.05	0.46	0.07	1.58	XXX	N
77790	TC			0	0.48	0.03	0.51	XXX	N
77799	00	C	Unlisted procedure, clinical brachytherapy	0	0	0	0	XXX	N
77799	26			0	0	0	0	XXX	N
77799	TC			0	0	0	0	XXX	N
78000	00	A	Thyroid uptake; single determination	0.19	1.01	0.07	1.27	XXX	N
78000	26			0.19	0.09	0.01	0.29	XXX	N
78000	TC			0	0.92	0.06	0.98	XXX	N
78001	00	A	Thyroid uptake; multiple determinations	0.26	1.36	0.10	1.72	XXX	N
78001	26			0.26	0.12	0.02	0.40	XXX	N
78001	TC			0	1.24	0.08	1.32	XXX	N
78003	00	A	Thyroid uptake; stimulation, suppression or discharge (not including initial uptake studies)	0.33	1.07	0.08	1.48	XXX	N
78003	26			0.33	0.15	0.02	0.50	XXX	N
78003	TC			0	0.92	0.06	0.98	XXX	N
78006	00	A	Thyroid imaging, with uptake; single determination	0.49	2.49	0.18	3.16	XXX	N
78006	26			0.49	0.22	0.03	0.74	XXX	N
78006	TC			0	2.27	0.15	2.42	XXX	N
78007	00	A	Thyroid imaging, with uptake; multiple determinations	0.50	2.68	0.19	3.37	XXX	N
78007	26			0.50	0.23	0.03	0.76	XXX	N
78007	TC			0	2.45	0.16	2.61	XXX	N
78010	00	A	Thyroid imaging; only	0.39	1.90	0.14	2.43	XXX	N
78010	26			0.39	0.17	0.03	0.59	XXX	N
78010	TC			0	1.73	0.11	1.84	XXX	N
78011	00	A	Thyroid imaging; with vascular flow	0.45	2.50	0.18	3.13	XXX	N
78011	26			0.45	0.21	0.03	0.69	XXX	N

CPT codes and descriptions only, © 1994 American Medical Association. Reimbursement information, © 1995 McGraw-Hill Inc.

Code/ CPT	Mod- ifier	Status	Description	Work value	Practice expense	Mal- practice	Total value	Global period	Up- date
78011	TC			0	2.29	0.15	2.44	XXX	N
78015	00	A	Thyroid carcinoma metastases imaging; limited area (eg, neck and chest only)	0.67	2.76	0.21	3.64	XXX	N
78015	26			0.67	0.31	0.05	1.03	XXX	N
78015	TC			0	2.45	0.16	2.61	XXX	N
78016	00	A	Thyroid carcinoma metastases imaging; with additional studies (eg, urinary recovery)	0.82	3.70	0.27	4.79	XXX	N
78016	26			0.82	0.38	0.06	1.26	XXX	N
78016	TC			0	3.32	0.21	3.53	XXX	N
78017	00	A	Thyroid carcinoma metastases imaging; multiple areas	0.87	3.94	0.28	5.09	XXX	N
78017	26			0.87	0.39	0.06	1.32	XXX	N
78017	TC			0	3.55	0.22	3.77	XXX	N
78018	00	A	Thyroid carcinoma metastases imaging; whole body	0.95	5.60	0.39	6.94	XXX	N
78018	26			0.95	0.43	0.06	1.44	XXX	N
78018	TC			0	5.17	0.33	5.50	XXX	N
78070	00	A	Parathyroid imaging	0.51	1.96	0.15	2.62	XXX	N
78070	26			0.51	0.23	0.04	0.78	XXX	N
78070	TC			0	1.73	0.11	1.84	XXX	N
78075	00	A	Adrenal imaging, cortex and/or medulla	0.74	5.51	0.38	6.63	XXX	N
78075	26			0.74	0.34	0.05	1.13	XXX	N
78075	TC			0	5.17	0.33	5.50	XXX	N
78099	00	C	Unlisted endocrine procedure, diagnostic nuclear medicine	0	0	0	0	XXX	N
78099	26			0	0	0	0	XXX	N
78099	TC			0	0	0	0	XXX	N
78102	00	A	Bone marrow imaging; limited area	0.55	2.19	0.17	2.91	XXX	N
78102	26			0.55	0.25	0.04	0.84	XXX	N
78102	TC			0	1.94	0.13	2.07	XXX	N
78103	00	A	Bone marrow imaging; multiple areas	0.75	3.36	0.24	4.35	XXX	N
78103	26			0.75	0.34	0.05	1.14	XXX	N
78103	TC			0	3.02	0.19	3.21	XXX	N
78104	00	A	Bone marrow imaging; whole body	0.80	4.25	0.30	5.35	XXX	N
78104	26			0.80	0.37	0.05	1.22	XXX	N
78104	TC			0	3.88	0.25	4.13	XXX	N
78110	00	A	Plasma volume, radiopharmaceutical volume-dilution technique (separate procedure); single sampling	0.19	0.99	0.07	1.25	XXX	N
78110	26			0.19	0.09	0.01	0.29	XXX	N
78110	TC			0	0.90	0.06	0.96	XXX	N
78111	00	A	Plasma volume, radiopharmaceutical volume-dilution technique (separate procedure); multiple samplings	0.22	2.55	0.18	2.95	XXX	N
78111	26			0.22	0.10	0.02	0.34	XXX	N
78111	TC			0	2.45	0.16	2.61	XXX	N
78120	00	A	Red cell volume determination (separate procedure); single sampling	0.23	1.76	0.13	2.12	XXX	N
78120	26			0.23	0.11	0.02	0.36	XXX	N
78120	TC			0	1.65	0.11	1.76	XXX	N
78121	00	A	Red cell volume determination (separate procedure); multiple samplings	0.32	2.92	0.19	3.43	XXX	N
78121	26			0.32	0.15	0.02	0.49	XXX	N
78121	TC			0	2.77	0.17	2.94	XXX	N

CPT codes and descriptions only, © 1994 American Medical Association. Reimbursement information, © 1995 McGraw-Hill Inc.

Code/ CPT	Mod-ifier	Status	Description	Work value	Practice expense	Mal-practice	Total value	Global period	Up-date
78122	00	A	Whole blood volume determination, including separate measurement of plasma volume and red cell volume (radiopharmaceutical volume-dilution technique)	0.45	4.59	0.31	5.35	XXX	N
78122	26			0.45	0.20	0.03	0.68	XXX	N
78122	TC			0	4.39	0.28	4.67	XXX	N
78130	00	A	Red cell survival study;	0.61	3.00	0.21	3.82	XXX	N
78130	26			0.61	0.28	0.04	0.93	XXX	N
78130	TC			0	2.72	0.17	2.89	XXX	N
78135	00	A	Red cell survival study; differential organ/tissue kinetics, (eg, splenic and/or hepatic sequestration)	0.64	4.93	0.34	5.91	XXX	N
78135	26			0.64	0.29	0.04	0.97	XXX	N
78135	TC			0	4.64	0.30	4.94	XXX	N
78140	00	A	Labeled red cell sequestration, differential organ/tissue, (eg, splenic and/or hepatic)	0.61	4.03	0.28	4.92	XXX	N
78140	26			0.61	0.28	0.04	0.93	XXX	N
78140	TC			0	3.75	0.24	3.99	XXX	N
78160	00	A	Plasma radioiron disappearance (turnover) rate	0.33	3.64	0.24	4.21	XXX	N
78160	26			0.33	0.15	0.02	0.50	XXX	N
78160	TC			0	3.49	0.22	3.71	XXX	N
78162	00	A	Radioiron oral absorption	0.45	3.25	0.22	3.92	XXX	N
78162	26			0.45	0.20	0.03	0.68	XXX	N
78162	TC			0	3.05	0.19	3.24	XXX	N
78170	00	A	Radioiron red cell utilization	0.41	5.24	0.35	6.00	XXX	N
78170	26			0.41	0.18	0.03	0.62	XXX	N
78170	TC			0	5.06	0.32	5.38	XXX	N
78172	00	C	Chelatable iron for estimation of total body iron	0.53*	1.35#	0.06*	1.94#	XXX	N
78172	26			0.53	0.25	0.04	0.82	XXX	N
78172	TC			0	1.09#	0.02*	1.12#	XXX	N
78185	00	A	Spleen imaging only, with or without vascular flow	0.40	2.43	0.18	3.01	XXX	N
78185	26			0.40	0.18	0.03	0.61	XXX	N
78185	TC			0	2.25	0.15	2.40	XXX	N
78190	00	A	Kinetics, study of platelet survival, with or without differential organ/tissue localization	1.09	5.93	0.42	7.44	XXX	N
78190	26			1.09	0.48	0.07	1.64	XXX	N
78190	TC			0	5.45	0.35	5.80	XXX	N
78191	00	A	Platelet survival study	0.61	7.27	0.48	8.36	XXX	N
78191	26			0.61	0.28	0.04	0.93	XXX	N
78191	TC			0	6.99	0.44	7.43	XXX	N
78195	00	A	Lymphatics and lymph glands imaging	0.70	4.20	0.30	5.20	XXX	N
78195	26			0.70	0.32	0.05	1.07	XXX	N
78195	TC			0	3.88	0.25	4.13	XXX	N
78199	00	C	Unlisted hematopoietic, reticuloendothelial and lymphatic procedure, diagnostic nuclear medicine	0	0	0	0	XXX	N
78199	26			0	0	0	0	XXX	N
78199	TC			0	0	0	0	XXX	N
78201	00	A	Liver imaging; static only	0.44	2.44	0.18	3.06	XXX	N
78201	26			0.44	0.19	0.03	0.66	XXX	N
78201	TC			0	2.25	0.15	2.40	XXX	N
78202	00	A	Liver imaging; with vascular flow	0.51	2.98	0.21	3.70	XXX	N
78202	26			0.51	0.23	0.04	0.78	XXX	N
78202	TC			0	2.75	0.17	2.92	XXX	N

CPT codes and descriptions only, © 1994 American Medical Association. Reimbursement information, © 1995 McGraw-Hill Inc.

Code/ CPT	Mod- ifier	Status	Description	Work value	Practice expense	Mal- practice	Total value	Global period	Up- date
78205	00	A	Liver imaging (SPECT)	0.71	5.96	0.41	7.08	XXX	N
78205	26			0.71	0.33	0.05	1.09	XXX	N
78205	TC			0	5.63	0.36	5.99	XXX	N
78215	00	A	Liver and spleen imaging; static only	0.49	3.02	0.20	3.71	XXX	N
78215	26			0.49	0.22	0.03	0.74	XXX	N
78215	TC			0	2.80	0.17	2.97	XXX	N
78216	00	A	Liver and spleen imaging; with vascular flow	0.57	3.58	0.25	4.40	XXX	N
78216	26			0.57	0.26	0.04	0.87	XXX	N
78216	TC			0	3.32	0.21	3.53	XXX	N
78220	00	A	Liver function study with hepatobiliary agents, with serial images	0.49	3.77	0.25	4.51	XXX	N
78220	26			0.49	0.22	0.03	0.74	XXX	N
78220	TC			0	3.55	0.22	3.77	XXX	N
78223	00	A	Hepatobiliary ductal system imaging, including gallbladder, with or without pharmacologic intervention, with or without quantitative measurement of gallbladder function	0.84	3.87	0.28	4.99	XXX	N
78223	26			0.84	0.38	0.06	1.28	XXX	N
78223	TC			0	3.49	0.22	3.71	XXX	N
78230	00	A	Salivary gland imaging;	0.45	2.28	0.17	2.90	XXX	N
78230	26			0.45	0.21	0.03	0.69	XXX	N
78230	TC			0	2.07	0.14	2.21	XXX	N
78231	00	A	Salivary gland imaging; with serial images	0.52	3.26	0.23	4.01	XXX	N
78231	26			0.52	0.24	0.04	0.80	XXX	N
78231	TC			0	3.02	0.19	3.21	XXX	N
78232	00	A	Salivary gland function study	0.47	3.59	0.24	4.30	XXX	N
78232	26			0.47	0.22	0.03	0.72	XXX	N
78232	TC			0	3.37	0.21	3.58	XXX	N
78258	00	A	Esophageal motility	0.74	3.09	0.22	4.05	XXX	N
78258	26			0.74	0.34	0.05	1.13	XXX	N
78258	TC			0	2.75	0.17	2.92	XXX	N
78261	00	A	Gastric mucosa imaging	0.69	4.23	0.30	5.22	XXX	N
78261	26			0.69	0.32	0.05	1.06	XXX	N
78261	TC			0	3.91	0.25	4.16	XXX	N
78262	00	A	Gastroesophageal reflux study	0.68	4.36	0.31	5.35	XXX	N
78262	26			0.68	0.31	0.05	1.04	XXX	N
78262	TC			0	4.05	0.26	4.31	XXX	N
78264	00	A	Gastric emptying study	0.78	4.29	0.30	5.37	XXX	N
78264	26			0.78	0.36	0.05	1.19	XXX	N
78264	TC			0	3.93	0.25	4.18	XXX	N
78270	00	A	Vitamin B-12 absorption study (eg, Schilling test); without intrinsic factor	0.20	1.57	0.11	1.88	XXX	N
78270	26			0.20	0.10	0.01	0.31	XXX	N
78270	TC			0	1.47	0.10	1.57	XXX	N
78271	00	A	Vitamin B-12 absorption study (eg, Schilling test); with intrinsic factor	0.20	1.67	0.11	1.98	XXX	N
78271	26			0.20	0.10	0.01	0.31	XXX	N
78271	TC			0	1.57	0.10	1.67	XXX	N
78272	00	A	Vitamin B-12 absorption studies combined, with and without intrinsic factor	0.27	2.34	0.17	2.78	XXX	N
78272	26			0.27	0.13	0.02	0.42	XXX	N
78272	TC			0	2.21	0.15	2.36	XXX	N

CPT codes and descriptions only, © 1994 American Medical Association. Reimbursement information, © 1995 McGraw-Hill Inc.

Code/ CPT	Mod-ifier	Status	Description	Work value	Practice expense	Mal-practice	Total value	Global period	Up-date
78278	00	A	Acute gastrointestinal blood loss imaging	0.99	5.09	0.37	6.45	XXX	N
78278	26			0.99	0.45	0.07	1.51	XXX	N
78278	TC			0	4.64	0.30	4.94	XXX	N
78282	00	C	Gastrointestinal protein loss	0.38*	1.33#	0.052*	1.76#	XXX	N
78282	26			0.38	0.17	0.03	0.58	XXX	N
78282	TC			0	1.16#	0.02*	1.18#	XXX	N
78290	00	A	Bowel imaging (eg, ectopic gastric mucosa, Meckel's localization, volvulus)	0.68	3.21	0.23	4.12	XXX	N
78290	26			0.68	0.31	0.05	1.04	XXX	N
78290	TC			0	2.90	0.18	3.08	XXX	N
78291	00	A	Peritoneal-venous shunt patency test (eg, for LeVeen, Denver shunt)	0.88	3.31	0.24	4.43	XXX	N
78291	26			0.88	0.39	0.06	1.33	XXX	N
78291	TC			0	2.92	0.18	3.10	XXX	N
78299	00	C	Unlisted gastrointestinal procedure, diagnostic nuclear medicine	0	0	0	0	XXX	N
78299	26			0	0	0	0	XXX	N
78299	TC			0	0	0	0	XXX	N
78300	00	A	Bone and/or joint imaging; limited area	0.62	2.66	0.20	3.48	XXX	N
78300	26			0.62	0.29	0.04	0.95	XXX	N
78300	TC			0	2.37	0.16	2.53	XXX	N
78305	00	A	Bone and/or joint imaging; multiple areas	0.83	3.87	0.28	4.98	XXX	N
78305	26			0.83	0.38	0.06	1.27	XXX	N
78305	TC			0	3.49	0.22	3.71	XXX	N
78306	00	A	Bone and/or joint imaging; whole body	0.86	4.46	0.32	5.64	XXX	N
78306	26			0.86	0.39	0.06	1.31	XXX	N
78306	TC			0	4.07	0.26	4.33	XXX	N
78315	00	A	Bone and/or joint imaging; three phase study	1.02	5.00	0.36	6.38	XXX	N
78315	26			1.02	0.45	0.07	1.54	XXX	N
78315	TC			0	4.55	0.29	4.84	XXX	N
78320	00	A	Bone and/or joint imaging; tomographic (SPECT)	1.04	6.09	0.43	7.56	XXX	N
78320	26			1.04	0.46	0.07	1.57	XXX	N
78320	TC			0	5.63	0.36	5.99	XXX	N
78350	00	A	Bone density (bone mineral content) study; single photon absorptiometry	0.22	0.82	0.07	1.11	XXX	N
78350	26			0.22	0.10	0.02	0.34	XXX	N
78350	TC			0	0.72	0.05	0.77	XXX	N
78351	00	N	Bone density (bone mineral content) study; dual photon absorptiometry	0.30	0.19	0.02	0.51	XXX	0
78399	00	C	Unlisted musculoskeletal procedure, diagnostic nuclear medicine	0	0	0	0	XXX	N
78399	26			0	0	0	0	XXX	N
78399	TC			0	0	0	0	XXX	N
78414	00	C	Determination of central c-v hemodynamics (non-imaging) (eg, ejection fraction with probe technique) with or without pharmacologic intervention or exercise, single or multiple determinations	0.45*	4.44#	0.15*	5.04#	XXX	N
78414	26			0.45	0.20	0.03	0.68	XXX	N
78414	TC			0	4.24#	0.12*	4.36#	XXX	N
78428	00	A	Cardiac shunt detection	0.78	2.51	0.19	3.48	XXX	N
78428	26			0.78	0.36	0.05	1.19	XXX	N
78428	TC			0	2.15	0.14	2.29	XXX	N

CPT codes and descriptions only, © 1994 American Medical Association. Reimbursement information, © 1995 McGraw-Hill Inc.

Code/ CPT	Mod- ifier	Status	Description	Work value	Practice expense	Mal- practice	Total value	Global period	Up- date
78445	00	A	Vascular flow imaging (ie, angiography, venography)	0.49	2.01	0.15	2.65	XXX	N
78445	26			0.49	0.24	0.04	0.77	XXX	N
78445	TC			0	1.77	0.11	1.88	XXX	N
78455	00	A	Venous thrombosis study (eg, radioactive fibrinogen)	0.73	4.13	0.29	5.15	XXX	N
78455	26			0.73	0.33	0.05	1.11	XXX	N
78455	TC			0	3.80	0.24	4.04	XXX	N
78457	00	A	Venous thrombosis imaging (eg, venogram); unilateral	0.77	2.88	0.22	3.87	XXX	N
78457	26			0.77	0.35	0.05	1.17	XXX	N
78457	TC			0	2.53	0.17	2.70	XXX	N
78458	00	A	Venous thrombosis imaging (eg, venogram); bilateral	0.90	4.23	0.30	5.43	XXX	N
78458	26			0.90	0.40	0.06	1.36	XXX	N
78458	TC			0	3.83	0.24	4.07	XXX	N
78460	00	A	Myocardial perfusion imaging; single study, at rest or stress (exercise and/or pharmacologic), qualitative or quantitative	0.86	2.64	0.21	3.71	XXX	N
78460	26			0.86	0.39	0.06	1.31	XXX	N
78460	TC			0	2.25	0.15	2.40	XXX	N
78461	00	A	Myocardial perfusion imaging; multiple studies, at rest and/or stress (exercise and/or pharmacologic), and redistribution and/or rest injection, qualitative or quantitative	1.23	5.04	0.37	6.64	XXX	N
78461	26			1.23	0.54	0.08	1.85	XXX	N
78461	TC			0	4.50	0.29	4.79	XXX	N
78464	00	A	Myocardial perfusion imaging; tomographic (SPECT), single study at rest or stress (exercise and/or pharmacologic), with or without quantitation	1.09	7.22	0.50	8.81	XXX	N
78464	26			1.09	0.48	0.07	1.64	XXX	N
78464	TC			0	6.74	0.43	7.17	XXX	N
78465	00	A	Myocardial perfusion imaging; tomographic (SPECT), multiple studies, at rest and/or stress (exercise and/or pharmacologic) and redistribution and/or rest injection, qualitative or quantitative	1.46	11.89	0.80	14.15	XXX	N
78465	26			1.46	0.65	0.10	2.21	XXX	N
78465	TC			0	11.24	0.70	11.94	XXX	N
78466	00	A	Myocardial imaging, infarct avid, planar; qualitative or quantitative	0.69	2.82	0.22	3.73	XXX	N
78466	26			0.69	0.32	0.05	1.06	XXX	N
78466	TC			0	2.50	0.17	2.67	XXX	N
78468	00	A	Myocardial imaging, infarct avid, planar; with ejection fraction by first pass technique	0.80	3.85	0.27	4.92	XXX	N
78468	26			0.80	0.36	0.05	1.21	XXX	N
78468	TC			0	3.49	0.22	3.71	XXX	N
78469	00	A	Myocardial imaging, infarct avid, planar; tomographic SPECT with or without quantitation	0.92	5.39	0.38	6.69	XXX	N
78469	26			0.92	0.41	0.06	1.39	XXX	N
78469	TC			0	4.98	0.32	5.30	XXX	N
78472	00	A	Cardiac blood pool imaging, gated equilibrium; single study at rest or stress (exercise and/or pharmacologic), wall motion study plus ejection fraction, with or without additional quantitative processing	0.98	5.69	0.41	7.08	XXX	N
78472	26			0.98	0.44	0.07	1.49	XXX	N
78472	TC			0	5.25	0.34	5.59	XXX	N

CPT codes and descriptions only, © 1994 American Medical Association. Reimbursement information, © 1995 McGraw-Hill Inc.

Code/ CPT	Mod- ifier	Status	Description	Work value	Practice expense	Mal- practice	Total value	Global period	Up- date
78473	00	A	Cardiac blood pool imaging, gated equilibrium; multiple studies, wall motion study plus ejection fraction, at rest and stress (exercise and/or pharmacologic), with or without additional quantification	1.47	8.52	0.59	10.58	XXX	N
78473	26			1.47	0.65	0.10	2.22	XXX	N
78473	TC			0	7.87	0.49	8.36	XXX	N
78478	00	A	Myocardial perfusion study with wall motion, qualitative or quantitative study (list separately in addition to code for primary procedure)(Use only for codes 78460, 78461, 78464, 78465)	0.62	1.76	0.14	2.52	XXX	N
78478	26			0.62	0.28	0.04	0.94	XXX	N
78478	TC			0	1.48	0.10	1.58	XXX	N
78480	00	A	Myocardial perfusion study with ejection fraction (list separately in addition to code for primary procedure) (Use only for codes 78460, 78461, 78464, 78465)	0.62	1.76	0.14	2.52	XXX	N
78480	26			0.62	0.28	0.04	0.94	XXX	N
78480	TC			0	1.48	0.10	1.58	XXX	N
78481	00	A	Cardiac blood pool imaging, first pass technique; single study, at rest or during stress (exercise and/or pharmacologic), wall motion study plus ejection fraction, with or without quantitative processing	0.98	5.42	0.39	6.79	XXX	N
78481	26			0.98	0.44	0.07	1.49	XXX	N
78481	TC			0	4.98	0.32	5.30	XXX	N
78483	00	A	Cardiac blood pool imaging, first pass technique; multiple studies, at rest and during stress (exercise and/or pharmacologic), wall motion study plus ejection fraction, with or without additional quantitative processing	1.47	8.15	0.57	10.19	XXX	N
78483	26			1.47	0.65	0.10	2.22	XXX	N
78483	TC			0	7.50	0.47	7.97	XXX	N
78499	00	C	Unlisted cardiovascular procedure, diagnostic nuclear medicine	0	0	0	0	XXX	N
78499	26			0	0	0	0	XXX	N
78499	TC			0	0	0	0	XXX	N
78580	00	A	Pulmonary perfusion imaging, particulate	0.74	3.61	0.26	4.61	XXX	N
78580	26			0.74	0.34	0.05	1.13	XXX	N
78580	TC			0	3.27	0.21	3.48	XXX	N
78584	00	A	Pulmonary perfusion imaging, particulate, with ventilation; single breath	0.99	3.50	0.26	4.75	XXX	N
78584	26			0.99	0.45	0.07	1.51	XXX	N
78584	TC			0	3.05	0.19	3.24	XXX	N
78585	00	A	Pulmonary perfusion imaging, particulate, with ventilation; rebreathing and washout, with or without single breath	1.09	5.85	0.41	7.35	XXX	N
78585	26			1.09	0.48	0.07	1.64	XXX	N
78585	TC			0	5.37	0.34	5.71	XXX	N
78586	00	A	Pulmonary ventilation imaging, aerosol; single projection	0.40	2.65	0.19	3.24	XXX	N
78586	26			0.40	0.18	0.03	0.61	XXX	N
78586	TC			0	2.47	0.16	2.63	XXX	N
78587	00	A	Pulmonary ventilation imaging, aerosol; multiple projections (eg, anterior, posterior, lateral views)	0.49	2.89	0.20	3.58	XXX	N
78587	26			0.49	0.22	0.03	0.74	XXX	N
78587	TC			0	2.67	0.17	2.84	XXX	N
78591	00	A	Pulmonary ventilation imaging, gaseous, single breath, single projection	0.40	2.90	0.20	3.50	XXX	N

CPT codes and descriptions only, © 1994 American Medical Association. Reimbursement information, © 1995 McGraw-Hill Inc.

Code/ CPT	Mod- ifier	Status	Description	Work value	Practice expense	Mal- practice	Total value	Global period	Up- date
78591	26			0.40	0.18	0.03	0.61	XXX	N
78591	TC			0	2.72	0.17	2.89	XXX	N
78593	00	A	Pulmonary ventilation imaging, gaseous, with rebreathing and washout with or without single breath; single projection	0.49	3.51	0.24	4.24	XXX	N
78593	26			0.49	0.22	0.03	0.74	XXX	N
78593	TC			0	3.29	0.21	3.50	XXX	N
78594	00	A	Pulmonary ventilation imaging, gaseous, with rebreathing and washout with or without single breath; multiple projections (eg, anterior, posterior, lateral views)	0.53	5.00	0.34	5.87	XXX	N
78594	26			0.53	0.25	0.04	0.82	XXX	N
78594	TC			0	4.75	0.30	5.05	XXX	N
78596	00	A	Pulmonary quantitative differential function (ventilation/perfusion) study	1.27	7.30	0.52	9.09	XXX	N
78596	26			1.27	0.56	0.09	1.92	XXX	N
78596	TC			0	6.74	0.43	7.17	XXX	N
78599	00	C	Unlisted respiratory procedure, diagnostic nuclear medicine	0	0	0	0	XXX	N
78599	26			0	0	0	0	XXX	N
78599	TC			0	0	0	0	XXX	N
78600	00	A	Brain imaging, limited procedure; static	0.44	2.95	0.20	3.59	XXX	N
78600	26			0.44	0.20	0.03	0.67	XXX	N
78600	TC			0	2.75	0.17	2.92	XXX	N
78601	00	A	Brain imaging, limited procedure; with vascular flow	0.51	3.48	0.24	4.23	XXX	N
78601	26			0.51	0.24	0.04	0.79	XXX	N
78601	TC			0	3.24	0.20	3.44	XXX	N
78605	00	A	Brain imaging, complete study; static	0.53	3.49	0.24	4.26	XXX	N
78605	26			0.53	0.25	0.04	0.82	XXX	N
78605	TC			0	3.24	0.20	3.44	XXX	N
78606	00	A	Brain imaging, complete study; with vascular flow	0.64	3.98	0.27	4.89	XXX	N
78606	26			0.64	0.29	0.04	0.97	XXX	N
78606	TC			0	3.69	0.23	3.92	XXX	N
78607	00	A	Brain imaging, complete study; tomographic (SPECT)	1.23	6.79	0.47	8.49	XXX	N
78607	26			1.23	0.54	0.08	1.85	XXX	N
78607	TC			0	6.25	0.39	6.64	XXX	N
78608	00	N	Brain imaging, positron emission tomography (PET); metabolic evaluation	0	0	0	0	XXX	0
78608	26			1.88*	0	0.01*	1.89#		
78608	TC			0	0	0	0		
78609	00	N	Brain imaging, positron emission tomography (PET); perfusion evaluation	0	0	0	0	XXX	0
78609	26			1.88*	0	0.01*	1.89#		
78609	TC			0	0	0	0		
78610	00	A	Brain imaging, vascular flow only	0.30	1.64	0.12	2.06	XXX	N
78610	26			0.30	0.14	0.02	0.46	XXX	N
78610	TC			0	1.50	0.10	1.60	XXX	N
78615	00	A	Cerebral blood flow	0.42	3.86	0.26	4.54	XXX	N
78615	26			0.42	0.19	0.03	0.64	XXX	N
78615	TC			0	3.67	0.23	3.90	XXX	N
78630	00	A	Cerebrospinal fluid flow, imaging (not including introduction of material); cisternography	0.68	5.11	0.36	6.15	XXX	N
78630	26			0.68	0.31	0.05	1.04	XXX	N
78630	TC			0	4.80	0.31	5.11	XXX	N

CPT codes and descriptions only, © 1994 American Medical Association. Reimbursement information, © 1995 McGraw-Hill Inc.

Code/ CPT	Mod- ifier	Status	Description	Work value	Practice expense	Mal- practice	Total value	Global period	Up- date
78635	00	A	Cerebrospinal fluid flow, imaging (not including introduction of material); ventriculography	0.61	2.70	0.20	3.51	XXX	N
78635	26			0.61	0.28	0.04	0.93	XXX	N
78635	TC			0	2.42	0.16	2.58	XXX	N
78645	00	A	Cerebrospinal fluid flow, imaging (not including introduction of material); shunt evaluation	0.57	3.53	0.25	4.35	XXX	N
78645	26			0.57	0.26	0.04	0.87	XXX	N
78645	TC			0	3.27	0.21	3.48	XXX	N
78647	00	A	Cerebrospinal fluid flow, imaging (not including introduction of material); tomographic (SPECT)	0.90	6.04	0.42	7.36	XXX	N
78647	26			0.90	0.41	0.06	1.37	XXX	N
78647	TC			0	5.63	0.36	5.99	XXX	N
78650	00	A	CSF leakage detection and localization	0.61	4.70	0.32	5.63	XXX	N
78650	26			0.61	0.28	0.04	0.93	XXX	N
78650	TC			0	4.42	0.28	4.70	XXX	N
78652	00	D	Cerebrospinal fluid scan(3D)	0.90*	3.02#	0.12*	4.04#	XXX	N
78652	26			0.90*	0.25#	0.02*	1.17#	XXX	N
78652	TC			0	2.77#	0.10*	2.87#	XXX	N
78655	00	A	Radiopharmaceutical identification of eye tumor	0.56	5.01	0.34	5.91	XXX	N
78655	26			0.56	0.26	0.04	0.86	XXX	N
78655	TC			0	4.75	0.30	5.05	XXX	N
78660	00	A	Radiopharmaceutical dacryocystography	0.53	2.27	0.17	2.97	XXX	N
78660	26			0.53	0.25	0.04	0.82	XXX	N
78660	TC			0	2.02	0.13	2.15	XXX	N
78699	00	C	Unlisted nervous system procedure, diagnostic nuclear medicine	0	0	0	0	XXX	N
78699	26			0	0	0	0	XXX	N
78699	TC			0	0	0	0	XXX	N
78700	00	A	Kidney imaging; static only	0.45	3.10	0.21	3.76	XXX	N
78700	26			0.45	0.20	0.03	0.68	XXX	N
78700	TC			0	2.90	0.18	3.08	XXX	N
78701	00	A	Kidney imaging; with vascular flow	0.49	3.61	0.24	4.34	XXX	N
78701	26			0.49	0.22	0.03	0.74	XXX	N
78701	TC			0	3.39	0.21	3.60	XXX	N
78704	00	A	Kidney imaging; with function study (ie, imaging renogram)	0.74	4.11	0.29	5.14	XXX	N
78704	26			0.74	0.34	0.05	1.13	XXX	N
78704	TC			0	3.77	0.24	4.01	XXX	N
78707	00	A	Kidney imaging; with vascular flow and function study	0.94	4.68	0.33	5.95	XXX	N
78707	26			0.94	0.42	0.06	1.42	XXX	N
78707	TC			0	4.26	0.27	4.53	XXX	N
78710	00	A	Kidney imaging; tomographic (SPECT)	0.66	5.93	0.41	7.00	XXX	N
78710	26			0.66	0.30	0.05	1.01	XXX	N
78710	TC			0	5.63	0.36	5.99	XXX	N
78715	00	A	Kidney vascular flow only	0.30	1.64	0.12	2.06	XXX	N
78715	26			0.30	0.14	0.02	0.46	XXX	N
78715	TC			0	1.50	0.10	1.60	XXX	N
78725	00	A	Kidney function study without pharmacologic intervention	0.38	1.87	0.14	2.39	XXX	N
78725	26			0.38	0.17	0.03	0.58	XXX	N
78725	TC			0	1.70	0.11	1.81	XXX	N
78726	00	A	Kidney function study including pharmacologic intervention	0.87	3.21	0.24	4.32	XXX	N
78726	26			0.87	0.39	0.06	1.32	XXX	N

CPT codes and descriptions only, © 1994 American Medical Association. Reimbursement information, © 1995 McGraw-Hill Inc.

Code/ CPT	Mod- ifier	Status	Description	Work value	Practice expense	Mal- practice	Total value	Global period	Up- date
78726	TC			0	2.82	0.18	3.00	XXX	N
78727	00	A	Kidney transplant evaluation	0.99	4.25	0.31	5.55	XXX	N
78727	26			0.99	0.45	0.07	1.51	XXX	N
78727	TC			0	3.80	0.24	4.04	XXX	N
78730	00	A	Urinary bladder residual study	0.36	1.55	0.11	2.02	XXX	N
78730	26			0.36	0.16	0.02	0.54	XXX	N
78730	TC			0	1.39	0.09	1.48	XXX	N
78740	00	A	Ureteral reflux study (radiopharmaceutical voiding cystogram)	0.57	2.28	0.17	3.02	XXX	N
78740	26			0.57	0.26	0.04	0.87	XXX	N
78740	TC			0	2.02	0.13	2.15	XXX	N
78760	00	A	Testicular imaging;	0.66	2.85	0.21	3.72	XXX	N
78760	26			0.66	0.30	0.04	1.00	XXX	N
78760	TC			0	2.55	0.17	2.72	XXX	N
78761	00	A	Testicular imaging; with vascular flow	0.71	3.38	0.24	4.33	XXX	N
78761	26			0.71	0.33	0.05	1.09	XXX	N
78761	TC			0	3.05	0.19	3.24	XXX	N
78799	00	C	Unlisted genitourinary procedure, diagnostic nuclear medicine	0	0	0	0	XXX	N
78799	26			0	0	0	0	XXX	N
78799	TC			0	0	0	0	XXX	N
78800	00	A	Radiopharmaceutical localization of tumor; limited area	0.65	3.54	0.24	4.43	XXX	N
78800	26			0.65	0.30	0.04	0.99	XXX	N
78800	TC			0	3.24	0.20	3.44	XXX	N
78801	00	A	Radiopharmaceutical localization of tumor; multiple areas	0.79	4.39	0.31	5.49	XXX	N
78801	26			0.79	0.36	0.05	1.20	XXX	N
78801	TC			0	4.03	0.26	4.29	XXX	N
78802	00	A	Radiopharmaceutical localization of tumor; whole body	0.86	5.66	0.40	6.92	XXX	N
78802	26			0.86	0.39	0.06	1.31	XXX	N
78802	TC			0	5.27	0.34	5.61	XXX	N
78803	00	A	Radiopharmaceutical localization of tumor; tomographic (SPECT)	1.09	6.73	0.46	8.28	XXX	N
78803	26			1.09	0.48	0.07	1.64	XXX	N
78803	TC			0	6.25	0.39	6.64	XXX	N
78805	00	A	Radiopharmaceutical localization of abscess; limited area	0.73	3.57	0.25	4.55	XXX	N
78805	26			0.73	0.33	0.05	1.11	XXX	N
78805	TC			0	3.24	0.20	3.44	XXX	N
78806	00	A	Radiopharmaceutical localization of abscess; whole body	0.73	6.51	0.45	7.69	XXX	N
78806	26			0.73	0.38	0.06	1.17	XXX	N
78806	TC			0	6.13	0.39	6.52	XXX	N
78807	00	A	Radiopharmaceutical localization of abscess; tomographic (SPECT)	1.09	6.73	0.46	8.28	XXX	N
78807	26			1.09	0.48	0.07	1.64	XXX	N
78807	TC			0	6.25	0.39	6.64	XXX	N
78890	00	B	Generation of automated data: interactive process involving nuclear physician and/or allied health professional personnel; simple manipulations and interpretation, not to exceed 30 minutes	0.05	1.26	0.08	1.39	XXX	0
78890	26			0.05	0.02	0	0.07	XXX	0
78890	TC			0	1.24	0.08	1.32	XXX	0

CPT codes and descriptions only, © 1994 American Medical Association. Reimbursement information, © 1995 McGraw-Hill Inc.

Code/ CPT	Mod- ifier	Status	Description	Work value	Practice expense	Mal- practice	Total value	Global period	Up- date
78891	00	B	Generation of automated data: interactive process involving nuclear physician and/or allied health professional personnel; complex manipulations and interpretation, exceeding 30 minutes	0.10	2.55	0.18	2.83	XXX	0
78891	26			0.10	0.05	0.01	0.16	XXX	0
78891	TC			0	2.50	0.17	2.67	XXX	0
78990	00	G	Provision of diagnostic radiopharmaceutical(s)	0	0.71#	0.02*	0.73#	XXX	0
78990	26			0	0.06#	0	0.06#		
78990	TC			0	0.65#	0.02*	0.67#		
78999	00	C	Unlisted miscellaneous procedure, diagnostic nuclear medicine	0	0	0	0	XXX	N
78999	26			0	0	0	0	XXX	N
78999	TC			0	0	0	0	XXX	N
79000	00	A	Radiopharmaceutical therapy, hyperthyroidism; initial, including evaluation of patient	1.80	3.31	0.29	5.40	XXX	N
79000	26			1.80	0.81	0.12	2.73	XXX	N
79000	TC			0	2.50	0.17	2.67	XXX	N
79001	00	A	Radiopharmaceutical therapy, hyperthyroidism; subsequent, each therapy	1.05	1.70	0.15	2.90	XXX	N
79001	26			1.05	0.46	0.07	1.58	XXX	N
79001	TC			0	1.24	0.08	1.32	XXX	N
79020	00	A	Radiopharmaceutical therapy, thyroid suppression (euthyroid cardiac disease), including evaluation of patient	1.81	3.31	0.29	5.41	XXX	N
79020	26			1.81	0.81	0.12	2.74	XXX	N
79020	TC			0	2.50	0.17	2.67	XXX	N
79030	00	A	Radiopharmaceutical ablation of gland for thyroid carcinoma	2.10	3.44	0.31	5.85	XXX	N
79030	26			2.10	0.94	0.14	3.18	XXX	N
79030	TC			0	2.50	0.17	2.67	XXX	N
79035	00	A	Radiopharmaceutical therapy for metastases of thyroid carcinoma	2.52	3.63	0.34	6.49	XXX	N
79035	26			2.52	1.13	0.17	3.82	XXX	N
79035	TC			0	2.50	0.17	2.67	XXX	N
79100	00	A	Radiopharmaceutical therapy, polycythemia vera, chronic leukemia, each treatment	1.32	3.08	0.26	4.66	XXX	N
79100	26			1.32	0.58	0.09	1.99	XXX	N
79100	TC			0	2.50	0.17	2.67	XXX	N
79200	00	A	Intracavitary radioactive colloid therapy	1.99	3.39	0.31	5.69	XXX	N
79200	26			1.99	0.89	0.14	3.02	XXX	N
79200	TC			0	2.50	0.17	2.67	XXX	N
79300	00	C	Interstitial radioactive colloid therapy	1.60*	5.77#	0.23*	7.59#	XXX	N
79300	26			1.60	0.71	0.11	2.42	XXX	N
79300	TC			0	5.06#	0.12*	5.17#	XXX	N
79400	00	A	Radiopharmaceutical therapy, nonthyroid, nonhematologic	1.96	3.37	0.30	5.63	XXX	N
79400	26			1.96	0.87	0.13	2.96	XXX	N
79400	TC			0	2.50	0.17	2.67	XXX	N
79420	00	C	Intravascular radiopharmaceutical therapy, particulate	1.51*	3.37#	0.15*	5.03#	XXX	N
79420	26			1.51	0.67	0.10	2.28	XXX	N
79420	TC			0	2.70#	0.05*	2.75#	XXX	N
79440	00	A	Intra-articular radiopharmaceutical therapy	1.99	3.39	0.31	5.69	XXX	N
79440	26			1.99	0.89	0.14	3.02	XXX	N
79440	TC			0	2.50	0.17	2.67	XXX	N

CPT codes and descriptions only, © 1994 American Medical Association. Reimbursement information, © 1995 McGraw-Hill Inc.

Code/ CPT	Mod-ifier	Status	Description	Work value	Practice expense	Mal-practice	Total value	Global period	Up-date
86291	00	X	Hepatitis B surface antibody (HBsAb)	0.15*	0.28#	0.01*	0.44#	XXX	0
86293	00	X	Hepatitis Be antigen (HBeAg)	0.15*	0.31#	0.02*	0.48#	XXX	0
86295	00	X	Hepatitis Be antibody (HBeAb)	0.15*	0.31#	0.02*	0.48#	XXX	0
86296	00	X	Hepatitis A antibody (HAAb); IgG and IgM	0.17*	0.37#	0.01*	0.55#	XXX	0
86299	00	X	Hepatitis A antibody (HAAb); IgM antibody	0.17*	0.33#	0.01*	0.51#	XXX	0
86302	00	X	Hepatitis C antibody;	0	0	0	0	XXX	0
86303	00	X	Hepatitis C antibody; confirmatory test (eg, immunoblot)	0	0	0	0	XXX	0
86306	00	X	Hepatitis, delta agent	0	0	0	0	XXX	0
86308	00	X	Heterophile antibodies; screening	0	0	0	0	XXX	0
86309	00	X	Heterophile antibodies; titer	0	0	0	0	XXX	0
86310	00	X	Heterophile antibodies; titers after absorption with beef cells and guinea pig kidney	0.11*	0.22#	0.01*	0.34#	XXX	0
86311	00	X	HIV, antigen	0	0	0	0	XXX	0
86313	00	X	Immunoassay for infectious agent antigen, qualitative or semiquantitative; multiple step method	0	0	0	0	XXX	0
86315	00	X	Immunoassay for infectious agent antigen, qualitative or semiquantitative; single step method (eg, reagent strip)	0	0	0	0	XXX	0
86316	00	X	Immunoassay for tumor antigen (eg, cancer antigen 125), each	0.18*	0.44#	0.03*	0.65#	XXX	0
86317	00	X	Immunoassay for infectious agent antibody, quantitative, not elsewhere specified	0.17*	0.35#	0.01*	0.53#	XXX	0
86318	00	X	Immunoassay for infectious agent antibody, qualitative or semiquantitative, single step method (eg, reagent strip)	0.17*	0.24#	0.01*	0.42#	XXX	0
86320	00	X	Immunoelectrophoresis; serum	0.37*	0.50#	0.03*	0.9#	XXX	0
86320	26			0.37	0.20	0.01	0.58	XXX	N
86325	00	X	Immunoelectrophoresis; other fluids (eg, urine, CSF) with concentration	0.37*	0.55#	0.03*	0.95#	XXX	0
86325	26			0.37	0.20	0.01	0.58	XXX	N
86327	00	X	Immunoelectrophoresis; crossed (2-dimensional assay)	0.37*	0.72#	0.04*	1.13#	XXX	0
86327	26			0.37	0.20	0.01	0.58	XXX	N
86329	00	X	Immunodiffusion; not elsewhere specified	0.20*	0.42#	0.03*	0.65#	XXX	0
86331	00	X	Immunodiffusion; gel diffusion, qualitative (Ouchterlony), each antigen or antibody	0.17*	0.39#	0.01*	0.57#	XXX	0
86332	00	X	Immune complex assay	0.31*	0.61#	0.03*	0.95#	XXX	0
86334	00	X	Immunofixation electrophoresis	0.37*	0.77#	0.04*	1.18#	XXX	0
86334	26			0.37	0.20	0.01	0.58	XXX	N
86337	00	X	Insulin antibodies	0.31*	0.61#	0.03*	0.95#	XXX	0
86340	00	X	Intrinsic factor antibodies	0.22*	0.44#	0.03*	0.69#	XXX	0
86341	00	X	Islet cell antibody	0	0	0	0	XXX	0
86343	00	X	Leukocyte histamine release test (LHR)	0.18*	0.37#	0.02*	0.57#	XXX	0
86344	00	X	Leukocyte phagocytosis	0.13*	0.24#	0.01*	0.38#	XXX	0
86353	00	X	Lymphocyte transformation, mitogen (phytomitogen) or antigen induced blastogenesis	0.52*	1.20#	0.05*	1.77#	XXX	0
86359	00	X	T cells; total count	0	0	0	0	XXX	0
86360	00	X	T cells; T4 and T8, including ratio	0	0	0	0	XXX	0
86376	00	X	Microsomal antibodies (eg, thyroid or liver-kidney), each	0.18*	0.41#	0.02*	0.61#	XXX	0
86378	00	X	Migration inhibitory factor test (MIF)	0.26*	0.52#	0.02*	0.80#	XXX	0
86382	00	X	Neutralization test, viral	0.24*	0.53#	0.03*	0.8#	XXX	0
86384	00	X	Nitroblue tetrazolium dye test (NTD)	0.15*	0.28#	0.01*	0.44#	XXX	0
86403	00	X	Particle agglutination; screen, each antibody	0.07*	0.28#	0.01*	0.36#	XXX	0
86406	00	X	Particle agglutination; titer, each antibody	0	0	0	0	XXX	0

CPT codes and descriptions only, © 1994 American Medical Association. Reimbursement information, © 1995 McGraw-Hill Inc.

Code/ CPT	Mod- ifier	Status	Description	Work value	Practice expense	Mal- practice	Total value	Global period	Up- date
86430	00	X	Rheumatoid factor; qualitative	0.07*	0.15#	0.01*	0.23#	XXX	0
86431	00	X	Rheumatoid factor; quantitative	0.11*	0.18#	0.02*	0.31#	XXX	0
86485	00	C	Skin test; candida	0	0	0	0	XXX	N
86490	00	A	Skin test; coccidioidomycosis	0	0.28	0.02	0.30	XXX	N
86510	00	A	Skin test; histoplasmosis	0	0.30	0.02	0.32	XXX	N
86580	00	A	Skin test; tuberculosis, intradermal	0	0.24	0.02	0.26	XXX	N
86585	00	A	Skin test; tuberculosis, tine test	0	0.19	0.01	0.20	XXX	N
86586	00	C	Skin test; unlisted antigen, each	0	0	0	0	XXX	N
86588	00	X	Streptococcus, screen, direct	0	0	0	0	XXX	0
86590	00	X	Streptokinase, antibody	0.11*	0.20#	0.01*	0.32#	XXX	0
86592	00	X	Syphilis test; qualitative (eg, VDRL, RPR, ART)	0.04*	0.11#	0	0.15#	XXX	0
86593	00	X	Syphilis test; quantitative	0.06*	0.13#	0	0.19#	XXX	0
86602	00	X	Antibody; actinomyces	0	0	0	0	XXX	0
86603	00	X	Antibody; adenovirus	0	0	0	0	XXX	0
86606	00	X	Antibody; Aspergillus	0	0	0	0	XXX	0
86609	00	X	Antibody; bacterium, not elsewhere specified	0	0	0	0	XXX	0
86612	00	X	Antibody; Blastomyces	0	0	0	0	XXX	0
86615	00	X	Antibody; Bordetella	0	0	0	0	XXX	0
86617	00	X	Antibody; Borrelia burgdorferi (Lyme disease) confirmatory test (eg, Western blot or immunoblot)	0	0	0	0	XXX	0
86618	00	X	Antibody; Borrelia burgdorferi (Lyme disease)	0	0	0	0	XXX	0
86619	00	X	Antibody; Borrelia (relapsing fever)	0	0	0	0	XXX	0
86622	00	X	Antibody; Brucella	0	0	0	0	XXX	0
86625	00	X	Antibody; Campylobacter	0	0	0	0	XXX	0
86628	00	X	Antibody; Candida	0	0	0	0	XXX	0
86631	00	X	Antibody; Chlamydia	0	0	0	0	XXX	0
86632	00	X	Antibody; Chlamydia, IgM	0	0	0	0	XXX	0
86635	00	X	Antibody; Coccidioides	0	0	0	0	XXX	0
86638	00	X	Antibody; Coxiella Brunetii (Q fever)	0	0	0	0	XXX	0
86641	00	X	Antibody; Cryptococcus	0	0	0	0	XXX	0
86644	00	X	Antibody; cytomegalovirus (CMV)	0	0	0	0	XXX	0
86645	00	X	Antibody; cytomegalovirus (CMV), IgM	0	0	0	0	XXX	0
86648	00	X	Antibody; Diphtheria	0	0	0	0	XXX	0
86651	00	X	Antibody; encephalitis, California (La Crosse)	0	0	0	0	XXX	0
86652	00	X	Antibody; encephalitis, Eastern equine	0	0	0	0	XXX	0
86653	00	X	Antibody; encephalitis, St. Louis	0	0	0	0	XXX	0
86654	00	X	Antibody; encephalitis, Western equine	0	0	0	0	XXX	0
86658	00	X	Antibody; enterovirus (eg, coxsackie, echo, polio)	0	0	0	0	XXX	0
86663	00	X	Antibody; Epstein-Barr (EB) virus, early antigen (EA)	0	0	0	0	XXX	0
86664	00	X	Antibody; Epstein-Barr (EB) virus, nuclear antigen (EBNA)	0	0	0	0	XXX	0
86665	00	X	Antibody; Epstein-Barr (EB) virus, viral capsid (VCA)	0	0	0	0	XXX	0
86668	00	X	Antibody; Francisella Tularensis	0	0	0	0	XXX	0
86671	00	X	Antibody; fungus, not elsewhere specified	0	0	0	0	XXX	0
86674	00	X	Antibody; Giardia Lamblia	0	0	0	0	XXX	0
86677	00	X	Antibody; Helicobacter Pylori	0	0	0	0	XXX	0
86682	00	X	Antibody; helminth, not elsewhere specified	0	0	0	0	XXX	0
86684	00	X	Antibody; Hemophilus influenza	0	0	0	0	XXX	0
86687	00	X	Antibody; HTLV I	0.06*	0.13#	0	0.19#	XXX	0

CPT codes and descriptions only, © 1994 American Medical Association. Reimbursement information, © 1995 McGraw-Hill Inc.

Code/ CPT	Mod- ifier	Status	Description	Work value	Practice expense	Mal- practice	Total value	Global period	Up- date
86688	00	X	Antibody; HTLV-II	0	0	0	0	XXX	0
86689	00	X	Antibody; HTLV or HIV antibody, confirmatory test (eg, Western Blot)	0.06*	0.13#	0	0.19#	XXX	0
86692	00	X	Antibody; hepatitis, delta agent	0	0	0	0	XXX	0
86694	00	X	Antibody; herpes simplex, non-specific type test	0	0	0	0	XXX	0
86695	00	X	Antibody; herpes simplex, type I	0	0	0	0	XXX	0
86698	00	X	Antibody; histoplasma	0	0	0	0	XXX	0
86701	00	X	Antibody; HIV-1	0	0	0	0	XXX	0
86702	00	X	Antibody; HIV-2	0	0	0	0	XXX	0
86703	00	X	Antibody; HIV-1 and HIV-2, single assay	0	0	0	0	XXX	0
86710	00	X	Antibody; influenza virus	0	0	0	0	XXX	0
86713	00	X	Antibody; Legionella	0	0	0	0	XXX	0
86717	00	X	Antibody; Leishmania	0	0	0	0	XXX	0
86720	00	X	Antibody; Leptospira	0	0	0	0	XXX	0
86723	00	X	Antibody; Listeria monocytogenes	0	0	0	0	XXX	0
86727	00	X	Antibody; lymphocytic choriomeningitis	0	0	0	0	XXX	0
86729	00	X	Antibody; Lymphogranuloma Venereum	0	0	0	0	XXX	0
86732	00	X	Antibody; mucormycosis	0	0	0	0	XXX	0
86735	00	X	Antibody; mumps	0.07*	0.15#	0.01*	0.23#	XXX	0
86738	00	X	Antibody; Mycoplasma	0	0	0	0	XXX	0
86741	00	X	Antibody; Neisseria meningitidis	0	0	0	0	XXX	0
86744	00	X	Antibody; Nocardia	0	0	0	0	XXX	0
86747	00	X	Antibody; parvovirus	0	0	0	0	XXX	0
86750	00	X	Antibody; Plasmodium (malaria)	0	0	0	0	XXX	0
86753	00	X	Antibody; protozoa, not elsewhere specified	0	0	0	0	XXX	0
86756	00	X	Antibody; respiratory syncytial virus	0	0	0	0	XXX	0
86759	00	X	Antibody; rotavirus	0	0	0	0	XXX	0
86762	00	X	Antibody; rubella	0	0	0	0	XXX	0
86765	00	X	Antibody; rubeola	0	0	0	0	XXX	0
86768	00	X	Antibody; Salmonella	0	0	0	0	XXX	0
86771	00	X	Antibody; Shigella	0	0	0	0	XXX	0
86774	00	X	Antibody; tetanus	0	0	0	0	XXX	0
86777	00	X	Antibody; Toxoplasma	0	0	0	0	XXX	0
86778	00	X	Antibody; Toxoplasma, IgM	0	0	0	0	XXX	0
86781	00	X	Antibody; Treponema Pallidum, confirmatory test (eg, FTA-abs)	0.13*	0.26#	0.01*	0.40#	XXX	0
86784	00	X	Antibody; trichinella	0	0	0	0	XXX	0
86787	00	X	Antibody; varicella-zoster	0	0	0	0	XXX	0
86790	00	X	Antibody; virus, not elsewhere specified	0	0	0	0	XXX	0
86793	00	X	Antibody; Yersinia	0	0	0	0	XXX	0
86800	00	X	Thyroglobulin antibody	0.24*	0.48#	0.02*	0.74#	XXX	0
86805	00	X	Lymphocytotoxicity assay, visual crossmatch; with titration	0.55*	1.07#	0.06*	1.68#	XXX	0
86806	00	X	Lymphocytotoxicity assay, visual crossmatch; without titration	0.48*	0.98#	0.05*	1.51#	XXX	0
86807	00	X	Serum screening for cytotoxic percent reactive antibody (PRA); standard method	0.37*	0.87#	0.04*	1.28#	XXX	0
86808	00	X	Serum screening for cytotoxic percent reactive antibody (PRA); quick method	0.26*	0.63#	0.03*	0.92#	XXX	0
86812	00	X	HLA typing; A, B, or C (eg, A10, B7, B27), single antigen	0.66*	1.55#	0.08*	2.29#	XXX	0

CPT codes and descriptions only, © 1994 American Medical Association. Reimbursement information, © 1995 McGraw-Hill Inc.

Code/ CPT	Mod- ifier	Status	Description	Work value	Practice expense	Mal- practice	Total value	Global period	Up- date
86813	00	X	HLA typing; A, B, or C, multiple antigens	0.52*	1.18#	0.05*	1.75#	XXX	0
86816	00	X	HLA typing; DR/DQ, single antigen	0.31*	0.76#	0.04*	1.11#	XXX	0
86817	00	X	HLA typing; DR/DQ, multiple antigens	0.66*	1.57#	0.08*	2.31#	XXX	0
86821	00	X	HLA typing; lymphocyte culture, mixed (MLC)	0.61*	1.44#	0.07*	2.12#	XXX	0
86822	00	X	HLA typing; lymphocyte culture, primed (PLC)	0.53*	1.07#	0.06*	1.66#	XXX	0
86849	00	X	Unlisted immunology procedure	0	0	0	0	XXX	0
86850	00	X	Antibody screen, RBC, each serum technique	0.07*	0.13#	0.01*	0.21#	XXX	0
86860	00	X	Antibody elution (RBC), each elution	0.26*	0.50#	0.02*	0.78#	XXX	0
86870	00	X	Antibody identification, RBC antibodies, each panel for each serum technique	0	0	0	0	XXX	0
86880	00	X	Antihuman globulin test (Coombs test); direct, each antiserum	0.07*	0.15#	0.01*	0.23#	XXX	0
86885	00	X	Antihuman globulin test (Coombs test); indirect, qualitative, each antiserum	0	0	0	0	XXX	0
86886	00	X	Antihuman globulin test (Coombs test); indirect, titer, each antiserum	0.07*	0.17#	0.01*	0.25#	XXX	0
86890	00	X	Autologous blood or component, collection processing and storage; predeposited	0	0	0	0	XXX	0
86891	00	X	Autologous blood or component, collection processing and storage; intra- or postoperative salvage	0.46*	1.07#	0.05*	1.58#	XXX	0
86900	00	X	Blood typing; ABO	0.06*	0.13#	0	0.19#	XXX	0
86901	00	X	Blood typing; Rh (D)	0.07*	0.13#	0.01*	0.21#	XXX	0
86903	00	X	Blood typing; antigen screening for compatible blood unit using reagent serum, per unit screened	0	0	0	0	XXX	0
86904	00	X	Blood typing; antigen screening for compatible unit using patient serum, per unit screened	0.11*	0.22#	0.01*	0.34#	XXX	0
86905	00	X	Blood typing; RBC antigens, other than ABO or Rh (D), each	0.04*	0.11#	0	0.15#	XXX	0
86906	00	X	Blood typing; Rh phenotyping, complete	0	0	0	0	XXX	0
86910	00	X	Blood typing, for paternity testing, per individual, ABO, Rh and MN;	0.42*	0.98#	0.05*	1.45#	XXX	0
86911	00	X	Blood typing, for paternity testing, per individual, ABO, Rh and MN; each additional antigen system	0	0	0	0	XXX	0
86915	00	X	Bone marrow, modification or treatment to eliminate cell (eg, T-cells, metastatic carcinoma)	0	0	0	0	XXX	0
86920	00	X	Compatibility test each unit; immediate spin technique	0.07*	0.28#	0.01*	0.36#	XXX	0
86921	00	X	Compatibility test each unit; incubation technique	0.13*	0.28#	0.01*	0.42#	XXX	0
86922	00	X	Compatibility test each unit; antiglobulin technique	0.13*	0.28#	0.01*	0.42#	XXX	0
86927	00	X	Fresh frozen plasma, thawing, each unit	0	0	0	0	XXX	0
86930	00	X	Frozen blood, preparation for freezing, each unit;	0.77*	1.81#	0.09*	2.67#	XXX	0
86931	00	X	Frozen blood, preparation for freezing, each unit; with thawing	0.77*	1.81#	0.09*	2.67#	XXX	0
86932	00	X	Frozen blood, preparation for freezing, each unit; with freezing and thawing	0.81*	1.86#	0.10*	2.77#	XXX	0
86940	00	X	Hemolysins and agglutinins, auto, screen, each;	0.09*	0.22#	0.01*	0.32#	XXX	0
86941	00	X	Hemolysins and agglutinins, auto, screen, each; incubated	0.15*	0.37#	0.01*	0.53#	XXX	0
86945	00	X	Irradiation of blood product, each unit	0.18*	0.41#	0.02*	0.61#	XXX	0
86950	00	X	Leukocyte transfusion	0.50*	1.16#	0.06*	1.72#	XXX	0
86965	00	X	Pooling of platelets or other blood products	0.13*	0.31#	0.02*	0.46#	XXX	0

CPT codes and descriptions only, © 1994 American Medical Association. Reimbursement information, © 1995 McGraw-Hill Inc.

Code/ CPT	Mod-ifier	Status	Description	Work value	Practice expense	Mal-practice	Total value	Global period	Up-date
86970	00	X	Pretreatment of RBC's for use in RBC antibody detection, identification, and/or compatibility testing; incubation with chemical agents or drugs, each	0.20*	0.50#	0.02*	0.72#	XXX	0
86971	00	X	Pretreatment of RBC's for use in RBC antibody detection, identification, and/or compatibility testing; incubation with enzymes, each	0.09*	0.26#	0.01*	0.36#	XXX	0
86972	00	X	Pretreatment of RBC's for use in RBC antibody detection, identification, and/or compatibility testing; by density gradient separation	0.11*	0.24#	0.01*	0.36#	XXX	0
86975	00	X	Pretreatment of serum for use in RBC antibody identification; incubation with drugs, each	0.28*	0.63#	0.02*	0.93#	XXX	0
86976	00	X	Pretreatment of serum for use in RBC antibody identification; by dilution	0.28*	0.63#	0.02*	0.93#	XXX	0
86977	00	X	Pretreatment of serum for use in RBC antibody identification; incubation with inhibitors, each	0.28*	0.63#	0.02*	0.93#	XXX	0
86978	00	X	Pretreatment of serum for use in RBC antibody identification; by differential red cell absorption using patient RBC's or RBC's of known phenotype, each absorption	0.33*	0.76#	0.04*	1.13#	XXX	0
86985	00	X	Splitting of blood or blood products, each unit	0	0	0	0	XXX	0
86999	00	X	Unlisted transfusion medicine procedure	0	0	0	0	XXX	0
87001	00	X	Animal inoculation, small animal; with observation	0.18*	0.41#	0.02*	0.61#	XXX	0
87003	00	X	Animal inoculation, small animal; with observation and dissection	0.22*	0.46#	0.03*	0.71#	XXX	0
87015	00	X	Concentration (any type), for parasites, ova, or tubercle bacillus (TB, AFB)	0.09*	0.18#	0.02*	0.29#	XXX	0
87040	00	X	Culture, bacterial, definitive; blood (includes anaerobic screen)	0.11*	0.20#	0.01*	0.32#	XXX	0
87045	00	X	Culture, bacterial, definitive; stool	0.13*	0.26#	0.01*	0.40#	XXX	0
87060	00	X	Culture, bacterial, definitive; throat or nose	0.06*	0.17#	0	0.23#	XXX	0
87070	00	X	Culture, bacterial, definitive; any other source	0.07*	0.17#	0.01*	0.25#	XXX	0
87072	00	X	Culture or direct bacterial identification method, each organism, by commercial kit, any source except urine	0.06*	0.17#	0	0.23#	XXX	0
87075	00	X	Culture, bacterial, any source; anaerobic (isolation)	0.11*	0.20#	0.01*	0.32#	XXX	0
87076	00	X	Culture, bacterial, any source; definitive identification, each anaerobic organism, including gas chromatography	0.15*	0.28#	0.01*	0.44#	XXX	0
87081	00	X	Culture, bacterial, screening only, for single organisms	0.06*	0.15#	0	0.21#	XXX	0
87082	00	X	Culture, presumptive, pathogenic organisms, screening only, by commercial kit (specify type); for single organisms	0.06*	0.15#	0	0.21#	XXX	0
87083	00	X	Culture, presumptive, pathogenic organisms, screening only, by commercial kit (specify type); multiple organisms	0.11*	0.20#	0.01*	0.32#	XXX	0
87084	00	X	Culture, presumptive, pathogenic organisms, screening only, by commercial kit (specify type); with colony estimation from density chart	0.13*	0.28#	0.01*	0.42#	XXX	0
87085	00	X	Culture, presumptive, pathogenic organisms, screening only, by commercial kit (specify type); with colony count	0.13*	0.28#	0.01*	0.42#	XXX	0
87086	00	X	Culture, bacterial, urine; quantitative, colony count	0.06*	0.18#	0.01*	0.25#	XXX	0
87087	00	X	Culture, bacterial, urine; commercial kit	0.09*	0.2#	0.02*	0.31#	XXX	0
87088	00	X	Culture, bacterial, urine; identification, in addition to quantitative or commercial kit	0.11*	0.20#	0.01*	0.32#	XXX	0
87101	00	X	Culture, fungi, isolation (with or without presumptive identification); skin	0.11*	0.24#	0.01*	0.36#	XXX	0

CPT codes and descriptions only, © 1994 American Medical Association. Reimbursement information, © 1995 McGraw-Hill Inc.

Code/ CPT	Mod-ifier	Status	Description	Work value	Practice expense	Mal-practice	Total value	Global period	Up-date
87102	00	X	Culture, fungi, isolation (with or without presumptive identification); other source (except blood)	0.11*	0.24#	0.01*	0.36#	XXX	0
87103	00	X	Culture, fungi, isolation (with or without presumptive identification); blood	0.18*	0.35#	0.02*	0.55#	XXX	0
87106	00	X	Culture, fungi, definitive identification of each fungus (use in addition to codes 87101, 87102, or 87103 when appropriate)	0.13*	0.31#	0.02*	0.46#	XXX	0
87109	00	X	Culture, mycoplasma, any source	0.15*	0.31#	0.02*	0.48#	XXX	0
87110	00	X	Culture, chlamydia	0.17*	0.39#	0.01*	0.57#	XXX	0
87116	00	X	Culture, tubercle or other acid-fast bacilli (eg, TB, AFB, mycobacteria); any source, isolation only	0.13*	0.31#	0.02*	0.46#	XXX	0
87117	00	X	Culture, tubercle or other acid-fast bacilli (eg, TB, AFB, mycobacteria); concentration plus isolation	0.15*	0.30#	0.01*	0.46#	XXX	0
87118	00	X	Culture, mycobacteria, definitive identification of each organism	0.13*	0.31#	0.02*	0.46#	XXX	0
87140	00	X	Culture, typing; fluorescent method, each antiserum	0.13*	0.30#	0.01*	0.44#	XXX	0
87143	00	X	Culture, typing; gas liquid chromatography (GLC) method	0.18*	0.39#	0.02*	0.59#	XXX	0
87145	00	X	Culture, typing; phage method	0.09*	0.22#	0.01*	0.32#	XXX	0
87147	00	X	Culture, typing; serologic method, agglutination grouping, per antiserum	0.15*	0.31#	0.02*	0.48#	XXX	0
87151	00	X	Culture, typing; serologic method, speciation	0.09*	0.17#	0.01*	0.27#	XXX	0
87155	00	X	Culture, typing; precipitin method, grouping, per antiserum	0.04*	0.13#	0	0.17#	XXX	0
87158	00	X	Culture, typing; other methods	0.04*	0.13#	0	0.17#	XXX	0
87163	00	X	Culture, any source, additional identification methods required (use in addition to primary culture code)	0.17*	0.35#	0.01*	0.53#	XXX	0
87164	00	X	Dark field examination, any source (eg, penile, vaginal, oral, skin); includes specimen collection	0.37*	0.28#	0.02*	0.67#	XXX	0
87164	26			0.37	0.20	0.01	0.58	XXX	N
87166	00	X	Dark field examination, any source (eg, penile, vaginal, oral, skin); without collection	0.13*	0.30#	0.01*	0.44#	XXX	0
87174	00	X	Endotoxin, bacterial (pyrogens); chemical	0.13*	0.28#	0.01*	0.42#	XXX	0
87175	00	X	Endotoxin, bacterial (pyrogens); biological assay (eg, Limulus lysate)	0.15*	0.31#	0.02*	0.48#	XXX	0
87176	00	X	Endotoxin, bacterial (pyrogens); homogenization, tissue, for culture	0.09*	0.18#	0.02*	0.29#	XXX	0
87177	00	X	Ova and parasites, direct smears, concentration and identification	0.11*	0.20#	0.01*	0.32#	XXX	0
87178	00	X	Microbial identification, nucleic acid probes, each probe used;	0.22*	0.41#	0.02*	0.65#	XXX	0
87179	00	X	Microbial identification, nucleic acid probes, each probe used; with amplification, eg, polymerase chain reaction (PCR)	0	0	0	0	XXX	0
87181	00	X	Sensitivity studies, antibiotic; agar diffusion method, per antibiotic	0.07*	0.15#	0.01*	0.23#	XXX	0
87184	00	X	Sensitivity studies, antibiotic; disk method, per plate (12 or less disks)	0.06*	0.17#	0	0.23#	XXX	0
87186	00	X	Sensitivity studies, antibiotic; microtiter, minimum inhibitory concentration (MIC), any number of antibiotics	0.07*	0.20#	0.02*	0.29#	XXX	0
87187	00	X	Sensitivity studies, antibiotic; minimum bactericidal concentration (MBC) (use in addition to 87186 or 87188)	0.06*	0.3#	0	0.36#	XXX	0
87188	00	X	Sensitivity studies, antibiotic; macrotube dilution method, each antibiotic	0.09*	0.22#	0.01*	0.32#	XXX	0

CPT codes and descriptions only, © 1994 American Medical Association. Reimbursement information, © 1995 McGraw-Hill Inc.

Code/ CPT	Mod-ifier	Status	Description	Work value	Practice expense	Mal-practice	Total value	Global period	Up-date
87190	00	X	Sensitivity studies, antibiotic; tubercle bacillus (TB, AFB), each drug	0.04*	0.09#	0	0.13#	XXX	0
87192	00	X	Sensitivity studies, antibiotic; fungi, each drug	0.09*	0.22#	0.01*	0.32#	XXX	0
87197	00	X	Serum bactericidal titer (Schlicter test)	0.17*	0.33#	0.01*	0.51#	XXX	0
87205	00	X	Smear, primary source, with interpretation; routine stain for bacteria, fungi, or cell types	0.06*	0.13#	0	0.19#	XXX	0
87206	00	X	Smear, primary source, with interpretation; fluorescent and/or acid fast stain for bacteria, fungi, or cell types	0.06*	0.20#	0.01*	0.27#	XXX	0
87207	00	X	Smear, primary source, with interpretation; special stain for inclusion bodies or intracellular parasites (eg, malaria, kala azar, herpes)	0.37*	0.28#	0.02*	0.67#	XXX	0
87207	26			0.37	0.20	0.01	0.58	XXX	N
87208	00	X	Smear, primary source, with interpretation; direct or concentrated, dry, for ova and parasites	0.09*	0.17#	0.01*	0.27#	XXX	0
87210	00	X	Smear, primary source, with interpretation; wet mount with simple stain, for bacteria, fungi, ova, and/or parasites	0.04*	0.11#	0	0.15#	XXX	0
87211	00	X	Smear, primary source, with interpretation; wet and dry mount, for ova and parasites	0.06*	0.11#	0	0.17#	XXX	0
87220	00	X	Tissue examination for fungi (eg, KOH slide)	0.07*	0.13#	0.01*	0.21#	XXX	0
87230	00	X	Toxin or antitoxin assay, tissue culture (eg, Clostridium difficile toxin)	0.18*	0.41#	0.02*	0.61#	XXX	0
87250	00	X	Virus identification; inoculation of embryonated eggs, or small animal, includes observation and dissection	0.22*	0.33#	0.02*	0.57#	XXX	0
87252	00	X	Virus identification; tissue culture inoculation and observation	0.24*	0.52#	0.02*	0.78#	XXX	0
87253	00	X	Virus identification; tissue culture, additional studies (eg, hemabsorption, neutralization) each isolate	0.17*	0.39#	0.01*	0.57#	XXX	0
87999	00	X	Unlisted microbiology procedure	0	0	0	0	XXX	0
88045	00	N	Necropsy (autopsy); coroner's call	0	0	0	0	XXX	0
88099	00	N	Unlisted necropsy (autopsy) procedure	0	0	0	0	XXX	0
88104	00	A	Cytopathology, fluids, washings or brushings, except cervical or vaginal; smears with interpretation	0.56	0.44	0.04	1.04	XXX	N
88104	26			0.56	0.23	0.02	0.81	XXX	N
88104	TC			0	0.21	0.02	0.23	XXX	N
88106	00	A	Cytopathology, fluids, washings or brushings, except cervical or vaginal; filter method only with interpretation	0.56	0.37	0.03	0.96	XXX	N
88106	26			0.56	0.20	0.01	0.77	XXX	N
88106	TC			0	0.17	0.02	0.19	XXX	N
88107	00	A	Cytopathology, fluids, washings or brushings, except cervical or vaginal; smears and filter preparation with interpretation	0.76	0.47	0.04	1.27	XXX	N
88107	26			0.76	0.24	0.02	1.02	XXX	N
88107	TC			0	0.23	0.02	0.25	XXX	N
88108	00	A	Cytopathology, fluids, washings or brushings, except cervical or vaginal; concentration technique, smears and interpretation (eg, Saccomanno technique)	0.56	0.47	0.04	1.07	XXX	N
88108	26			0.56	0.24	0.02	0.82	XXX	N
88108	TC			0	0.23	0.02	0.25	XXX	N
88125	00	A	Cytopathology, forensic (eg, sperm)	0.26	0.11	0	0.37	XXX	N
88125	26			0.26	0.07	0	0.33	XXX	N
88125	TC			0	0.04	0	0.04	XXX	N

CPT codes and descriptions only, © 1994 American Medical Association. Reimbursement information, © 1995 McGraw-Hill Inc.

Code/ CPT	Mod- ifier	Status	Description	Work value	Practice expense	Mal- practice	Total value	Global period	Up- date
88130	00	X	Sex chromatin identification; Barr bodies	0.13*	0.31#	0.01*	0.45#	XXX	0
88140	00	X	Sex chromatin identification; peripheral blood smear, polymorphonuclear "drumsticks"	0.09*	0.22#	0.01*	0.32#	XXX	0
88150	00	X	Cytopathology, smears, cervical or vaginal, up to three smears; screening by technician under physician supervision	0.06*	0.11#	0	0.17#	XXX	0
88151	26			0.42	0.32	0.04	0.78	XXX	N
88155	00	X	Cytopathology, smears, cervical or vaginal, up to three smears; with definitive hormonal evaluation (eg, maturation index, karyopyknotic index, estrogenic index)	0.06*	0.15#	0	0.21#	XXX	0
88156	00	X	Cytopathology, smears, cervical or vaginal, (the Bethesda System (TBS)), up to three smears; screening by technician under physician supervision	0	0	0	0	XXX	0
88157	00	X	Cytopathology, smears, cervical or vaginal, (the Bethesda System (TBS)), up to three smears; requiring interpretation by physician	0	0	0	0	XXX	0
88157	26			0.42	0.32	0.04	0.78	XXX	N
88160	00	A	Cytopathology, smears, any other source; screening and interpretation	0.50	0.33	0.03	0.86	XXX	N
88160	26			0.50	0.17	0.01	0.68	XXX	N
88160	TC			0	0.16	0.02	0.18	XXX	N
88161	00	A	Cytopathology, smears, any other source; preparation, screening and interpretation	0.50	0.39	0.03	0.92	XXX	N
88161	26			0.50	0.20	0.01	0.71	XXX	N
88161	TC			0	0.19	0.02	0.21	XXX	N
88162	00	A	Cytopathology, smears, any other source; extended study involving over 5 slides and/or multiple stains	0.76	0.79	0.05	1.60	XXX	N
88162	26			0.76	0.41	0.03	1.20	XXX	N
88162	TC			0	0.38	0.02	0.40	XXX	N
88170	00	A	Fine needle aspiration with or without preparation of smears; superficial tissue (eg, thyroid, breast, prostate)	0.50	0.99	0.09	1.58	XXX	N
88170	26			0.50	0.52	0.05	1.07	XXX	N
88170	TC			0	0.47	0.04	0.51	XXX	N
88171	00	A	Fine needle aspiration with or without preparation of smears; deep tissue under radiologic guidance	1.05	1.35	0.09	2.49	XXX	N
88171	26			1.05	0.71	0.05	1.81	XXX	N
88171	TC			0	0.64	0.04	0.68	XXX	N
88172	00	A	Evaluation of fine needle aspirate with or without preparation of smears; immediate cytohistologic study to determine adequacy of specimen(s)	0.60	0.71	0.05	1.36	XXX	N
88172	26			0.60	0.36	0.03	0.99	XXX	N
88172	TC			0	0.35	0.02	0.37	XXX	N
88173	00	A	Evaluation of fine needle aspirate with or without preparation of smears; interpretation and report	1.08	0.87	0.05	2.00	XXX	N
88173	26			1.08	0.45	0.03	1.56	XXX	N
88173	TC			0	0.42	0.02	0.44	XXX	N
88180	00	A	Flow cytometry; each cell surface marker	0.36	0.33	0.03	0.72	XXX	N
88180	26			0.36	0.17	0.01	0.54	XXX	N
88180	TC			0	0.16	0.02	0.18	XXX	N
88182	00	A	Flow cytometry; cell cycle or DNA analysis	0.77	0.89	0.07	1.73	XXX	N
88182	26			0.77	0.45	0.03	1.25	XXX	N
88182	TC			0	0.44	0.04	0.48	XXX	N

CPT codes and descriptions only, © 1994 American Medical Association. Reimbursement information, © 1995 McGraw-Hill Inc.

Code/ CPT	Mod- ifier	Status	Description	Work value	Practice expense	Mal- practice	Total value	Global period	Up- date
88199	00	C	Unlisted cytopathology procedure	0	0	0	0	XXX	N
88230	00	X	Tissue culture for chromosome analysis; lymphocyte	1.01*	2.40#	0.07*	3.48#	XXX	0
88233	00	X	Tissue culture for chromosome analysis; skin or other solid tissue biopsy	1.22*	2.84#	0.08*	4.14#	XXX	0
88235	00	X	Tissue culture for chromosome analysis; amniotic fluid or chorionic villus cells	1.27*	2.97#	0.08*	4.32#	XXX	0
88237	00	X	Tissue culture for chromosome analysis; bone marrow (myeloid) cells	1.11*	2.58#	0.07*	3.76#	XXX	0
88239	00	X	Tissue culture for chromosome analysis; other tissue	1.27*	2.97#	0.08*	4.32#	XXX	0
88245	00	X	Chromosome analysis for breakage syndromes; score 25 cells (SCE study), count 5 cells, 1 karyotype, with banding (eg, Bloom syndrome)	1.29*	3.04#	0.09*	4.42#	XXX	0
88248	00	X	Chromosome analysis for breakage syndromes; score 100 cells, count 20 cells, 2 karyotypes, with banding (eg, ataxia telangiectasia, Fanconi anemia)	1.27*	2.97#	0.08*	4.32#	XXX	0
88250	00	X	Chromosome analysis for fragile X associated with fragile X-linked mental retardation, score 100 cells, count 20 cells, 2 karyotypes, with banding	1.38*	3.23#	0.09*	4.70#	XXX	0
88260	00	X	Chromosome analysis; count 5 cells, screening, with banding	0.98*	2.30#	0.07*	3.35#	XXX	0
88261	00	X	Chromosome analysis; count 5 cells, 1 karyotype, with banding	1.64*	3.82#	0.10*	5.56#	XXX	0
88262	00	X	Chromosome analysis; count 15–20 cells, 2 karyotypes, with banding	1.59*	3.67#	0.10*	5.36#	XXX	0
88263	00	X	Chromosome analysis; count 45 cells for mosaicism, 2 karyotypes, with banding	1.33*	3.10#	0.08*	4.51#	XXX	0
88267	00	X	Chromosome analysis, amniotic fluid or chorionic villus, count 15 cells, 1 karyotype, with banding	2.42*	5.64#	0.15*	8.21#	XXX	0
88269	00	X	Chromosome analysis, in situ for amniotic fluid cells, count cells from 6–12 colonies, 1 karyotype, with banding	1.48*	2.95#	0.08*	4.51#	XXX	0
88280	00	X	Chromosome analysis; additional karyotypes, each study	0.31*	0.72#	0.02*	1.05#	XXX	0
88283	00	X	Chromosome analysis; additional specialized banding technique (eg, NOR, C-banding)	0.61*	1.42#	0.04*	2.07#	XXX	0
88285	00	X	Chromosome analysis; additional cells counted, each study	0.17*	0.39#	0	0.56#	XXX	0
88289	00	X	Chromosome analysis; additional high resolution study	0.31*	0.72#	0.02*	1.05#	XXX	0
88299	00	C	Unlisted cytogenetic study	0	0	0	0	XXX	N
88300	00	A	LEVEL I—Surgical pathology, gross examination only	0.08	0.20	0.01	0.29	XXX	N
88300	26			0.08	0.10	0.01	0.19	XXX	N
88300	TC			0	0.10	0	0.10	XXX	N
88302	00	A	LEVEL II—Surgical pathology, gross and microscopic examination Appendix, Incidental Fallopian Tube, Sterilization Fingers/Toes, Amputation, Traumatic Foreskin, Newborn Hernia Sac, Any Location Hydrocele Sac Nerve Skin, Plastic Repair Sympathetic Ganglion Testis, Castration Vaginal Mucosa, Incidental Vas Deferens, Sterilization	0.13	0.43	0.04	0.60	XXX	N
88302	26			0.13	0.20	0.02	0.35	XXX	N
88302	TC			0	0.23	0.02	0.25	XXX	N

CPT codes and descriptions only, © 1994 American Medical Association. Reimbursement information, © 1995 McGraw-Hill Inc.

Code/ CPT	Mod-ifier	Status	Description	Work value	Practice expense	Mal-practice	Total value	Global period	Up-date
88304	00	A	LEVEL III—Surgical pathology, gross and microscopic examination Abortion, Induced Abscess Aneurysm—Arterial/Ventricular Anus, Tag Appendix, Other than Incidental Artery, Atheromatous Plaque Bartholin's Gland Cyst Bone Fragment(s), Other than Pathologic Fracture Bursa/Synovial Cyst Carpal Tunnel Tissue Cartilage, Shavings Cholesteatoma Colon, Colostomy Stoma Conjunctiva—Biopsy/Pterygium Cornea Diverticulum—Esophagus/Small Bowel Dupuytren's Contracture Tissue Femoral Head, Other than Fracture Fissure/Fistula Foreskin, Other than Newborn Gallbladder Ganglion Cyst Hematoma Hemorrhoids Hydatid of Morgagni Intervertebral Disc Joint, Loose Body Meniscus Mucocele, Salivary Neuroma—Morton's/Traumatic Pilonidal Cyst/Sinus Polyps, Inflammatory—Nasal/Sinusoidal Skin—Cyst/Tag/Debridement Soft Tissue, Debridement Soft Tissue, Lipoma Spermatocele Tendon/Tendon Sheath Testicular Appendage Thrombus or Embolus Tonsil and/or Adenoids Varicocele Vas Deferens, Other than Sterilization Vein, Varicosity	0.22	0.62	0.04	0.88	XXX	N
88304	26			0.22	0.29	0.02	0.53	XXX	N
88304	TC			0	0.33	0.02	0.35	XXX	N
88305	00	A	LEVEL IV—Surgical pathology, gross and microscopic examination Abortion—Spontaneous/Missed Artery, Biopsy Bone Marrow, Biopsy Bone Exostosis Brain/Meninges, Other than for Tumor Resection Breast, Biopsy Breast, Reduction Mammoplasty Bronchus, Biopsy Cell Block, Any Source Cervix, Biopsy Colon, Biopsy Duodenum, Biopsy Endocervix, Curettings/Biopsy Endometrium, Curettings/Biopsy Esophagus, Biopsy Extremity, Amputation, Traumatic Fallopian Tube, Biopsy Fallopian Tube, Ectopic Pregnancy Femoral Head, Fracture Fingers/Toes, Amputation, Non-traumatic Gingiva/Oral Mucosa, Biopsy Heart Valve Joint, Resection Kidney, Biopsy Larynx, Biopsy Leiomyoma(s), Uterine Myomectomy—without Uterus Lip, Biopsy/Wedge Resection Lung, Transbronchial Biopsy Lymph Node, Biopsy Muscle, Biopsy Nasal Mucosa, Biopsy Nasopharynx/Oropharynx, Biopsy Nerve, Biopsy Odontogenic/Dental Cyst Omentum, Biopsy Ovary with or without Tube, Non-neoplastic Ovary, Biopsy/Wedge Resection Parathyroid Gland Peritoneum, Biopsy Pituitary Tumor Placenta, Other than Third Trimester Pleura/Pericardium—Biopsy/Tissue Polyp, Cervical/Endometrial Polyp, Colorectal Polyp, Stomach/Small Bowel Prostate, Needle Biopsy Prostate, TUR Salivary Gland, Biopsy Sinus, Paranasal Skin, Other than Cyst/Tag/Debridement/Plastic Repair Small Intestine, Soft Tissue, Other than Tumor/Mass/Lipoma/Debridement, Biopsy Testis, Other than Tumor/Biopsy/Castration Thyroglossal Duct/Brachial Cleft Tongue, Biopsy Tonsil, Trachea, Ureter, Biopsy Urethra, Urinary Bladder, Uterus, with or without Tubes & Ovaries, for Vagina, Vulva/Labia, Biopsy	0.75	1.03	0.08	1.86	XXX	N
88305	26			0.75	0.53	0.04	1.32	XXX	N
88305	TC			0	0.50	0.04	0.54	XXX	N

CPT codes and descriptions only, © 1994 American Medical Association. Reimbursement information, © 1995 McGraw-Hill Inc.

Code/ CPT	Mod-ifier	Status	Description	Work value	Practice expense	Mal-practice	Total value	Global period	Up-date
88307	00	A	LEVEL V—Surgical pathology, gross and microscopic examination Adrenal, Resection Bone—Biopsy/Curettings Bone Fragment(s), Pathologic Fracture Brain, Biopsy Brain/Meninges, Tumor Resection Breast, Mastectomy—Partial/Simple Cervix, Conization Colon, Segmental Resection, Other than for Tumor Extremity, Amputation, Non-traumatic Eye, Enucleation Kidney, Partial/Total Nephrectomy Larynx, Partial/Total Resection Liver, Biopsy—Needle/Wedge Liver, Partial Resection Lung, Wedge Biopsy Lymph Nodes, Regional Resection Mediastinum, Mass Myocardium, Biopsy Odontogenic Tumor Ovary with or without Tube, Neoplastic Pancreas, Biopsy Placenta, Third Trimester Prostate, Except Radical Resection Salivary Gland Small Intestine, Resection, Other than for Tumor Soft Tissue Mass (except Lipoma)—Biopsy/Simple Excision Stomach—Subtotal/Total Resection, Other than for Tumor Testis, Biopsy Thymus, Tumor Thyroid, Total/Lobe Ureter, Resection Urinary Bladder, TUR Uterus, with or without Tubes & Ovaries, Other than Neoplastic/Prolapse	1.59	1.52	0.12	3.23	XXX	N
88307	26			1.59	0.78	0.06	2.43	XXX	N
88307	TC			0	0.74	0.06	0.80	XXX	N
88309	00	A	LEVEL VI—Surgical pathology, gross and microscopic examination Bone Resection Breast, Mastectomy—with Regional Lymph Nodes Colon, Segmental Resection for Tumor Colon, Total Resection Esophagus, Partial/Total Resection Extremity, Disarticulation Fetus, with Dissection Larynx, Partial/Total Resection—with Regional Lymph Nodes Lung—Total/Lobe/Segment Resection Pancreas, Total/Subtotal Resection Prostate, Radical Resection Small Intestine, Resection for Tumor Soft Tissue Tumor, Extensive Resection Stomach—Subtotal/Total Resection for Tumor Testis, Tumor Tongue/Tonsil—Resection for Tumor Urinary Bladder, Partial/Total Resection Uterus, with or without Tubes & Ovaries, Neoplastic Vulva, Total/Subtotal Resection	2.28	1.92	0.13	4.33	XXX	N
88309	26			2.28	0.99	0.07	3.34	XXX	N
88309	TC			0	0.93	0.06	0.99	XXX	N
88311	00	A	Decalcification procedure (List separately in addition to code for surgical pathology examination)	0.24	0.21	0.01	0.46	XXX	N
88311	26			0.24	0.11	0.01	0.36	XXX	N
88311	TC			0	0.10	0	0.10	XXX	N
88312	00	A	Special stains (List separately in addition to code for surgical pathology examination); Group I for microorganisms (eg, Gridley, acid fast, methenamine silver), each	0.54	0.26	0.01	0.81	XXX	N
88312	26			0.54	0.14	0.01	0.69	XXX	N
88312	TC			0	0.12	0	0.12	XXX	N
88313	00	A	Special stains (List separately in addition to code for surgical pathology examination); Group II, all other, (eg, iron, trichrome), except immunocytochemistry and immunoperoxidase stains, each	0.24	0.21	0.01	0.46	XXX	N
88313	26			0.24	0.11	0.01	0.36	XXX	N
88313	TC			0	0.10	0	0.10	XXX	N

CPT codes and descriptions only, © 1994 American Medical Association. Reimbursement information, © 1995 McGraw-Hill Inc.

Code/ CPT	Mod-ifier	Status	Description	Work value	Practice expense	Mal-practice	Total value	Global period	Up-date
88314	00	A	Special stains (List separately in addition to code for surgical pathology examination); histochemical staining with frozen section(s)	0.45	0.62	0.04	1.11	XXX	N
88314	26			0.45	0.35	0.02	0.82	XXX	N
88314	TC			0	0.27	0.02	0.29	XXX	N
88318	00	A	Determinative histochemistry to identify chemical components (eg, copper, zinc)	0.42	0.24	0.01	0.67	XXX	N
88318	26			0.42	0.12	0.01	0.55	XXX	N
88318	TC			0	0.12	0	0.12	XXX	N
88319	00	A	Determinative histochemistry or cytochemistry to identify enzyme constituents, each	0.53	0.49	0.04	1.06	XXX	N
88319	26			0.53	0.26	0.02	0.81	XXX	N
88319	TC			0	0.23	0.02	0.25	XXX	N
88321	00	A	Consultation and report on referred slides prepared elsewhere	1.30	0.41	0.03	1.74	XXX	N
88323	00	A	Consultation and report on referred material requiring preparation of slides	1.35	0.72	0.05	2.12	XXX	N
88323	26			1.35	0.39	0.03	1.77	XXX	N
88323	TC			0	0.33	0.02	0.35	XXX	N
88325	00	A	Consultation, comprehensive, with review of records and specimens, with report on referred material	2.22	0.47	0.04	2.73	XXX	N
88329	00	A	Pathology consultation during surgery;	0.67	0.37	0.03	1.07	XXX	N
88331	00	A	Pathology consultation during surgery; with frozen section(s), single specimen	1.19	1.10	0.08	2.37	XXX	N
88331	26			1.19	0.56	0.04	1.79	XXX	N
88331	TC			0	0.54	0.04	0.58	XXX	N
88332	00	A	Pathology consultation during surgery; each additional tissue block with frozen section(s)	0.59	0.56	0.04	1.19	XXX	N
88332	26			0.59	0.29	0.02	0.90	XXX	N
88332	TC			0	0.27	0.02	0.29	XXX	N
88342	00	A	Immunocytochemistry (including tissue immunoperoxidase), each antibody	0.85	0.64	0.04	1.53	XXX	N
88342	26			0.85	0.33	0.02	1.20	XXX	N
88342	TC			0	0.31	0.02	0.33	XXX	N
88346	00	A	Immunofluorescent study, each antibody; direct method	0.86	0.58	0.04	1.48	XXX	N
88346	26			0.86	0.31	0.02	1.19	XXX	N
88346	TC			0	0.27	0.02	0.29	XXX	N
88347	00	A	Immunofluorescent study, each antibody; indirect method	0.86	0.42	0.04	1.32	XXX	N
88347	26			0.86	0.15	0.02	1.03	XXX	N
88347	TC			0	0.27	0.02	0.29	XXX	N
88348	00	A	Electron microscopy; diagnostic	1.51	2.28	0.16	3.95	XXX	N
88348	26			1.51	1.19	0.08	2.78	XXX	N
88348	TC			0	1.09	0.08	1.17	XXX	N
88349	00	A	Electron microscopy; scanning	0.76	1.55	0.12	2.43	XXX	N
88349	26			0.76	0.79	0.06	1.61	XXX	N
88349	TC			0	0.76	0.06	0.82	XXX	N
88355	00	A	Morphometric analysis; skeletal muscle	1.85	1.74	0.13	3.72	XXX	N
88355	26			1.85	0.92	0.07	2.84	XXX	N
88355	TC			0	0.82	0.06	0.88	XXX	N
88356	00	A	Morphometric analysis; nerve	3.02	2.66	0.18	5.86	XXX	N
88356	26			3.02	1.39	0.10	4.51	XXX	N

CPT codes and descriptions only, © 1994 American Medical Association. Reimbursement information, © 1995 McGraw-Hill Inc.

Code/ CPT	Mod- ifier	Status	Description	Work value	Practice expense	Mal- practice	Total value	Global period	Up- date
88356	TC			0	1.27	0.08	1.35	XXX	N
88358	00	A	Morphometric analysis; tumor	2.82	2.32	0.16	5.30	XXX	N
88358	26			2.82	1.16	0.08	4.06	XXX	N
88358	TC			0	1.16	0.08	1.24	XXX	N
88362	00	A	Nerve teasing preparations	2.17	1.97	0.13	4.27	XXX	N
88362	26			2.17	1.00	0.07	3.24	XXX	N
88362	TC			0	0.97	0.06	1.03	XXX	N
88365	00	A	Tissue in situ hybridization, interpretation and report	0.93	0.75	0.05	1.73	XXX	N
88365	26			0.93	0.38	0.03	1.34	XXX	N
88365	TC			0	0.37	0.02	0.39	XXX	N
88371	00	X	Protein analysis of tissue by Western Blot, with interpretation and report;	0	0	0	0	XXX	0
88371	26			0.37	0.20	0.01	0.58	XXX	N
88372	00	X	Protein analysis of tissue by Western Blot, with interpretation and report; immunological probe for band identification, each	0	0	0	0	XXX	0
88372	26			0.37	0.20	0.01	0.58	XXX	N
88399	00	C	Unlisted surgical pathology procedure	0	0	0	0	XXX	N
89050	00	X	Cell count, miscellaneous body fluids (eg, CSF, joint fluid), except blood;	0.06*	0.11#	0	0.17#	XXX	0
89051	00	X	Cell count, miscellaneous body fluids (eg, CSF, joint fluid), except blood; with differential count	0.07*	0.15#	0.01*	0.23#	XXX	0
89060	00	X	Crystal identification by light microscopy with or without polarizing lens analysis, any body fluid (except urine)	0.37*	0.28#	0.01*	0.66#	XXX	0
89060	26			0.37	0.20	0.01	0.58	XXX	N
89100	00	A	Duodenal intubation and aspiration; single specimen (eg, simple bile study or afferent loop culture) plus appropriate test procedure	0.60	0.42	0.03	1.05	XXX	N
89105	00	A	Duodenal intubation and aspiration; collection of multiple fractional specimens with pancreatic or gallbladder stimulation, single or double lumen tube	0.50	0.39	0.03	0.92	XXX	N
89125	00	X	Fat stain, feces, urine, or sputum	0.07*	0.17#	0	0.24#	XXX	0
89130	00	A	Gastric intubation and aspiration, diagnostic, each specimen, for chemical analyses or cytopathology;	0.45	0.41	0.03	0.89	XXX	N
89132	00	A	Gastric intubation and aspiration, diagnostic, each specimen, for chemical analyses or cytopathology; after stimulation	0.19	0.19	0.02	0.40	XXX	N
89135	00	A	Gastric intubation, aspiration, and fractional collections (eg, gastric secretory study); one hour	0.79	0.58	0.04	1.41	XXX	N
89136	00	A	Gastric intubation, aspiration, and fractional collections (eg, gastric secretory study); two hours	0.21	0.22	0.02	0.45	XXX	N
89140	00	A	Gastric intubation, aspiration, and fractional collections (eg, gastric secretory study); two hours including gastric stimulation (eg, histalog, pentagastrin)	0.94	0.81	0.07	1.82	XXX	N
89141	00	A	Gastric intubation, aspiration, and fractional collections (eg, gastric secretory study); three hours, including gastric stimulation	0.85	0.73	0.06	1.64	XXX	N
89160	00	X	Meat fibers, feces	0.04*	0.07#	0	0.11#	XXX	0
89190	00	X	Nasal smear for eosinophils	0.06*	0.11#	0	0.17#	XXX	0
89300	00	X	Semen analysis; presence and/or motility of sperm including Huhner test	0.13*	0.26#	0	0.39#	XXX	0
89310	00	X	Semen analysis; motility and count	0.09*	0.24#	0.01*	0.34#	XXX	0

CPT codes and descriptions only, © 1994 American Medical Association. Reimbursement information, © 1995 McGraw-Hill Inc.

Code/ CPT	Mod- ifier	Status	Description	Work value	Practice expense	Mal- practice	Total value	Global period	Up- date
89320	00	X	Semen analysis; complete (volume, count, motility and differential)	0.11*	0.28#	0	0.39#	XXX	0
89325	00	X	Sperm antibodies	0.09*	0.24#	0.01*	0.34#	XXX	0
89329	00	X	Sperm evaluation; hamster penetration test	0.42*	0.74#	0.02*	1.18#	XXX	0
89330	00	X	Sperm evaluation; cervical mucus penetration test, with or without spinnbarkeit test	0.09*	0.24#	0.01*	0.34#	XXX	0
89350	00	A	Sputum, obtaining specimen, aerosol induced technique (separate procedure)	0	0.39	0.03	0.42	XXX	N
89355	00	X	Starch granules, feces	0.06*	0.11#	0	0.17#	XXX	0
89360	00	A	Sweat collection by iontophoresis	0	0.43	0.03	0.46	XXX	N
89365	00	X	Water load test	0.13*	0.30#	0	0.43#	XXX	0
89399	00	C	Unlisted miscellaneous pathology test	0	0	0	0	XXX	N

CPT codes and descriptions only, © 1994 American Medical Association. Reimbursement information, © 1995 McGraw-Hill Inc.

CHAPTER 5

Medicine

The editors have elected to indicate that a relative value is not available for procedures with a "0" in the individual units column.

I. Separate Procedures: Procedures identified as "separate procedures" are frequently included in the global value of other procedures. Listing of a "separate procedure" code and full value is appropriate if the procedure is not included in the global value of another. Listing of "separate procedure" codes is not appropriate when procedure is included in the global value of another.

II. Unusual Service or Procedure: A service may necessitate skills and time of the physician over and above listed services and values. If substantiated "by report" (BR), additional values may be warranted. Use modifier -22 to indicate these procedures.

III. Unlisted Service or Procedure: When a service or procedure provided is not adequately identified, use of the unlisted procedure code for the related anatomical area is appropriate. Most codes of this nature have 99 for the last two digits. Value should be substantiated "by report" (BR).

IV. Procedures without Specified Unit Values: Procedures which have RNE or BR in the units column should be substantiated "by report."

V. By Report: Value of a procedure should be established for any "by report" circumstance by identifying a similar service and justifying value difference. When a report is indicated, the report should include the following:

1. Accurate procedure definition or description;
2. Justification for procedural variance, when appropriate;
3. Similar procedure and value; and
4. Justification for value difference.

VI. Reduced Values: Under some circumstances, value for a procedure may be reduced or eliminated. Use modifier -52 to identify reduced value services.

VII. Multiple Modifiers: If circumstances require the use of more than one modifier with any one procedure code, modifier -99 should be added to the procedure code. Other modifiers are then attached to the procedure code and listed separately with appropriate values for each.

VIII. Materials Supplied by Physician: Supplies and materials provided by the physician (i.e., sterile trays, drugs, etc.) are considered to be bundled by Medicare. Supplies should not be billed separately except for permanent condition supplies, home use, and surgical trays

CPT codes and descriptions only, © 1994 American Medical Association. Reimbursement information, © 1995 McGraw-Hill Inc.

for designated procedures. For use within the private sector, identify supplies by using code 99070. Supplies and materials provided by the physician (i.e., sterile trays, drugs, etc.) over and above those usually indicated with the office visit or other services rendered may be listed separately. This rule varies by contract.

IX. **Professional Component:** The unit value listed next to the modifier column (modifier -26) is used to designate professional services. Modifier -26 is added to the procedure code to indicate the use of this value. The professional component includes examination of the patient, when indicated, performance and/or supervision of the procedure or lab test, interpretation and/or written report concerning the examination or lab test, and consultation with referring physicians.

CPT codes and descriptions only, © 1994 American Medical Association. Reimbursement information, © 1995 McGraw-Hill Inc.

Editor's Note: The variable costs associated with immunizations have caused some difficulty in establishing a fair relative value. The editors have elected to insert unit values which do *not* include the cost of the injectable. For billing purposes, one can conform to CPT instructions and add the cost of the injectable to the administration value or break from CPT and code the injectable separately.

MEDICINE VALUES

Code/ CPT	Mod- ifier	Status	Description	Work value	Practice expense	Mal- practice	Total value	Global period	Up- date
90700	00	E	Immunization, active; diphtheria, tetanus toxoids, and acellular pertussis vaccine (DTaP)	0.24*	0.29#	0.02*	0.55#	XXX	0
90701	00	E	Immunization, active; diphtheria and tetanus toxoids and pertussis vaccine (DTP)	0.24*	0.29#	0.02*	0.55#	XXX	0
90702	00	E	Immunization, active; diphtheria and tetanus toxoids (DT)	0.12*	0.14#	0.01*	0.27#	XXX	0
90703	00	E	Immunization, active; tetanus toxoid	0.12*	0.14#	0.01*	0.27#	XXX	0
90704	00	E	Immunization, active; mumps virus vaccine, live	0.15*	0.18#	0.01*	0.34#	XXX	0
90705	00	E	Immunization, active; measles virus vaccine, live, attenuated	0.15*	0.18#	0.01*	0.34#	XXX	0
90706	00	E	Immunization, active; rubella virus vaccine, live	0.15*	0.18#	0.01*	0.34#	XXX	0
90707	00	E	Immunization, active; measles, mumps and rubella virus vaccine, live	0.32*	0.38#	0.03*	0.73#	XXX	0
90708	00	E	Immunization, active; measles and rubella virus vaccine, live	0.21*	0.25#	0.02*	0.48#	XXX	0
90709	00	E	Immunization, active; rubella and mumps virus vaccine, live	0.21*	0.25#	0.02*	0.48#	XXX	0
90710	00	E	Immunization, active; measles, mumps, rubella, and varicella vaccine	0.24*	0.29#	0.02*	0.55#	XXX	0
90711	00	E	Immunization, active; diphtheria, tetanus, and pertussis (DTP) and injectable poliomyelitis vaccine	0.24*	0.29#	0.02*	0.55#	XXX	0
90712	00	E	Immunization, active; poliovirus vaccine, live, oral (any type(s))	0.24*	0.29#	0.02*	0.55#	XXX	0
90713	00	E	Immunization, active; poliomyelitis vaccine	0.15*	0.18#	0.01*	0.34#	XXX	0
90714	00	E	Immunization, active; typhoid vaccine	0.12*	0.14#	0.01*	0.27#	XXX	0
90716	00	E	Immunization, active; varicella (chicken pox) vaccine	0.15*	0.18#	0.01*	0.34#	XXX	0
90717	00	E	Immunization, active; yellow fever vaccine	0.12*	0.14#	0.01*	0.27#	XXX	0
90718	00	E	Immunization, active; tetanus and diphtheria toxoids absorbed, for adult use (Td)	0.15*	0.18#	0.01*	0.34#	XXX	0
90719	00	E	Immunization, active; diphtheria toxoid	0.12*	0.14#	0.01*	0.27#	XXX	0
90720	00	E	Immunization, active; diphtheria, tetanus, and pertussis (DTP) and Hemophilus influenza B (HIB) vaccine	0.27*	0.32#	0.02*	0.61#	XXX	0
90724	00	X	Immunization, active; influenza virus vaccine	0.18*	0.21#	0.02*	0.41#	XXX	0
90725	00	N	Immunization, active; cholera vaccine	0.12*	0.14#	0.01*	0.27#	XXX	0
90726	00	E	Immunization, active; rabies vaccine	0.15*	0.18#	0.01*	0.34#	XXX	0
90727	00	E	Immunization, active; plague vaccine	0.15*	0.18#	0.01*	0.34#	XXX	0
90728	00	E	Immunization, active; BCG vaccine	0.15*	0.18#	0.01*	0.34#	XXX	0
90730	00	E	Immunization, active; hepatitis A vaccine	0.28*	0.33#	0.02*	0.63#	XXX	0
90731	00	X	Immunization, active; hepatitis B vaccine	0.28*	0.33#	0.02*	0.63#	XXX	0
90732	00	X	Immunization, active; pneumococcal vaccine, polyvalent	0.18*	0.21#	0.02*	0.41#	XXX	0
90733	00	E	Immunization, active; meningococcal polysaccharide vaccine (any group(s))	0.18*	0.21#	0.02*	0.41#	XXX	0
90735	00	E	Immunization, active; encephalitis virus vaccine	0.18*	0.21#	0.02*	0.41#	XXX	0
90737	00	E	Immunization, active; Hemophilus influenza B	0.27*	0.32#	0.02*	0.61#	XXX	0

CPT codes and descriptions only, © 1994 American Medical Association. Reimbursement information, © 1995 McGraw-Hill Inc.

Code/ CPT	Mod-ifier	Status	Description	Work value	Practice expense	Mal-practice	Total value	Global period	Up-date
90741	00	E	Immunization, passive; immune serum globulin, human (ISG)	0.12*	0.14#	0.01*	0.27#	XXX	0
90742	00	E	Immunization, passive; specific hyperimmune serum globulin (eg, hepatitis B, measles, pertussis, rabies, Rho(D), tetanus, vaccinia, varicella-zoster)	0.27*	0.32#	0.02*	0.61#	XXX	0
90749	00	C	Unlisted immunization procedure	0	0	0	0	XXX	N
90780	00	A	IV infusion for therapy/diagnosis, administered by physician or under direct supervision of physician; up to one hour	0	1.06	0.08	1.14	XXX	N
90781	00	A	IV infusion for therapy/diagnosis, administered by physician or under direct supervision of physician; each additional hour, up to eight (8) hours	0	0.53	0.04	0.57	XXX	N
90782	00	T	Therapeutic or diagnostic injection (specify material injected); subcutaneous or intramuscular	0	0.10	0.01	0.11	XXX	N
90783	00	T	Therapeutic or diagnostic injection (specify material injected); intra-arterial	0	0.39	0.03	0.42	XXX	N
90784	00	T	Therapeutic or diagnostic injection (specify material injected); intravenous	0	0.45	0.04	0.49	XXX	N
90788	00	T	Intramuscular injection of antibiotic (specify)	0	0.11	0.01	0.12	XXX	N
90799	00	C	Unlisted therapeutic or diagnostic injection	0	0	0	0	XXX	N
90801	00	A	Psychiatric diagnostic interview examination including history, mental status, or disposition (may include communication with family or other sources, ordering and medical interpretation of laboratory or other medical diagnostic studies. In certain circumstances other informants will be seen in lieu of the patient)	2.19	0.67	0.09	2.95	XXX	N
90820	00	A	Interactive medical psychiatric diagnostic interview examination	2.25	0.38	0.05	2.68	XXX	N
90825	00	A	Psychiatric evaluation of hospital records, other psychiatric reports, psychometric and/or projective tests, and other accumulated data for medical diagnostic purposes	0.97	0.31	0.04	1.32	XXX	N
90830	00	A	Psychological testing (includes psychodiagnostic assessment of personality, psychopathology, emotionality, intellectual abilities, eg, WAIS-R, Rorschach, MMPI) with interpretation and report, per hour	0	1.68	0.20	1.88	XXX	N
90835	00	A	Narcosynthesis for psychiatric diagnostic and therapeutic purposes (eg, sodium amobarbital (Amytal) interview)	2.82	0.50	0.07	3.39	XXX	N
90841	00	G	Individual medical psychotherapy by a physician, with continuing medical diagnostic evaluation, and drug management when indicated, including insight oriented, behavior modifying or supportive psychotherapy; time unspecified	1.41*	0.53#	0.07*	2.01#	XXX	0
90842	00	A	Individual medical psychotherapy by a physician, with continuing medical diagnostic evaluation, and drug management when indicated, including insight oriented, behavior modifying or supportive psychotherapy; approximately 75 to 80 minutes	2.74	1.04	0.15	3.93	XXX	N
90843	00	A	Individual medical psychotherapy by a physician, with continuing medical diagnostic evaluation, and drug management when indicated, including insight oriented, behavior modifying or supportive psychotherapy; approximately 20 to 30 minutes	1.10	0.35	0.05	1.50	XXX	N
90844	00	A	Individual medical psychotherapy by a physician, with continuing medical diagnostic evaluation, and drug management when indicated, including insight oriented, behavior modifying or supportive psychotherapy; approximately 45 to 50 minutes	1.72	0.54	0.08	2.34	XXX	N

CPT codes and descriptions only, © 1994 American Medical Association. Reimbursement information, © 1995 McGraw-Hill Inc.

Code/ CPT	Mod- ifier	Status	Description	Work value	Practice expense	Mal- practice	Total value	Global period	Up- date
90845	00	A	Medical psychoanalysis	1.78	0.41	0.05	2.24	XXX	N
90846	00	A	Family medical psychotherapy (without the patient present)	1.82	0.62	0.08	2.52	XXX	N
90847	00	A	Family medical psychotherapy (conjoint psychotherapy) by a physician, with continuing medical diagnostic evaluation, and drug management when indicated	2.19	0.58	0.08	2.85	XXX	N
90849	00	R	Multiple-family group medical psychotherapy by a physician, with continuing medical diagnostic evaluation, and drug management when indicated	0.59	0.26	0.03	0.88	XXX	N
90853	00	A	Group medical psychotherapy (other than of a multiple-family group) by a physician, with continuing medical diagnostic evaluation and drug management when indicated	0.43	0.26	0.03	0.72	XXX	N
90855	00	A	Interactive individual medical psychotherapy	1.81	0.59	0.09	2.49	XXX	N
90857	00	A	Interactive group medical psychotherapy	0.43	0.15	0.02	0.60	XXX	N
90862	00	A	Pharmacologic management, including prescription, use, and review of medication with no more than minimal medical psychotherapy	0.95	0.37	0.05	1.37	XXX	N
90870	00	A	Electroconvulsive therapy (includes necessary monitoring); single seizure	1.88	0.55	0.08	2.51	0	N
90871	00	A	Electroconvulsive therapy (includes necessary monitoring); multiple seizures, per day	2.72	0.83	0.13	3.68	0	N
90880	00	A	Medical hypnotherapy	2.19	0.64	0.07	2.90	XXX	N
90882	00	N	Environmental intervention for medical management purposes on a psychiatric patient's behalf with agencies, employers, or institutions	0.02*	0.01#	0.01	0.04#	XXX	0
90887	00	A	Interpretation or explanation of results of psychiatric, other medical examinations and procedures, or other accumulated data to family or other responsible persons, or advising them how to assist patient	1.48	0.33	0.04	1.85	XXX	N
90889	00	B	Preparation of report of patient's psychiatric status, history, treatment, or progress (other than for legal or consultative purposes) for other physicians, agencies, or insurance carriers	0.02*	0.01#	0.01	0.04#	XXX	0
90899	00	C	Unlisted psychiatric service or procedure	0	0	0	0	XXX	N
90900	00	A	Biofeedback training; by electromyogram application (eg, in tension headache, muscle spasm)	0.89	0.90	0.08	1.87	0	N
90902	00	A	Biofeedback training; in conduction disorder (eg, arrhythmia)	0.89	0.63	0.05	1.57	0	N
90904	00	A	Biofeedback training; regulation of blood pressure (eg, in essential hypertension)	0.89	0.35	0.03	1.27	0	N
90906	00	A	Biofeedback training; regulation of skin temperature or peripheral blood flow	0.89	1.60	0.11	2.60	0	N
90908	00	A	Biofeedback training; by electroencephalogram application (eg, in anxiety, insomnia)	0.89	0.86	0.06	1.81	0	N
90910	00	A	Biofeedback training; by electro-oculogram application (eg, in blepharospasm)	0.89	0.67	0.10	1.66	0	N
90911	00	A	Biofeedback training; anorectal, including EMG and/or manometry	2.15	1.13	0.27	3.55	0	N
90915	00	A	Biofeedback training; other	0.89	0.76	0.06	1.71	0	N
90918	00	A	End stage renal disease (ESRD) related services per full month; for patients under 2 years of age to include monitoring for the adequacy of nutrition, assessment of growth and development, and counseling of parents	9.77	2.18	0.14	12.09	XXX	N

CPT codes and descriptions only, © 1994 American Medical Association. Reimbursement information, © 1995 McGraw-Hill Inc.

Code/ CPT	Mod- ifier	Status	Description	Work value	Practice expense	Mal- practice	Total value	Global period	Up- date
90919	00	A	End stage renal disease (ESRD) related services per full month; between the second and twelfth birthdays to include monitoring for the adequacy of nutrition, assessment of growth and development, and counseling of parents	7.13	2.18	0.14	9.45	XXX	N
90920	00	A	End stage renal disease (ESRD) related services per full month; through age nineteen to include monitoring for the adequacy of nutrition, assessment of growth and development, and counseling of parents	5.86	2.18	0.14	8.18	XXX	N
90921	00	A	End stage renal disease (ESRD) related services per full month; for patients twenty years of age and over	3.06	2.18	0.14	5.38	XXX	N
90922	00	A	End stage renal disease (ESRD) related services (less than full month), per day	0.10	0.07	0.01	0.18	XXX	N
90935	00	A	Hemodialysis procedure with single physician evaluation	1.22	1.49	0.10	2.81	0	N
90937	00	A	Hemodialysis procedure requiring repeated evaluation(s) with or without substantial revision of dialysis prescription	2.11	2.65	0.18	4.94	0	N
90945	00	A	Dialysis procedure other than hemodialysis (eg, peritoneal, hemofiltration), with single physician evaluation	1.28	1.27	0.08	2.63	0	N
90947	00	A	Dialysis procedure other than hemodialysis (eg, peritoneal, hemofiltration) requiring repeated evaluations, with or without substantial revision of dialysis prescription	2.16	2.09	0.14	4.39	0	N
90989	00	X	Dialysis training, patient, including helper where applicable, any mode, completed course	2.95*	2.10#	0.13*	5.18#	XXX	0
90993	00	X	Dialysis training, patient, including helper where applicable, any mode, course not completed, per training session	0.71*	0.51#	0.03*	1.25#	XXX	0
90997	00	A	Hemoperfusion (eg, with activated charcoal or resin)	1.84	2.35	0.16	4.35	0	N
90999	00	C	Unlisted dialysis procedure, inpatient or outpatient	0	0	0	0	XXX	N
91000	00	A	Esophageal intubation and collection of washings for cytology, including preparation of specimens (separate procedure)	0.99	0.66	0.06	1.71	0	N
91000	26			0.99	0.59	0.05	1.63	0	N
91000	TC			0	0.07	0.01	0.08	0	N
91010	00	A	Esophageal motility study;	1.65	2.28	0.17	4.10	0	N
91010	26			1.65	1.50	0.11	3.26	0	N
91010	TC			0	0.78	0.06	0.84	0	N
91011	00	A	Esophageal motility study; with mecholyl or similar stimulant	1.98	2.66	0.18	4.82	0	N
91011	26			1.98	1.68	0.11	3.77	0	N
91011	TC			0	0.98	0.07	1.05	0	N
91012	00	A	Esophageal motility study; with acid perfusion studies	1.92	3.12	0.23	5.27	0	N
91012	26			1.92	2.02	0.15	4.09	0	N
91012	TC			0	1.10	0.08	1.18	0	N
91020	00	A	Esophagogastric manometric studies	1.89	2.50	0.18	4.57	0	N
91020	26			1.89	1.77	0.12	3.78	0	N
91020	TC			0	0.73	0.06	0.79	0	N
91030	00	A	Esophagus, acid perfusion (Bernstein) test for esophagitis	1.20	0.56	0.05	1.81	0	N
91030	26			1.20	0.35	0.03	1.58	0	N
91030	TC			0	0.21	0.02	0.23	0	N
91032	00	A	Esophagus, acid reflux test, with intraluminal pH electrode for detection of gastroesophageal reflux;	1.59	1.96	0.16	3.71	0	N
91032	26			1.59	1.25	0.10	2.94	0	N
91032	TC			0	0.71	0.06	0.77	0	N

CPT codes and descriptions only, © 1994 American Medical Association. Reimbursement information, © 1995 McGraw-Hill Inc.

Code/ CPT	Mod-ifier	Status	Description	Work value	Practice expense	Mal-practice	Total value	Global period	Up-date
91033	00	A	Esophagus, acid reflux test, with intraluminal pH electrode for detection of gastroesophageal reflux; prolonged recording	1.71	2.97	0.25	4.93	0	N
91033	26			1.71	1.69	0.14	3.54	0	N
91033	TC			0	1.28	0.11	1.39	0	N
91052	00	A	Gastric analysis test with injection of stimulant of gastric secretion (eg, histamine, insulin, pentagastrin, calcium and secretin)	1.71	0.82	0.07	2.60	0	N
91052	26			1.71	0.50	0.04	2.25	0	N
91052	TC			0	0.32	0.03	0.35	0	N
91055	00	A	Gastric intubation, washings, and preparing slides for cytology (separate procedure)	1.28	0.80	0.06	2.14	0	N
91055	26			1.28	0.51	0.04	1.83	0	N
91055	TC			0	0.29	0.02	0.31	0	N
91060	00	A	Gastric saline load test	0.45	0.71	0.06	1.22	0	N
91060	26			0.45	0.50	0.04	0.99	0	N
91060	TC			0	0.21	0.02	0.23	0	N
91065	00	A	Breath hydrogen test (eg, for detection of lactase deficiency)	0.45	0.83	0.05	1.33	0	N
91065	26			0.45	0.49	0.03	0.97	0	N
91065	TC			0	0.34	0.02	0.36	0	N
91100	00	A	Intestinal bleeding tube, passage, positioning and monitoring	1.08	0.56	0.05	1.69	0	N
91105	00	A	Gastric intubation, and aspiration or lavage for treatment (eg, for ingested poisons)	0.37	0.46	0.04	0.87	0	N
91122	00	A	Anorectal manometry	1.77	1.73	0.22	3.72	0	S
91122	26			1.77	1.06	0.13	2.96	0	S
91122	TC			0	0.67	0.09	0.76	0	S
91299	00	C	Unlisted diagnostic gastroenterology procedure	0	0	0	0	XXX	N
91299	26			0	0	0	0	XXX	N
91299	TC			0	0	0	0	XXX	N
92002	00	A	Ophthalmological services: medical examination and evaluation with initiation of diagnostic and treatment program; intermediate, new patient	1.01	0.49	0.02	1.52	XXX	P
92004	00	A	Ophthalmological services: medical examination and evaluation with initiation of diagnostic and treatment program; comprehensive, new patient, one or more visits	1.61	0.57	0.02	2.20	XXX	P
92012	00	A	Ophthalmological services: medical examination and evaluation, with initiation or continuation of diagnostic and treatment program; intermediate, established patient	0.82	0.44	0.02	1.28	XXX	N
92014	00	A	Ophthalmological services: medical examination and evaluation, with initiation or continuation of diagnostic and treatment program; comprehensive, established patient, one or more visits	1.06	0.54	0.02	1.62	XXX	N
92015	00	N	Determination of refractive state	0.38	0.32	0.02	0.72	XXX	0
92018	00	A	Ophthalmological examination and evaluation, under general anesthesia, with or without manipulation of globe for passive range of motion or other manipulation to facilitate diagnostic examination; complete	1.51	0.47	0.03	2.01	XXX	N
92019	00	A	Ophthalmological examination and evaluation, under general anesthesia, with or without manipulation of globe for passive range of motion or other manipulation to facilitate diagnostic examination; limited	1.31	0.47	0.03	1.81	XXX	N
92020	00	A	Gonioscopy with medical diagnostic evaluation (separate procedure)	0.37	0.29	0.01	0.67	XXX	N

CPT codes and descriptions only, © 1994 American Medical Association. Reimbursement information, © 1995 McGraw-Hill Inc.

Code/ CPT	Mod- ifier	Status	Description	Work value	Practice expense	Mal- practice	Total value	Global period	Up- date
92060	00	A	Sensorimotor examination with multiple measurements of ocular deviation and medical diagnostic evaluation (eg, restrictive or paretic muscle with diplopia) (separate procedure)	0.50	0.39	0.02	0.91	XXX	N
92060	26			0.50	0.21	0.01	0.72	XXX	N
92060	TC			0	0.18	0.01	0.19	XXX	N
92065	00	A	Orthoptic and/or pleoptic training, with continuing medical direction and evaluation	0.37	0.36	0.01	0.74	XXX	N
92065	26			0.37	0.20	0.01	0.58	XXX	N
92065	TC			0	0.16	0	0.16	XXX	N
92070	00	A	Fitting of contact lens for treatment of disease, including supply of lens	0.70	1.20	0.06	1.96	XXX	N
92081	00	A	Visual field examination, unilateral or bilateral, with medical diagnostic evaluation; limited examination (eg, tangent screen, Autoplot, arc perimeter, or single stimulus level automated test, such as Octopus 3 or 7 equivalent)	0.36	0.32	0.01	0.69	XXX	N
92081	26			0.36	0.17	0.01	0.54	XXX	N
92081	TC			0	0.15	0	0.15	XXX	N
92082	00	A	Visual field examination, unilateral or bilateral, with medical diagnostic evaluation; intermediate examination (eg, at least 2 isopters on Goldmann perimeter, or semiquantitative, automated suprathreshold screening program, Humphrey suprathreshold automatic diagnostic test, Octopus program 33)	0.44	0.49	0.02	0.95	XXX	N
92082	26			0.44	0.30	0.01	0.75	XXX	N
92082	TC			0	0.19	0.01	0.20	XXX	N
92083	00	A	Visual field examination, unilateral or bilateral, with medical diagnostic evaluation; extended examination (eg, Goldmann visual fields with at least 3 isopters plotted and static determination within the central 30, or quantitative, automated threshold perimetry, Octopus program G-1, 32 or 42, Humphrey visual field analyzer full threshold programs 30-2, 24-2, or 30/60-2)	0.50	0.83	0.04	1.37	XXX	N
92083	26			0.50	0.55	0.03	1.08	XXX	N
92083	TC			0	0.28	0.01	0.29	XXX	N
92100	00	A	Serial tonometry (separate procedure) with multiple measurements of intraocular pressure over an extended time period with medical diagnostic evaluation, same day (eg, diurnal curve or medical treatment of acute elevation of intraocular pressure)	0.92	0.25	0.01	1.18	XXX	N
92120	00	A	Tonography with medical diagnostic evaluation, recording indentation tonometer method or perilimbal suction method	0.81	0.31	0.02	1.14	XXX	N
92130	00	A	Tonography with water provocation	0.81	0.49	0.02	1.32	XXX	N
92140	00	A	Provocative tests for glaucoma, with medical diagnostic evaluation, without tonography	0.50	0.30	0.01	0.81	XXX	N
92225	00	A	Ophthalmoscopy, extended, with retinal drawing (eg, for retinal detachment, melanoma), with medical diagnostic evaluation; initial	0.58	0.45	0.02	1.05	XXX	N
92226	00	A	Ophthalmoscopy, extended, with retinal drawing (eg, for retinal detachment, melanoma), with medical diagnostic evaluation; subsequent	0.50	0.40	0.02	0.92	XXX	N
92230	00	A	Fluorescein angioscopy with medical diagnostic evaluation	0.60	0.69	0.04	1.33	XXX	N
92235	00	A	Fluorescein angiography (includes multiframe imaging) with medical diagnostic evaluation	0.81	1.58	0.09	2.48	XXX	N
92235	26			0.81	0.59	0.03	1.43	XXX	N

CPT codes and descriptions only, © 1994 American Medical Association. Reimbursement information, © 1995 McGraw-Hill Inc.

Code/ CPT	Mod-ifier	Status	Description	Work value	Practice expense	Mal-practice	Total value	Global period	Up-date
92235	TC			0	0.99	0.06	1.05	XXX	N
92250	00	A	Fundus photography with medical diagnostic evaluation	0.44	0.42	0.02	0.88	XXX	N
92250	26			0.44	0.25	0.01	0.70	XXX	N
92250	TC			0	0.17	0.01	0.18	XXX	N
92260	00	A	Ophthalmodynamometry	0.50	0.54	0.03	1.07	XXX[	
92265	00	A	Needle oculoelectromyography, one or more extraocular muscles, one or both eyes, with medical diagnostic evaluation	0.81	0.29	0.02	1.12	XXX	N
92265	26			0.81	0.07	0	0.88	XXX	N
92265	TC			0	0.22	0.02	0.24	XXX	N
92270	00	A	Electro-oculography, with medical diagnostic evaluation	0.81	0.67	0.05	1.53	XXX	N
92270	26			0.81	0.37	0.03	1.21	XXX	N
92270	TC			0	0.30	0.02	0.32	XXX	N
92275	00	A	Electroretinography, with medical diagnostic evaluation	1.01	0.90	0.05	1.96	XXX	N
92275	26			1.01	0.51	0.03	1.55	XXX	N
92275	TC			0	0.39	0.02	0.41	XXX	N
92280	00	A	Visually evoked potential (response) study, with medical diagnostic evaluation	0.35	0.83	0.05	1.23	XXX	N
92280	26			0.35	0.58	0.04	0.97	XXX	N
92280	TC			0	0.25	0.01	0.26	XXX	N
92283	00	A	Color vision examination, extended, eg, anomaloscope or equivalent	0.26	0.29	0.01	0.56	XXX	N
92283	26			0.26	0.17	0.01	0.44	XXX	N
92283	TC			0	0.12	0	0.12	XXX	N
92284	00	A	Dark adaptation examination, with medical diagnostic evaluation	0.37	0.45	0.02	0.84	XXX	N
92284	26			0.37	0.28	0.01	0.66	XXX	N
92284	TC			0	0.17	0.01	0.18	XXX	N
92285	00	A	External ocular photography with medical diagnostic evaluation for documentation of medical progress (eg, close-up photography, slit lamp photography, goniophotography, stereo-photography)	0.20	0.29	0.01	0.50	XXX	N
92285	26			0.20	0.18	0.01	0.39	XXX	N
92285	TC			0	0.11	0	0.11	XXX	N
92286	00	A	Special anterior segment photography with medical diagnostic evaluation; with specular endothelial microscopy and cell count	0.66	1.22	0.07	1.95	XXX	N
92286	26			0.66	0.83	0.05	1.54	XXX	N
92286	TC			0	0.39	0.02	0.41	XXX	N
92287	00	A	Special anterior segment photography with medical diagnostic evaluation; with fluorescein angiography	0.81	1.52	0.08	2.41	XXX	N
92310	00	N	Prescription of optical and physical characteristics of and fitting of contact lens, with medical supervision of adaptation; corneal lens, both eyes, except for aphakia	1.17	1.32	0	2.49	XXX	0
92311	00	A	Prescription of optical and physical characteristics of and fitting of contact lens, with medical supervision of adaptation; corneal lens for aphakia, one eye	1.08	0.90	0.03	2.01	XXX	N
92312	00	A	Prescription of optical and physical characteristics of and fitting of contact lens, with medical supervision of adaptation; corneal lens for aphakia, both eyes	1.26	1.16	0.03	2.45	XXX	N
92313	00	A	Prescription of optical and physical characteristics of and fitting of contact lens, with medical supervision of adaptation; corneoscleral lens	0.92	0.88	0.03	1.83	XXX	N

CPT codes and descriptions only, © 1994 American Medical Association. Reimbursement information, © 1995 McGraw-Hill Inc.

Code/ CPT	Mod- ifier	Status	Description	Work value	Practice expense	Mal- practice	Total value	Global period	Up- date
92314	00	N	Prescription of optical and physical characteristics of contact lens, with medical supervision of adaptation and direction of fitting by independent technician; corneal lens, both eyes, except for aphakia	0.69	0.78	0	1.47	XXX	0
92315	00	A	Prescription of optical and physical characteristics of contact lens, with medical supervision of adaptation and direction of fitting by independent technician; corneal lens for aphakia, one eye	0.45	0.66	0.03	1.14	XXX	N
92316	00	A	Prescription of optical and physical characteristics of contact lens, with medical supervision of adaptation and direction of fitting by independent technician; corneal lens for aphakia, both eyes	0.68	0.95	0.04	1.67	XXX	N
92317	00	A	Prescription of optical and physical characteristics of contact lens, with medical supervision of adaptation and direction of fitting by independent technician; corneoscleral lens	0.45	0.39	0.02	0.86	XXX	N
92325	00	A	Modification of contact lens (separate procedure), with medical supervision of adaptation	0	0.38	0.01	0.39	XXX	N
92326	00	A	Replacement of contact lens	0	1.56	0.06	1.62	XXX	N
92330	00	A	Prescription, fitting, and supply of ocular prosthesis (artificial eye), with medical supervision of adaptation	1.08	1.13	0.09	2.30	XXX	N
92335	00	A	Prescription of ocular prosthesis (artificial eye) and direction of fitting and supply by independent technician, with medical supervision of adaptation	0.45	1.97	0.11	2.53	XXX	N
92340	00	N	Fitting of spectacles, except for aphakia; monofocal	0.37	0.42	0	0.79	XXX	0
92341	00	N	Fitting of spectacles, except for aphakia; bifocal	0.47	0.53	0	1.00	XXX	0
92342	00	N	Fitting of spectacles, except for aphakia; multifocal, other than bifocal	0.53	0.60	0	1.13	XXX	0
92352	00	A	Fitting of spectacle prosthesis for aphakia; monofocal	0.37	0.30	0.01	0.68	XXX	N
92353	00	A	Fitting of spectacle prosthesis for aphakia; multifocal	0.50	0.40	0.01	0.91	XXX	N
92354	00	A	Fitting of spectacle mounted low vision aid; single element system	0	8.44	0.10	8.54	XXX	N
92355	00	A	Fitting of spectacle mounted low vision aid; telescopic or other compound lens system	0	4.13	0.01	4.14	XXX	N
92358	00	A	Prosthesis service for aphakia, temporary (disposable or loan, including materials)	0	0.92	0.05	0.97	XXX	N
92370	00	N	Repair and refitting spectacles; except for aphakia	0.32	0.36	0	0.68	XXX	0
92371	00	A	Repair and refitting spectacles; spectacle prosthesis for aphakia	0	0.59	0.02	0.61	XXX	N
92390	00	N	Supply of spectacles, except prosthesis for aphakia and low vision aids	0	0	0	0	XXX	0
92391	00	N	Supply of contact lenses, except prosthesis for aphakia	0	0	0	0	XXX	0
92392	00	G	Supply of low vision aids (A low vision aid is any lens or device used to aid or improve visual function in a person whose vision cannot be normalized by conventional spectacle correction. Includes reading additions up to 4D.)	0	3.85	0.02	3.87	XXX	0
92393	00	G	Supply of ocular prosthesis (artificial eye)	0	11.96	0.67	12.63	XXX	0
92395	00	G	Supply of permanent prosthesis for aphakia; spectacles	0	1.31	0.10	1.41	XXX	0
92396	00	G	Supply of permanent prosthesis for aphakia; contact lenses	0	2.19	0.08	2.27	XXX	0
92499	00	C	Unlisted ophthalmological service or procedure	0	0	0	0	XXX	N
92499	26			0	0	0	0	XXX	N
92499	TC			0	0	0	0	XXX	N
92502	00	A	Otolaryngologic examination under general anesthesia	1.51	1.12	0.12	2.75	0	N
92504	00	A	Binocular microscopy (separate diagnostic procedure)	0.18	0.26	0.02	0.46	XXX	N

CPT codes and descriptions only, © 1994 American Medical Association. Reimbursement information, © 1995 McGraw-Hill Inc.

Code/ CPT	Mod- ifier	Status	Description	Work value	Practice expense	Mal- practice	Total value	Global period	Up- date
92506	00	A	Medical evaluation, speech, language and/or hearing problems	0.86	0.52	0.05	1.43	XXX	N
92507	00	A	Speech, language or hearing therapy, with continuing medical supervision; individual	0.52	0.33	0.03	0.88	XXX	N
92508	00	A	Speech, language or hearing therapy, with continuing medical supervision; group	0.26	0.18	0.02	0.46	XXX	N
92511	00	A	Nasopharyngoscopy with endoscope (separate procedure)	0.84	0.85	0.09	1.78	0	S
92512	00	A	Nasal function studies (eg, rhinomanometry)	0.55	0.47	0.05	1.07	XXX	N
92516	00	A	Facial nerve function studies	0.43	0.39	0.04	0.86	XXX	N
92520	00	A	Laryngeal function studies	0.76	0.53	0.05	1.34	XXX	N
92531	00	B	Spontaneous nystagmus, including gaze	0.15*	0.14#	0.01*	0.30#	XXX	0
92532	00	B	Positional nystagmus	0.20*	0.18#	0.02*	0.40#	XXX	0
92533	00	B	Caloric vestibular test, each irrigation (binaural, bithermal stimulation constitutes four tests)	0.12*	0.11#	0.01*	0.24#	XXX	0
92534	00	B	Optokinetic nystagmus	0.06*	0.05#	0.01*	0.12#	XXX	0
92541	00	A	Spontaneous nystagmus test, including gaze and fixation nystagmus, with recording	0.40	0.67	0.07	1.14	XXX	N
92541	26			0.40	0.45	0.05	0.90	XXX	N
92541	TC			0	0.22	0.02	0.24	XXX	N
92542	00	A	Positional nystagmus test, minimum of 4 positions, with recording	0.33	0.61	0.07	1.01	XXX	N
92542	26			0.33	0.36	0.04	0.73	XXX	N
92542	TC			0	0.25	0.03	0.28	XXX	N
92543	00	A	Caloric vestibular test, each irrigation (binaural, bithermal stimulation constitutes four tests), with recording	0.38	0.82	0.09	1.29	XXX	N
92543	26			0.38	0.42	0.05	0.85	XXX	N
92543	TC			0	0.40	0.04	0.44	XXX	N
92544	00	A	Optokinetic nystagmus test, bidirectional, foveal or peripheral stimulation, with recording	0.26	0.47	0.05	0.78	XXX	N
92544	26			0.26	0.27	0.03	0.56	XXX	N
92544	TC			0	0.20	0.02	0.22	XXX	N
92545	00	A	Oscillating tracking test, with recording	0.23	0.40	0.04	0.67	XXX	N
92545	26			0.23	0.20	0.02	0.45	XXX	N
92545	TC			0	0.20	0.02	0.22	XXX	N
92546	00	A	Torsion swing test, with recording	0.29	0.53	0.05	0.87	XXX	N
92546	26			0.29	0.30	0.03	0.62	XXX	N
92546	TC			0	0.23	0.02	0.25	XXX	N
92547	00	A	Use of vertical electrodes in any or all of above tests counts as one additional test	0	0.53	0.06	0.59	XXX	N
92551	00	N	Screening test, pure tone, air only	0.21*	0.19#	0.02*	0.42#	XXX	0
92552	00	A	Pure tone audiometry (threshold); air only	0	0.42	0.04	0.46	XXX	N
92553	00	A	Pure tone audiometry (threshold); air and bone	0	0.63	0.07	0.70	XXX	N
92555	00	A	Speech audiometry; threshold only	0	0.36	0.04	0.40	XXX	N
92556	00	A	Speech audiometry; threshold and discrimination	0	0.54	0.06	0.60	XXX	N
92557	00	A	Basic comprehensive audiometry (92553 and 92556 combined), (pure tone, air and bone, and speech, threshold and discrimination)	0	1.13	0.13	1.26	XXX	N
92559	00	N	Audiometric testing of groups	0.21*	0.19#	0.02*	0.42#	XXX	0
92560	00	N	Bekesy audiometry; screening	0.12*	0.11#	0.01*	0.24#	XXX	0
92561	00	A	Bekesy audiometry; diagnostic	0	0.68	0.07	0.75	XXX	N
92562	00	A	Loudness balance test, alternate binaural or monaural	0	0.39	0.04	0.43	XXX	N
92563	00	A	Tone decay test	0	0.36	0.04	0.40	XXX	N

CPT codes and descriptions only, © 1994 American Medical Association. Reimbursement information, © 1995 McGraw-Hill Inc.

Code/ CPT	Mod-ifier	Status	Description	Work value	Practice expense	Mal-practice	Total value	Global period	Up-date
92564	00	A	Short increment sensitivity index (SISI)	0	0.45	0.05	0.50	XXX	N
92565	00	A	Stenger test, pure tone	0	0.38	0.04	0.42	XXX	N
92567	00	A	Tympanometry (impedance testing)	0	0.50	0.06	0.56	XXX	N
92568	00	A	Acoustic reflex testing	0	0.36	0.04	0.40	XXX	N
92569	00	A	Acoustic reflex decay test	0	0.39	0.04	0.43	XXX	N
92571	00	A	Filtered speech test	0	0.37	0.04	0.41	XXX	N
92572	00	A	Staggered spondaic word test	0	0.08	0.01	0.09	XXX	N
92573	00	A	Lombard test	0	0.33	0.04	0.37	XXX	N
92574	00	A	Swinging story test	0	1.16	0.09	1.25	XXX	N
92575	00	A	Sensorineural acuity level test	0	0.29	0.03	0.32	XXX	N
92576	00	A	Synthetic sentence identification test	0	0.42	0.05	0.47	XXX	N
92577	00	A	Stenger test, speech	0	0.68	0.08	0.76	XXX	N
92578	00	A	Delayed auditory feedback test	0	0.52	0.05	0.57	XXX	N
92580	00	A	Electrodermal audiometry	0	0.64	0.07	0.71	XXX	N
92582	00	A	Conditioning play audiometry	0	0.69	0.07	0.76	XXX	N
92583	00	A	Select picture audiometry	0	0.85	0.09	0.94	XXX	N
92584	00	A	Electrocochleography	0	2.36	0.25	2.61	XXX	N
92585	00	A	Brainstem evoked response recording (evoked response (EEG) audiometry)	0.50	3.25	0.31	4.06	XXX	N
92585	26			0.50	1.49	0.14	2.13	XXX	N
92585	TC			0	1.76	0.17	1.93	XXX	N
92587	00	A	Evoked otoacoustic emissions; limited (single stimulus level, either transient or distortion products)	0.13	1.35	0.13	1.61	XXX	N
92587	26			0.13	0.11	0.01	0.25	XXX	N
92587	TC			0	1.24	0.12	1.36	XXX	N
92588	00	A	Evoked otoacoustic emissions; comprehensive or diagnostic evaluation (comparison of transient and distortion product otoacoustic emissions at multiple levels and frequencies)	0.36	1.70	0.16	2.22	XXX	N
92588	26			0.36	0.30	0.02	0.68	XXX	N
92588	TC			0	1.40	0.14	1.54	XXX	N
92589	00	A	Central auditory function test(s) (specify)	0	0.51	0.06	0.57	XXX	N
92590	00	N	Hearing aid examination and selection; monaural	0.65*	0.59#	0.06*	1.30#	XXX	0
92591	00	N	Hearing aid examination and selection; binaural	0.97*	0.88#	0.10*	1.95#	XXX	0
92592	00	N	Hearing aid check; monaural	0.24*	0.22#	0.02*	0.48#	XXX	0
92593	00	N	Hearing aid check; binaural	0.35*	0.32#	0.03*	0.7#	XXX	0
92594	00	N	Electroacoustic evaluation for hearing aid; monaural	0.24*	0.22#	0.02*	0.48#	XXX	0
92595	00	N	Electroacoustic evaluation for hearing aid; binaural	0.35*	0.32#	0.03*	0.70#	XXX	0
92596	00	A	Ear protector attenuation measurements	0	0.56	0.06	0.62	XXX	N
92599	00	C	Unlisted otorhinolaryngological service or procedure	0	0	0	0	XXX	N
92599	26			0	0	0	0	XXX	N
92599	TC			0	0	0	0	XXX	N
92950	00	A	Cardiopulmonary resuscitation (eg, in cardiac arrest)	3.80	2.27	0.17	6.24	0	N
92953	00	A	Temporary transcutaneous pacing	0.23	1.11	0.15	1.49	0	N
92960	00	A	Cardioversion, elective, electrical conversion of arrhythmia, external	2.25	1.88	0.16	4.29	0	N
92970	00	A	Cardioassist-method of circulatory assist; internal	3.52	3.47	0.41	7.40	0	N
92971	00	A	Cardioassist-method of circulatory assist; external	1.77	1.11	0.08	2.96	0	N
92975	00	A	Thrombolysis, coronary; by intracoronary infusion, including selective coronary angiography	7.25	5.71	0.42	13.38	0	N

CPT codes and descriptions only, © 1994 American Medical Association. Reimbursement information, © 1995 McGraw-Hill Inc.

Code/ CPT	Mod- ifier	Status	Description	Work value	Practice expense	Mal- practice	Total value	Global period	Up- date
92977	00	A	Thrombolysis, coronary; by intravenous infusion	0	7.68	0.54	8.22	XXX	N
92980	00	A	Transcatheter placement of an intracoronary stent(s), percutaneous, with or without other therapeutic intervention, any method; single vessel	14.84	16.41	1.22	32.47	0	N
92981	00	A	Transcatheter placement of an intracoronary stent(s), percutaneous, with or without other therapeutic intervention, any method; each additional vessel	4.17	5.51	0.44	10.12	ZZZ	N
92982	00	A	Percutaneous transluminal coronary balloon angioplasty; single vessel	10.98	14.05	1.22	26.25	0	N
92984	00	A	Percutaneous transluminal coronary balloon angioplasty; each additional vessel	2.97	4.32	0.44	7.73	ZZZ	N
92986	00	A	Percutaneous balloon valvuloplasty; aortic valve	20.34	12.04	0.90	33.28	90	N
92990	00	A	Percutaneous balloon valvuloplasty; pulmonary valve	16.22	9.59	0.71	26.52	90	N
92992	00	C	Atrial septectomy or septostomy; transvenous method, balloon, Rashkind type (includes cardiac catheterization)	2.00*	1.18#	0.09*	3.27#	90	S
92993	00	C	Atrial septectomy or septostomy; blade method (Park septostomy) (includes cardiac catheterization)	2.12*	1.25#	0.09*	3.46#	90	S
92995	00	A	Percutaneous transluminal coronary atherectomy, with or without balloon angioplasty; single vessel	12.09	15.47	1.22	28.78	0	N
92996	00	A	Percutaneous transluminal coronary atherectomy, with or without balloon angioplasty; each additional vessel	3.26	4.48	0.44	8.18	ZZZ	N
93000	00	A	Electrocardiogram, routine ECG with at least 12 leads; with interpretation and report	0.17	0.59	0.04	0.80	XXX	N
93005	00	A	Electrocardiogram, routine ECG with at least 12 leads; tracing only, without interpretation and report	0	0.43	0.03	0.46	XXX	N
93010	00	A	Electrocardiogram, routine ECG with at least 12 leads; interpretation and report only	0.17	0.16	0.01	0.34	XXX	N
93012	00	A	Telephonic transmission of post-symptom electrocardiogram rhythm strip(s), per 30 day period of time; tracing only	0	2.25	0.22	2.47	XXX	N
93014	00	A	Telephonic transmission of post-symptom electrocardiogram rhythm strip(s), per 30 day period of time; physician review with interpretation and report only	0.52	0.40	0.05	0.97	XXX	N
93015	00	A	Cardiovascular stress test using maximal or submaximal treadmill or bicycle exercise, continous electrocardiographic monitoring, and/or pharmacological stress; with physician supervision, with interpretation and report	0.75	2.37	0.18	3.30	XXX	N
93016	00	A	Cardiovascular stress test using maximal or submaximal treadmill or bicycle exercise, continous electrocardiographic monitoring, and/or pharmacological stress; physician supervision only, without interpretation and report	0.45	0.39	0.03	0.87	XXX	N
93017	00	A	Cardiovascular stress test using maximal or submaximal treadmill or bicycle exercise, continous electrocardiographic monitoring, and/or pharmacological stress; tracing only, without interpretation and report	0	1.60	0.12	1.72	XXX	N
93018	00	A	Cardiovascular stress test using maximal or submaximal treadmill or bicycle exercise, continous electrocardiographic monitoring, and/or pharmacological stress; interpretation and report only	0.30	0.38	0.03	0.71	XXX	N
93024	00	A	Ergonovine provocation test	1.17	2.56	0.23	3.96	XXX	N
93024	26			1.17	1.49	0.14	2.80	XXX	N
93024	TC			0	1.07	0.09	1.16	XXX	N

CPT codes and descriptions only, © 1994 American Medical Association. Reimbursement information, © 1995 McGraw-Hill Inc.

Code/ CPT	Mod-ifier	Status	Description	Work value	Practice expense	Mal-practice	Total value	Global period	Up-date
93040	00	A	Rhythm ECG, one to three leads; with interpretation and report	0.16	0.26	0.02	0.44	XXX	N
93041	00	A	Rhythm ECG, one to three leads; tracing only without interpretation and report	0	0.14	0.01	0.15	XXX	N
93042	00	A	Rhythm ECG, one to three leads; interpretation and report only	0.16	0.12	0.01	0.29	XXX	N
93201	00	A	Phonocardiogram with or without ECG lead; with supervision during recording with interpretation and report (when equipment is supplied by the physician)	0.42	1.03	0.09	1.54	XXX	N
93202	00	A	Phonocardiogram with or without ECG lead; tracing only, without interpretation and report (eg, when equipment is supplied by the hospital, clinic)	0	0.75	0.07	0.82	XXX	N
93204	00	A	Phonocardiogram with or without ECG lead; interpretation and report	0.42	0.28	0.02	0.72	XXX	N
93205	00	A	Phonocardiogram with ECG lead, with indirect carotid artery and/or jugular vein tracing, and/or apex cardiogram; with interpretation and report	0.46	0.88	0.07	1.41	XXX	N
93208	00	A	Phonocardiogram with ECG lead, with indirect carotid artery and/or jugular vein tracing, and/or apex cardiogram; tracing only, without interpretation and report	0	0.33	0.03	0.36	XXX	N
93209	00	A	Phonocardiogram with ECG lead, with indirect carotid artery and/or jugular vein tracing, and/or apex cardiogram; interpretation and report only	0.46	0.55	0.04	1.05	XXX	N
93210	00	A	Phonocardiogram, intracardiac	0.92	1.73	0.13	2.78	XXX	N
93210	26			0.92	0.82	0.06	1.80	XXX	N
93210	TC			0	0.91	0.07	0.98	XXX	N
93220	00	A	Vectorcardiogram (VCG), with or without ECG; with interpretation and report	0.26	0.93	0.07	1.26	XXX	N
93221	00	A	Vectorcardiogram (VCG), with or without ECG; tracing only, without interpretation and report	0	0.58	0.04	0.62	XXX	N
93222	00	A	Vectorcardiogram (VCG), with or without ECG; interpretation and report only	0.26	0.35	0.03	0.64	XXX	N
93224	00	A	Electrocardiographic monitoring for 24 hours by continuous original ECG waveform recording and storage, with visual superimposition scanning; includes recording, scanning analysis with report, physician review and interpretation	0.52	3.95	0.31	4.78	XXX	N
93225	00	A	Electrocardiographic monitoring for 24 hours by continuous original ECG waveform recording and storage, with visual superimposition scanning; recording (includes hook-up, recording, and disconnection)	0	1.18	0.09	1.27	XXX	N
93226	00	A	Electrocardiographic monitoring for 24 hours by continuous original ECG waveform recording and storage, with visual superimposition scanning; scanning analysis with report	0	2.08	0.16	2.24	XXX	N
93227	00	A	Electrocardiographic monitoring for 24 hours by continuous original ECG waveform recording and storage, with visual superimposition scanning; physician review and interpretation	0.52	0.69	0.06	1.27	XXX	N
93230	00	A	Electrocardiographic monitoring for 24 hours by continuous original ECG waveform recording and storage without superimposition scanning utilizing a device capable of producing a full miniaturized printout; includes recording, microprocessor-based analysis with report, physician review and interpretation	0.52	4.32	0.34	5.18	XXX	N

CPT codes and descriptions only, © 1994 American Medical Association. Reimbursement information, © 1995 McGraw-Hill Inc.

Code/ CPT	Mod-ifier	Status	Description	Work value	Practice expense	Mal-practice	Total value	Global period	Up-date
93231	00	A	Electrocardiographic monitoring for 24 hours by continuous original ECG waveform recording and storage without superimposition scanning utilizing a device capable of producing a full miniaturized printout; recording (includes hook-up, recording, and disconnection)	0	1.45	0.11	1.56	XXX	N
93232	00	A	Electrocardiographic monitoring for 24 hours by continuous original ECG waveform recording and storage without superimposition scanning utilizing a device capable of producing a full miniaturized printout; microprocessor-based analysis with report	0	2.07	0.15	2.22	XXX	N
93233	00	A	Electrocardiographic monitoring for 24 hours by continuous original ECG waveform recording and storage without superimposition scanning utilizing a device capable of producing a full miniaturized printout; physician review and interpretation	0.52	0.80	0.08	1.40	XXX	N
93235	00	A	Electrocardiographic monitoring for 24 hours by continuous computerized monitoring and non-continuous recording, and real-time data analysis utilizing a device capable of producing intermittent full-sized waveform tracings, possibly patient activated; includes monitoring and real time data analysis with report, physician review and interpretation	0.45	3.17	0.23	3.85	XXX	N
93236	00	A	Electrocardiographic monitoring for 24 hours by continuous computerized monitoring and non-continuous recording, and real-time data analysis utilizing a device capable of producing intermittent full-sized waveform tracings, possibly patient activated; monitoring and real-time data analysis with report	0	2.50	0.17	2.67	XXX	N
93237	00	A	Electrocardiographic monitoring for 24 hours by continuous computerized monitoring and non-continuous recording, and real-time data analysis utilizing a device capable of producing intermittent full-sized waveform tracings, possibly patient activated; physician review and interpretation	0.45	0.67	0.06	1.18	XXX	N
93255	00	D	Apexcardiography	0.59*	0.35#	0.03*	0.97#	XXX	N
93255	26			0	0	0	0		
93268	00	A	Patient demand single or multiple event recording with presymptom memory loop, per 30 day period of time; includes transmission, physician review and interpretation	0.52	3.83	0.36	4.71	XXX	N
93268	TC			0	0	0	0	XXX	N
93270	00	A	Patient demand single or multiple event recording with presymptom memory loop, per 30 day period of time; recording (includes hook-up, recording and disconnection)	0	1.18	0.09	1.27	XXX	N
93271	00	A	Patient demand single or multiple event recording with presymptom memory loop, per 30 day period of time; monitoring, receipt of transmissions, and analysis	0	2.25	0.22	2.47	XXX	N
93272	00	A	Patient demand single or multiple event recording with presymptom memory loop, per 30 day period of time; physician review and interpretation only	0.52	0.40	0.05	0.97	XXX	N
93278	00	A	Signal-averaged electrocardiography (SAECG), with or without ECG	0.35	1.65	0.18	2.18	XXX	N
93278	26			0.35	0.55	0.06	0.96	XXX	N
93278	TC			0	1.10	0.12	1.22	XXX	N
93307	00	A	Echocardiography, real-time with image documentation (2D) with or without M-mode recording; complete	0.78	4.68	0.36	5.82	XXX	N
93307	26			0.78	1.00	0.09	1.87	XXX	N
93307	TC			0	3.68	0.27	3.95	XXX	N

CPT codes and descriptions only, © 1994 American Medical Association. Reimbursement information, © 1995 McGraw-Hill Inc.

Code/ CPT	Mod- ifier	Status	Description	Work value	Practice expense	Mal- practice	Total value	Global period	Up- date
93308	00	A	Echocardiography, real-time with image documentation (2D) with or without M-mode recording; follow-up or limited study	0.53	2.53	0.19	3.25	XXX	N
93308	26			0.53	0.68	0.05	1.26	XXX	N
93308	TC			0	1.85	0.14	1.99	XXX	N
93312	00	A	Echocardiography, real time with image documentation (2D) (with or without M-Mode recording), transesophageal; including probe placement, image acquisition, interpretation and report	1.57	4.95	0.45	6.97	XXX	N
93312	26			1.57	1.35	0.12	3.04	XXX	N
93312	TC			0	3.60	0.33	3.93	XXX	N
93313	00	A	Echocardiography, real time with image documentation (2D) (with or without M-Mode recording), transesophageal; placement of transesophageal probe only	0.95	0.67	0.06	1.68	XXX	N
93314	00	A	Echocardiography, real time with image documentation (2D) (with or without M-Mode recording), transesophageal; image acquisition, interpretation and report only	0.95	4.27	0.39	5.61	XXX	N
93314	26			0.95	0.67	0.06	1.68	XXX	N
93314	TC			0	3.60	0.33	3.93	XXX	N
93320	00	A	Doppler echocardiography, pulsed wave and/or continuous wave with spectral display; complete	0.38	2.16	0.18	2.72	XXX	N
93320	26			0.38	0.53	0.05	0.96	XXX	N
93320	TC			0	1.63	0.13	1.76	XXX	N
93321	00	A	Doppler echocardiography, pulsed wave and/or continuous wave with spectral display; follow-up or limited study	0.15	1.28	0.11	1.54	XXX	N
93321	26			0.15	0.22	0.02	0.39	XXX	N
93321	TC			0	1.06	0.09	1.15	XXX	N
93325	00	A	Doppler color flow velocity mapping (list separately in addition to code for echocardiography 76825, 76826, 76827, 76828, 93307, 93308, 93312, 93314, 93320, 93321)	0.07	2.80	0.25	3.12	XXX	N
93325	26			0.07	0.04	0.01	0.12	XXX	N
93325	TC			0	2.76	0.24	3.00	XXX	N
93350	00	A	Echocardiography, real-time with image documentation (2D), with or without M-mode recording, during rest and cardiovascular stress test using maximal or submaximal treadmill, bicycle exercise and/or pharmacologically induced stress, including electrocardiographic monitoring, with interpretation and report	0.78	3.63	0.24	4.65	XXX	N
93350	26			0.78	1.95	0.10	2.83	XXX	N
93350	TC			0	1.68	0.14	1.82	XXX	N
93501	00	A	Right heart catheterization	3.02	19.72	1.54	24.28	0	N
93501	26			3.02	3.61	0.34	6.97	0	N
93501	TC			0	16.11	1.20	17.31	0	N
93503	00	A	Insertion and placement of flow directed catheter (eg, Swan-Ganz) for monitoring purposes	2.43	2.37	0.36	5.16	0	N
93505	00	A	Endomyocardial biopsy	4.56	4.92	0.46	9.94	0	N
93505	26			4.56	3.03	0.28	7.87	0	N
93505	TC			0	1.89	0.18	2.07	0	N
93510	00	A	Left heart catheterization, retrograde, from the brachial artery, axillary artery or femoral artery; percutaneous	4.33	38.28	2.86	45.47	0	N
93510	26			4.33	3.06	0.23	7.62	0	N
93510	TC			0	35.22	2.63	37.85	0	N

CPT codes and descriptions only, © 1994 American Medical Association. Reimbursement information, © 1995 McGraw-Hill Inc.

Code/ CPT	Mod- ifier	Status	Description	Work value	Practice expense	Mal- practice	Total value	Global period	Up- date
93511	00	A	Left heart catheterization, retrograde, from the brachial artery, axillary artery or femoral artery; by cutdown	5.03	36.91	2.76	44.70	0	N
93511	26			5.03	2.62	0.20	7.85	0	N
93511	TC			0	34.29	2.56	36.85	0	N
93514	00	A	Left heart catheterization by left ventricular puncture	7.05	38.84	2.94	48.83	0	S
93514	26			7.05	4.55	0.38	11.98	0	S
93514	TC			0	34.29	2.56	36.85	0	S
93524	00	A	Combined transseptal and retrograde left heart catheterization	6.95	49.45	3.69	60.09	0	N
93524	26			6.95	4.65	0.34	11.94	0	N
93524	TC			0	44.80	3.35	48.15	0	N
93526	00	A	Combined right heart catheterization and retrograde left heart catheterization	5.99	51.48	3.83	61.30	0	N
93526	26			5.99	5.45	0.39	11.83	0	N
93526	TC			0	46.03	3.44	49.47	0	N
93527	00	A	Combined right heart catheterization and transseptal left heart catheterization through intact septum (with or without retrograde left heart catheterization)	7.28	51.94	3.85	63.07	0	N
93527	26			7.28	7.14	0.50	14.92	0	N
93527	TC			0	44.80	3.35	48.15	0	N
93528	00	A	Combined right heart catheterization with left ventricular puncture (with or without retrograde left heart catheterization)	9	49.23	3.68	61.91	0	N
93528	26			9	4.43	0.33	13.76	0	N
93528	TC			0	44.80	3.35	48.15	0	N
93529	00	A	Combined right heart catheterization and left heart catheterization through existing septal opening (with or without retrograde left heart catheterization)	4.80	47.73	3.57	56.10	0	N
93529	26			4.80	2.93	0.22	7.95	0	N
93529	TC			0	44.80	3.35	48.15	0	N
93536	00	A	Percutaneous insertion of intra-aortic balloon catheter	4.85	6.38	0.71	11.94	0	N
93539	00	A	Injection procedure during cardiac catheterization; for selective opacification of arterial conduits (eg, internal mammary), whether native or used for bypass	0.29	1.46	0.20	1.95	0	N
93540	00	A	Injection procedure during cardiac catheterization; for selective opacification of aortocoronary venous bypass grafts, one or more coronary arteries	0.43	1.46	0.20	2.09	0	N
93541	00	A	Injection procedure during cardiac catheterization; for pulmonary angiography	0.29	1.18	0.16	1.63	0	N
93542	00	A	Injection procedure during cardiac catheterization; for selective right ventricular or right atrial angiography	0.29	1.18	0.16	1.63	0	N
93543	00	A	Injection procedure during cardiac catheterization; for selective left ventricular or left atrial angiography	0.29	0.88	0.11	1.28	0	N
93544	00	A	Injection procedure during cardiac catheterization; for aortography	0.29	0.87	0.11	1.27	0	N
93545	00	A	Injection procedure during cardiac catheterization; for selective coronary angiography (injection of radiopaque material may be by hand)	0.29	1.77	0.24	2.30	0	N
93555	00	A	Imaging supervision, interpretation and report for injection procedure(s) during cardiac catheterization; ventricular and/or atrial angiography	0.81	6.25	0.42	7.48	XXX	N
93555	26			0.81	0.27	0.04	1.12	XXX	N
93555	TC			0	5.98	0.38	6.36	XXX	N

CPT codes and descriptions only, © 1994 American Medical Association. Reimbursement information, © 1995 McGraw-Hill Inc.

Code/ CPT	Mod- ifier	Status	Description	Work value	Practice expense	Mal- practice	Total value	Global period	Up- date
93556	00	A	Imaging supervision, interpretation and report for injection procedure(s) during cardiac catheterization; pulmonary angiography, aortography, and/or selective coronary angiography including venous bypass grafts and arterial conduits (whether native or used in bypass)	0.83	9.88	0.65	11.36	XXX	N
93556	26			0.83	0.45	0.07	1.35	XXX	N
93556	TC			0	9.43	0.58	10.01	XXX	N
93561	00	A	Indicator dilution studies such as dye or thermal dilution, including arterial and/or venous catheterization; with cardiac output measurement (separate procedure)	1.15	1.25	0.16	2.56	0	N
93561	26			1.15	0.75	0.09	1.99	0	N
93561	TC			0	0.50	0.07	0.57	0	N
93562	00	A	Indicator dilution studies such as dye or thermal dilution, including arterial and/or venous catheterization; subsequent measurement of cardiac output	0.37	0.76	0.10	1.23	0	N
93562	26			0.37	0.46	0.06	0.89	0	N
93562	TC			0	0.30	0.04	0.34	0	N
93600	00	A	Bundle of His recording	2.12	4.57	0.38	7.07	0	N
93600	26			2.12	2.71	0.24	5.07	0	N
93600	TC			0	1.86	0.14	2.00	0	N
93602	00	A	Intra-atrial recording	2.12	2.83	0.22	5.17	0	N
93602	26			2.12	1.77	0.14	4.03	0	N
93602	TC			0	1.06	0.08	1.14	0	N
93603	00	A	Right ventricular recording	2.12	3.79	0.28	6.19	0	N
93603	26			2.12	2.19	0.16	4.47	0	N
93603	TC			0	1.60	0.12	1.72	0	N
93607	00	A	Left ventricular recording	3.26	3.63	0.28	7.17	0	N
93607	26			3.26	2.21	0.17	5.64	0	N
93607	TC			0	1.42	0.11	1.53	0	N
93609	00	A	Intraventricular and/or intra-atrial mapping of tachycardia site(s) with catheter manipulation to record from multiple sites to identify origin of tachycardia	10.07	6.43	0.47	16.97	0	N
93609	26			10.07	3.84	0.28	14.19	0	N
93609	TC			0	2.59	0.19	2.78	0	N
93610	00	A	Intra-atrial pacing	3.02	3.60	0.27	6.89	0	N
93610	26			3.02	2.31	0.17	5.50	0	N
93610	TC			0	1.29	0.10	1.39	0	N
93612	00	A	Intraventricular pacing	3.02	3.88	0.29	7.19	0	N
93612	26			3.02	2.34	0.17	5.53	0	N
93612	TC			0	1.54	0.12	1.66	0	N
93615	00	A	Esophageal recording of atrial electrogram with or without ventricular electrogram(s);	0.99	0.65	0.04	1.68	0	N
93615	26			0.99	0.35	0.02	1.36	0	N
93615	TC			0	0.30	0.02	0.32	0	N
93616	00	A	Esophageal recording of atrial electrogram with or without ventricular electrogram(s); with pacing	1.49	1.66	0.10	3.25	0	N
93616	26			1.49	1.36	0.08	2.93	0	N
93616	TC			0	0.30	0.02	0.32	0	N
93618	00	A	Induction of arrhythmia by electrical pacing	4.26	9.24	0.72	14.22	0	N
93618	26			4.26	5.46	0.44	10.16	0	N
93618	TC			0	3.78	0.28	4.06	0	N

CPT codes and descriptions only, © 1994 American Medical Association. Reimbursement information, © 1995 McGraw-Hill Inc.

Code/ CPT	Mod- ifier	Status	Description	Work value	Practice expense	Mal- practice	Total value	Global period	Up- date
93619	00	A	Comprehensive electrophysiologic evaluation with right atrial pacing and recording, right ventricular pacing and recording, His bundle recording, including insertion and repositioning of multiple electrode catheters; without induction of arrhythmia (This code is to be used when 93600 is combined with 93602, 93603, 93610, 93612)	7.32	16.92	1.40	25.64	0	N
93619	26			7.32	9.58	0.86	17.76	0	N
93619	TC			0	7.34	0.54	7.88	0	N
93620	00	A	Comprehensive electrophysiologic evaluation with right atrial pacing and recording, right ventricular pacing and recording, His bundle recording, including insertion and repositioning of multiple electrode catheters; with induction of arrhythmia (This code is to be used when 93618 is combined with 93619)	11.59	22.07	1.55	35.21	0	N
93620	26			11.59	13.53	0.95	26.07	0	N
93620	TC			0	8.54	0.60	9.14	0	N
93621	00	C	Comprehensive electrophysiologic evaluation with right atrial pacing and recording, right ventricular pacing and recording, His bundle recording, including insertion and repositioning of multiple electrode catheters; with left atrial recordings from coronary sinus or left atrium, with or without pacing	0	0	0	0	0	N
93621	26			12.66	14.94	1.11	28.71	0	N
93621	TC			0	0	0	0	0	N
93622	00	C	Comprehensive electrophysiologic evaluation with right atrial pacing and recording, right ventricular pacing and recording, His bundle recording, including insertion and repositioning of multiple electrode catheters; with left ventricular recordings, with or without pacing	0	0	0	0	0	N
93622	26			12.74	14.74	1.07	28.55	0	N
93622	TC			0	0	0	0	0	N
93623	00	C	Programmed stimulation and pacing after intravenous drug infusion (Use this code with 93620, 93621, 93622)	0	0	0	0	0	N
93623	26			2.85	2.78	0.20	5.83	0	N
93623	TC			0	0	0	0	0	N
93624	00	A	Electrophysiologic follow-up study with pacing and recording to test effectiveness of therapy, including induction or attempted induction of arrhythmia	4.81	4.88	0.35	10.04	0	N
93624	26			4.81	2.99	0.21	8.01	0	N
93624	TC			0	1.89	0.14	2.03	0	N
93631	00	A	Intra-operative epicardial and endocardial pacing and mapping to localize the site of tachycardia or zone of slow conduction for surgical correction	7.60	11.62	1.37	20.59	0	N
93631	26			7.60	5.76	0.67	14.03	0	N
93631	TC			0	5.86	0.70	6.56	0	N
93640	00	A	Electrophysiologic evaluation of cardioverter-defibrillator leads (includes defibrillation threshold testing and sensing function) at time of initial implantation or replacement;	3.52	12.66	1.09	17.27	0	N
93640	26			3.52	5.82	0.61	9.95	0	N
93640	TC			0	6.84	0.48	7.32	0	N
93641	00	A	Electrophysiologic evaluation of cardioverter-defibrillator leads (includes defibrillation threshold testing and sensing function) at time of initial implantation or replacement; with testing of cardioverter-defibrillator pulse generator	5.93	13.85	1.09	20.87	0	N
93641	26			5.93	7.01	0.61	13.55	0	N

CPT codes and descriptions only, © 1994 American Medical Association. Reimbursement information, © 1995 McGraw-Hill Inc.

Code/ CPT	Mod- ifier	Status	Description	Work value	Practice expense	Mal- practice	Total value	Global period	Up- date
93641	TC			0	6.84	0.48	7.32	0	N
93642	00	A	Electrophysiologic evaluation of cardioverter-defibrillator (includes defibrillation threshold evaluation, induction of arrhythmia, evaluation of sensing and pacing for arrhythmia termination, and programming or reprogramming of sensing or therapeutic parameters)	4.89	13.33	1.09	19.31	0	N
93642	26			4.89	6.49	0.61	11.99	0	N
93642	TC			0	6.84	0.48	7.32	0	N
93650	00	A	Intracardiac catheter ablation of atrioventricular node function, atrioventricular conduction for creation of complete heart block, with or without temporary pacemaker placement	10.51	14.17	1.34	26.02	0	N
93651	00	A	Intracardiac catheter ablation of arrhythmogenic focus; for treatment of supraventricular tachycardia by ablation of fast or slow atrioventricular pathways, accessory atrioventricular connections or other atrial foci, singly or in combination	16.25	17.83	1.34	35.42	0	N
93652	00	A	Intracardiac catheter ablation of arrhythmogenic focus; for treatment of ventricular tachycardia	17.68	17.83	1.34	36.85	0	N
93660	00	C	Autonomic nervous system evaluation of cardiovascular function with tilt table evaluation, with or without pharmacological intervention	0	0	0	0	0	N
93660	26			1.89	1.44	0.17	3.50	0	N
93660	TC			0	0	0	0	0	N
93720	00	A	Plethysmography, total body; with interpretation and report	0.17	0.91	0.10	1.18	XXX	N
93721	00	A	Plethysmography, total body; tracing only, without interpretation and report	0	0.67	0.07	0.74	XXX	N
93722	00	A	Plethysmography, total body; interpretation and report only	0.17	0.24	0.03	0.44	XXX	N
93724	00	A	Electronic analysis of antitachycardia pacemaker system (includes electrocardiographic recording, programming of device, induction and termination of tachycardia via implanted pacemaker, and interpretation of recordings)	4.89	6.66	0.50	12.05	0	N
93724	26			4.89	2.88	0.22	7.99	0	N
93724	TC			0	3.78	0.28	4.06	0	N
93731	00	A	Electronic analysis of dual-chamber pacemaker system (includes evaluation of programmable parameters at rest and during activity where applicable, using electrocardiographic recording and interpretation of recordings at rest and during exercise, analysis of event markers and device response); without reprogramming	0.45	0.79	0.07	1.31	XXX	N
93731	26			0.45	0.32	0.03	0.80	XXX	N
93731	TC			0	0.47	0.04	0.51	XXX	N
93732	00	A	Electronic analysis of dual-chamber pacemaker system (includes evaluation of programmable parameters at rest and during activity where applicable, using electrocardiographic recording and interpretation of recordings at rest and during exercise, analysis of event markers and device response); with reprogramming	0.92	0.91	0.08	1.91	XXX	N
93732	26			0.92	0.42	0.04	1.38	XXX	N
93732	TC			0	0.49	0.04	0.53	XXX	N
93733	00	A	Electronic analysis of dual chamber internal pacemaker system (may include rate, pulse amplitude and duration, configuration of wave form, and/or testing of sensory function of pacemaker), telephonic analysis	0.17	0.91	0.08	1.16	XXX	N
93733	26			0.17	0.22	0.02	0.41	XXX	N

CPT codes and descriptions only, © 1994 American Medical Association. Reimbursement information, © 1995 McGraw-Hill Inc.

Code/ CPT	Mod- ifier	Status	Description	Work value	Practice expense	Mal- practice	Total value	Global period	Up- date
93733	TC			0	0.69	0.06	0.75	XXX	N
93734	00	A	Electronic analysis of single chamber pacemaker system (includes evaluation of programmable parameters at rest and during activity where applicable, using electrocardiographic recording and interpretation of recordings at rest and during exercise, analysis of event markers and device response); without reprogramming	0.38	0.64	0.06	1.08	XXX	N
93734	26			0.38	0.31	0.03	0.72	XXX	N
93734	TC			0	0.33	0.03	0.36	XXX	N
93735	00	A	Electronic analysis of single chamber pacemaker system (includes evaluation of programmable parameters at rest and during activity where applicable, using electrocardiographic recording and interpretation of recordings at rest and during exercise, analysis of event markers and device response); with reprogramming	0.74	0.85	0.08	1.67	XXX	N
93735	26			0.74	0.43	0.04	1.21	XXX	N
93735	TC			0	0.42	0.04	0.46	XXX	N
93736	00	A	Electronic analysis of single chamber internal pacemaker system (may include rate, pulse amplitude and duration, configuration of wave form, and/or testing of sensory function of pacemaker), telephonic analysis	0.15	0.82	0.09	1.06	XXX	N
93736	26			0.15	0.22	0.03	0.40	XXX	N
93736	TC			0	0.60	0.06	0.66	XXX	N
93737	00	A	Electronic analysis of cardioverter/defibrillator only (interrogation, evaluation of pulse generator status); without reprogramming	0.45	0.74	0.06	1.25	XXX	N
93737	26			0.45	0.27	0.02	0.74	XXX	N
93737	TC			0	0.47	0.04	0.51	XXX	N
93738	00	A	Electronic analysis of cardioverter/defibrillator only (interrogation, evaluation of pulse generator status); with reprogramming	0.92	0.88	0.07	1.87	XXX	N
93738	26			0.92	0.39	0.03	1.34	XXX	N
93738	TC			0	0.49	0.04	0.53	XXX	N
93740	00	A	Temperature gradient studies	0.16	0.45	0.04	0.65	XXX	N
93740	26			0.16	0.30	0.03	0.49	XXX	N
93740	TC			0	0.15	0.01	0.16	XXX	N
93760	00	N	Thermogram; cephalic	1.41*	0.83#	0.06*	2.30#	XXX	0
93760	26			0	0	0	0		
93762	00	N	Thermogram; peripheral	1.77*	1.04#	0.08*	2.89#	XXX	0
93762	26			0	0	0	0		
93770	00	A	Determination of venous pressure	0.16	0.20	0.02	0.38	XXX	N
93770	26			0.16	0.17	0.02	0.35	XXX	N
93770	TC			0	0.03	0	0.03	XXX	N
93784	00	N	Ambulatory blood pressure monitoring, utilizing a system such as magnetic tape and/or computer disk, for 24 hours or longer; including recording, scanning analysis, interpretation and report	1.89*	1.12#	0.08*	3.09#	XXX	0
93786	00	N	Ambulatory blood pressure monitoring, utilizing a system such as magnetic tape and/or computer disk, for 24 hours or longer; recording only	0.65*	0.38#	0.03*	1.06#	XXX	0
93788	00	N	Ambulatory blood pressure monitoring, utilizing a system such as magnetic tape and/or computer disk, for 24 hours or longer; scanning analysis with report	0.59*	0.35#	0.03*	0.97#	XXX	0

CPT codes and descriptions only, © 1994 American Medical Association. Reimbursement information, © 1995 McGraw-Hill Inc.

Code/ CPT	Mod- ifier	Status	Description	Work value	Practice expense	Mal- practice	Total value	Global period	Up- date
93790	00	N	Ambulatory blood pressure monitoring, utilizing a system such as magnetic tape and/or computer disk, for 24 hours or longer; physician review with interpretation and report	0.71*	0.42#	0.03*	1.16#	XXX	0
93797	00	A	Physician services for outpatient cardiac rehabilitation; without continuous ECG monitoring (per session)	0.18	0.30	0.02	0.50	0	N
93798	00	A	Physician services for outpatient cardiac rehabilitation; with continuous ECG monitoring (per session)	0.28	0.47	0.04	0.79	0	N
93799	00	C	Unlisted cardiovascular service or procedure	0	0	0	0	XXX	N
93799	26			0	0	0	0	XXX	N
93799	TC			0	0	0	0	XXX	N
93875	00	A	Noninvasive physiologic studies of extracranial arteries, complete bilateral study (eg, periorbital flow direction with arterial compression, ocular pneumoplethysmography, Doppler ultrasound spectral analysis)	0.22	1.44	0.18	1.84	XXX	N
93875	26			0.22	0.39	0.06	0.67	XXX	N
93875	TC			0	1.05	0.12	1.17	XXX	N
93880	00	A	Duplex scan of extracranial arteries; complete bilateral study	0.60	3.94	0.44	4.98	XXX	N
93880	26			0.60	0.39	0.04	1.03	XXX	N
93880	TC			0	3.55	0.40	3.95	XXX	N
93882	00	A	Duplex scan of extracranial arteries; unilateral or limited study	0.40	2.62	0.29	3.31	XXX	N
93882	26			0.40	0.26	0.03	0.69	XXX	N
93882	TC			0	2.36	0.26	2.62	XXX	N
93886	00	A	Transcranial Doppler study of the intracranial arteries; complete study	0.94	4.44	0.50	5.88	XXX	N
93886	26			0.94	0.42	0.05	1.41	XXX	N
93886	TC			0	4.02	0.45	4.47	XXX	N
93888	00	A	Transcranial Doppler study of the intracranial arteries; limited study	0.62	2.96	0.34	3.92	XXX	N
93888	26			0.62	0.28	0.03	0.93	XXX	N
93888	TC			0	2.68	0.31	2.99	XXX	N
93922	00	A	Noninvasive physiologic studies of upper or lower extremity arteries, single level, bilateral (eg, ankle/brachial indices, Doppler waveform analysis, volume plethysmography, transcutaneous oxygen tension measurement)	0.25	1.39	0.19	1.83	XXX	N
93922	26			0.25	0.29	0.05	0.59	XXX	N
93922	TC			0	1.10	0.14	1.24	XXX	N
93923	00	A	Non-invasive physiologic studies of upper or lower extremity arteries, multiple levels or with provocative functional maneuvers, complete bilateral study (eg, segmental blood pressure measurements, segmental Doppler waveform analysis, segmental volume plethysmography, segmental transcutaneous oxygen tension measurements, measurements with postural provocative tests, measurements with reactive hyperemia)	0.45	2.63	0.35	3.43	XXX	N
93923	26			0.45	0.55	0.09	1.09	XXX	N
93923	TC			0	2.08	0.26	2.34	XXX	N
93924	00	A	Non-invasive physiologic studies of lower extremity arteries, at rest and following treadmill stress testing, complete bilateral study	0.50	2.85	0.39	3.74	XXX	N
93924	26			0.50	0.59	0.10	1.19	XXX	N
93924	TC			0	2.26	0.29	2.55	XXX	N

CPT codes and descriptions only, © 1994 American Medical Association. Reimbursement information, © 1995 McGraw-Hill Inc.

Code/ CPT	Mod- ifier	Status	Description	Work value	Practice expense	Mal- practice	Total value	Global period	Up- date
93925	00	A	Duplex scan of lower extremity arteries or arterial bypass grafts; complete bilateral study	0.58	3.96	0.44	4.98	XXX	N
93925	26			0.58	0.39	0.04	1.01	XXX	N
93925	TC			0	3.57	0.40	3.97	XXX	N
93926	00	A	Duplex scan of lower extremity arteries or arterial bypass grafts; unilateral or limited study	0.39	2.64	0.30	3.33	XXX	N
93926	26			0.39	0.26	0.03	0.68	XXX	N
93926	TC			0	2.38	0.27	2.65	XXX	N
93930	00	A	Duplex scan of upper extremity arteries or arterial bypass grafts; complete bilateral study	0.46	4.18	0.47	5.11	XXX	N
93930	26			0.46	0.39	0.05	0.90	XXX	N
93930	TC			0	3.79	0.42	4.21	XXX	N
93931	00	A	Duplex scan of upper extremity arteries or arterial bypass grafts; unilateral or limited study	0.31	2.78	0.31	3.40	XXX	N
93931	26			0.31	0.26	0.03	0.60	XXX	N
93931	TC			0	2.52	0.28	2.80	XXX	N
93965	00	A	Non-invasive physiologic studies of extremity veins, complete bilateral study (eg, Doppler waveform analysis with responses to compression and other maneuvers, phleborheography, impedance plethysmography)	0.35	1.49	0.19	2.03	XXX	N
93965	26			0.35	0.45	0.06	0.86	XXX	N
93965	TC			0	1.04	0.13	1.17	XXX	N
93970	00	A	Duplex scan of extremity veins including responses to compression and other maneuvers; complete bilateral study	0.68	4.33	0.51	5.52	XXX	N
93970	26			0.68	0.40	0.05	1.13	XXX	N
93970	TC			0	3.93	0.46	4.39	XXX	N
93971	00	A	Duplex scan of extremity veins including responses to compression and other maneuvers; unilateral or limited study	0.45	2.89	0.34	3.68	XXX	N
93971	26			0.45	0.27	0.03	0.75	XXX	N
93971	TC			0	2.62	0.31	2.93	XXX	N
93975	00	A	Duplex scan of arterial inflow and venous outflow of abdominal, pelvic, and/or retroperitoneal organs; complete study	1.80	4.90	0.55	7.25	XXX	N
93975	26			1.80	0.42	0.05	2.27	XXX	N
93975	TC			0	4.48	0.50	4.98	XXX	N
93976	00	A	Duplex scan of arterial inflow and venous outflow of abdominal, pelvic, and/or retroperitoneal organs; limited study	1.21	3.27	0.37	4.85	XXX	N
93976	26			1.21	0.28	0.03	1.52	XXX	N
93976	TC			0	2.99	0.34	3.33	XXX	N
93978	00	A	Duplex scan of aorta, inferior vena cava, iliac vasculature, or bypass grafts; complete study	0.65	4.06	0.47	5.18	XXX	N
93978	26			0.65	0.39	0.05	1.09	XXX	N
93978	TC			0	3.67	0.42	4.09	XXX	N
93979	00	A	Duplex scan of aorta, inferior vena cava, iliac vasculature, or bypass grafts; unilateral or limited study	0.44	2.70	0.31	3.45	XXX	N
93979	26			0.44	0.26	0.03	0.73	XXX	N
93979	TC			0	2.44	0.28	2.72	XXX	N
93980	00	A	Duplex scan of arterial inflow and venous outflow of penile vessels; complete study	1.82	4.15	0.45	6.42	XXX	N
93980	26			1.82	0.82	0.07	2.71	XXX	N
93980	TC			0	3.33	0.38	3.71	XXX	N

CPT codes and descriptions only, © 1994 American Medical Association. Reimbursement information, © 1995 McGraw-Hill Inc.

Code/ CPT	Mod- ifier	Status	Description	Work value	Practice expense	Mal- practice	Total value	Global period	Up- date
93981	00	A	Duplex scan of arterial inflow and venous outflow of penile vessels; follow-up or limited study	0.64	3.47	0.39	4.50	XXX	N
93981	26			0.64	0.40	0.03	1.07	XXX	N
93981	TC			0	3.07	0.36	3.43	XXX	N
93990	00	A	Duplex scan of hemodialysis access (including arterial inflow, body of access and venous outflow)	0.25	2.57	0.29	3.11	XXX	N
93990	26			0.25	0.19	0.02	0.46	XXX	N
93990	TC			0	2.38	0.27	2.65	XXX	N
94010	00	A	Spirometry, including graphic record, total and timed vital capacity, expiratory flow rate measurement(s), and/or maximal voluntary ventilation	0.17	0.68	0.05	0.90	XXX	N
94010	26			0.17	0.28	0.02	0.47	XXX	N
94010	TC			0	0.40	0.03	0.43	XXX	N
94060	00	A	Bronchospasm evaluation: spirometry as in 94010, before and after bronchodilator (aerosol or parenteral) or exercise	0.31	1.27	0.09	1.67	XXX	N
94060	26			0.31	0.38	0.03	0.72	XXX	N
94060	TC			0	0.89	0.06	0.95	XXX	N
94070	00	A	Prolonged postexposure evaluation of bronchospasm with multiple spirometric determinations after test dose of bronchodilator (aerosol only) antigen, exercise, cold air, methocholine or other chemical agent, with spirometry as in 94010	0.60	1.77	0.13	2.50	XXX	N
94070	26			0.60	0.38	0.03	1.01	XXX	N
94070	TC			0	1.39	0.10	1.49	XXX	N
94150	00	A	Vital capacity, total (separate procedure)	0.11	0.20	0.02	0.33	XXX	N
94150	26			0.11	0.12	0.01	0.24	XXX	N
94150	TC			0	0.08	0.01	0.09	XXX	N
94160	00	A	Vital capacity screening tests: total capacity, with timed forced expiratory volume (state duration), and peak flow rate	0.18	0.37	0.02	0.57	XXX	N
94160	26			0.18	0.19	0.01	0.38	XXX	N
94160	TC			0	0.18	0.01	0.19	XXX	N
94200	00	A	Maximum breathing capacity, maximal voluntary ventilation	0.11	0.38	0.03	0.52	XXX	N
94200	26			0.11	0.14	0.01	0.26	XXX	N
94200	TC			0	0.24	0.02	0.26	XXX	N
94240	00	A	Functional residual capacity or residual volume: helium method, nitrogen open circuit method, or other method	0.26	0.88	0.07	1.21	XXX	N
94240	26			0.26	0.23	0.02	0.51	XXX	N
94240	TC			0	0.65	0.05	0.70	XXX	N
94250	00	A	Expired gas collection, quantitative, single procedure (separate procedure)	0.11	0.27	0.02	0.40	XXX	N
94250	26			0.11	0.14	0.01	0.26	XXX	N
94250	TC			0	0.13	0.01	0.14	XXX	N
94260	00	A	Thoracic gas volume	0.13	0.72	0.06	0.91	XXX	N
94260	26			0.13	0.20	0.02	0.35	XXX	N
94260	TC			0	0.52	0.04	0.56	XXX	N
94350	00	A	Determination of maldistribution of inspired gas: multiple breath nitrogen washout curve including alveolar nitrogen or helium equilibration time	0.26	0.73	0.05	1.04	XXX	N
94350	26			0.26	0.21	0.01	0.48	XXX	N
94350	TC			0	0.52	0.04	0.56	XXX	N
94360	00	A	Determination of resistance to airflow, oscillatory or plethysmographic methods	0.26	1.11	0.07	1.44	XXX	N

CPT codes and descriptions only, © 1994 American Medical Association. Reimbursement information, © 1995 McGraw-Hill Inc.

Code/ CPT	Mod-ifier	Status	Description	Work value	Practice expense	Mal-practice	Total value	Global period	Up-date
94360	26			0.26	0.19	0.01	0.46	XXX	N
94360	TC			0	0.92	0.06	0.98	XXX	N
94370	00	A	Determination of airway closing volume, single breath tests	0.26	0.40	0.03	0.69	XXX	N
94370	26			0.26	0.14	0.01	0.41	XXX	N
94370	TC			0	0.26	0.02	0.28	XXX	N
94375	00	A	Respiratory flow volume loop	0.31	0.67	0.04	1.02	XXX	N
94375	26			0.31	0.21	0.01	0.53	XXX	N
94375	TC			0	0.46	0.03	0.49	XXX	N
94400	00	A	Breathing response to CO_2 (CO_2 response curve)	0.40	0.77	0.19	1.36	XXX	N
94400	26			0.40	0.47	0.13	1.00	XXX	N
94400	TC			0	0.30	0.06	0.36	XXX	N
94450	00	A	Breathing response to hypoxia (hypoxia response curve)	0.40	0.61	0.05	1.06	XXX	N
94450	26			0.40	0.24	0.02	0.66	XXX	N
94450	TC			0	0.37	0.03	0.40	XXX	N
94620	00	A	Pulmonary stress testing, simple or complex	0.88	2.05	0.15	3.08	XXX	N
94620	26			0.88	0.70	0.05	1.63	XXX	N
94620	TC			0	1.35	0.10	1.45	XXX	N
94640	00	A	Nonpressurized inhalation treatment for acute airway obstruction	0	0.39	0.03	0.42	XXX	N
94642	00	C	Aerosol inhalation of pentamidine for pneumocystis carinii pneumonia treatment or prophylaxis	0	0	0	0	XXX	N
94642	26			0	0	0	0		
94650	00	A	Intermittent positive pressure breathing (IPPB) treatment, air or oxygen, with or without nebulized medication; initial demonstration and/or evaluation	0	0.37	0.03	0.40	XXX	N
94651	00	A	Intermittent positive pressure breathing (IPPB) treatment, air or oxygen, with or without nebulized medication; subsequent	0	0.36	0.03	0.39	XXX	N
94652	00	A	Intermittent positive pressure breathing (IPPB) treatment, air or oxygen, with or without nebulized medication; newborn infants	0	0.41	0.08	0.49	XXX	N
94656	00	A	Ventilation assist and management, initiation of pressure or volume preset ventilators for assisted or controlled breathing; first day	1.22	1.13	0.12	2.47	XXX	N
94657	00	A	Ventilation assist and management, initiation of pressure or volume preset ventilators for assisted or controlled breathing; subsequent days	0.83	0.62	0.05	1.50	XXX	N
94660	00	A	Continuous positive airway pressure ventilation (CPAP), initiation and management	0.76	0.71	0.06	1.53	XXX	N
94662	00	A	Continuous negative pressure ventilation (CNP), initiation and management	0.76	0.30	0.02	1.08	XXX	N
94664	00	A	Aerosol or vapor inhalations for sputum mobilization, bronchodilation, or sputum induction for diagnostic purposes; initial demonstration and/or evaluation	0	0.50	0.04	0.54	XXX	N
94665	00	A	Aerosol or vapor inhalations for sputum mobilization, bronchodilation, or sputum induction for diagnostic purposes; subsequent	0	0.46	0.05	0.51	XXX	N
94667	00	A	Manipulation chest wall, such as cupping, percussing, and vibration to facilitate lung function; initial demonstration and/or evaluation	0	0.55	0.05	0.60	XXX	N
94668	00	A	Manipulation chest wall, such as cupping, percussing, and vibration to facilitate lung function; subsequent	0	0.34	0.03	0.37	XXX	N
94680	00	A	Oxygen uptake, expired gas analysis; rest and exercise, direct, simple	0.26	0.82	0.10	1.18	XXX	N

CPT codes and descriptions only, © 1994 American Medical Association. Reimbursement information, © 1995 McGraw-Hill Inc.

Code/ CPT	Mod-ifier	Status	Description	Work value	Practice expense	Mal-practice	Total value	Global period	Up-date
94680	26			0.26	0.33	0.03	0.62	XXX	N
94680	TC			0	0.49	0.07	0.56	XXX	N
94681	00	A	Oxygen uptake, expired gas analysis; including CO_2 output, percentage oxygen extracted	0.20	1.64	0.17	2.01	XXX	N
94681	26			0.20	0.32	0.04	0.56	XXX	N
94681	TC			0	1.32	0.13	1.45	XXX	N
94690	00	A	Oxygen uptake, expired gas analysis; rest, indirect (separate procedure)	0.07	0.56	0.04	0.67	XXX	N
94690	26			0.07	0.05	0	0.12	XXX	N
94690	TC			0	0.51	0.04	0.55	XXX	N
94720	00	A	Carbon monoxide diffusing capacity, any method	0.26	1.03	0.08	1.37	XXX	N
94720	26			0.26	0.23	0.02	0.51	XXX	N
94720	TC			0	0.80	0.06	0.86	XXX	N
94725	00	A	Membrane diffusion capacity	0.26	1.84	0.14	2.24	XXX	N
94725	26			0.26	0.18	0.01	0.45	XXX	N
94725	TC			0	1.66	0.13	1.79	XXX	N
94750	00	A	Pulmonary compliance study, any method	0.23	0.83	0.06	1.12	XXX	N
94750	26			0.23	0.28	0.02	0.53	XXX	N
94750	TC			0	0.55	0.04	0.59	XXX	N
94760	00	A	Noninvasive ear or pulse oximetry for oxygen saturation; single determination	0	0.25	0.02	0.27	XXX	N
94761	00	A	Noninvasive ear or pulse oximetry for oxygen saturation; multiple determinations (eg, during exercise)	0	0.64	0.06	0.70	XXX	N
94762	00	A	Noninvasive ear or pulse oximetry for oxygen saturation; by continuous overnight monitoring (separate procedure)	0	1.08	0.10	1.18	XXX	N
94770	00	A	Carbon dioxide, expired gas determination by infrared analyzer	0.20	0.40	0.11	0.71	XXX	N
94770	26			0.20	0.11	0.03	0.34	XXX	N
94770	TC			0	0.29	0.08	0.37	XXX	N
94772	00	C	Circadian respiratory pattern recording (pediatric pneumogram), 12 to 24 hour continuous recording, infant	0	0	0	0	XXX	N
94772	26			0	0	0	0	XXX	N
94772	TC			0	0	0	0	XXX	N
94799	00	C	Unlisted pulmonary service or procedure	0	0	0	0	XXX	N
94799	26			0	0	0	0	XXX	N
94799	TC			0	0	0	0	XXX	N
95004	00	A	Percutaneous tests (scratch, puncture, prick) with allergenic extracts, immediate type reaction, specify number of tests	0	0.09	0.01	0.10	XXX	N
95010	00	A	Percutaneous tests (scratch, puncture, prick) sequential and incremental, with drugs, biologicals or venoms, immediate type reaction, specify number of tests	0.15	0.11	0.01	0.27	XXX	N
95015	00	A	Intracutaneous (intradermal) tests, sequential and incremental, with drugs, biologicals, or venoms, immediate type reaction, specify number of tests	0.15	0.11	0.01	0.27	XXX	N
95024	00	A	Intracutaneous (intradermal) tests with allergenic extracts, immediate type reaction, specify number of tests	0	0.14	0.01	0.15	XXX	N
95027	00	A	Skin end point titration	0	0.14	0.01	0.15	XXX	N
95028	00	A	Intracutaneous (intradermal) tests with allergenic extracts, delayed type reaction, including reading, specify number of tests	0	0.22	0.01	0.23	XXX	N
95044	00	A	Patch or application test(s) (specify number of tests)	0	0.19	0.01	0.20	XXX	N
95052	00	A	Photo patch test(s) (specify number of tests)	0	0.24	0.01	0.25	XXX	N

CPT codes and descriptions only, © 1994 American Medical Association. Reimbursement information, © 1995 McGraw-Hill Inc.

Code/ CPT	Mod-ifier	Status	Description	Work value	Practice expense	Mal-practice	Total value	Global period	Up-date
95056	00	A	Photo tests	0	0.17	0.01	0.18	XXX	N
95060	00	A	Ophthalmic mucous membrane tests	0	0.33	0.02	0.35	XXX	N
95065	00	A	Direct nasal mucous membrane test	0	0.19	0.01	0.20	XXX	N
95070	00	A	Inhalation bronchial challenge testing (not including necessary pulmonary function tests); with histamine, methacholine, or similar compounds	0	2.17	0.02	2.19	XXX	N
95071	00	A	Inhalation bronchial challenge testing (not including necessary pulmonary function tests); with antigens or gases, specify	0	2.78	0.02	2.80	XXX	N
95075	00	A	Ingestion challenge test (sequential and incremental ingestion of test items, eg, food, drug or other substance such as metabisulfite)	0.95	1.97	0.02	2.94	XXX	N
95078	00	A	Provocative testing (eg, Rinkel test)	0	0.24	0.02	0.26	XXX	N
95115	00	A	Professional services for allergen immunotherapy not including provision of allergenic extracts; single injection	0	0.37	0.02	0.39	XXX	N
95117	00	A	Professional services for allergen immunotherapy not including provision of allergenic extracts; multiple injections	0	0.48	0.02	0.50	XXX	N
95120	00	G	Professional services for allergen immunotherapy in prescribing physician's office or institution, including provision of allergenic extract; single injection	0.18*	0.13#	0.01*	0.32#	XXX	0
95125	00	G	Professional services for allergen immunotherapy in prescribing physician's office or institution, including provision of allergenic extract; multiple injections (specify number of injections)	0.27*	0.19#	0.01*	0.47#	XXX	0
95130	00	G	Professional services for allergen immunotherapy in prescribing physician's office or institution, including provision of allergenic extract; single stinging insect venom	0.29*	0.21#	0.01*	0.51#	XXX	0
95131	00	G	Professional services for allergen immunotherapy in prescribing physician's office or institution, including provision of allergenic extract; two stinging insect venoms	0.41*	0.29#	0.02*	0.72#	XXX	0
95132	00	G	Professional services for allergen immunotherapy in prescribing physician's office or institution, including provision of allergenic extract; three stinging insect venoms	0.47*	0.34#	0.02*	0.83#	XXX	0
95133	00	G	Professional services for allergen immunotherapy in prescribing physician's office or institution, including provision of allergenic extract; four stinging insect venoms	0.53*	0.38#	0.02*	0.93#	XXX	0
95134	00	G	Professional services for allergen immunotherapy in prescribing physician's office or institution, including provision of allergenic extract; five stinging insect venoms	0.59*	0.42#	0.03*	1.04#	XXX	0
95144	00	A	Professional services for the supervision and provision of antigens for allergen immunotherapy, single or multiple antigens, single dose vials (specify number of vials)	0.06	0.13	0.01	0.20	XXX	N
95145	00	A	Professional services for the supervision and provision of antigens for allergen immunotherapy (specify number of doses); single stinging insect venom, multiple dose vials	0.06	0.34	0.03	0.43	XXX	N
95146	00	A	Professional services for the supervision and provision of antigens for allergen immunotherapy (specify number of doses); two single stinging insect venoms, multiple dose vials	0.06	0.61	0.03	0.70	XXX	N
95147	00	A	Professional services for the supervision and provision of antigens for allergen immunotherapy (specify number of doses); three single stinging insect venoms, multiple dose vials	0.06	0.91	0.03	1.00	XXX	N
95148	00	A	Professional services for the supervision and provision of antigens for allergen immunotherapy (specify number of doses); four single stinging insect venoms, multiple dose vials	0.06	0.91	0.03	1.00	XXX	N

CPT codes and descriptions only, © 1994 American Medical Association. Reimbursement information, © 1995 McGraw-Hill Inc.

Code/ CPT	Mod- ifier	Status	Description	Work value	Practice expense	Mal- practice	Total value	Global period	Up- date
95149	00	A	Professional services for the supervision and provision of antigens for allergen immunotherapy (specify number of doses); five single stinging insect venoms, multiple dose vials	0.06	1.14	0.03	1.23	XXX	N
95165	00	A	Professional services for the supervision and provision of antigens for allergen immunotherapy; single or multiple antigens, multiple dose vial(s), (specify number of doses)	0.06	0.10	0.01	0.17	XXX	N
95170	00	A	Professional services for the supervision and provision of antigens for allergen immunotherapy; whole body extract of biting insect or other arthropod (specify number of doses)	0.06	0.35	0.03	0.44	XXX	N
95180	00	A	Rapid desensitization procedure, each hour (eg, insulin, penicillin, horse serum)	2.01	0.14	0.01	2.16	XXX	N
95199	00	C	Unlisted allergy/clinical immunologic service or procedure	0	0	0	0	XXX	N
95805	00	A	Multiple sleep latency testing (MSLT), recording, analysis and interpretation of physiological measurements of sleep during multiple nap opportunities	1.88	5.51	0.45	7.84	XXX	N
95805	26			1.88	0.56	0.07	2.51	XXX	N
95805	TC			0	4.95	0.38	5.33	XXX	N
95807	00	A	Sleep study, 3 or more parameters of sleep other than sleep staging, attended by a technologist	1.66	6.77	0.52	8.95	XXX	N
95807	26			1.66	1.82	0.14	3.62	XXX	N
95807	TC			0	4.95	0.38	5.33	XXX	N
95808	00	A	Polysomnography; sleep staging with 1–3 additional parameters of sleep, attended by a technologist	2.65	6.77	0.52	9.94	XXX	N
95808	26			2.65	1.82	0.14	4.61	XXX	N
95808	TC			0	4.95	0.38	5.33	XXX	N
95810	00	A	Polysomnography; sleep staging with 4 or more additional parameters of sleep, attended by a technologist	3.53	6.77	0.52	10.82	XXX	N
95810	26			3.53	1.82	0.14	5.49	XXX	N
95810	TC			0	4.95	0.38	5.33	XXX	N
95812	00	A	Electroencephalogram (EEG) extended monitoring; up to one hour	1.08	1.85	0.15	3.08	XXX	N
95812	26			1.08	0.50	0.04	1.62	XXX	N
95812	TC			0	1.35	0.11	1.46	XXX	N
95813	00	A	Electroencephalogram (EEG) extended monitoring; greater than one hour	1.73	1.85	0.15	3.73	XXX	N
95813	26			1.73	0.50	0.04	2.27	XXX	N
95813	TC			0	1.35	0.11	1.46	XXX	N
95816	00	A	Electroencephalogram (EEG) including recording awake and drowsy, with hyperventilation and/or photic stimulation	1.08	1.54	0.13	2.75	XXX	N
95816	26			1.08	0.28	0.03	1.39	XXX	N
95816	TC			0	1.26	0.10	1.36	XXX	N
95817	00	D	Electroencephalogram (EEG)	1.41*	1#	0.07*	2.48#	XXX	N
95817	26			0.47*	0.33#	0.02*	0.82#	XXX	N
95819	00	A	Electroencephalogram (EEG) including recording awake and asleep, with hyperventilation and/or photic stimulation	1.08	1.80	0.14	3.02	XXX	N
95819	26			1.08	0.50	0.04	1.62	XXX	N
95819	TC			0	1.30	0.10	1.40	XXX	N
95821	00	D	Portable EEG	1.53*	1.09#	0.08*	2.70#	XXX	N
95821	26			0.47*	0.33#	0.02*	0.82#	XXX	N
95822	00	A	Electroencephalogram (EEG); sleep only	1.08	2.28	0.18	3.54	XXX	N
95822	26			1.08	0.56	0.04	1.68	XXX	N

CPT codes and descriptions only, © 1994 American Medical Association. Reimbursement information, © 1995 McGraw-Hill Inc.

Code/ CPT	Mod- ifier	Status	Description	Work value	Practice expense	Mal- practice	Total value	Global period	Up- date
95822	TC			0	1.72	0.14	1.86	XXX	N
95823	00	D	Activation EEG	1.12*	0.80#	0.06*	1.98#	XXX	N
95823	26			0.24*	0.17#	0.01*	0.42#	XXX	N
95824	00	A	Electroencephalogram (EEG); cerebral death evaluation only	0.74	0.98	0.07	1.79	XXX	N
95824	26			0.74	0.58	0.04	1.36	XXX	N
95824	TC			0	0.40	0.03	0.43	XXX	N
95826	00	D	Depth electroencephalogram	1.41*	1.00#	0.07*	2.48#	XXX	N
95826	26			0.29*	0.21#	0.02*	0.52#	XXX	N
95827	00	A	Electroencephalogram (EEG); all night sleep only	1.08	3.06	0.24	4.38	XXX	N
95827	26			1.08	0.88	0.07	2.03	XXX	N
95827	TC			0	2.18	0.17	2.35	XXX	N
95829	00	A	Electrocorticogram at surgery (separate procedure)	6.21	0.59	0.05	6.85	XXX	N
95829	26			6.21	0.45	0.03	6.69	XXX	N
95829	TC			0	0.14	0.02	0.16	XXX	N
95830	00	A	Insertion by physician of sphenoidal electrodes for electroencephalographic (EEG) recording	1.70	0.78	0.07	2.55	XXX	N
95831	00	A	Muscle testing, manual (separate procedure); extremity (excluding hand) or trunk, with report	0.28	0.29	0.03	0.60	XXX	N
95832	00	A	Muscle testing, manual (separate procedure); hand (with or without comparison with normal side)	0.29	0.25	0.02	0.56	XXX	N
95833	00	A	Muscle testing, manual (separate procedure); total evaluation of body, excluding hands	0.47	0.38	0.05	0.90	XXX	N
95834	00	A	Muscle testing, manual (separate procedure); total evaluation of body, including hands	0.60	0.61	0.06	1.27	XXX	N
95842	00	D	Muscle testing, electrical: reaction of degeneration, chronaxie, galvanic/tetanus ratio, one or more extremities, one or more methods (CCR 95999) (95845 has been deleted. To report, use 95999)	0.44*	0.31#	0.02*	0.77#	XXX	N
95851	00	A	Range of motion measurements and report (separate procedure); each extremity (excluding hand) or each trunk section (spine)	0.28	0.24	0.02	0.54	XXX	N
95852	00	A	Range of motion measurements and report (separate procedure); hand, with or without comparison with normal side	0.19	0.15	0.02	0.36	XXX	N
95857	00	A	Tensilon test for myasthenia gravis;	0.53	0.50	0.04	1.07	XXX	N
95858	00	A	Tensilon test for myasthenia gravis; with electromyographic recording	1.56	1.02	0.09	2.67	XXX	N
95858	26			1.56	0.64	0.05	2.25	XXX	N
95858	TC			0	0.38	0.04	0.42	XXX	N
95860	00	A	Needle electromyography, one extremity and related paraspinal areas	0.96	1.09	0.09	2.14	XXX	N
95860	26			0.96	0.73	0.06	1.75	XXX	N
95860	TC			0	0.36	0.03	0.39	XXX	N
95861	00	A	Needle electromyography, two extremities and related paraspinal areas	1.54	1.97	0.16	3.67	XXX	N
95861	26			1.54	1.27	0.10	2.91	XXX	N
95861	TC			0	0.70	0.06	0.76	XXX	N
95863	00	A	Needle electromyography, three extremities and related paraspinal areas	1.87	2.30	0.18	4.35	XXX	N
95863	26			1.87	1.41	0.11	3.39	XXX	N
95863	TC			0	0.89	0.07	0.96	XXX	N

CPT codes and descriptions only, © 1994 American Medical Association. Reimbursement information, © 1995 McGraw-Hill Inc.

Code/ CPT	Mod-ifier	Status	Description	Work value	Practice expense	Mal-practice	Total value	Global period	Up-date
95864	00	A	Needle electromyography, four extremities and related paraspinal areas	1.99	3.45	0.27	5.71	XXX	N
95864	26			1.99	1.75	0.14	3.88	XXX	N
95864	TC			0	1.70	0.13	1.83	XXX	N
95867	00	A	Needle electromyography, cranial nerve supplied muscles, unilateral	0.62	1.13	0.09	1.84	XXX	N
95867	26			0.62	0.58	0.05	1.25	XXX	N
95867	TC			0	0.55	0.04	0.59	XXX	N
95868	00	A	Needle electromyography, cranial nerve supplied muscles, bilateral	1.50	1.92	0.15	3.57	XXX	N
95868	26			1.50	1.26	0.10	2.86	XXX	N
95868	TC			0	0.66	0.05	0.71	XXX	N
95869	00	A	Needle electromyography, limited study of specific muscles (eg, thoracic spinal muscles)	0.37	0.53	0.05	0.95	XXX	N
95869	26			0.37	0.33	0.03	0.73	XXX	N
95869	TC			0	0.20	0.02	0.22	XXX	N
95872	00	A	Needle electromyography, single fiber, any technique	1.50	1.25	0.11	2.86	XXX	N
95872	26			1.50	0.68	0.06	2.24	XXX	N
95872	TC			0	0.57	0.05	0.62	XXX	N
95875	00	A	Ischemic limb exercise with needle electromyography, with lactic acid determination	1.34	0.60	0.10	2.04	XXX	N
95875	26			1.34	0.22	0.04	1.60	XXX	N
95875	TC			0	0.38	0.06	0.44	XXX	N
95880	00	A	Assessment of aphasia (includes assessment of expressive and receptive speech and language function, language comprehension, speech production ability, reading, spelling, writing, eg, by Boston Diagnostic Aphasia Examination) with interpretation and report, per hour	0	1.68	0.20	1.88	XXX	N
95881	00	A	Developmental testing (includes assessment of motor, language, social, adaptive and/or cognitive functioning by standardized developmental instruments, eg, Bayley Scales of Infant Development) with interpretation and report, per hour	0	1.68	0.20	1.88	XXX	N
95882	00	A	Neurobehavioral status exam (clinical assessment of thinking, reasoning and judgement, eg, acquired knowledge, attention, memory, visual spatial abilities, language functions, planning) with interpretation and report, per hour	0	1.68	0.20	1.88	XXX	N
95883	00	A	Neuropsychological testing battery (eg, Halstead-Reitan, LURIA, WAIS-R) with report, per hour	0	1.68	0.20	1.88	XXX	N
95900	00	A	Nerve conduction, velocity and/or latency study; motor, each nerve	0.42	0.62	0.05	1.09	XXX	N
95900	26			0.42	0.35	0.03	0.80	XXX	N
95900	TC			0	0.27	0.02	0.29	XXX	N
95904	00	A	Nerve conduction, velocity and/or latency study; sensory, each nerve	0.34	0.55	0.05	0.94	XXX	N
95904	26			0.34	0.34	0.03	0.71	XXX	N
95904	TC			0	0.21	0.02	0.23	XXX	N
95920	00	A	Intraoperative neurophysiology testing, per hour	2.11	2.67	0.20	4.98	XXX	N
95920	26			2.11	1.43	0.12	3.66	XXX	N
95920	TC			0	1.24	0.08	1.32	XXX	N
95925	00	A	Somatosensory testing (eg, cerebral evoked potentials), one or more nerves	0.81	2.28	0.19	3.28	XXX	N
95925	26			0.81	0.96	0.08	1.85	XXX	N

CPT codes and descriptions only, © 1994 American Medical Association. Reimbursement information, © 1995 McGraw-Hill Inc.

Code/ CPT	Mod- ifier	Status	Description	Work value	Practice expense	Mal- practice	Total value	Global period	Up- date
95925	TC			0	1.32	0.11	1.43	XXX	N
95933	00	A	Orbicularis oculi (blink) reflex, by electrodiagnostic testing	0.59	1.25	0.10	1.94	XXX	N
95933	26			0.59	0.50	0.04	1.13	XXX	N
95933	TC			0	0.75	0.06	0.81	XXX	N
95935	00	A	"H" or "F" reflex study, by electrodiagnostic testing	0.59	0.54	0.05	1.18	XXX	N
95935	26			0.59	0.34	0.03	0.96	XXX	N
95935	TC			0	0.20	0.02	0.22	XXX	N
95937	00	A	Neuromuscular junction testing (repetitive stimulation, paired stimuli), each nerve, any one method	0.60	0.77	0.07	1.44	XXX	N
95937	26			0.60	0.45	0.04	1.09	XXX	N
95937	TC			0	0.32	0.03	0.35	XXX	N
95950	00	A	Monitoring for identification and lateralization of cerebral seizure focus by attached electrodes; electroencephalographic (eg, 8 channel EEG) recording and interpretation, each 24 hours	1.51	7.25	0.60	9.36	XXX	N
95950	26			1.51	1.21	0.10	2.82	XXX	N
95950	TC			0	6.04	0.50	6.54	XXX	N
95951	00	A	Monitoring for identification and lateralization of cerebral seizure focus by attached electrodes; combined electroencephalographic (EEG) and video recording and interpretation, each 24 hours	3.80	8.83	0.64	13.27	XXX	N
95951	26			3.80	1.50	0.11	5.41	XXX	N
95951	TC			0	7.33	0.53	7.86	XXX	N
95953	00	A	Monitoring for localization of cerebral seizure focus by computerized portable 16 or more channel EEG; electroencephalographic (EEG) recording and interpretation, each 24 hours	3.08	7.25	0.60	10.93	XXX	N
95953	26			3.08	1.21	0.10	4.39	XXX	N
95953	TC			0	6.04	0.50	6.54	XXX	N
95954	00	A	Pharmacological or physical activation requiring physician attendance during EEG recording of activation phase (eg, thiopental activation test)	2.45	2.32	0.28	5.05	XXX	N
95954	26			2.45	1.87	0.22	4.54	XXX	N
95954	TC			0	0.45	0.06	0.51	XXX	N
95955	00	A	Electroencephalogram (EEG) during nonintracranial surgery (eg, carotid surgery)	1.01	2.90	0.30	4.21	XXX	N
95955	26			1.01	1.03	0.11	2.15	XXX	N
95955	TC			0	1.87	0.19	2.06	XXX	N
95956	00	A	Monitoring for localization of cerebral seizure focus by cable or radio, 16 or more channel telemetry, electroencephalographic (EEG) recording and interpretation, each 24 hours	3.08	7.54	0.61	11.23	XXX	N
95956	26			3.08	1.50	0.11	4.69	XXX	N
95956	TC			0	6.04	0.50	6.54	XXX	N
95957	00	A	Digital analysis of electroencephalogram (EEG) (eg, for epileptic spike analysis) (list separately in addition to code for primary procedure)	1.98	2.25	0.18	4.41	XXX	N
95957	26			1.98	0.63	0.05	2.66	XXX	N
95957	TC			0	1.62	0.13	1.75	XXX	N
95958	00	A	Wada activation test for hemispheric function, including electroencephalographic (EEG) monitoring	4.25	4.89	0.52	9.66	XXX	N
95958	26			4.25	3.23	0.38	7.86	XXX	N
95958	TC			0	1.66	0.14	1.80	XXX	N

CPT codes and descriptions only, © 1994 American Medical Association. Reimbursement information, © 1995 McGraw-Hill Inc.

Code/ CPT	Mod- ifier	Status	Description	Work value	Practice expense	Mal- practice	Total value	Global period	Up- date
95961	00	A	Functional cortical mapping by stimulation of electrodes on brain surface, or of depth electrodes, to provoke seizures or identify vital cortex; initial hour of physician attendance	2.97	2.67	0.20	5.84	XXX	N
95961	26			2.97	1.43	0.12	4.52	XXX	N
95961	TC			0	1.24	0.08	1.32	XXX	N
95962	00	A	Functional cortical mapping by stimulation of electrodes on brain surface, or of depth electrodes, to provoke seizures or identify vital cortex; each additional hour of physician attendance	3.21	2.67	0.20	6.08	XXX	N
95962	26			3.21	1.43	0.12	4.76	XXX	N
95962	TC			0	1.24	0.08	1.32	XXX	N
95999	00	C	Unlisted neurological or neuromuscular diagnostic procedure	0	0	0	0	XXX	N
96400	00	A	Chemotherapy administration, subcutaneous or intramuscular, with or without local anesthesia	0	0.13	0.01	0.14	XXX	N
96405	00	A	Chemotherapy administration, intralesional; up to and including 7 lesions	0.52	0.38	0.03	0.93	0	S
96406	00	A	Chemotherapy administration, intralesional; more than 7 lesions	0.80	0.56	0.04	1.40	0	S
96408	00	A	Chemotherapy administration, intravenous; push technique	0	0.92	0.06	0.98	XXX	N
96410	00	A	Chemotherapy administration, intravenous; infusion technique, up to one hour	0	1.47	0.09	1.56	XXX	N
96412	00	A	Chemotherapy administration, intravenous; infusion technique, one to 8 hours, each additional hour	0	1.10	0.08	1.18	XXX	N
96414	00	A	Chemotherapy administration, intravenous; infusion technique, initiation of prolonged infusion (more than 8 hours), requiring the use of a portable or implantable pump	0	1.27	0.09	1.36	XXX	N
96420	00	A	Chemotherapy administration, intra-arterial; push technique	0	1.19	0.09	1.28	XXX	N
96422	00	A	Chemotherapy administration, intra-arterial; infusion technique, up to one hour	0	1.17	0.09	1.26	XXX	N
96423	00	A	Chemotherapy administration, intra-arterial; infusion technique, one to 8 hours, each additional hour	0	0.46	0.03	0.49	XXX	N
96425	00	A	Chemotherapy administration, intra-arterial; infusion technique, initiation of prolonged infusion (more than 8 hours), requiring the use of a portable or implantable pump	0	1.36	0.09	1.45	XXX	N
96440	00	A	Chemotherapy administration into pleural cavity, requiring and including thoracentesis	2.37	0.81	0.06	3.24	0	N
96445	00	A	Chemotherapy administration into peritoneal cavity, requiring and including peritoneocentesis	2.20	0.98	0.09	3.27	0	N
96450	00	A	Chemotherapy administration, into CNS (eg, intrathecal), requiring and including lumbar puncture	1.89	0.87	0.06	2.82	0	N
96520	00	A	Refilling and maintenance of portable pump	0	0.85	0.06	0.91	XXX	N
96530	00	A	Refilling and maintenance of implantable pump or reservoir	0	1.01	0.07	1.08	XXX	N
96542	00	A	Chemotherapy injection, subarachnoid or intraventricular via subcutaneous reservoir, single or multiple agents	1.42	1.09	0.13	2.64	XXX	N
96545	00	B	Provision of chemotherapy agent	0.41*	0.31#	0.04*	0.76#	XXX	0
96549	00	C	Unlisted chemotherapy procedure	0	0	0	0	XXX	N
96900	00	A	Actinotherapy (ultraviolet light)	0	0.38	0.03	0.41	XXX	N
96910	00	A	Photochemotherapy; tar and ultraviolet B (Goeckerman treatment) or petrolatum and ultraviolet B	0	0.55	0.04	0.59	XXX	N
96912	00	A	Photochemotherapy; psoralens and ultraviolet A (PUVA)	0	0.63	0.05	0.68	XXX	N

CPT codes and descriptions only, © 1994 American Medical Association. Reimbursement information, © 1995 McGraw-Hill Inc.

Code/ CPT	Mod- ifier	Status	Description	Work value	Practice expense	Mal- practice	Total value	Global period	Up- date
96913	00	A	Photochemotherapy (Goeckerman and/or PUVA) for severe photoresponsive dermatoses requiring at least four to eight hours of care under direct supervision of the physician (includes application of medication and dressings)	0	1.29	0.10	1.39	XXX	N
96999	00	C	Unlisted special dermatological service or procedure	0	0	0	0	XXX	N
97010	00	A	Application of a modality to one or more areas; hot or cold packs	0.11	0.21	0.02	0.34	XXX	N
97012	00	A	Application of a modality to one or more areas; traction, mechanical	0.25	0.19	0.02	0.46	XXX	N
97014	00	A	Application of a modality to one or more areas; electrical stimulation (unattended)	0.18	0.20	0.02	0.40	XXX	N
97016	00	A	Application of a modality to one or more areas; vasopneumatic devices	0.18	0.25	0.02	0.45	XXX	N
97018	00	A	Application of a modality to one or more areas; paraffin bath	0.11	0.24	0.03	0.38	XXX	N
97020	00	A	Application of a modality to one or more areas; microwave	0.11	0.20	0.02	0.33	XXX	N
97022	00	A	Application of a modality to one or more areas; whirlpool	0.25	0.19	0.02	0.46	XXX	N
97024	00	A	Application of a modality to one or more areas; diathermy	0.11	0.21	0.02	0.34	XXX	N
97026	00	A	Application of a modality to one or more areas; infrared	0.11	0.19	0.02	0.32	XXX	N
97028	00	A	Application of a modality to one or more areas; ultraviolet	0.20	0.19	0.01	0.40	XXX	N
97032	00	A	Application of a modality to one or more areas; electrical stimulation (manual), each 15 minutes	0.25	0.14	0.01	0.40	XXX	N
97033	00	A	Application of a modality to one or more areas; iontophoresis, each 15 minutes	0.26	0.14	0.02	0.42	XXX	N
97034	00	A	Application of a modality to one or more areas; contrast baths, each 15 minutes	0.21	0.10	0.01	0.32	XXX	N
97035	00	A	Application of a modality to one or more areas; ultrasound, each 15 minutes	0.21	0.11	0.01	0.33	XXX	N
97036	00	A	Application of a modality to one or more areas; Hubbard tank, each 15 minutes	0.38	0.21	0.02	0.61	XXX	N
97039	00	A	Unlisted modality (specify type and time if constant attendance)	0.29	0.24	0.03	0.56	XXX	N
97110	00	A	Therapeutic procedure, one or more areas, each 15 minutes; therapeutic exercises to develop strength and endurance, range of motion and flexibility	0.45	0.13	0.02	0.60	XXX	N
97112	00	A	Therapeutic procedure, one or more areas, each 15 minutes; neuromuscular reeducation of movement, balance, coordination, kinesthetic sense, posture, and proprioception	0.45	0.13	0.01	0.59	XXX	N
97113	00	A	Therapeutic procedure, one or more areas, each 15 minutes; aquatic therapy with therapeutic exercises	0.44	0.20	0.02	0.66	XXX	N
97114	00	D	Functional activity therapy	0.29*	0.22#	0.03*	0.54#	XXX	N
97116	00	A	Therapeutic procedure, one or more areas, each 15 minutes; gait training	0.40	0.11	0.01	0.52	XXX	N
97118	00	D	Manual electric stimulation	0.29*	0.22#	0.03*	0.54#	XXX	N
97120	00	D	Electric current therapy	0.29*	0.22#	0.03*	0.54#	XXX	N
97122	00	A	Therapeutic procedure, one or more areas, each 15 minutes; traction, manual	0.45	0.11	0.01	0.57	XXX	N
97124	00	A	Therapeutic procedure, one or more areas, each 15 minutes; massage, including effleurage, petrissage and/or tapotement (stroking, compression, percussion)	0.35	0.11	0.01	0.47	XXX	N
97126	00	D	Contrast baths therapy	0.29*	0.22#	0.03*	0.54#	XXX	N
97128	00	D	Ultrasound therapy	0.29*	0.22#	0.03*	0.54#	XXX	N
97139	00	A	Therapeutic procedure, one or more areas, each 15 minutes; unlisted therapeutic procedure (specify)	0.21	0.16	0.02	0.39	XXX	N

CPT codes and descriptions only, © 1994 American Medical Association. Reimbursement information, © 1995 McGraw-Hill Inc.

Code/ CPT	Mod- ifier	Status	Description	Work value	Practice expense	Mal- practice	Total value	Global period	Up- date
97145	00	D	Extended physiotherapy	0.09*	0.07#	0.01*	0.17#	XXX	N
97150	00	A	Therapeutic procedure(s), group (2 or more individuals)	0.27	0.20	0.02	0.49	XXX	N
97220	00	D	Hydrotherapy	0.24*	0.18#	0.02*	0.44#	XXX	N
97221	00	D	Extended hydrotherapy	0.09*	0.07#	0.01*	0.17#	XXX	N
97240	00	D	Hydrotherapy	0.47*	0.36#	0.04*	0.87#	XXX	N
97241	00	D	Extended hydrotherapy	0.12*	0.09#	0.01*	0.22#	XXX	N
97250	00	A	Myofascial release/soft tissue mobilization, one or more regions	0.45	0.35	0.04	0.84	0	N
97260	00	A	Manipulation (cervical, thoracic, lumbosacral, sacroiliac, hand, wrist) (separate procedure), performed by physician; one area	0.19	0.20	0.02	0.41	0	N
97261	00	A	Manipulation (cervical, thoracic, lumbosacral, sacroiliac, hand, wrist) (separate procedure), performed by physician; each additional area	0.12	0.11	0.01	0.24	0	N
97265	00	A	Joint mobilization, one or more areas (peripheral or spinal)	0.45	0.35	0.04	0.84	XXX	N
97500	00	A	Orthotics training (dynamic bracing, splinting), upper and/or lower extremities; initial 30 minutes, each visit	0.31	0.27	0.04	0.62	XXX	N
97501	00	A	Orthotics training (dynamic bracing, splinting), upper and/or lower extremities; each additional 15 minutes	0.17	0.15	0.02	0.34	XXX	N
97520	00	A	Prosthetic training; initial 30 minutes, each visit	0.37	0.30	0.04	0.71	XXX	N
97521	00	A	Prosthetic training; each additional 15 minutes	0.22	0.17	0.02	0.41	XXX	N
97530	00	A	Therapeutic activities, direct (one on one) patient contact by the provider (use of dynamic activities to improve functional performance), each 15 minutes	0.44	0.17	0.02	0.63	XXX	N
97531	00	D	Added kinetic therapy	0.10*	0.07#	0.01*	0.18#	XXX	N
97540	00	A	Training in activities of daily living (self care skills and/or daily life management skills); initial 30 minutes, each visit	0.44	0.37	0.03	0.84	XXX	N
97541	00	A	Training in activities of daily living (self care skills and/or daily life management skills); each additional 15 minutes	0.21	0.16	0.01	0.38	XXX	N
97545	00	R	Work hardening/conditioning; initial 2 hours	1.41*	1.07#	0.12*	2.60#	XXX	N
97546	00	R	Work hardening/conditioning; each additional hour	0.71*	0.54#	0.06*	1.31#	XXX	N
97700	00	A	Office visit, including one of the following tests or measurements, with report a. Orthotic "check-out" b. Prosthetic "check-out" c. Activities of daily living "check-out"; initial 30 minutes, each visit	0.39	0.35	0.04	0.78	XXX	N
97701	00	A	Office visit, including one of the following tests or measurements, with report a. Orthotic "check-out" b. Prosthetic "check-out" c. Activities of daily living "check-out"; each additional 15 minutes	0.19	0.17	0.02	0.38	XXX	N
97720	00	D	Extremity testing	0.18*	0.14#	0.02*	0.34#	XXX	N
97721	00	D	Supplemental limb testing	0.06*	0.05#	0.01*	0.12#	XXX	N
97750	00	A	Physical performance test or measurement (eg, musculoskeletal, functional capacity), with written report, each 15 minutes	0.45	0.24	0.03	0.72	XXX	N
97752	00	D	Muscle testing with exercise	0.83*	0.63#	0.07*	1.53#	XXX	N
97752	26			0.59*	0.45#	0.05*	1.09#	XXX	N
97752	TC			0	0	0	0	XXX	N
97770	00	R	Development of cognitive skills to improve attention, memory, problem solving, includes compensatory training and/or sensory integrative activities, direct (one on one) patient contact by the provider, each 15 minutes	0.44	0.28	0.03	0.75	XXX	N
97799	00	C	Unlisted physical medicine/rehabilitation service or procedure	0	0	0	0	XXX	N

CPT codes and descriptions only, © 1994 American Medical Association. Reimbursement information, © 1995 McGraw-Hill Inc.

Code/ CPT	Mod-ifier	Status	Description	Work value	Practice expense	Mal-practice	Total value	Global period	Up-date
98925	00	A	Osteopathic manipulative treatment (OMT); one to two body regions involved	0.45	0.25	0.02	0.72	0	N
98926	00	A	Osteopathic manipulative treatment (OMT); three to four body regions involved	0.65	0.40	0.03	1.08	0	N
98927	00	A	Osteopathic manipulative treatment (OMT); five to six body regions involved	0.87	0.38	0.03	1.28	0	N
98928	00	A	Osteopathic manipulative treatment (OMT); seven to eight body regions involved	1.03	0.42	0.04	1.49	0	N
98929	00	A	Osteopathic manipulative treatment (OMT); nine to ten body regions involved	1.19	0.39	0.03	1.61	0	N
99000	00	B	Handling and/or conveyance of specimen for transfer from the physician's office to a laboratory	0.18*	0.14#	0.02*	0.34#	XXX	0
99001	00	B	Handling and/or conveyance of specimen for transfer from the patient in other than a physician's office to a laboratory (distance may be indicated)	0.09*	0.07#	0.01*	0.17#	XXX	0
99002	00	B	Handling, conveyance, and/or any other service in connection with the implementation of an order involving devices (eg, designing, fitting, packaging, handling, delivery or mailing) when devices such as orthotics, protectives, prosthetics are fabricated by an outside laboratory or shop but which items have been designed, and are to be fitted and adjusted by the attending physician	0.09*	0.07#	0.01*	0.17#	XXX	0
99024	00	B	Postoperative follow-up visit, included in global service	0	0	0	0	XXX	0
99025	00	B	Initial (new patient) visit when starred (*) surgical procedure constitutes major service at that visit	0.24*	0.18#	0.02*	0.44#	XXX	0
99050	00	B	Services requested after office hours in addition to basic service	0.24*	0.18#	0.02*	0.44#	XXX	0
99052	00	B	Services requested between 10:00 PM and 8:00 AM in addition to basic service	0.47*	0.36#	0.04*	0.87#	XXX	0
99054	00	B	Services requested on Sundays and holidays in addition to basic service	0.47*	0.36#	0.04*	0.87#	XXX	0
99056	00	B	Services provided at request of patient in a location other than physician's office which are normally provided in the office	0.24*	0.18#	0.02*	0.44#	XXX	0
99058	00	B	Office services provided on an emergency basis	0.24*	0.18#	0.02*	0.44#	XXX	0
99070	00	B	Supplies and materials (except spectacles), provided by the physician over and above those usually included with the office visit or other services rendered (list drugs, trays, supplies, or materials provided)	0	0	0	0	XXX	0
99071	00	B	Educational supplies, such as books, tapes, and pamphlets, provided by the physician for the patient's education at cost to physician	0	0	0	0	XXX	0
99075	00	N	Medical testimony	2.06*	1.56#	0.18*	3.80#	XXX	0
99078	00	B	Physician educational services rendered to patients in a group setting (eg, prenatal, obesity, or diabetic instructions)	0	0	0	0	XXX	0
99080	00	B	Special reports such as insurance forms, more than the information conveyed in the usual medical communications or standard reporting form	0	0	0	0	XXX	0
99082	00	C	Unusual travel (eg, transportation and escort of patient)	0	0	0	0	XXX	N
99090	00	B	Analysis of information data stored in computers (eg, ECGs, blood pressures, hematologic data)	1.30*	0.98#	0.12*	2.40#	XXX	0
99100	00	B	Anesthesia for patient of extreme age, under one year and over seventy	0	0	0	0	XXX	0
99116	00	B	Anesthesia complicated by utilization of total body hypothermia	0	0	0	0	XXX	0

CPT codes and descriptions only, © 1994 American Medical Association. Reimbursement information, © 1995 McGraw-Hill Inc.

Code/ CPT	Mod-ifier	Status	Description	Work value	Practice expense	Mal-practice	Total value	Global period	Up-date
99135	00	B	Anesthesia complicated by utilization of controlled hypotension	0	0	0	0	XXX	0
99140	00	B	Anesthesia complicated by emergency conditions (specify)	0	0	0	0	XXX	0
99175	00	A	Ipecac or similar administration for individual emesis and continued observation until stomach adequately emptied of poison	0	1.33	0.10	1.43	XXX	N
99178	00	C	Administration and medical interpretation of developmental tests	0	0	0	0	XXX	N
99183	00	A	Physician attendance and supervision of hyperbaric oxygen therapy, per session	2.34	1.67	0.11	4.12	XXX	N
99185	00	A	Hypothermia; regional	0	0.61	0.04	0.65	XXX	N
99186	00	A	Hypothermia; total body	0	1.70	0.52	2.22	XXX	N
99190	00	X	Assembly and operation of pump with oxygenator or heat exchanger (with or without ECG and/or pressure monitoring); each hour	5.07*	4.63#	0.28*	9.98#	XXX	0
99191	00	X	Assembly and operation of pump with oxygenator or heat exchanger (with or without ECG and/or pressure monitoring); ¾ hour	3.77*	3.44#	0.21*	7.42#	XXX	0
99192	00	X	Assembly and operation of pump with oxygenator or heat exchanger (with or without ECG and/or pressure monitoring); ½ hour	2.51*	2.29#	0.14*	4.94#	XXX	0
99195	00	A	Phlebotomy, therapeutic (separate procedure)	0	0.42	0.03	0.45	XXX	N
99199	00	C	Unlisted special service or report	0	0	0	0	XXX	N

CPT codes and descriptions only, © 1994 American Medical Association. Reimbursement information, © 1995 McGraw-Hill Inc.

CHAPTER 6

Evaluation & Management

The editors have elected to indicate that a relative value is not available for procedures with a "0" in the individual units column.

I. **General:** Visits, examinations, consultations, and similar services as listed in this section reflect the wide variations required in time and skill. The following alphabetical list of definitions is included to aid in the determination of the correct code for the service provided. Documentation for each aspect of the service performed should be included in the patient record to substantiate the level of service. The listed relativities for each code group apply only when these services are performed by or under the responsible supervision of a physician.

Chief Complaint: A concise statement describing the symptom, problem, condition, diagnosis, or other factor that is the reason for the encounter.

Classification of Service: Each code in this section is grouped into a category. The groupings are defined by place (e.g. office, hospital, nursing home, etc.) and type of service (e.g. consultation, preventive, etc.). Some of the codes are grouped into subcategories (e.g. new patient, established patient, initial, etc.). Each code in the group represents a different level of service defined by the clinical components of a patient encounter for E/M (see Levels of Service).

Components: Each level of service recognizes seven components. The components include history, physical examination, medical decision making, counseling, coordination of care, nature of presenting problem, and time. (See Levels of Service, Key Components, History, Physical Examination, Medical Decision Making, Counseling, Problem, and Time.)

Concurrent Care: The provision of similar services (e.g. hospital visits) to the same patient by more than one physician on the same day. CPT has deleted modifier -75 and does not require any special reporting for concurrent care.

Consultation: There are three categories for consultation: outpatient, inpatient, and confirmatory. Any physician may use an appropriate consultation code on any patient for any problem including one which has been previously evaluated by the consulting physician provided the following criteria are met.

1. The attending physician or appropriate source requests that the physician render advice or opinion regarding the evaluation and/or management of a specific problem.
2. The need for the consultation, the consultant's opinion, and any services ordered or performed must be well documented in the patients record.
3. The information is communicated to the requesting physician or appropriate source.

Counseling: A discussion with the patient and/or family concerning one or more of the following:

CPT codes and descriptions only, © 1994 American Medical Association.

Reimbursement information, © 1995 McGraw-Hill Inc.

- Diagnostic results, impressions, and/or recommended diagnostic studies;
- Prognosis;
- Risks and benefits of management options;
- Instructions for management and/or follow-up;
- Importance of compliance with chosen management;
- Risk factor reduction; and
- Patient and family education.
- (See Key components and Time.)

Established Patient: A patient who has received professional services from a physician or another physician in the same specialty within the same group within the last three years. In the instance a physician is covering for or on call for another physician, the patient is classified as an established patient if the other physician or a member of the providing physician specialty group has provided services for the patient within the last three years.

Family History: A review of medical events in the patient's family that includes significant information about:

- the health status or cause of death of parents, siblings, and children;
- specific diseases related to problems identified in the Chief Complaint or History of the Present Illness, and/or System Review;
- diseases of family members which may be hereditary or place the patient at risk.

History: This key component relates to the type of history obtained during a patient encounter. The four types of history are defined as follows:

Problem focused—brief history of present illness or problem as related to the chief complaint.

Expanded problem focused—brief history of present illness relating to chief complaint and pertinent system review.

Detailed—extended history of present illness related to chief complaint, an extended system review, and pertinent past, family and/or social history.

Comprehensive—extended history of present illness related to chief complaint, complete system review, and complete past, family and social history.

History of Present Illness: A chronological description of the development of the patient's present illness from the first sign and/or symptom to the present. This includes a description of location, quality, severity, timing, context, modifying factors, and associated signs and symptoms significantly related to the presenting problem(s).

Key Components: Those components which are used primarily to determine the appropriate code level. These components include Medical Decision Making, Physical Examination, and History (see History, Physical Examination, Medical Decision Making). Time is not considered a key component unless counseling constitutes more than 50% of the face-to-face patient/physician encounter, then time is considered the key component (see Time, Counseling).

Levels of Service: Each category and subcategory contains three to five levels of service indicated by code. The services include examinations, evaluations, treatments, conferences with/or concerning patients, preventative pediatric and adult health supervision, and similar services. Each level of service recognizes seven clinical components. Three of these components are considered key components (see Components of Service, History, Physical Examination, and Medical Decision Making). Each level of service may be used by all physicians.

Medical Decision Making: The complexity of establishing a diagnosis or selecting a management option. Medical decision making is divided into four categories. The level of medical decision making is determined using documentation in the patient record for three subcategories including: number of possible diagnoses and/or the number of management options considered; the amount and/or complexity of medical records, diagnostic tests, and/or other information which must be obtained, reviewed, and analyzed; and the risk of significant complications, morbidity and/or mortality, as well as comorbidities, associated with the patient's presenting problem(s), the diagnostic procedure(s), and/or the possible management options. The following four classifications for level of medical decision making are used in determining the proper code.

Straightforward: minimal number of possible diagnoses or management options, minimal or no amount and/or complexity of data to be reviewed, and minimal risk of complications and/or morbidity or mortality.

Low Complexity: limited number of possible diagnoses or management options, limited amount and/or complexity of data to be reviewed, and low risk of complications and/or morbidity or mortality.

Moderate Complexity: multiple number of possible diagnoses or management options, moderate amount and/or complexity of data to be reviewed, and moderate risk of complications and/or morbidity or mortality.

High Complexity: extensive number of possible di-

CPT codes and descriptions only, © 1994 American Medical Association. Reimbursement information, © 1995 McGraw-Hill Inc.

agnoses or management options, extensive amount and/or complexity of data to be reviewed, and high risk of complications and/or morbidity or mortality.

Nature of Presenting Problem: A presenting problem is a disease, condition, illness, injury, symptom, sign, finding, complaint, or other reason for encounter, with or without a diagnosis being established at the time of the encounter. The E/M codes recognize five types of presenting problems that are defined as follows:

Minimal: A problem that may not require the presence of the physician, but service is provided under the physician's supervision.

Self-limited or minor: A problem that runs a definite and prescribed course, is transient in nature, and is not likely to permanently alter health status OR has a good prognosis with management/compliance.

Low severity: A problem where the risk of morbidity without treatment is low; there is little to no risk of mortality without treatment; full recovery without functional impairment is expected.

Moderate severity: A problem where the risk of morbidity without treatment is moderate; there is moderate risk of mortality without treatment; uncertain prognosis OR increased probability of prolonged functional impairment.

High severity: A problem where the risk of morbidity without treatment is high to extreme; there is a moderate to high risk of mortality without treatment OR high probability of severe, prolonged functional impairment.

New Patient: A patient who has not received any professional services from a physician or another physician in the same specialty within the same group within the past three years. In the instance where a physician is on call for or covering for another physician, the patient is classified as a new patient if the other physician or a member of the providing physician's specialty group has not provided any professional service for the patient within three years. (See Established Patient.)

Past History: A review of the patient's past experiences with illnesses, injuries, and treatments that include significant information about:

- prior major illnesses and injuries;
- prior operations;
- prior hospitalizations;
- current medications;
- allergies (eg, drug, food);
- age appropriate immunization status;
- age appropriate feeding/dietary status.

Physical Examination: This key component relates to the type of physical examination performed during a patient encounter. The four defined types of physical examination are:

Problem focused—an examination limited to the affected body area or organ system.

Expanded problem focused—an examination of the affected body area or organ system and other symptomatic or related organ systems.

Detailed—an extended examination of the affected body area(s) and other symptomatic or related organ system(s).

Comprehensive—a complete single system specialty examination or a complete multi-system examination.

Problem: Problem describes the nature of the problem presented as the reason for the encounter. Problem is considered to be a contributing factor and therefore is not used as a primary factor in determining level of service. Problem is classified in the following five categories:

Minimal: A problem that may not require the presence of the physician, but service is provided under the supervision of the physician.

Self-limited or minor: A problem that runs a definite and prescribed course, is transient in nature, and is not likely to permanently alter health status or has a good prognosis with management compliance.

Low severity: A problem where the risk of morbidity without treatment is low; there is little to no risk of mortality without treatment; full recovery without functional impairment is expected.

Moderate severity: A problem where the risk of morbidity without treatment is moderate; there is moderate risk of mortality without treatment; uncertain prognosis or increased probability of prolonged functional impairment.

High severity: A problem where the risk of morbidity without treatment is high to extreme; there is moderate to high risk of mortality without treatment or high probability of severe, prolonged functional impairment.

Review of Systems: An inventory of body systems obtained through a series of questions seeking to identify signs and/or symptoms which the patient may be experiencing or has experienced. For the purposes of CPT the following elements of a system review have been identified:

- Constitutional symptoms (fever, weight loss, etc.)
- Eyes
- Ears, Nose, Mouth, Throat

CPT codes and descriptions only, © 1994 American Medical Association. Reimbursement information, © 1995 McGraw-Hill Inc.

- Cardiovascular
- Respiratory
- Gastrointestinal
- Genitourinary
- Musculoskeletal
- Integumentary (skin and/or breast)
- Neurological
- Psychiatric
- Endocrine
- Hematologic/Lymphatic
- Allergic/Immunologic

Social History: An age appropriate review of past and current activities that includes significant information about:

- marital status and/or living arrangements;
- current employment;
- occupational history;
- use of drugs, alcohol, and tobacco;
- level of education;
- sexual history;
- other relevant social factors.

Time: Time for an outpatient is considered to be face-to-face time spent with the patient and does not include time spent in such things as record review or dictating. The time for an inpatient is considered to be the time spent "on the floor" and does include record review, dictating, and other services rendered while in the hospital unit of the patient. Times given are considered to be an average and should not be used to determine the length of time spent in the encounter. Time is considered to be a contributory factor and as such is not used to define the level of service unless 50% or more of the service performed is spent in counseling or coordinating care. In cases where 50% of the service is counseling or coordinating care, time is considered the overriding component and is used as the primary component for defining the level of service. Careful documentation of time is essential in cases where time is the defining component.

II. **Unusual Service or Procedure:** A service may necessitate skills and time of the physician over and above listed services and values. If substantiated "by report" (BR), additional values may be warranted. Use modifier -22 to indicate these procedures.

III. **Unlisted Service or Procedure:** When a service or procedure provided is not adequately identified, use of the unlisted procedure code for the related anatomical area is appropriate. Most codes of this nature have 99 for the last two digits. Value should be substantiated "by report" (BR). (See By Report.)

IV. **Prolonged Evaluation and Management Service:** When a service provided is prolonged or otherwise greater than that usually required for the E/M service, use of prolonged service codes is appropriate. Medicare will only pay for face-to-face prolonged care. A report may be required.

V. **Unrelated E/M Service by the Same Physician During a Postoperative Period:** If a service which is not related to the original procedure and is performed during the follow-up period for that period may be billed at 100% of the listed value. Use modifier -24 to indicate this service is unrelated.

VI. **Significant, Separately Identifiable E/M Service by the Same Physician on the Day of a Procedure:** In cases where an E/M service is performed on the same day of a procedure above and beyond normal pre- and post-operative care associated with the procedure performed may be billed at 100% of the listed value. Services of this nature must be substantiated by report. Use modifier -25 to indicate this type of service. **Medicare will pay for this service if it is used in conjunction with a same date procedure with a 0 or 10 day global period.**

VII. **E/M Service Resulting in Initial Decision for Surgery:** If an evaluation and management encounter results in the initial decision to perform surgery, modifier -57 may be attached to the E/M service code. At such time as the decision for surgery is made, meaning recommended to the patient and agreed to by the patient, the preoperative time begins, and other E/M services related to the procedure are included in the global value of the procedure. The modifier does not reduce or increase the value of the service and should be billed at 100% of the listed value. **Medicare will pay for this modifier if the service is provided on the day of, or the day before, a 90 day global procedure.**

VIII. **Unrelated E/M Service During a Designated Preoperative Period:** An evaluation and management service which is unrelated to a planned procedure provided during a designated preoperative period may be repeated using modifier -59. Modifier -59 should be billed at 100%. (Note: This modifier is not CPT compatible.) **Medicare will not pay.**

IX. **Procedures without Specified Units Values:** Procedures which have RNE or BR in the units column, should be substantiated "by report."

X. **By Report:** Value of a procedure should be established for any "by report" circumstance by identifying a similar service and justifying value difference. When

CPT codes and descriptions only, © 1994 American Medical Association. Reimbursement information, © 1995 McGraw-Hill Inc.

a report is indicated, the report should include the following:

1. Accurate procedure definition or description;
2. Operative report;
3. Justification for procedural variance, when appropriate;
4. Similar procedure and value; and
5. Justification for value difference.

XI. **Reduced Values:** Under some circumstances, value for a procedure may be reduced or eliminated. Use modifier -52 to identify reduced value services.

XII. **Multiple Modifiers:** If circumstances require the use of more than one modifier with any one procedure code, modifier -99 should be added to the procedure code. Other modifiers are then attached to the procedure code and listed separately with appropriate values for each.

XIII. **Materials Supplied by Physician:** Supplies and materials provided by the physician (i.e., sterile trays, drugs, etc.) are considered to be bundled by Medicare. Supplies should not be billed separately except for permanent condition supplies, home use, and surgical trays for designated procedures. For use within the private sector, identify supplies by using code 99070. Supplies and materials provided by the physician (i.e., sterile trays, drugs, etc.) over and above those usually indicated with the office visit or other services rendered may be listed separately. This rule varies by contract.

CPT codes and descriptions only, © 1994 American Medical Association. Reimbursement information, © 1995 McGraw-Hill Inc.

EVALUATION & MANAGEMENT VALUES

Code/ CPT	Mod- ifier	Status	Description	Work value	Practice expense	Mal- practice	Total value	Global period	Up- date
99201	00	A	Office or other outpatient visit for the evaluation and management of a new patient, which requires these three key components: a problem focused history; a problem focused examination; and straightforward medical decision making. Counseling and/or coordination of care with other providers or agencies are provided consistent with the nature of the problem(s) and the patient's and/or family's needs. Usually, the presenting problems are self limited or minor. Physicians typically spend 10 minutes face-to-face with the patient and/or family.	0.38	0.37	0.04	0.79	XXX	P
99202	00	A	Office or other outpatient visit for the evaluation and management of a new patient, which requires these three key components: an expanded problem focused history; an expanded problem focused examination; and straightforward medical decision making. Counseling and/or coordination of care with other providers or agencies are provided consistent with the nature of the problem(s) and the patient's and/or family's needs. Usually, the presenting problem(s) are of low to moderate severity. Physicians typically spend 20 minutes face-to-face with the patient and/or family.	0.75	0.45	0.05	1.25	XXX	P
99203	00	A	Office or other outpatient visit for the evaluation and management of a new patient, which requires these three key components: a detailed history; a detailed examination; and medical decision making of low complexity. Counseling and/or coordination of care with other providers or agencies are provided consistent with the nature of the problem(s) and the patient's and/or family's needs. Usually, the presenting problem(s) are of moderate severity. Physicians typically spend 30 minutes face-to-face with the patient and/or family.	1.14	0.52	0.06	1.72	XXX	P
99204	00	A	Office or other outpatient visit for the evaluation and management of a new patient, which requires these three key components: a comprehensive history; a comprehensive examination; and medical decision making of moderate complexity. Counseling and/or coordination of care with other providers or agencies are provided consistent with the nature of the problem(s) and the patient's and/or family's needs. Usually, the presenting problem(s) are of moderate to high severity. Physicians typically spend 45 minutes face-to-face with the patient and/or family.	1.71	0.78	0.08	2.57	XXX	P

CPT codes and descriptions only, © 1994 American Medical Association. Reimbursement information, © 1995 McGraw-Hill Inc.

Code/ CPT	Mod- ifier	Status	Description	Work value	Practice expense	Mal- practice	Total value	Global period	Up- date
99205	00	A	Office or other outpatient visit for the evaluation and management of a new patient, which requires these three key components: a comprehensive history; a comprehensive examination; and medical decision making of high complexity. Counseling and/or coordination of care with other providers or agencies are provided consistent with the nature of the problem(s) and the patient's and/or family's needs. Usually, the presenting problem(s) are of moderate to high severity. Physicians typically spend 60 minutes face-to-face with the patient and/or family.	2.28	0.85	0.09	3.22	XXX	P
99211	00	A	Office or other outpatient visit for the evaluation and management of an established patient, that may not require the presence of a physician. Usually, the presenting problem(s) are minimal. Typically, 5 minutes are spent performing or supervising these services.	0.17	0.19	0.02	0.38	XXX	P
99212	00	A	Office or other outpatient visit for the evaluation and management of an established patient, which requires at least two of these three key components: a problem focused history; a problem focused examination; straightforward medical decision making. Counseling and/or coordination of care with other providers or agencies are provided consistent with the nature of the problem(s) and the patient's and/or family's needs. Usually, the presenting problem(s) are self limited or minor. Physicians typically spend 10 minutes face-to-face with the patient and/or family.	0.38	0.28	0.02	0.68	XXX	P
99213	00	A	Office or other outpatient visit for the evaluation and management of an established patient, which requires at least two of these three key components: an expanded problem focused history; an expanded problem focused examination; medical decision making of low complexity. Counseling and coordination of care with other providers or agencies are provided consistent with the nature of the problem(s) and the patient's and/or family's needs. Usually, the presenting problem(s) are of low to moderate severity. Physicians typically spend 15 minutes face-to-face with the patient and/or family.	0.55	0.38	0.03	0.96	XXX	P
99214	00	A	Office or other outpatient visit for the evaluation and management of an established patient, which requires at least two of these three key components: a detailed history; a detailed examination; medical decision making of moderate complexity. Counseling and/or coordination of care with other providers or agencies are provided consistent with the nature of the problem(s) and the patient's and/or family's needs. Usually, the presenting problem(s) are of moderate to high severity. Physicians typically spend 25 minutes face-to-face with the patient and/or family.	0.94	0.50	0.04	1.48	XXX	P
99215	00	A	Office or other outpatient visit for the evaluation and management of an established patient, which requires at least two of these three key components: a comprehensive history; a comprehensive examination; medical decision making of high complexity. Counseling and/or coordination of care with other providers or agencies are provided consistent with the nature of the problem(s) and the patient's and/or family's needs.	1.51	0.76	0.07	2.34	XXX	P

CPT codes and descriptions only, © 1994 American Medical Association. Reimbursement information, © 1995 McGraw-Hill Inc.

Code/ CPT	Mod- ifier	Status	Description	Work value	Practice expense	Mal- practice	Total value	Global period	Up- date
			Usually, the presenting problem(s) are of moderate to high severity. Physicians typically spend 40 minutes face-to-face with the patient and/or family.						
99217	00	A	Observation care discharge day management	1.09	0.52	0.04	1.65	XXX	N
99218	00	A	Initial observation care, per day, for the evaluation and management of a patient which requires these three key components: a detailed or comprehensive history; a detailed or comprehensive examination; and medical decision making that is straightforward or of low complexity. Counseling and/or coordination of care with other providers or agencies are provided consistent with the nature of the problem(s) and the patient's and/or family's needs. Usually, the problem(s) requiring admission to "observation status" are of low severity.	1.08	0.68	0.06	1.82	XXX	N
99219	00	A	Initial observation care, per day, for the evaluation and management of a patient, which requires these three key components: a comprehensive history; a comprehensive examination; and medical decision making of moderate complexity. Counseling and/or coordination of care with other providers or agencies are provided consistent with the nature of the problem(s) and the patient's and/or family's needs. Usually, the problem(s) requiring admission to "observation status" are of moderate severity.	1.75	1.05	0.09	2.89	XXX	N
99220	00	A	Initial observation care, per day, for the evaluation and management of a patient, which requires these three key components: a comprehensive history; a comprehensive examination; and medical decision making of high complexity. Counseling and/or coordination of care with other providers or agencies are provided consistent with the nature of the problem(s) and the patient's and/or family's needs. Usually, the problem(s) requiring admission to "observation status" are of high severity.	2.41	1.14	0.09	3.64	XXX	N
99221	00	A	Initial hospital care, per day, for the evaluation and management of a patient which requires these three key components: a detailed or comprehensive history; a detailed or comprehensive examination; and medical decision making that is straightforward or of low complexity. Counseling and/or coordination of care with other providers or agencies are provided consistent with the nature of the problem(s) and the patient's and/or family's needs. Usually, the problem(s) requiring admission are of low severity. Physicians typically spend 30 minutes at the bedside and on the patient's hospital floor or unit.	1.06	0.67	0.06	1.79	XXX	N
99222	00	A	Initial hospital care, per day, for the evaluation and management of a patient, which requires these three key components: a comprehensive history; a comprehensive examination; and medical decision making of moderate complexity. Counseling and/or coordination of care with other providers or agencies are provided consistent with the nature of the problem(s) and the patient's and/or family's needs. Usually, the problem(s) requiring admission are of moderate severity. Physicians typically spend 50 minutes at the bedside and on the patient's hospital floor or unit.	1.84	1.04	0.09	2.97	XXX	N

CPT codes and descriptions only, © 1994 American Medical Association. Reimbursement information, © 1995 McGraw-Hill Inc.

Code/ CPT	Mod- ifier	Status	Description	Work value	Practice expense	Mal- practice	Total value	Global period	Up- date
99223	00	A	Initial hospital care, per day, for the evaluation and management of a patient, which requires these three key components: a comprehensive history; a comprehensive examination; and medical decision making of high complexity. Counseling and/or coordination of care with other providers or agencies are provided consistent with the nature of the problem(s) and the patient's and/or family's needs. Usually, the problem(s) requiring admission are of high severity. Physicians typically spend 70 minutes at the bedside and on the patient's hospital floor or unit.	2.57	1.13	0.08	3.78	XXX	N
99231	00	A	Subsequent hospital care, per day, for the evaluation and management of a patient, which requires at least two of these three key components: a problem focused interval history; a problem focused examination; medical decision making that is straightforward or of low complexity. Counseling and/or coordination of care with other providers or agencies are provided consistent with the nature of the problem(s) and the patient's and/or family's needs. Usually, the patient is stable, recovering or improving. Physicians typically spend 15 minutes at the bedside and on the patient's hospital floor or unit.	0.51	0.38	0.03	0.92	XXX	N
99232	00	A	Subsequent hospital care, per day, for the evaluation and management of a patient, which requires at least two of these three key components: an expanded problem focused interval history; an expanded problem focused examination; medical decision making of moderate complexity. Counseling and/or coordination of care with other providers or agencies are provided consistent with the nature of the problem(s) and the patient's and/or family's needs. Usually, the patient is responding inadequately to therapy or has developed a minor complication. Physicians typically spend 25 minutes at the bedside and on the patient's hospital floor or unit.	0.88	0.45	0.04	1.37	XXX	N
99233	00	A	Subsequent hospital care, per day, for the evaluation and management of a patient, which requires at least two of these three key components: a detailed interval history; a detailed examination; medical decision making of high complexity. Counseling and/or coordination of care with other providers or agencies are provided consistent with the nature of the problem(s) and the patient's and/or family's needs. Usually, the patient is unstable or has developed a significant complication or a significant new problem. Physicians typically spend 35 minutes at the bedside and on the patient's hospital floor or unit.	1.25	0.60	0.05	1.90	XXX	N
99238	00	A	Hospital discharge day management (This code is to be utilized by the physician to report all services provided to a patient on the date of discharge, if other than the initial date of inpatient status. To report services to a patient who is admitted as an inpatient, and discharged on the same date, use only the codes for Initial Hospital Inpatient Services, 99221-99223. To report concurrent care services provided by a physician(s) other than the attending physician, use subsequent hospital care codes (99231-99233) on the day of discharge.) (For Observation Care Discharge, use 99217)	1.06	0.51	0.04	1.61	XXX	N
99241	00	A	Office consultation for a new or established patient, which requires these three key components: a problem focused	0.54	0.64	0.08	1.26	XXX	N

CPT codes and descriptions only, © 1994 American Medical Association. Reimbursement information, © 1995 McGraw-Hill Inc.

Code/ CPT	Mod- ifier	Status	Description	Work value	Practice expense	Mal- practice	Total value	Global period	Up- date
			history; a problem focused examination; and straightforward medical decision making. Counseling and/or coordination of care with other providers or agencies are provided consistent with the nature of the problem(s) and the patient's and/or family's needs. Usually, the presenting problem(s) are self limited or minor. Physicians typically spend 15 minutes face-to-face with the patient and/or family.						
99242	00	A	Office consultation for a new or established patient, which requires these three key components: an expanded problem focused history; an expanded problem focused examination; and straightforward medical decision making. Counseling and/or coordination of care with other providers or agencies are provided consistent with the nature of the problem(s) and the patient(s) and/or family's needs. Usually, the presenting problem(s) are of low severity. Physicians typically spend 30 minutes face-to-face with the patient and/or family.	1.11	0.77	0.09	1.97	XXX	N
99243	00	A	Office consultation for a new or established patient, which requires these three key components: a detailed history; a detailed examination; and medical decision making of low complexity. Counseling and/or coordination of care with other providers or agencies are provided consistent with the nature of the problem(s) and the patient's and/or family's needs. Usually, the presenting problem(s) are of moderate severity. Physicians typically spend 40 minutes face-to-face with the patient and/or family.	1.47	0.97	0.10	2.54	XXX	N
99244	00	A	Office consultation for a new or established patient, which requires these three key components: a comprehensive history; a comprehensive examination; and medical decision making of moderate complexity. Counseling and/or coordination of care with other providers or agencies are provided consistent with the nature of the problem(s) and the patient's and/or family's needs. Usually, the presenting problem(s) are of moderate to high severity. Physicians typically spend 60 minutes face-to-face with the patient and/or family.	2.23	1.23	0.11	3.57	XXX	N
99245	00	A	Office consultation for a new or established patient, which requires these three key components: a comprehensive history; a comprehensive examination; and medical decision making of high complexity. Counseling and/or coordination of care with other providers or agencies are provided consistent with the nature of the problem(s) and the patient's and/or family's needs. Usually, the presenting problem(s) are of moderate to high severity. Physicians typically spend 80 minutes face-to-face with the patient and/or family.	2.96	1.69	0.16	4.81	XXX	N
99251	00	A	Initial inpatient consultation for a new or established patient, which requires these three key components: a problem focused history; a problem focused examination; and straightforward medical decision making. Counseling and/or coordination of care with other providers or agencies are provided consistent with the nature of the problem(s) and the patient's and/or family's needs. Usually, the presenting problem(s) are self limited or minor. Physicians typically spend 20 minutes at the bedside and on the patient's hospital floor or unit.	0.54	0.67	0.08	1.29	XXX	N

CPT codes and descriptions only, © 1994 American Medical Association. Reimbursement information, © 1995 McGraw-Hill Inc.

Code/ CPT	Mod- ifier	Status	Description	Work value	Practice expense	Mal- practice	Total value	Global period	Up- date
99252	00	A	Initial inpatient consultation for a new or established patient, which requires these three key components: an expanded problem focused history; an expanded problem focused examination; and straightforward medical decision making. Counseling and/or coordination of care with other providers or agencies are provided consistent with the nature of the problem(s) and the patient's and/or family's needs. Usually, the presenting problem(s) are of low severity. Physicians typically spend 40 minutes at the bedside and on the patient's hospital floor or unit.	1.13	0.76	0.09	1.98	XXX	N
99253	00	A	Initial inpatient consultation for a new or established patient, which requires these three key components: a detailed history; a detailed examination; and medical decision making of low complexity. Counseling and/or coordination of care with other providers or agencies are provided consistent with the nature of the problem(s) and the patient's and/or family's needs. Usually, the presenting problem(s) are of moderate severity. Physicians typically spend 55 minutes at the bedside and on the patient's hospital floor or unit.	1.56	0.95	0.10	2.61	XXX	N
99254	00	A	Initial inpatient consultation for a new or established patient, which requires three key components: a comprehensive history; a comprehensive examination; and medical decision making of moderate complexity. Counseling and/or coordination of care with other providers or agencies are provided consistent with the nature of the problem(s) and the patient's and/or family's needs. Usually, the presenting problem(s) are of moderate to high severity. Physicians typically spend 80 minutes at the bedside and on the patient's hospital floor or unit.	2.27	1.20	0.11	3.58	XXX	N
99255	00	A	Initial inpatient consultation for a new or established patient, which requires these three key components: a comprehensive history; a comprehensive examination; and medical decision making of high complexity. Counseling and/or coordination of care with other providers or agencies are provided consistent with the nature of the problem(s) and the patient's and/or family's needs. Usually, the presenting problem(s) are of moderate to high severity. Physicians typically spend 110 minutes at the bedside and on the patient's hospital floor or unit.	3.14	1.57	0.14	4.85	XXX	N
99261	00	A	Follow-up inpatient consultation for an established patient, which requires at least two of these three key components: a problem focused interval history; a problem focused examination; medical decision making that is straightforward or of low complexity. Counseling and/or coordination of care with other providers or agencies are provided consistent with nature of the problem(s) and the patient's and/or family's needs. Usually, the patient is stable, recovering or improving. Physicians typically spend 10 minutes at the bedside and on the patient's hospital floor or unit.	0.36	0.33	0.03	0.72	XXX	N
99262	00	A	Follow-up inpatient consultation for an established patient which requires at least two of these three key components: an expanded problem focused interval history; an expanded problem focused examination; medical decision making of moderate complexity. Counseling and/or coordination of care with other providers or agencies are provided consistent with the	0.74	0.46	0.04	1.24	XXX	N

CPT codes and descriptions only, © 1994 American Medical Association. Reimbursement information, © 1995 McGraw-Hill Inc.

Code/ CPT	Mod- ifier	Status	Description	Work value	Practice expense	Mal- practice	Total value	Global period	Up- date
			nature of the problem(s) and the patient's and/or family's needs. Usually, the patient is responding inadequately to therapy or has developed a minor complication. Physicians typically spend 20 minutes at the bedside and on the patient's hospital floor or unit.						
99263	00	A	Follow-up inpatient consultation for an established patient which requires at least two of these three key components: a detailed interval history; a detailed examination; medical decision making of high complexity. Counseling and/or coordination of care with other providers or agencies are provided consistent with the nature of the problem(s) and the patient's and/or family's needs. Usually, the patient is unstable or has developed a significant complication or a significant new problem. Physicians typically spend 30 minutes at the bedside and on the patient's hospital floor or unit.	1.16	0.67	0.04	1.87	XXX	N
99271	00	A	Confirmatory consultation for a new or established patient, which requires these three key components: a problem focused history; a problem focused examination; and straightforward medical decision making. Counseling and/or coordination of care with other providers or agencies are provided consistent with the nature of the problem(s) and the patient's and/or family's needs. Usually, the presenting problem(s) are self limited or minor.	0.45	0.58	0.07	1.10	XXX	N
99272	00	A	Confirmatory consultation for a new or established patient, which requires these three key components: an expanded problem focused history; an expanded problem focused examination; and straightforward medical decision making. Counseling and/or coordination of care with other providers or agencies are provided consistent with the nature of the problem(s) and the patient's and/or family's needs. Usually, the presenting problem(s) are of low severity.	0.84	0.71	0.09	1.64	XXX	N
99273	00	A	Confirmatory consultation for a new or established patient, which requires these three key components: a detailed history; a detailed examination; and medical decision making of low complexity. Counseling and/or coordination of care with other providers or agencies are provided consistent with the nature of the problem(s) and the patient's and/or family's needs. Usually, the presenting problem(s) are of moderate severity.	1.19	1.02	0.11	2.32	XXX	N
99274	00	A	Confirmatory consultation for a patient, which requires these three key components: a comprehensive history; a comprehensive examination; and medical decision making of moderate complexity. Counseling and/or coordination of care with other providers or agencies are provided consistent with the nature of the problem(s) and the patient's and/or family's needs. Usually, the presenting problem(s) are of moderate to high severity.	1.73	1.22	0.11	3.06	XXX	N
99275	00	A	Confirmatory consultation for a patient, which requires these three key components: a comprehensive history; a comprehensive examination; and medical decision making of high complexity. Counseling and/or coordination of care with other providers or agencies are provided consistent with the nature of the problem(s) and the patient's and/or family's needs. Usually, the presenting problem(s) are of moderate to high severity.	2.31	1.74	0.17	4.22	XXX	N

CPT codes and descriptions only, © 1994 American Medical Association. Reimbursement information, © 1995 McGraw-Hill Inc.

Code/ CPT	Mod- ifier	Status	Description	Work value	Practice expense	Mal- practice	Total value	Global period	Up- date
99281	00	A	Emergency department visit for the evaluation and management of a patient, which requires these three key components: a problem focused history; a problem focused examination; and straightforward medical decision making. Counseling and/or coordination of care with other providers or agencies are provided consistent with the nature of the problem(s) and the patient's and/or family's needs. Usually, the presenting problem(s) are self limited or minor.	0.28	0.28	0.01	0.57	XXX	P
99282	00	A	Emergency department visit for the evaluation and management of a patient, which requires these three key components: an expanded problem focused history; an expanded problem focused examination; and medical decision making of low complexity. Counseling and/or coordination of care with other providers or agencies are provided consistent with the nature of the problem(s) and the patient's and/or family's needs. Usually, the presenting problem(s) are of low to moderate severity.	0.47	0.38	0.03	0.88	XXX	P
99283	00	A	Emergency department visit for the evaluation and management of a patient, which requires these three key components: an expanded problem focused history; an expanded problem focused examination; and medical decision making of moderate complexity. Counseling and/or coordination of care with other providers or agencies are provided consistent with the nature of the problem(s) and the patient's and/or family's needs. Usually, the presenting problem(s) are of moderate severity.	1.07	0.49	0.04	1.60	XXX	P
99284	00	A	Emergency department visit for the evaluation and management of a patient, which requires these three key components: a detailed history; a detailed examination; and medical decision making of moderate complexity. Counseling and/or coordination of care with other providers or agencies are provided consistent with the nature of the problem(s) and the patient's and/or family's needs. Usually, the presenting problem(s) are of high severity, and require urgent evaluation by the physician but do not pose an immediate significant threat to life or physiologic function.	1.68	0.70	0.06	2.44	XXX	P
99285	00	A	Emergency department visit for the evaluation and management of a patient, which requires these three key components within the constraints imposed by the urgency of the patient's clinical condition and mental status: a comprehensive history; a comprehensive examination; and medical decision making of high complexity. Counseling and/or coordination of care with other providers or agencies are provided consistent with the nature of the problem(s) and the patient's and/or family's needs. Usually, the presenting problem(s) are of high severity and pose an immediate significant threat to life or physiologic function.	2.63	1.13	0.08	3.84	XXX	P
99288	00	B	Physician direction of emergency medical systems (EMS) emergency care, advanced life support	2.36*	1.78#	0.21*	4.35#	XXX	0
99291	00	A	Critical care, evaluation and management of the critically ill or critically injured patient, requiring the constant attendance of the physician; first hour	3.64	1.43	0.11	5.18	XXX	N

CPT codes and descriptions only, © 1994 American Medical Association. Reimbursement information, © 1995 McGraw-Hill Inc.

Code/ CPT	Mod-ifier	Status	Description	Work value	Practice expense	Mal-practice	Total value	Global period	Up-date
99292	00	A	Critical care, evaluation and management of the critically ill or critically injured patient, requiring the constant attendance of the physician; each additional 30 minutes	1.84	0.63	0.04	2.51	XXX	N
99295	00	A	Initial neonatal intensive care, per day, for the evaluation and management of a critically ill neonate or infant This care is provided on the date of admission of a neonate who requires cardiopulmonary monitoring and support. Such care includes the following, as necessary: initiation of mechanical ventilation or continuous positive airway pressure (CPAP); surfactant administration; pharmacologic control of the circulatory system; intravascular fluid administration; transfusion of blood components; vascular punctures; and blood gas interpretation.	16.03	5.08	1.55	22.66	XXX	N
99296	00	A	Subsequent neonatal intensive care, per day, for the evaluation and management of a critically ill and unstable neonate or infant A critically ill and unstable neonate represents a neonate whose cardiopulmonary and metabolic status is unstable; whose neurologic status may be unstable; who requires frequent ventilator changes, inotropic and chronotropic support; who requires frequent IV changes and whose condition is changing almost minute to minute. Such an infant requires almost constant attention by a physician. This description represents care provided on dates subsequent to the admission date. Such care includes the following, as necessary: mechanical ventilation or CPAP; surfactant administration; pharmacologic control of the circulatory system; total parenteral nutrition; seizure management; invasive or non-invasive electronic monitoring of vital signs, and/or monitoring of blood gases or oxygen saturation.	7.40	2.46	0.77	10.63	XXX	N
99297	00	A	Subsequent neonatal intensive care, per day, for the evaluation and management of a critically ill and stable neonate or infant A critically ill and stable neonate may represent an infant who is still intubated and requires invasive cardiopulmonary monitoring but whose vital signs are stable; who is not seizing; whose metabolic status is stable but who is still NPO and receiving parenteral nutrition and IV medications; and who is not yet over the acute phase of the initial problem. This description represents care provided on dates subsequent to the admission date. Such care includes the following, as necessary: ventilatory support and treatment; total parenteral nutrition; invasive or non-invasive electronic monitoring of vital signs; apnea management and/or monitoring of blood gases or oxygen saturation.	3.84	1.23	0.38	5.45	XXX	N
99301	00	A	Evaluation and management of a new or established patient involving an annual nursing facility assessment which requires these three key components: a detailed interval history; a comprehensive examination; and medical decision making that is straightforward or of low complexity. Counseling and/or coordination of care with other providers or agencies are provided consistent with the nature of the problem(s) and the patient's and/or family's needs. Usually, the patient is stable, recovering or improving. The review and affirmation of the medical plan of care is required. Physicians typically spend 30 minutes at the bedside and on the patient's facility floor or unit.	1.07	0.45	0.03	1.55	XXX	P

CPT codes and descriptions only, © 1994 American Medical Association. Reimbursement information, © 1995 McGraw-Hill Inc.

Code/ CPT	Mod- ifier	Status	Description	Work value	Practice expense	Mal- practice	Total value	Global period	Up- date
99302	00	A	Evaluation and management of a new or established patient involving a nursing facility assessment which requires these three key components: a detailed interval history; a comprehensive examination; and medical decision making of moderate to high complexity. Counseling and/or coordination of care with other providers or agencies are provided consistent with the nature of the problem(s) and the patient's and/or family's needs. Usually, the patient has developed a significant complication or a significant new problem and has had a major permanent change in status. The creation of a new medical plan of care is required. Physicians typically spend 40 minutes at the bedside and on the patient's facility floor or unit.	1.67	0.50	0.04	2.21	XXX	P
99303	00	A	Evaluation and management of a new or established patient involving a nursing facility assessment at the time of initial admission or readmission to the facility, which requires these three key components: a comprehensive history; a comprehensive examination; and medical decision making of moderate to high complexity. Counseling and/or coordination of care with other providers or agencies are provided consistent with the nature of the problem(s) and the patient's and/or family's needs. The creation of a medical plan of care is required. Physicians typically spend 50 minutes at the bedside and on the patient's facility floor or unit.	2.29	0.95	0.07	3.31	XXX	P
99311	00	A	Subsequent nursing facility care, per day, for the evaluation and management of a new or established patient, which requires at least two of these three key components: a problem focused interval history; a problem focused examination; medical decision making that is straightforward or of low complexity. Counseling and/or coordination of care with other providers or agencies are provided consistent with the nature of the problem(s) and the patient's and/or family's needs. Usually, the patient is stable, recovering or improving. Physicians typically spend 15 minutes at the bedside and on the patient's facility floor or unit.	0.54	0.34	0.03	0.91	XXX	P
99312	00	A	Subsequent nursing facility care, per day, for the evaluation and management of a new or established patient, which requires at least two of these three key components: an expanded problem focused interval history; an expanded problem focused examination; medical decision making of moderate complexity. Counseling and/or coordination of care with other providers or agencies are provided consistent with the nature of the problem(s) and the patient's and/or family's needs. Usually, the patient is responding inadequately to therapy or has developed a minor complication. Physicians typically spend 25 minutes at the bedside and on the patient's facility floor or unit.	0.89	0.41	0.03	1.33	XXX	P
99313	00	A	Subsequent nursing facility care, per day, for the evaluation and management of a new or established patient, which requires at least two of these three key components: a detailed interval history; a detailed examination; medical decision making of moderate to high complexity. Counseling and/or coordination of care with other	1.19	0.46	0.04	1.69	XXX	P

CPT codes and descriptions only, © 1994 American Medical Association. Reimbursement information, © 1995 McGraw-Hill Inc.

Code/ CPT	Mod- ifier	Status	Description	Work value	Practice expense	Mal- practice	Total value	Global period	Up- date
			providers or agencies are provided consistent with the nature of the problem(s) and the patient's and/or family's needs. Usually, the patient has developed a significant complication or a significant new problem. Physicians typically spend 35 minutes at the bedside and on the patient's facility floor or unit.						
99321	00	A	Domiciliary or rest home visit for the evaluation and management of a new patient which requires these three key components: a problem focused history; a problem focused examination; and medical decision making that is straightforward or of low complexity. Counseling and/or coordination of care with other providers or agencies are provided consistent with the nature of the problem(s) and the patient's and/or family's needs. Usually, the presenting problem(s) are of low severity.	0.71	0.37	0.03	1.11	XXX	P
99322	00	A	Domiciliary or rest home visit for the evaluation and management of a new patient, which requires these three key components: an expanded problem focused history; an expanded problem focused examination; and medical decision making of moderate complexity. Counseling and/or coordination of care with other providers or agencies are provided consistent with the nature of the problem(s) and the patient's and/or family's needs. Usually, the presenting problem(s) are of moderate severity.	1.01	0.51	0.05	1.57	XXX	P
99323	00	A	Domiciliary or rest home visit for the evaluation and management of a new patient, which requires these three key components: a detailed history; a detailed examination; and medical decision making of high complexity. Counseling and/or coordination of care with other providers or agencies are provided consistent with the nature of the problem(s) and the patient's and/or family's needs. Usually, the presenting problem(s) are of high complexity.	1.28	0.73	0.06	2.07	XXX	P
99331	00	A	Domiciliary or rest home visit for the evaluation and management of an established patient, which requires at least two of these three key components: a problem focused interval history; a problem focused examination; medical decision making that is straightforward or of low complexity. Counseling and/or coordination of care with other providers or agencies are provided consistent with the nature of the problem(s) and the patient's and/or family's needs. Usually, the patient is stable, recovering or improving.	0.60	0.28	0.02	0.90	XXX	P
99332	00	A	Domiciliary or rest home visit for the evaluation and management of an established patient, which requires at least two of these three key components: an expanded problem focused interval history; an expanded problem focused examination; medical decision making of moderate complexity. Counseling and/or coordination of care with other providers or agencies are provided consistent with the nature of the problem(s) and the patient's and/or family's needs. Usually, the patient is responding inadequately to therapy or has developed a minor complication.	0.80	0.36	0.03	1.19	XXX	P

CPT codes and descriptions only, © 1994 American Medical Association. Reimbursement information, © 1995 McGraw-Hill Inc.

Code/ CPT	Mod-ifier	Status	Description	Work value	Practice expense	Mal-practice	Total value	Global period	Up-date
99333	00	A	Domiciliary or rest home visit for the evaluation and management of an established patient, which requires at least two of these three key components: a detailed interval history; a detailed examination; medical decision making of high complexity. Counseling and/or coordination of care with other providers or agencies are provided consistent with the nature of the problem(s) and the patient's and/or family's needs. Usually, the patient is unstable or has developed a significant complication or a significant new problem.	1	0.44	0.02	1.46	XXX	P
99341	00	A	Home visit for the evaluation and management of a new patient, which requires these three key components: a problem focused history; a problem focused examination; and medical decision making that is straightforward or of low complexity. Counseling and/or coordination of care with other providers or agencies are provided consistent with the nature of the problem(s) and the patient's and/or family's needs. Usually, the presenting problem(s) are of low severity.	1.12	0.53	0.05	1.70	XXX	P
99342	00	A	Home visit for the evaluation and management of a new patient, which requires these three key components: an expanded problem focused history; an expanded problem focused examination; and medical decision making of moderate complexity. Counseling and/or coordination of care with other providers or agencies are provided consistent with the nature of the problem(s) and the patient's and/or family's needs. Usually, the presenting problem(s) are of moderate severity.	1.58	0.60	0.05	2.23	XXX	P
99343	00	A	Home visit for the evaluation and management of a new patient, which requires these three key components: a detailed history; a detailed examination; and medical decision making of high complexity. Counseling and/or coordination of care with other providers or agencies are provided consistent with the nature of the problem(s) and the patient's and/or family's needs. Usually, the presenting problem(s) are of high severity.	2.09	0.77	0.06	2.92	XXX	P
99351	00	A	Home visit for the evaluation and management of an established patient, which requires at least two of these three key components: a problem focused interval history; a problem focused examination; medical decision making that is straightforward or of low complexity. Counseling and/or coordination of care with other providers or agencies are provided consistent with the nature of the problem(s) and the patient's and/or family's needs. Usually, the patient is stable, recovering or improving.	0.83	0.45	0.04	1.32	XXX	P
99352	00	A	Home visit for the evaluation and management of an established patient, which requires at least two of these three key components: an expanded problem focused interval history; an expanded problem focused examination; medical decision making of moderate complexity. Counseling and/or coordination of care with other providers or agencies are provided consistent with the nature of the problem(s) and the patient's and/or family's needs. Usually, the patient is responding inadequately to therapy or has developed a minor complication.	1.12	0.53	0.04	1.69	XXX	P
99353	00	A	Home visit for the evaluation and management of an established patient, which requires at least two of these three key components: a detailed interval history; a	1.48	0.61	0.05	2.14	XXX	P

CPT codes and descriptions only, © 1994 American Medical Association. Reimbursement information, © 1995 McGraw-Hill Inc.

Code/ CPT	Mod- ifier	Status	Description	Work value	Practice expense	Mal- practice	Total value	Global period	Up- date
			detailed examination; medical decision making of high complexity. Counseling and/or coordination of care with other providers or agencies are provided consistent with the nature of the problem(s) and the patient's and/or family's needs. Usually, the patient is unstable or has developed a significant complication or a significant new problem.						
99354	00	A	Prolonged physician service in the office or other outpatient setting requiring direct (face-to-face) patient contact beyond the usual service (eg, prolonged care and treatment of an acute asthmatic patient in an outpatient setting); first hour	1.51	0.76	0.07	2.34	XXX	P
99355	00	A	Prolonged physician service in the office or other outpatient setting requiring direct (face-to-face) patient contact beyond the usual service (eg, prolonged care and treatment of an acute asthmatic patient in an outpatient setting); each additional 30 minutes	1.51	0.76	0.07	2.34	XXX	P
99356	00	A	Prolonged physician service in the inpatient setting, requiring direct (face-to-face) patient contact beyond the usual service (eg, maternal fetal monitoring for high risk delivery or other physiological monitoring, prolonged care of an acutely ill inpatient); first hour	1.44	0.85	0.08	2.37	XXX	N
99357	00	A	Prolonged physician service in the inpatient setting, requiring direct (face-to-face) patient contact beyond the usual service (eg, maternal fetal monitoring for high risk delivery or other physiological monitoring, prolonged care of an acutely ill inpatient); each additional 30 minutes	1.44	0.85	0.08	2.37	XXX	N
99358	00	B	Prolonged evaluation and management service before and/or after direct (face-to-face) patient care (eg, review of extensive records and tests, communication with other professionals and/or the patient/family); first hour	0.94*	0.71#	0.08*	1.73#	XXX	0
99359	00	B	Prolonged evaluation and management service before and/or after direct (face-to-face) patient care (eg, review of extensive records and tests, communication with other professionals and/or the patient/family); each additional 30 minutes	0.47*	0.36#	0.04*	0.87#	XXX	0
99360	00	X	Physician standby service, requiring prolonged physician attendance, each 30 minutes (eg, operative standby, standby for frozen section, for cesarean/high risk delivery for newborn care, for monitoring EEG)	0.88*	0.66#	0.08*	1.62#	XXX	0
99361	00	B	Medical conference by a physician with interdisciplinary team of health professionals or representatives of community agencies to coordinate activities of patient care (patient not present); approximately 30 minutes	0.59*	0.45#	0.05*	1.09#	XXX	0
99362	00	B	Medical conference by a physician with interdisciplinary team of health professionals or representatives of community agencies to coordinate activities of patient care (patient not present); approximately 60 minutes	1.06*	0.80#	0.09*	1.95#	XXX	0
99371	00	B	Telephone call by a physician to patient or for consultation or medical management or for coordinating medical management with other health care professionals (eg, nurses, therapists, social workers, nutritionists, physicians, pharmacists); simple or brief (eg, to report on tests and/or laboratory results, to clarify or alter previous instructions, to integrate new information from other health professionals into the medical treatment plan, or to adjust therapy)	0.12*	0.09#	0.01*	0.22#	XXX	0

CPT codes and descriptions only, © 1994 American Medical Association. Reimbursement information, © 1995 McGraw-Hill Inc.

Code/ CPT	Mod- ifier	Status	Description	Work value	Practice expense	Mal- practice	Total value	Global period	Up- date
99372	00	B	Telephone call by a physician to patient or for consultation or medical management or for coordinating medical management with other health care professionals (eg, nurses, therapists, social workers, nutritionists, physicians, pharmacists); intermediate (eg, to provide advice to an established patient on a new problem, to initiate therapy that can be handled by telephone, to discuss test results in detail, to coordinate medical management of a new problem in an established patient, to discuss and evaluate new information and details, or to initiate new plan of care)	0.24*	0.18#	0.02*	0.44#	XXX	0
99373	00	B	Telephone call by a physician to patient or for consultation or medical management or for coordinating medical management with other health care professionals (eg, nurses, therapists, social workers, nutritionists, physicians, pharmacists); complex or lengthy (eg, lengthy counseling session with anxious or distraught patient, detailed or prolonged discussion with family members regarding seriously ill patient, lengthy communication necessary to coordinate complex services of several different health professionals working on different aspects of the total patient care plan)	0.35*	0.27#	0.03*	0.65#	XXX	0
99375	00	A	Physician supervision of patients under care of home health agencies, hospice or nursing facility patients (patient not present) requiring complex or multidisciplinary care modalities involving regular physician development and/or revision of care plans, review of subsequent reports of patient status, review of related laboratory and other studies, communication (including telephone calls) with other health care professionals involved in patient's care, integration of new information into the medical treatment plan and/or adjustment of medical therapy, within a 30-day period; 30-60 minutes	1.06	0.51	0.04	1.61	XXX	P
99376	00	B	Physician supervision of patients under care of home health agencies, hospice or nursing facility patients (patient not present) requiring complex or multidisciplinary care modalities involving regular physician development and/or revision of care plans, review of subsequent reports of patient status, review of related laboratory and other studies, communication (including telephone calls) with other health care professionals involved in patient's care, integration of new information into the medical treatment plan and/or adjustment of medical therapy, within a 30-day period; greater than 60 minutes	1.18*	0.89#	0.10*	2.17#	XXX	0
99381	00	N	Initial preventive medicine evaluation and management of an individual including a comprehensive history, a comprehensive examination, counseling/anticipatory guidance/risk factor reduction interventions, and the ordering of appropriate laboratory/diagnostic procedures, new patient; infant (age under 1 year)	1.19	1.23	0.08	2.50	XXX	0
99382	00	N	Initial preventive medicine evaluation and management of an individual including a comprehensive history, a comprehensive examination, counseling/anticipatory guidance/risk factor reduction interventions, and the ordering of appropriate laboratory/diagnostic procedures, new patient; early childhood (age 1 through 4 years)	1.36	1.41	0.09	2.86	XXX	0
99383	00	N	Initial preventive medicine evaluation and management of an individual including a comprehensive history, a comprehensive examination, counseling/anticipatory	1.36	1.41	0.09	2.86	XXX	0

CPT codes and descriptions only, © 1994 American Medical Association. Reimbursement information, © 1995 McGraw-Hill Inc.

Code/ CPT	Mod- ifier	Status	Description	Work value	Practice expense	Mal- practice	Total value	Global period	Up- date
			guidance/risk factor reduction interventions, and the ordering of appropriate laboratory/diagnostic procedures, new patient; late childhood (age 5 through 11 years)						
99384	00	N	Initial preventive medicine evaluation and management of an individual including a comprehensive history, a comprehensive examination, counseling/anticipatory guidance/risk factor reduction interventions, and the ordering of appropriate laboratory/diagnostic procedures, new patient; adolescent (age 12 through 17 years)	1.53	1.59	0.10	3.22	XXX	0
99385	00	N	Initial preventive medicine evaluation and management of an individual including a comprehensive history, a comprehensive examination, counseling/anticipatory guidance/risk factor reduction interventions, and the ordering of appropriate laboratory/diagnostic procedures, new patient; 18-39 years	1.53	1.40	0.09	3.02	XXX	0
99386	00	N	Initial preventive medicine evaluation and management of an individual including a comprehensive history, a comprehensive examination, counseling/anticipatory guidance/risk factor reduction interventions, and the ordering of appropriate laboratory/diagnostic procedures, new patient; 40-64 years	1.88	1.72	0.10	3.70	XXX	0
99387	00	N	Initial preventive medicine evaluation and management of an individual including a comprehensive history, a comprehensive examination, counseling/anticipatory guidance/risk factor reduction interventions, and the ordering of appropriate laboratory/diagnostic procedures, new patient; 65 years and over	2.06	1.88	0.11	4.05	XXX	0
99391	00	N	Periodic preventive medicine reevaluation and management of an individual including a comprehensive history, comprehensive examination, counseling/anticipatory guidance/risk factor reduction interventions, and the ordering of appropriate laboratory/diagnostic procedures, established patient; infant (age under 1 year)	1.02	1.06	0.07	2.15	XXX	0
99392	00	N	Periodic preventive medicine reevaluation and management of an individual including a comprehensive history, comprehensive examination, counseling/anticipatory guidance/risk factor reduction interventions, and the ordering of appropriate laboratory/diagnostic procedures, established patient; early childhood (age 1 through 4 years)	1.19	1.23	0.08	2.50	XXX	0
99393	00	N	Periodic preventive medicine reevaluation and management of an individual including a comprehensive history, comprehensive examination, counseling/anticipatory guidance/risk factor reduction interventions, and the ordering of appropriate laboratory/diagnostic procedures, established patient; late childhood (age 5 through 11 years)	1.19	1.23	0.08	2.50	XXX	0
99394	00	N	Periodic preventive medicine reevaluation and management of an individual including a comprehensive history, comprehensive examination, counseling/anticipatory guidance/risk factor reduction interventions, and the ordering of appropriate laboratory/diagnostic procedures, established patient; adolescent (age 12 through 17 years)	1.36	1.41	0.09	2.86	XXX	0

CPT codes and descriptions only, © 1994 American Medical Association. Reimbursement information, © 1995 McGraw-Hill Inc.

Code/ CPT	Mod-ifier	Status	Description	Work value	Practice expense	Mal-practice	Total value	Global period	Up-date
99395	00	N	Periodic preventive medicine reevaluation and management of an individual including a comprehensive history, comprehensive examination, counseling/anticipatory guidance/risk factor reduction interventions, and the ordering of appropriate laboratory/diagnostic procedures, established patient; 18-39 years	1.36	1.25	0.08	2.69	XXX	0
99396	00	N	Periodic preventive medicine reevaluation and management of an individual including a comprehensive history, comprehensive examination, counseling/anticipatory guidance/risk factor reduction interventions, and the ordering of appropriate laboratory/diagnostic procedures, established patient; 40-64 years	1.53	1.40	0.09	3.02	XXX	0
99397	00	N	Periodic preventive medicine reevaluation and management of an individual including a comprehensive history, comprehensive examination, counseling/anticipatory guidance/risk factor reduction interventions, and the ordering of appropriate laboratory/diagnostic procedures, established patient; 65 years and over	1.71	1.56	0.10	3.37	XXX	0
99401	00	N	Preventive medicine counseling and/or risk factor reduction intervention(s) provided to an individual (separate procedure); approximately 15 minutes	0.48	0.45	0.03	0.96	XXX	0
99402	00	N	Preventive medicine counseling and/or risk factor reduction intervention(s) provided to an individual (separate procedure); approximately 30 minutes	0.98	0.89	0.05	1.92	XXX	0
99403	00	N	Preventive medicine counseling and/or risk factor reduction intervention(s) provided to an individual (separate procedure); approximately 45 minutes	1.46	1.34	0.08	2.88	XXX	0
99404	00	N	Preventive medicine counseling and/or risk factor reduction intervention(s) provided to an individual (separate procedure); approximately 60 minutes	1.95	1.78	0.11	3.84	XXX	0
99411	00	N	Preventive medicine counseling and/or risk factor reduction intervention(s) provided to individuals in a group setting (separate procedure); approximately 30 minutes	0.53*	0.40#	0.05*	0.98#	XXX	0
99412	00	N	Preventive medicine counseling and/or risk factor reduction intervention(s) provided to individuals in a group setting (separate procedure); approximately 60 minutes	1.06*	0.80#	0.09*	1.95#	XXX	0
99420	00	N	Administration and interpretation of health risk assessment instrument (eg, health hazard appraisal)	0	0	0	0	XXX	0
99429	00	N	Unlisted preventive medicine service	0	0	0	0	XXX	0
99431	00	A	History and examination of the normal newborn infant, initiation of diagnostic and treatment programs and preparation of hospital records. (This code should also be used for birthing room deliveries.)	1.17	1.21	0.08	2.46	XXX	N
99432	00	A	Normal newborn care in other than hospital or birthing room setting, including physical examination of baby and conference(s) with parent(s)	1.26	1.31	0.08	2.65	XXX	N
99433	00	A	Subsequent hospital care, for the evaluation and management of a normal newborn, per day	0.62	0.64	0.04	1.30	XXX	N
99440	00	A	Newborn resuscitation: care of the high risk newborn at delivery, including, for example, inhalation therapy, aspiration, administration of medication for initial stabilization	2.93	3.04	0.19	6.16	XXX	N

CPT codes and descriptions only, © 1994 American Medical Association. Reimbursement information, © 1995 McGraw-Hill Inc.

Code/ CPT	Mod- ifier	Status	Description	Work value	Practice expense	Mal- practice	Total value	Global period	Up- date
99450	00	N	Basic life and/or disability examination that includes: ■ measurement of height, weight and blood pressure; ■ completion of a medical history following a life insurance pro forma; ■ collection of blood sample and/or urinalysis complying with "chain of custody" protocols; and ■ completion of necessary documentation/certificates	0	0	0	0	XXX	N
99455	00	R	Work related or medical disability examination by the treating physician that includes: ■ completion of a medical history commensurate with the patient's condition; ■ performance of an examination commensurate with the patient's condition; ■ formulation of a diagnosis, assessment of capabilities and stability, and calculation of impairment; ■ development of future medical treatment plan; and ■ completion of necessary documentation/certificates and report.	0	0	0	0	XXX	0
99456	00	R	Work related or medical disability examination by other than the treating physician that includes: ■ completion of a medical history commensurate with the patient's condition; ■ performance of an examination commensurate with the patient's condition; ■ formulation of a diagnosis, assessment of capabilities and stability, and calculation of impairment; ■ development of future medical treatment plan; and ■ completion of necessary documentation/certificates and report.	0	0	0	0	XXX	N
99499	00	C	Unlisted evaluation and management service	0	0	0	0	XXX	N

CPT codes and descriptions only, © 1994 American Medical Association. Reimbursement information, © 1995 McGraw-Hill Inc.

CHAPTER 7

HCPCS

RVP now includes a listing of HCPCS Level II as they relate to physician services. The following is a list of these codes as developed by the Health Care Financing Administration (HCFA) for 1990. The editors are researching a methodology for value of all HCPCS codes. Many of these procedures have relative values or value guidelines for use with the conversion factor used for Medicine. Other codes list or include the cost of medical equipment and supplies. These codes are supplied in the comprehensive listing for your convenience. Values cannot be determined under the current relative value structure. The editors are researching fees for these procedures with the intention of publishing a fee range for each medical equipment or supply code in the future. The editors have elected to indicate that a relative value is not available for procedures with a "0" in the individual units column. These codes should be treated as a "by report" code and substantiating documentation should accompany the code submission.

"Physician's Current Procedural Terminology," Fourth Edition, Copyright 1990 by the American Medical Association ("CPT-4") is a listing of descriptive terms and numeric identifying codes and modifiers for reporting medical services and procedures performed by physicians. This Health Care Financing Administration common procedure coding system ("HCPCS") includes CPT-4 descriptive terms and numeric identifying codes and modifiers for reporting medical services and procedures and other materials contained in CPT-4 which are copyrighted by the American Medical Association. Participants will be authorized to use copies of CPT-4 material in HCPCS only for the purposes directly related to participating in HCFA programs and permission for any other use must be obtained from the AMA.

HCPCS Disclaimer

The HCPCS coding system is designed to promote uniform medical services reporting and statistical data collection. Inclusion of a service, product, or supply does not constitute endorsement by the HCPCS editorial panel that it is noninvestigational or is commonly and customarily recognized as appropriate for medical care and treatment. Inclusion or exclusion of a procedure, product, or supply does not imply any health insurance coverage or reimbursement policy.

Note concerning the detailed portion of the HCPCS record:

The following fields are updated annually as necessary: Maintenance Date (M/D), Action Code (A/C), Coverage (COV), Control Statement (CNST), Cross Reference (X/R), the Independent Laboratory Certification (ILC), Coverage Issues Manual (CIM), and Medicare Carriers Manual (MCM). All Medicare carriers update their individual systems and records with current coverage information throughout the year. That information is not reflected on the aggregate HCPCS listing that follows. Absence of a code in FD-08 (COV) does not mean the item is automatically covered but that the carrier has the authority to determine coverage and payment policy.

CPT codes and descriptions only, © 1994 American Medical Association. Reimbursement information, © 1995 McGraw-Hill Inc.

HCPCS VALUES

Code/ CPT	Mod- ifier	Status	Description	Work value	Practice expense	Mal- practice	Total value	Global period	Up- date
A0010		D	Ambsvc bls bas rte em tr 1wy	0	0	0	0	XXX	0
A0020		D	Basic support amb one way	0	0	0	0	XXX	0
A0021		G	Outside state ambulance serv	0	0	0	0	XXX	0
A0030		X	Air ambulance service	0	0	0	0	XXX	0
A0040		X	Helicopter ambulance service	0	0	0	0	XXX	0
A0050		X	Water amb service emergency	0	0	0	0	XXX	0
A0060		D	Ambulance waiting time	0	0	0	0	XXX	0
A0070		D	Amb 02 & suppls life sustain	0	0	0	0	XXX	0
A0080		G	Noninterest escort in non er	0	0	0	0	XXX	0
A0090		G	Interest escort in non er	0	0	0	0	XXX	0
A0100		G	Nonemergency transport taxi	0	0	0	0	XXX	0
A0110		G	Nonemergency transport bus	0	0	0	0	XXX	0
A0120		G	Noner transport mini-bus	0	0	0	0	XXX	0
A0130		G	Noner transport wheelch van	0	0	0	0	XXX	0
A0140		G	Nonemergency transport air	0	0	0	0	XXX	0
A0150		D	Noner transport ambulance	0	0	0	0	XXX	0
A0160		G	Noner transport case worker	0	0	0	0	XXX	0
A0170		G	Noner transport parking fees	0	0	0	0	XXX	0
A0180		G	Noner transport lodgng recip	0	0	0	0	XXX	0
A0190		G	Noner transport meals recip	0	0	0	0	XXX	0
A0200		G	Noner transport lodgng escrt	0	0	0	0	XXX	0
A0210		G	Noner transport meals escort	0	0	0	0	XXX	0
A0215		D	Ambulance service & supplies	0	0	0	0	XXX	0
A0220		D	Amb adv support incl service	0	0	0	0	XXX	0
A0221		D	Amb adv support one way	0	0	0	0	XXX	0
A0222		D	Return trip ambulance	0	0	0	0	XXX	0
A0223		D	Amb adv support sep supplies	0	0	0	0	XXX	0
A0225		X	Neonatal emergency transport	0	0	0	0	XXX	0
A0300		X	Ambulance basic non-emer all	0	0	0	0	XXX	0
A0302		X	Ambulance basic emergeny all	0	0	0	0	XXX	0
A0304		X	Amb adv non-er no serv all	0	0	0	0	XXX	0
A0306		X	Amb adv non-er spec serv all	0	0	0	0	XXX	0
A0308		X	Amb adv er no spec serv all	0	0	0	0	XXX	0
A0310		X	Amb adv er spec serv all	0	0	0	0	XXX	0
A0320		X	Amb basic non-er + supplies	0	0	0	0	XXX	0
A0322		X	Amb basic emerg + supplies	0	0	0	0	XXX	0
A0324		X	Adv non-er serv sep mileage	0	0	0	0	XXX	0
A0326		X	Adv non-er no serv sep mile	0	0	0	0	XXX	0
A0328		X	Adv er no serv sep mileage	0	0	0	0	XXX	0

CPT codes and descriptions only, © 1994 American Medical Association. Reimbursement information, © 1995 McGraw-Hill Inc.

Code/ CPT	Mod-ifier	Status	Description	Work value	Practice expense	Mal-practice	Total value	Global period	Up-date
A0330		X	Adv er spec serv sep mile	0	0	0	0	XXX	0
A0340		X	Amb basic non-er + mileage	0	0	0	0	XXX	0
A0342		X	Ambul basic emer + mileage	0	0	0	0	XXX	0
A0344		X	Amb adv non-er no serv +mile	0	0	0	0	XXX	0
A0346		X	Amb adv non-er serv + mile	0	0	0	0	XXX	0
A0348		X	Adv emer no spec serv + mile	0	0	0	0	XXX	0
A0350		X	Adv emer spec serv + mileage	0	0	0	0	XXX	0
A0360		X	Basic non-er sep mile & supp	0	0	0	0	XXX	0
A0362		X	Basic emer sep mile & supply	0	0	0	0	XXX	0
A0364		X	Adv non-er no serv sep mi&su	0	0	0	0	XXX	0
A0366		X	Adv non-er serv sep mil&supp	0	0	0	0	XXX	0
A0368		X	Adv er no serv sep mile&supp	0	0	0	0	XXX	0
A0370		X	Adv er spec serv sep mi&supp	0	0	0	0	XXX	0
A0380		X	Basic life support mileage	0	0	0	0	XXX	0
A0382		X	Basic support routine suppls	0	0	0	0	XXX	0
A0384		X	Bls defibrillation supplies	0	0	0	0	XXX	0
A0390		X	Advanced life support mileag	0	0	0	0	XXX	0
A0392		X	Als defibrillation supplies	0	0	0	0	XXX	0
A0394		X	Als IV drug therapy supplies	0	0	0	0	XXX	0
A0396		X	Als esophageal intub suppls	0	0	0	0	XXX	0
A0398		X	Als routine disposble suppls	0	0	0	0	XXX	0
A0420		X	Ambulance waiting 1/2 hr	0	0	0	0	XXX	0
A0422		X	Ambulance 02 life sustaining	0	0	0	0	XXX	0
A0424		X	Extra ambulance attendant	0	0	0	0	XXX	0
A0888		N	Noncovered ambulance mileage	0	0	0	0	XXX	0
A0999		X	Unlisted ambulance service	0	0	0	0	XXX	0
A2000		A	Chiropractor manip of spine	0.45	0.29	0.01	0.75	XXX	N
A4190		P	Transparent film each	0	0	0	0	XXX	0
A4200		P	Gauze pad medicated/non-med	0	0	0	0	XXX	0
A4202		P	Elastic gauze roll	0	0	0	0	XXX	0
A4203		P	Non-elastic gauze roll	0	0	0	0	XXX	0
A4204		P	Absorptve dressing	0	0	0	0	XXX	0
A4205		P	Nonabsorptive dressing	0	0	0	0	XXX	0
A4206		P	1 CC sterile syringe&needle	0	0	0	0	XXX	0
A4207		P	2 CC sterile syringe&needle	0	0	0	0	XXX	0
A4208		P	3 CC sterile syringe&needle	0	0	0	0	XXX	0
A4209		P	5+ CC sterile syringe&needle	0	0	0	0	XXX	0
A4210		N	Nonneedle injection device	0	0	0	0	XXX	0
A4211		P	Supp for self-adm injections	0	0	0	0	XXX	0
A4212		P	Non coring needle or stylet	0	0	0	0	XXX	0
A4213		P	20+ CC syringe only	0	0	0	0	XXX	0
A4214		P	30 CC sterile water/saline	0	0	0	0	XXX	0
A4215		P	Sterile needle	0	0	0	0	XXX	0
A4220		P	Infusion pump refill kit	0	0	0	0	XXX	0
A4244		P	Alcohol or peroxide per pint	0	0	0	0	XXX	0
A4245		P	Alcohol wipes per box	0	0	0	0	XXX	0
A4246		P	Betadine/phisohex solution	0	0	0	0	XXX	0
A4247		P	Betadine/iodine swabs/wipes	0	0	0	0	XXX	0
A4250		R	Urine reagent strips/tablets	0	0	0	0	XXX	N
A4253		P	Blood glucose/reagent strips	0	0	0	0	XXX	0

CPT codes and descriptions only, © 1994 American Medical Association. Reimbursement information, © 1995 McGraw-Hill Inc.

Code/ CPT	Mod- ifier	Status	Description	Work value	Practice expense	Mal- practice	Total value	Global period	Up- date
A4256		P	Calibrator solution/chips	0	0	0	0	XXX	0
A4259		P	Lancets per box	0	0	0	0	XXX	0
A4260		N	Levonorgestrel implant	0	0	0	0	XXX	0
A4262		B	Temporary tear duct plug	0	0	0	0	XXX	0
A4263		A	Permanent tear duct plug	0	0.95	0	0.95	XXX	N
A4265		P	Paraffin	0	0	0	0	XXX	0
A4270		B	Disposable endoscope sheath	0	0	0	0	XXX	0
A4300		A	Cath impl vasc access portal	0	0.95	0	0.95	XXX	N
A4305		P	Drug delivery system =50 ML	0	0	0	0	XXX	0
A4306		P	Drug delivery system =5 ML	0	0	0	0	XXX	0
A4310		P	Insert tray w/o bag/cath	0	0	0	0	XXX	0
A4311		P	Catheter w/o bag 2-way latex	0	0	0	0	XXX	0
A4312		P	Cath w/o bag 2-way silicone	0	0	0	0	XXX	0
A4313		P	Catheter w/bag 3-way	0	0	0	0	XXX	0
A4314		P	Cath w/drainage 2-way latex	0	0	0	0	XXX	0
A4315		P	Cath w/drainage 2-way silcne	0	0	0	0	XXX	0
A4316		P	Cath w/drainage 3-way	0	0	0	0	XXX	0
A4320		P	Irrigation tray	0	0	0	0	XXX	0
A4322		P	Irrigation syringe	0	0	0	0	XXX	0
A4323		P	Saline irrigation solution	0	0	0	0	XXX	0
A4326		P	Male external catheter	0	0	0	0	XXX	0
A4327		P	Fem urinary collect dev cup	0	0	0	0	XXX	0
A4328		P	Fem urinary collect pouch	0	0	0	0	XXX	0
A4329		P	External catheter start set	0	0	0	0	XXX	0
A4330		P	Stool collection pouch	0	0	0	0	XXX	0
A4335		P	Incontinence supply	0	0	0	0	XXX	0
A4338		P	Indwelling catheter latex	0	0	0	0	XXX	0
A4340		P	Indwelling catheter special	0	0	0	0	XXX	0
A4344		P	Cath indw foley 2 way silicn	0	0	0	0	XXX	0
A4346		P	Cath indw foley 3 way	0	0	0	0	XXX	0
A4347		P	Male external catheter	0	0	0	0	XXX	0
A4351		P	Straight tip urine catheter	0	0	0	0	XXX	0
A4352		P	Coude tip urinary catheter	0	0	0	0	XXX	0
A4354		P	Cath insertion tray w/bag	0	0	0	0	XXX	0
A4355		P	Bladder irrigation tubing	0	0	0	0	XXX	0
A4356		P	Ext ureth clmp or compr dvc	0	0	0	0	XXX	0
A4357		P	Bedside drainage bag	0	0	0	0	XXX	0
A4358		P	Urinary leg bag	0	0	0	0	XXX	0
A4359		P	Urinary suspensory w/o leg b	0	0	0	0	XXX	0
A4361		P	Ostomy face plate	0	0	0	0	XXX	0
A4362		P	Solid skin barrier	0	0	0	0	XXX	0
A4363		P	Liquid skin barrier	0	0	0	0	XXX	0
A4364		P	Ostomy/cath adhesive	0	0	0	0	XXX	0
A4367		P	Ostomy belt	0	0	0	0	XXX	0
A4397		P	Irrigation supply sleeve	0	0	0	0	XXX	0
A4398		P	Irrigation supply bags	0	0	0	0	XXX	0
A4399		P	Irrigation supply cone/cathe	0	0	0	0	XXX	0
A4400		P	Ostomy irrigation set	0	0	0	0	XXX	0
A4402		P	Lubricant per ounce	0	0	0	0	XXX	0
A4404		P	Ostomy ring each	0	0	0	0	XXX	0

CPT codes and descriptions only, © 1994 American Medical Association. Reimbursement information, © 1995 McGraw-Hill Inc.

Code/ CPT	Mod- ifier	Status	Description	Work value	Practice expense	Mal- practice	Total value	Global period	Up- date
A4421		P	Ostomy supply misc	0	0	0	0	XXX	0
A4454		P	Tape all types all sizes	0	0	0	0	XXX	0
A4455		P	Adhesive remover per ounce	0	0	0	0	XXX	0
A4460		P	Elastic compression bandage	0	0	0	0	XXX	0
A4465		P	Non-elastic extremity binder	0	0	0	0	XXX	0
A4470		P	Gravlee jet washer	0	0	0	0	XXX	0
A4480		P	Vabra aspirator	0	0	0	0	XXX	0
A4490		N	Above knee surgical stocking	0	0	0	0	XXX	0
A4495		N	Thigh length surg stocking	0	0	0	0	XXX	0
A4500		N	Below knee surgical stocking	0	0	0	0	XXX	0
A4510		N	Full length surg stocking	0	0	0	0	XXX	0
A4550		A	Surgical trays	0	0.95	0	0.95	XXX	N
A4554		N	Disposable underpads	0	0	0	0	XXX	0
A4556		P	Electrodes	0	0	0	0	XXX	0
A4557		P	Lead wires	0	0	0	0	XXX	0
A4558		P	Conductive paste or gel	0	0	0	0	XXX	0
A4560		X	Pessary	0	0	0	0	XXX	0
A4565		X	Slings	0	0	0	0	XXX	0
A4570		X	Splint	0	0	0	0	XXX	0
A4572		X	Rib belt	0	0	0	0	XXX	0
A4580		X	Cast supplies (plaster)	0	0	0	0	XXX	0
A4581		X	Risser jacket supplies	0	0	0	0	XXX	0
A4590		X	Special casting material	0	0	0	0	XXX	0
A4610		X	Med supplies for use in DME	0	0	0	0	XXX	0
A4611		X	Heavy duty battery	0	0	0	0	XXX	0
A4612		X	Battery cables	0	0	0	0	XXX	0
A4613		X	Battery charger	0	0	0	0	XXX	0
A4615		X	Cannula nasal	0	0	0	0	XXX	0
A4616		X	Tubing (oxygen) per foot	0	0	0	0	XXX	0
A4617		X	Mouth piece	0	0	0	0	XXX	0
A4618		X	Breathing circuits	0	0	0	0	XXX	0
A4619		X	Face tent	0	0	0	0	XXX	0
A4620		X	Variable concentration mask	0	0	0	0	XXX	0
A4621		X	Tracheotomy mask or collar	0	0	0	0	XXX	0
A4622		X	Tracheostomy or larngectomy	0	0	0	0	XXX	0
A4623		X	Tracheostomy inner cannula	0	0	0	0	XXX	0
A4624		X	Tracheal suction tube	0	0	0	0	XXX	0
A4625		X	Tracheostomy care kit	0	0	0	0	XXX	0
A4626		X	Tracheostomy cleaning brush	0	0	0	0	XXX	0
A4627		X	Spacer bag/reservoir	0	0	0	0	XXX	0
A4630		X	Repl bat t.e.n.s. own by pt	0	0	0	0	XXX	0
A4631		X	Wheelchair battery	0	0	0	0	XXX	0
A4635		X	Underarm crutch pad	0	0	0	0	XXX	0
A4636		X	Handgrip for cane etc	0	0	0	0	XXX	0
A4637		X	Repl tip cane/crutch/walker	0	0	0	0	XXX	0
A4640		X	Alternating pressure pad	0	0	0	0	XXX	0
A4641		E	Diagnostic imaging agent	0	0	0	0	XXX	0
A4642		X	Satumomab pendetide per dose	0	0	0	0	XXX	0
A4643		X	High dose contrast MRI	0	0	0	0	XXX	0
A4644		E	Contrast 100-199 MGs iodine	0	0	0	0	XXX	0

CPT codes and descriptions only, © 1994 American Medical Association. Reimbursement information, © 1995 McGraw-Hill Inc.

Code/ CPT	Mod- ifier	Status	Description	Work value	Practice expense	Mal- practice	Total value	Global period	Up- date
A4645		E	Contrast 200-299 MGs iodine	0	0	0	0	XXX	0
A4646		E	Contrast 300-399 MGs iodine	0	0	0	0	XXX	0
A4647		B	Supp- paramagnetic contr mat	0	0	0	0	XXX	0
A4649		B	Surgical supplies	0	0	0	0	XXX	0
A4650		X	Supp esrd centrifuge	0	0	0	0	XXX	0
A4655		X	Esrd syringe/needle	0	0	0	0	XXX	0
A4660		X	Esrd blood pressure device	0	0	0	0	XXX	0
A4663		X	Esrd blood pressure cuff	0	0	0	0	XXX	0
A4670		N	Auto blood pressure monitor	0	0	0	0	XXX	0
A4680		X	Activated carbon filters	0	0	0	0	XXX	0
A4690		X	Dialyzers	0	0	0	0	XXX	0
A4700		X	Standard dialysate solution	0	0	0	0	XXX	0
A4705		X	Bicarb dialysate solution	0	0	0	0	XXX	0
A4712		X	Sterile water	0	0	0	0	XXX	0
A4714		X	Treated water for dialysis	0	0	0	0	XXX	0
A4730		X	Fistula cannulation set dial	0	0	0	0	XXX	0
A4735		X	Local/topical anesthetics	0	0	0	0	XXX	0
A4740		X	Esrd shunt accessory	0	0	0	0	XXX	0
A4750		X	Arterial or venous tubing	0	0	0	0	XXX	0
A4755		X	Arterial and venous tubing	0	0	0	0	XXX	0
A4760		X	Standard testing solution	0	0	0	0	XXX	0
A4765		X	Dialysate concentrate	0	0	0	0	XXX	0
A4770		X	Blood testing supplies	0	0	0	0	XXX	0
A4771		X	Blood clotting time tube	0	0	0	0	XXX	0
A4772		X	Dextrostick/glucose strips	0	0	0	0	XXX	0
A4773		X	Hemostix	0	0	0	0	XXX	0
A4774		X	Ammonia test paper	0	0	0	0	XXX	0
A4780		X	Esrd sterilizing agent	0	0	0	0	XXX	0
A4790		X	Esrd cleansing agents	0	0	0	0	XXX	0
A4800		X	Heparin/antidote dialysis	0	0	0	0	XXX	0
A4820		X	Supplies hemodialysis kit	0	0	0	0	XXX	0
A4850		X	Rubber tipped hemostats	0	0	0	0	XXX	0
A4860		X	Disposable catheter caps	0	0	0	0	XXX	0
A4870		X	Plumbing/electrical work	0	0	0	0	XXX	0
A4880		X	Water storage tanks	0	0	0	0	XXX	0
A4890		N	Contracts/repair/maintenance	0	0	0	0	XXX	0
A4900		X	Capd supply kit	0	0	0	0	XXX	0
A4901		X	Ccpd supply kit	0	0	0	0	XXX	0
A4905		X	Ipd supply kit	0	0	0	0	XXX	0
A4910		X	Esrd nonmedical supplies	0	0	0	0	XXX	0
A4912		X	Gomco drain bottle	0	0	0	0	XXX	0
A4913		X	Esrd supply	0	0	0	0	XXX	0
A4914		X	Preparation kit	0	0	0	0	XXX	0
A4918		X	Venous pressure clamp	0	0	0	0	XXX	0
A4919		X	Supp dialysis dialyzer holde	0	0	0	0	XXX	0
A4920		X	Harvard pressure clamp	0	0	0	0	XXX	0
A4921		X	Measuring cylinder	0	0	0	0	XXX	0
A4927		X	Gloves	0	0	0	0	XXX	0
A5051		P	Pouch clsd w barr attached	0	0	0	0	XXX	0
A5052		P	Clsd ostomy pouch w/o barr	0	0	0	0	XXX	0

CPT codes and descriptions only, © 1994 American Medical Association. Reimbursement information, © 1995 McGraw-Hill Inc.

Code/ CPT	Mod- ifier	Status	Description	Work value	Practice expense	Mal- practice	Total value	Global period	Up- date
A5053		P	Clsd ostomy pouch faceplate	0	0	0	0	XXX	0
A5054		P	Clsd ostomy pouch w/flange	0	0	0	0	XXX	0
A5055		P	Stoma cap	0	0	0	0	XXX	0
A5061		P	Pouch drainable w barrier at	0	0	0	0	XXX	0
A5062		P	Drnble ostomy pouch w/o barr	0	0	0	0	XXX	0
A5063		P	Drain ostomy pouch w/flange	0	0	0	0	XXX	0
A5064		P	Drain ostomy pouch w/fceplte	0	0	0	0	XXX	0
A5065		P	Drain ostomy pouch on fcplte	0	0	0	0	XXX	0
A5071		P	Urinary pouch w/barrier	0	0	0	0	XXX	0
A5072		P	Urinary pouch w/o barrier	0	0	0	0	XXX	0
A5073		P	Urinary pouch on barr w/flng	0	0	0	0	XXX	0
A5074		P	Urinary pouch w/faceplate	0	0	0	0	XXX	0
A5075		P	Urinary pouch on faceplate	0	0	0	0	XXX	0
A5081		P	Continent stoma plug	0	0	0	0	XXX	0
A5082		P	Continent stoma catheter	0	0	0	0	XXX	0
A5093		P	Ostomy accessory convex inse	0	0	0	0	XXX	0
A5102		P	Bedside btle rigid/expanable	0	0	0	0	XXX	0
A5105		P	Urinary suspensory	0	0	0	0	XXX	0
A5112		P	Urinary leg bag	0	0	0	0	XXX	0
A5113		P	Latex leg strap	0	0	0	0	XXX	0
A5114		P	Foam/fabric leg strap	0	0	0	0	XXX	0
A5119		P	Skin barrier wipes box pr 50	0	0	0	0	XXX	0
A5121		P	Solid skin barrier 6x6	0	0	0	0	XXX	0
A5122		P	Solid skin barrier 8x8	0	0	0	0	XXX	0
A5123		P	Skin barrier with flange	0	0	0	0	XXX	0
A5126		P	Adhesive disc/foam pad	0	0	0	0	XXX	0
A5131		P	Appliance cleaner	0	0	0	0	XXX	0
A5149		P	Incontinence/ostomy supply	0	0	0	0	XXX	0
A5500		X	Diab shoe for density insert	0	0	0	0	XXX	0
A5501		X	Diabetic custom molded shoe	0	0	0	0	XXX	0
A5502		X	Diabetic shoe density insert	0	0	0	0	XXX	0
A5503		X	Diabetic shoe w/roller/rockr	0	0	0	0	XXX	0
A5504		X	Diabetic shoe with wedge	0	0	0	0	XXX	0
A5505		X	Diab shoe w/metatarsal bar	0	0	0	0	XXX	0
A5506		X	Diabetic shoe w/off set heel	0	0	0	0	XXX	0
A5507		X	Modification diabetic shoe	0	0	0	0	XXX	0
A9150		E	Misc/exper non-prescript dru	0	0	0	0	XXX	0
A9160		N	Podiatrist non-covered servi	0	0	0	0	XXX	0
A9170		N	Chiropractor non-covered ser	0	0	0	0	XXX	0
A9180		D	Naturopaths	0	0	0	0	XXX	0
A9190		N	Misc/expe personal comfort i	0	0	0	0	XXX	0
A9270		N	Non-covered item or service	0	0	0	0	XXX	0
A9290		D	Descrip not indicat hosp vis	0	0	0	0	XXX	0
A9300		N	Exercise equipment	0	0	0	0	XXX	0
D0110		R	Initial oral examination	0	0	0	0	YYY	N
D0120		R	Periodic oral examination	0	0	0	0	YYY	N
D0130		R	Emergency oral examination	0	0	0	0	YYY	N
D0210		R	Intraor complete film series	0	0	0	0	YYY	N
D0220		R	Intraoral periapical first f	0	0	0	0	YYY	N
D0230		R	Intraoral periapical ea add	0	0	0	0	YYY	N

CPT codes and descriptions only, © 1994 American Medical Association. Reimbursement information, © 1995 McGraw-Hill Inc.

Code/ CPT	Mod-ifier	Status	Description	Work value	Practice expense	Mal-practice	Total value	Global period	Up-date
D0240		R	Intraoral occlusal film	0	0	0	0	YYY	N
D0250		R	Extraoral first film	0	0	0	0	YYY	N
D0260		R	Extraoral ea additional film	0	0	0	0	YYY	N
D0270		R	Dental bitewing single film	0	0	0	0	YYY	N
D0272		R	Dental bitewings two films	0	0	0	0	YYY	N
D0274		R	Dental bitewings four films	0	0	0	0	YYY	N
D0290		R	Dental film skull/facial bon	0	0	0	0	YYY	N
D0310		R	Dental saliography	0	0	0	0	YYY	N
D0320		R	Dental tmj arthrogram incl i	0	0	0	0	YYY	N
D0321		R	Dental other tmj films	0	0	0	0	YYY	N
D0322		R	Dental tomographic survey	0	0	0	0	YYY	N
D0330		R	Dental panoramic film	0	0	0	0	YYY	N
D0340		R	Dental cephalometric film	0	0	0	0	YYY	N
D0415		R	Bacteriologic study	0	0	0	0	YYY	N
D0425		R	Caries susceptibility test	0	0	0	0	YYY	N
D0460		R	Pulp vitality test	0	0	0	0	YYY	N
D0470		R	Diagnostic casts	0	0	0	0	YYY	N
D0471		R	Diagnostic photographs	0	0	0	0	YYY	N
D0501		R	Histopathologic examinations	0	0	0	0	YYY	N
D0502		R	Other oral pathology procedu	0	0	0	0	YYY	N
D0999		R	Unspecified diagnostic proce	0	0	0	0	YYY	N
D1110		R	Dental prophylaxis adult	0	0	0	0	YYY	N
D1120		R	Dental prophylaxis child	0	0	0	0	YYY	N
D1201		R	Topical fluor w prophy child	0	0	0	0	YYY	N
D1203		R	Topical fluor w/o prophy chi	0	0	0	0	YYY	N
D1204		R	Topical fluor w/o prophy adu	0	0	0	0	YYY	N
D1205		R	Topical fluoride w/ prophy a	0	0	0	0	YYY	N
D1310		R	Nutri counsel-control caries	0	0	0	0	YYY	N
D1330		R	Oral hygiene instruction	0	0	0	0	YYY	N
D1351		R	Dental sealant per tooth	0	0	0	0	YYY	N
D1510		R	Space maintainer fxd unilat	0	0	0	0	YYY	N
D1515		R	Fixed bilat space maintainer	0	0	0	0	YYY	N
D1520		R	Remove unilat space maintain	0	0	0	0	YYY	N
D1525		R	Remove bilat space maintain	0	0	0	0	YYY	N
D1550		R	Recement space maintainer	0	0	0	0	YYY	N
D2110		R	Amalgam one surface primary	0	0	0	0	YYY	N
D2120		R	Amalgam two surfaces primary	0	0	0	0	YYY	N
D2130		R	Amalgam three surfaces prima	0	0	0	0	YYY	N
D2131		R	Amalgam four/more surf prima	0	0	0	0	YYY	N
D2140		R	Amalgam one surface permanen	0	0	0	0	YYY	N
D2150		R	Amalgam two surfaces permane	0	0	0	0	YYY	N
D2160		R	Amalgam three surfaces perma	0	0	0	0	YYY	N
D2161		R	Amalgam 4 or surfaces perm	0	0	0	0	YYY	N
D2210		R	Silcate cement per restorat	0	0	0	0	YYY	N
D2330		R	Resin one surface-anterior	0	0	0	0	YYY	N
D2331		R	Resin two surfaces-anterior	0	0	0	0	YYY	N
D2332		R	Resin three surfaces-anterio	0	0	0	0	YYY	N
D2335		R	Resin 4/ surf or w incis an	0	0	0	0	YYY	N
D2336		R	Composite resin crown	0	0	0	0	YYY	N
D2380		R	Resin one surf poster primar	0	0	0	0	YYY	N

CPT codes and descriptions only, © 1994 American Medical Association. Reimbursement information, © 1995 McGraw-Hill Inc.

Code/ CPT	Mod- ifier	Status	Description	Work value	Practice expense	Mal- practice	Total value	Global period	Up- date
D2381		R	Resin two surf poster primar	0	0	0	0	YYY	N
D2382		R	Resin three/more surf post p	0	0	0	0	YYY	N
D2385		R	Resin one surf poster perman	0	0	0	0	YYY	N
D2386		R	Resin two surf poster perman	0	0	0	0	YYY	N
D2387		R	Resin three/more surf post p	0	0	0	0	YYY	N
D2410		R	Dental gold foil one surface	0	0	0	0	YYY	N
D2420		R	Dental gold foil two surface	0	0	0	0	YYY	N
D2430		R	Dental gold foil three surfa	0	0	0	0	YYY	N
D2510		R	Dental inlay metalic 1 surf	0	0	0	0	YYY	N
D2520		R	Dental inlay metallic 2 surf	0	0	0	0	YYY	N
D2530		R	Dental inlay metallic 3 surf	0	0	0	0	YYY	N
D2540		R	Dental onlay metallic	0	0	0	0	YYY	N
D2610		R	Inlay porcelain/ceramic 1 su	0	0	0	0	YYY	N
D2620		R	Inlay porcelain/ceramic 2 su	0	0	0	0	YYY	N
D2630		R	Inlay porcelain/ceramic 3 su	0	0	0	0	YYY	N
D2640		R	Onlay w inlay porcelain/cera	0	0	0	0	YYY	N
D2650		R	Inlay composite/resin one su	0	0	0	0	YYY	N
D2651		R	Inlay composite/resin two su	0	0	0	0	YYY	N
D2652		R	Inlay composite/resin 3 surf	0	0	0	0	YYY	N
D2660		R	Onlay w inlay composite/resi	0	0	0	0	YYY	N
D2710		R	Crown resin laboratory	0	0	0	0	YYY	N
D2720		R	Crown resin w/ high noble me	0	0	0	0	YYY	N
D2721		R	Crown resin w/ base metal	0	0	0	0	YYY	N
D2722		R	Crown resin w/ noble metal	0	0	0	0	YYY	N
D2740		R	Crown porcelain/ceramic subs	0	0	0	0	YYY	N
D2750		R	Crown porcelain w/ h noble m	0	0	0	0	YYY	N
D2751		R	Crown porcelain fused base m	0	0	0	0	YYY	N
D2752		R	Crown porcelain w/ noble met	0	0	0	0	YYY	N
D2790		R	Crown full cast high noble m	0	0	0	0	YYY	N
D2791		R	Crown full cast base metal	0	0	0	0	YYY	N
D2792		R	Crown full cast noble metal	0	0	0	0	YYY	N
D2810		R	Crown 3/4 cast metallic	0	0	0	0	YYY	N
D2910		R	Dental recement inlay	0	0	0	0	YYY	N
D2920		R	Dental recement crown	0	0	0	0	YYY	N
D2930		R	Prefab stnlss steel crwn pri	0	0	0	0	YYY	N
D2931		R	Prefab stnlss steel crown pe	0	0	0	0	YYY	N
D2932		R	Prefabricated resin crown	0	0	0	0	YYY	N
D2933		R	Prefab stainless steel crown	0	0	0	0	YYY	N
D2940		R	Dental sedative filling	0	0	0	0	YYY	N
D2950		R	Core build-up incl any pins	0	0	0	0	YYY	N
D2951		R	Tooth pin retention	0	0	0	0	YYY	N
D2952		R	Post and core cast + crown	0	0	0	0	YYY	N
D2954		R	Prefab post/core + crown	0	0	0	0	YYY	N
D2960		R	Laminate labial veneer	0	0	0	0	YYY	N
D2961		R	Lab labial veneer resin	0	0	0	0	YYY	N
D2962		R	Lab labial veneer porcelain	0	0	0	0	YYY	N
D2970		R	Temporary- fractured tooth	0	0	0	0	YYY	N
D2980		R	Crown repair	0	0	0	0	YYY	N
D2999		R	Dental unspec restorative pr	0	0	0	0	YYY	N
D3110		R	Pulp cap direct	0	0	0	0	YYY	N

CPT codes and descriptions only, © 1994 American Medical Association. Reimbursement information, © 1995 McGraw-Hill Inc.

Code/ CPT	Mod- ifier	Status	Description	Work value	Practice expense	Mal- practice	Total value	Global period	Up- date
D3120		R	Pulp cap indirect	0	0	0	0	YYY	N
D3220		R	Therapeutic pulpotomy	0	0	0	0	YYY	N
D3310		R	Anterior	0	0	0	0	YYY	N
D3320		R	Root canal therapy 2 canals	0	0	0	0	YYY	N
D3330		R	Root canal therapy 3 canals	0	0	0	0	YYY	N
D3346		R	Repeat root canal thrapy ant	0	0	0	0	YYY	N
D3347		R	Repeat root canal bicuspid	0	0	0	0	YYY	N
D3348		R	Repeat root canal molar	0	0	0	0	YYY	N
D3351		R	Apexification/recalc initial	0	0	0	0	YYY	N
D3352		R	Apexification/recalc interim	0	0	0	0	YYY	N
D3353		R	Apexification/recalc final	0	0	0	0	YYY	N
D3410		R	Apicoect/perirad surg anter	0	0	0	0	YYY	N
D3421		R	Root surgery bicuspid	0	0	0	0	YYY	N
D3425		R	Root surgery molar	0	0	0	0	YYY	N
D3426		R	Root surgery ea add root	0	0	0	0	YYY	N
D3430		R	Retrograde filling	0	0	0	0	YYY	N
D3450		R	Root amputation	0	0	0	0	YYY	N
D3460		R	Endodontic endosseous implan	0	0	0	0	YYY	N
D3470		R	Intentional replantation	0	0	0	0	YYY	N
D3910		R	Isolation- tooth w rubb dam	0	0	0	0	YYY	N
D3920		R	Tooth splitting	0	0	0	0	YYY	N
D3950		R	Canal prep/fitting of dowel	0	0	0	0	YYY	N
D3960		R	Bleaching of discolored toot	0	0	0	0	YYY	N
D3999		R	Endodontic procedure	0	0	0	0	YYY	N
D4210		R	Gingivectomy/plasty per quad	0	0	0	0	YYY	S
D4211		R	Gingivectomy/plasty per toot	0	0	0	0	YYY	N
D4220		R	Gingival curettage per quadr	0	0	0	0	YYY	N
D4240		R	Gingival flap proc w/ planin	0	0	0	0	YYY	S
D4249		R	Crown lengthening	0	0	0	0	YYY	N
D4250		R	Mucogingival surg per quadra	0	0	0	0	YYY	N
D4260		R	Osseous surgery per quadrant	0	0	0	0	YYY	S
D4261		R	Bone replace graft single si	0	0	0	0	YYY	S
D4262		R	Bone replace graft mult site	0	0	0	0	YYY	N
D4268		R	Guided tissue regeneration	0	0	0	0	YYY	N
D4270		R	Pedicle soft tissue graft pr	0	0	0	0	YYY	S
D4271		R	Free soft tissue graft proc	0	0	0	0	YYY	S
D4320		R	Provision splnt intracoronal	0	0	0	0	YYY	N
D4321		R	Provisional splint extracoro	0	0	0	0	YYY	N
D4341		R	Periodontal scaling & root	0	0	0	0	YYY	N
D4345		R	Periodontal scaling w/inflam	0	0	0	0	YYY	N
D4910		R	Periodontal maint procedures	0	0	0	0	YYY	N
D4920		R	Unscheduled dressing change	0	0	0	0	YYY	N
D4999		R	Unspecified periodontal proc	0	0	0	0	YYY	N
D5110		R	Dentures complete upper	0	0	0	0	YYY	N
D5120		R	Dentures complete lower	0	0	0	0	YYY	N
D5130		R	Dentures immediate upper	0	0	0	0	YYY	N
D5140		R	Dentures immediate lower	0	0	0	0	YYY	N
D5211		R	Dentures upp part resin base	0	0	0	0	YYY	N
D5212		R	Lower part denture acrylic	0	0	0	0	YYY	N
D5213		R	Upper part denture base cast	0	0	0	0	YYY	N

CPT codes and descriptions only, © 1994 American Medical Association. Reimbursement information, © 1995 McGraw-Hill Inc.

Code/ CPT	Mod- ifier	Status	Description	Work value	Practice expense	Mal- practice	Total value	Global period	Up- date
D5214		R	Lower part denture base cast	0	0	0	0	YYY	N
D5281		R	Removable partial denture	0	0	0	0	YYY	N
D5410		R	Dentur adjust complete upper	0	0	0	0	YYY	N
D5411		R	Denture adjust complete lowr	0	0	0	0	YYY	N
D5421		R	Dentures adjust part upper	0	0	0	0	YYY	N
D5422		R	Dentures adjust part lower	0	0	0	0	YYY	N
D5510		R	Dentur repr broken compl bas	0	0	0	0	YYY	N
D5520		R	Replace denture teeth complt	0	0	0	0	YYY	N
D5610		R	Repair resin saddle or base	0	0	0	0	YYY	N
D5620		R	Rep part denture cast frame	0	0	0	0	YYY	N
D5630		R	Rep partial denture clasp	0	0	0	0	YYY	N
D5640		R	Replace part denture teeth	0	0	0	0	YYY	N
D5650		R	Add tooth to partial denture	0	0	0	0	YYY	N
D5660		R	Add clasp to partial denture	0	0	0	0	YYY	N
D5710		R	Dentur rebase complete upper	0	0	0	0	YYY	N
D5711		R	Repl base comp lower denture	0	0	0	0	YYY	N
D5720		R	Repl base part upper denture	0	0	0	0	YYY	N
D5721		R	Repl base part lower denture	0	0	0	0	YYY	N
D5730		R	Dentur relin upp compl chrsd	0	0	0	0	YYY	N
D5731		R	Resurface l comp denture chr	0	0	0	0	YYY	N
D5740		R	Resurface u part denture chr	0	0	0	0	YYY	N
D5741		R	Resurface l part denture chr	0	0	0	0	YYY	N
D5750		R	Resurface u comp denture lab	0	0	0	0	YYY	N
D5751		R	Resurface l comp denture lab	0	0	0	0	YYY	N
D5760		R	Resurface u part denture lab	0	0	0	0	YYY	N
D5761		R	Resurface l part denture lab	0	0	0	0	YYY	N
D5810		R	Denturs interim complete upp	0	0	0	0	YYY	N
D5811		R	Temp complete denture lower	0	0	0	0	YYY	N
D5820		R	Temp partial denture upper	0	0	0	0	YYY	N
D5821		R	Temp partial denture lower	0	0	0	0	YYY	N
D5850		R	Tissue conditioning	0	0	0	0	YYY	N
D5851		R	Tissue conditioning lower	0	0	0	0	YYY	N
D5860		R	Overdenture complete	0	0	0	0	YYY	N
D5861		R	Overdenture partial	0	0	0	0	YYY	N
D5862		R	Precision attachment	0	0	0	0	YYY	N
D5899		R	Removable prosthodontic proc	0	0	0	0	YYY	N
D5911		R	Facial moulage sectional	0	0	0	0	YYY	N
D5912		R	Facial moulage complete	0	0	0	0	YYY	N
D5913		R	Nasal prosthesis	0	0	0	0	YYY	N
D5914		R	Auricular prosthesis	0	0	0	0	YYY	N
D5915		R	Orbital prosthesis	0	0	0	0	YYY	N
D5916		R	Ocular prosthesis	0	0	0	0	YYY	N
D5919		R	Facial prosthesis	0	0	0	0	YYY	N
D5922		R	Nasal septal prosthesis	0	0	0	0	YYY	N
D5923		R	Ocular prosthesis interim	0	0	0	0	YYY	N
D5924		R	Cranial prosthesis	0	0	0	0	YYY	N
D5925		R	Facial augmentation implant	0	0	0	0	YYY	N
D5926		R	Replacement nasal prosthesis	0	0	0	0	YYY	N
D5927		R	Auricular replacement	0	0	0	0	YYY	N
D5928		R	Orbital replacement	0	0	0	0	YYY	N

CPT codes and descriptions only, © 1994 American Medical Association. Reimbursement information, © 1995 McGraw-Hill Inc.

Code/ CPT	Mod- ifier	Status	Description	Work value	Practice expense	Mal- practice	Total value	Global period	Up- date
D5929		R	Facial replacement	0	0	0	0	YYY	N
D5931		R	Surgical obturator	0	0	0	0	YYY	N
D5932		R	Postsurgical obturator	0	0	0	0	YYY	N
D5933		R	Refitting of obturator	0	0	0	0	YYY	N
D5934		R	Mandibular flange prosthesis	0	0	0	0	YYY	N
D5935		R	Mandibular denture prosth	0	0	0	0	YYY	N
D5936		R	Temp obturator prosthesis	0	0	0	0	YYY	N
D5937		R	Trismus appliance	0	0	0	0	YYY	N
D5951		R	Feeding aid	0	0	0	0	YYY	N
D5952		R	Pediatric speech aid	0	0	0	0	YYY	N
D5953		R	Adult speech aid	0	0	0	0	YYY	N
D5954		R	Superimposed prosthesis	0	0	0	0	YYY	N
D5955		R	Palatal lift prosthesis	0	0	0	0	YYY	N
D5958		R	Intraoral con def inter plt	0	0	0	0	YYY	N
D5959		R	Intraoral con def mod palat	0	0	0	0	YYY	N
D5960		R	Modify speech aid prosthesis	0	0	0	0	YYY	N
D5982		R	Surgical stent	0	0	0	0	YYY	N
D5983		R	Radiation applicator	0	0	0	0	YYY	N
D5984		R	Radiation shield	0	0	0	0	YYY	N
D5985		R	Radiation cone locator	0	0	0	0	YYY	N
D5986		R	Fluoride applicator	0	0	0	0	YYY	N
D5987		R	Commissure splint	0	0	0	0	YYY	N
D5988		R	Surgical splint	0	0	0	0	YYY	N
D5999		R	Maxillofacial prosthesis	0	0	0	0	YYY	N
D6030		R	Prosthodont endosseous impl	0	0	0	0	YYY	N
D6040		R	Subperiosteal implant	0	0	0	0	YYY	N
D6050		R	Transosseous implant	0	0	0	0	YYY	N
D6055		R	Implant connecting bar	0	0	0	0	YYY	N
D6080		R	Implant maintenance	0	0	0	0	YYY	N
D6090		R	Repair implant	0	0	0	0	YYY	N
D6100		R	Removal of implant	0	0	0	0	YYY	N
D6199		R	Implant procedure	0	0	0	0	YYY	N
D6210		R	Prosthodont high noble metal	0	0	0	0	YYY	N
D6211		R	Bridge base metal cast	0	0	0	0	YYY	N
D6212		R	Bridge noble metal cast	0	0	0	0	YYY	N
D6240		R	Bridge porcelain high noblc	0	0	0	0	YYY	N
D6241		R	Bridge porcelain base metal	0	0	0	0	YYY	N
D6242		R	Bridge porcelain nobel metal	0	0	0	0	YYY	N
D6250		R	Bridge resin w/high noble	0	0	0	0	YYY	N
D6251		R	Bridge resin base metal	0	0	0	0	YYY	N
D6252		R	Bridge resin w/noble metal	0	0	0	0	YYY	N
D6520		R	Dental retainer two surfaces	0	0	0	0	YYY	N
D6530		R	Retainer metallic 3+ surface	0	0	0	0	YYY	N
D6540		R	Retainer metallic cusps	0	0	0	0	YYY	N
D6545		R	Retainer acid etch bridge	0	0	0	0	YYY	N
D6720		R	Retain crown resin w hi nble	0	0	0	0	YYY	N
D6721		R	Crown resin w/base metal	0	0	0	0	YYY	N
D6722		R	Crown resin w/noble metal	0	0	0	0	YYY	N
D6750		R	Crown porcelain high noble	0	0	0	0	YYY	N
D6751		R	Crown porcelain base metal	0	0	0	0	YYY	N

CPT codes and descriptions only, © 1994 American Medical Association. Reimbursement information, © 1995 McGraw-Hill Inc.

Code/ CPT	Mod- ifier	Status	Description	Work value	Practice expense	Mal- practice	Total value	Global period	Up- date
D6752		R	Crown porcelain noble metal	0	0	0	0	YYY	N
D6780		R	Crown 3/4 high noble metal	0	0	0	0	YYY	N
D6790		R	Crown full high noble metal	0	0	0	0	YYY	N
D6791		R	Crown full base metal cast	0	0	0	0	YYY	N
D6792		R	Crown full noble metal cast	0	0	0	0	YYY	N
D6930		R	Dental recement bridge	0	0	0	0	YYY	N
D6940		R	Stress breaker	0	0	0	0	YYY	N
D6950		R	Precision attachment	0	0	0	0	YYY	N
D6970		R	Post & core plus retainer	0	0	0	0	YYY	N
D6971		R	Cast post bridge retainer	0	0	0	0	YYY	N
D6972		R	Prefab post & core plus reta	0	0	0	0	YYY	N
D6973		R	Core build up for retainer	0	0	0	0	YYY	N
D6975		R	Coping metal	0	0	0	0	YYY	N
D6980		R	Bridge repair	0	0	0	0	YYY	N
D6999		R	Fixed prosthodontic proc	0	0	0	0	YYY	N
D7110		R	Oral surgery single tooth	0	0	0	0	YYY	S
D7120		R	Each add tooth extraction	0	0	0	0	YYY	S
D7130		R	Tooth root removal	0	0	0	0	YYY	S
D7210		R	Rem imp tooth w mucoper flp	0	0	0	0	YYY	S
D7220		R	Impact tooth remov soft tiss	0	0	0	0	YYY	S
D7230		R	Impact tooth remov part bony	0	0	0	0	YYY	S
D7240		R	Impact tooth remov comp bony	0	0	0	0	YYY	S
D7241		R	Impact tooth rem bony w/comp	0	0	0	0	YYY	S
D7250		R	Tooth root removal	0	0	0	0	YYY	S
D7260		R	Oral antral fistula closure	0	0	0	0	YYY	S
D7270		R	Tooth reimplantation	0	0	0	0	YYY	S
D7271		R	Tooth implantation	0	0	0	0	YYY	N
D7272		R	Tooth transplantation	0	0	0	0	YYY	N
D7280		R	Exposure impact tooth orthod	0	0	0	0	YYY	N
D7281		R	Exposure tooth aid eruption	0	0	0	0	YYY	N
D7285		R	Biopsy of oral tissue hard	0	0	0	0	YYY	S
D7286		R	Biopsy of oral tissue soft	0	0	0	0	YYY	S
D7290		R	Repositioning of teeth	0	0	0	0	YYY	S
D7291		R	Transseptal fiberotomy	0	0	0	0	YYY	N
D7310		R	Alveoplasty w/ extraction	0	0	0	0	YYY	S
D7320		R	Alveoplasty w/o extraction	0	0	0	0	YYY	S
D7340		R	Vestibuloplasty ridge extens	0	0	0	0	YYY	S
D7350		R	Vestibuloplasty exten graft	0	0	0	0	YYY	S
D7410		R	Rad exc lesion up to 1.25 cm	0	0	0	0	YYY	S
D7420		R	Lesion 1.25 cm	0	0	0	0	YYY	S
D7430		R	Exc benign tumor to 1.25 cm	0	0	0	0	YYY	S
D7431		R	Benign tumor exc 1.25 cm	0	0	0	0	YYY	S
D7440		R	Malig tumor exc to 1.25 cm	0	0	0	0	YYY	N
D7441		R	Malig tumor 1.25 cm	0	0	0	0	YYY	S
D7450		R	Rem odontogen cyst to 1.25cm	0	0	0	0	YYY	S
D7451		R	Rem odontogen cyst 1.25 cm	0	0	0	0	YYY	S
D7460		R	Rem nonodonto cyst to 1.25cm	0	0	0	0	YYY	S
D7461		R	Rem nonodonto cyst 1.25 cm	0	0	0	0	YYY	S
D7465		R	Lesion destruction	0	0	0	0	YYY	N
D7470		R	Rem exostosis maxilla/mandib	0	0	0	0	YYY	S

CPT codes and descriptions only, © 1994 American Medical Association. Reimbursement information, © 1995 McGraw-Hill Inc.

Code/ CPT	Mod- ifier	Status	Description	Work value	Practice expense	Mal- practice	Total value	Global period	Up- date
D7480		R	Partial ostectomy	0	0	0	0	YYY	S
D7490		R	Mandible resection	0	0	0	0	YYY	S
D7510		R	I&d absc intraoral soft tiss	0	0	0	0	YYY	S
D7520		R	I&d abscess extraoral	0	0	0	0	YYY	S
D7530		R	Removal fb skin/areolar tiss	0	0	0	0	YYY	S
D7540		R	Removal of fb reaction	0	0	0	0	YYY	S
D7550		R	Removal of sloughed off bone	0	0	0	0	YYY	S
D7560		R	Maxillary sinusotomy	0	0	0	0	YYY	S
D7610		R	Maxilla open reduct simple	0	0	0	0	YYY	S
D7620		R	Clsd reduct simpl maxilla fx	0	0	0	0	YYY	S
D7630		R	Open red simpl mandible fx	0	0	0	0	YYY	S
D7640		R	Clsd red simpl mandible fx	0	0	0	0	YYY	S
D7650		R	Open red simp malar/zygom fx	0	0	0	0	YYY	S
D7660		R	Clsd red simp malar/zygom fx	0	0	0	0	YYY	S
D7670		R	Open red simple alveolus fx	0	0	0	0	YYY	S
D7680		R	Reduct simple facial bone fx	0	0	0	0	YYY	S
D7710		R	Maxilla open reduct compound	0	0	0	0	YYY	S
D7720		R	Clsd reduct compd maxilla fx	0	0	0	0	YYY	S
D7730		R	Open reduct compd mandble fx	0	0	0	0	YYY	S
D7740		R	Clsd reduct compd mandble fx	0	0	0	0	YYY	S
D7750		R	Open red comp malar/zygma fx	0	0	0	0	YYY	S
D7760		R	Clsd red comp malar/zygma fx	0	0	0	0	YYY	N
D7770		R	Open reduc compd alveolus fx	0	0	0	0	YYY	N
D7780		R	Reduct compnd facial bone fx	0	0	0	0	YYY	S
D7810		R	Tmj open reduct-dislocation	0	0	0	0	YYY	S
D7820		R	Closed tmp manipulation	0	0	0	0	YYY	S
D7830		R	Tmj manipulation under anest	0	0	0	0	YYY	N
D7840		R	Removal of tmj condyle	0	0	0	0	YYY	S
D7850		R	Tmj meniscectomy	0	0	0	0	YYY	N
D7852		R	Tmj repair of joint disc	0	0	0	0	YYY	N
D7854		R	Tmj excisn of joint membrane	0	0	0	0	YYY	N
D7856		R	Tmj cutting of a muscle	0	0	0	0	YYY	N
D7858		R	Tmj reconstruction	0	0	0	0	YYY	N
D7860		R	Tmj cutting into joint	0	0	0	0	YYY	S
D7865		R	Tmj reshaping components	0	0	0	0	YYY	N
D7870		R	Tmj aspiration joint fluid	0	0	0	0	YYY	N
D7872		R	Tmj diagnostic arthroscopy	0	0	0	0	YYY	N
D7873		R	Tmj arthroscopy lysis adhesn	0	0	0	0	YYY	N
D7874		R	Tmj arthroscopy disc reposit	0	0	0	0	YYY	N
D7875		R	Tmj arthroscopy synovectomy	0	0	0	0	YYY	N
D7876		R	Tmj arthroscopy discectomy	0	0	0	0	YYY	N
D7877		R	Tmj arthroscopy debridement	0	0	0	0	YYY	N
D7880		R	Occlusal orthotic appliance	0	0	0	0	YYY	S
D7899		R	Tmj unspecified therapy	0	0	0	0	YYY	N
D7910		R	Dent sutur recent wnd to 5cm	0	0	0	0	YYY	N
D7911		R	Dental suture wound to 5 cm	0	0	0	0	YYY	S
D7912		R	Suture complicate wnd 5 cm	0	0	0	0	YYY	S
D7920		R	Dental skin graft	0	0	0	0	YYY	S
D7940		R	Reshaping bone orthognathic	0	0	0	0	YYY	S
D7941		R	Bone cutting ramus closed	0	0	0	0	YYY	N

CPT codes and descriptions only, © 1994 American Medical Association. Reimbursement information, © 1995 McGraw-Hill Inc.

Code/ CPT	Mod- ifier	Status	Description	Work value	Practice expense	Mal- practice	Total value	Global period	Up- date
D7942		R	Bone cutting ramus open	0	0	0	0	YYY	N
D7943		R	Cutting ramus open w/graft	0	0	0	0	YYY	S
D7944		R	Bone cutting segmented	0	0	0	0	YYY	N
D7945		R	Bone cutting body mandible	0	0	0	0	YYY	S
D7946		R	Reconstruction maxilla total	0	0	0	0	YYY	S
D7947		R	Reconstruct maxilla segment	0	0	0	0	YYY	N
D7948		R	Reconstruct midface no graft	0	0	0	0	YYY	S
D7949		R	Reconstruct midface w/graft	0	0	0	0	YYY	N
D7950		R	Mandible graft	0	0	0	0	YYY	S
D7955		R	Repair maxillofacial defects	0	0	0	0	YYY	S
D7960		R	Frenulectomy/frenulotomy	0	0	0	0	YYY	S
D7970		R	Excision hyperplastic tissue	0	0	0	0	YYY	N
D7971		R	Excision pericoronal gingiva	0	0	0	0	YYY	N
D7980		R	Sialolithotomy	0	0	0	0	YYY	S
D7981		R	Excision of salivary gland	0	0	0	0	YYY	S
D7982		R	Sialodochoplasty	0	0	0	0	YYY	S
D7983		R	Closure of salivary fistula	0	0	0	0	YYY	N
D7990		R	Emergency tracheotomy	0	0	0	0	YYY	S
D7991		R	Dental coronoidectomy	0	0	0	0	YYY	S
D7993		R	Implant facial bones	0	0	0	0	YYY	N
D7994		R	Implant chin	0	0	0	0	YYY	N
D7999		R	Oral surgery procedure	0	0	0	0	YYY	S
D8110		R	Orthodontic rem appliance tx	0	0	0	0	YYY	N
D8120		R	Fixed appliance therapy guid	0	0	0	0	YYY	N
D8210		R	Orthodontic rem appliance tx	0	0	0	0	YYY	N
D8220		R	Fixed appliance therapy habt	0	0	0	0	YYY	N
D8360		R	Orthodontic rem appliance tx	0	0	0	0	YYY	N
D8370		R	Fixed appliance interceptive	0	0	0	0	YYY	N
D8460		R	Trans dentit class I maloccl	0	0	0	0	YYY	N
D8470		R	Class ii malocclusion trnstn	0	0	0	0	YYY	N
D8480		R	Class iii malocclusion trnst	0	0	0	0	YYY	N
D8560		R	Class i tx atyp/ext skel cas	0	0	0	0	YYY	N
D8570		R	Class ii malocclusion perman	0	0	0	0	YYY	N
D8580		R	Class iii malocclusion permn	0	0	0	0	YYY	N
D8650		R	Tx atypical/extend skel case	0	0	0	0	YYY	N
D8750		R	Post-treatment stabilization	0	0	0	0	YYY	N
D8999		R	Orthodontic procedure	0	0	0	0	YYY	N
D9110		R	Dent procedure general minor	0	0	0	0	YYY	N
D9210		R	Dent anesthesia w/o surgery	0	0	0	0	YYY	N
D9211		R	Regional block anesthesia	0	0	0	0	YYY	N
D9212		R	Trigeminal block anesthesia	0	0	0	0	YYY	N
D9215		R	Local anesthesia	0	0	0	0	YYY	N
D9220		R	General anesthesia	0	0	0	0	YYY	N
D9221		R	General anesthesia ea ad 15m	0	0	0	0	YYY	N
D9230		R	Analgesia	0	0	0	0	YYY	N
D9240		R	Intravenous sedation	0	0	0	0	YYY	N
D9310		R	Dental consultation	0	0	0	0	YYY	N
D9410		R	Dental house call	0	0	0	0	YYY	N
D9420		R	Hospital call	0	0	0	0	YYY	N
D9430		R	Office visit during hours	0	0	0	0	YYY	N

CPT codes and descriptions only, © 1994 American Medical Association. Reimbursement information, © 1995 McGraw-Hill Inc.

Code/ CPT	Mod- ifier	Status	Description	Work value	Practice expense	Mal- practice	Total value	Global period	Up- date
D9440		R	Office visit after hours	0	0	0	0	YYY	N
D9610		R	Dent therapeutic drug inject	0	0	0	0	YYY	N
D9630		R	Other drugs/medicaments	0	0	0	0	YYY	N
D9910		R	Dent appl desensitizing med	0	0	0	0	YYY	N
D9920		R	Behavior management	0	0	0	0	YYY	N
D9930		R	Treatment of complications	0	0	0	0	YYY	N
D9940		R	Occlusal guards	0	0	0	0	YYY	N
D9941		R	Fabrication of mouthguards	0	0	0	0	YYY	N
D9950		R	Occlusion analysis	0	0	0	0	YYY	N
D9951		R	Limited occlusal adjustment	0	0	0	0	YYY	N
D9952		R	Complete occlusal adjustment	0	0	0	0	YYY	N
D9999		R	Adjunctive procedure	0	0	0	0	YYY	N
G0001		X	Drawing blood for specimen	0	0	0	0	XXX	0
G0002		A	Temporary urinary catheter	0.50	0.70	0.02	1.22	0	S
G0003		D	ECG 24hr attended monitoring	0	0	0	0	XXX	N
G0003	26	D	ECG 24hr attended monitoring	0	0	0	0	XXX	N
G0003	TC	D	ECG 24hr attended monitoring	0	0	0	0	XXX	N
G0004		A	ECG transm phys review & int	0.52	7.31	0.65	8.48	XXX	N
G0005		A	ECG 24 hour recording	0	1.18	0.09	1.27	XXX	N
G0006		A	ECG transmission & analysis	0	5.73	0.51	6.24	XXX	N
G0007		A	ECG phy review & interpret	0.52	0.40	0.05	0.97	XXX	N
G0008		X	Admin influenza virus vac	0	0	0	0	XXX	0
G0009		X	Admin pneumococcal vaccine	0	0	0	0	XXX	0
G0010		X	Admin hepatitis b vaccine	0	0	0	0	XXX	0
G0015		A	Post symptom ECG tracing	0	5.73	0.51	6.24	XXX	N
G0016		A	Post symptom ECG md review	0.52	0.40	0.05	0.97	XXX	N
G0020		C	Prepare face/oral prosthesis	0	0	0	0	10	S
G0021		C	Prepare orbital prosthesis	0	0	0	0	90	S
G0025		A	Collagen skin test kit	0	0.95	0	0.95	XXX	N
H5300		A	Occupational therapy	0.32	0.24	0.03	0.59	XXX	N
J0110		E	Administration injection	0	0	0	0	XXX	0
J0120		E	Tetracyclin injection	0	0	0	0	XXX	0
J0150		E	Injection adenosine 6 MG	0	0	0	0	XXX	0
J0170		E	Adrenalin epinephrin inject	0	0	0	0	XXX	0
J0190		E	Biperiden 2 MG injection	0	0	0	0	XXX	0
J0205		E	Alglucerase injection	0	0	0	0	XXX	0
J0210		E	Methyldopate hcl injection	0	0	0	0	XXX	0
J0220		D	Allergy desensitization aqeo	0	0	0	0	XXX	0
J0230		D	Allergy desensitization allp	0	0	0	0	XXX	0
J0240		D	Allergy desensitiz emulsific	0	0	0	0	XXX	0
J0256		E	Alpha 1-proteinase 500 MG	0	0	0	0	XXX	0
J0280		E	Aminophyllin 250 MG inj	0	0	0	0	XXX	0
J0290		E	Ampicillin 500 MG inj	0	0	0	0	XXX	0
J0295		E	Ampicillin sodium per 1.5 gm	0	0	0	0	XXX	0
J0300		E	Amobarbital 125 MG inj	0	0	0	0	XXX	0
J0330		E	Succinycholine chloride inj	0	0	0	0	XXX	0
J0340		E	Nandrolon phenpropionate inj	0	0	0	0	XXX	0
J0350		E	Injection anistreplase 30 u	0	0	0	0	XXX	0
J0360		E	Hydralazine hcl injection	0	0	0	0	XXX	0
J0380		E	Metaraminol injection	0	0	0	0	XXX	0

CPT codes and descriptions only, © 1994 American Medical Association. Reimbursement information, © 1995 McGraw-Hill Inc.

Code/ CPT	Mod- ifier	Status	Description	Work value	Practice expense	Mal- practice	Total value	Global period	Up- date
J0390		E	Chloroquine injection	0	0	0	0	XXX	0
J0400		E	Trimethaphan injection	0	0	0	0	XXX	0
J0460		E	Atropine sulfate injection	0	0	0	0	XXX	0
J0470		E	Dimecaprol injection	0	0	0	0	XXX	0
J0475		E	Baclofen 10 MG injection	0	0	0	0	XXX	0
J0500		E	Dicyclomine injection	0	0	0	0	XXX	0
J0510		E	Benzquinamide injection	0	0	0	0	XXX	0
J0515		E	Benztropine injection	0	0	0	0	XXX	0
J0520		E	Bethanechol chloride inject	0	0	0	0	XXX	0
J0530		E	Penicillin g benzathine inj	0	0	0	0	XXX	0
J0540		E	Penicillin g benzathine inj	0	0	0	0	XXX	0
J0550		E	Penicillin g benzathine inj	0	0	0	0	XXX	0
J0560		E	Penicillin g benzathine inj	0	0	0	0	XXX	0
J0570		E	Penicillin g benzathine inj	0	0	0	0	XXX	0
J0580		E	Penicillin g benzathine inj	0	0	0	0	XXX	0
J0585		E	Botulinum toxin a per 100 u	0	0	0	0	XXX	0
J0590		E	Ethylnorepinephrine hcl inj	0	0	0	0	XXX	0
J0600		E	Edetate calcium disodium inj	0	0	0	0	XXX	0
J0610		E	Calcium gluconate injection	0	0	0	0	XXX	0
J0620		E	Calcium glycer & lact/10 ML	0	0	0	0	XXX	0
J0630		E	Calcitonin salmon injection	0	0	0	0	XXX	0
J0635		E	Calcitriol injection	0	0	0	0	XXX	0
J0640		E	Leucovorin calcium injection	0	0	0	0	XXX	0
J0670		E	Mepivacaine injection	0	0	0	0	XXX	0
J0680		E	Deslanoside injection	0	0	0	0	XXX	0
J0690		E	Cefazolin sodium injection	0	0	0	0	XXX	0
J0694		E	Cefoxitin sodium injection	0	0	0	0	XXX	0
J0695		E	Cefonocid sodium injection	0	0	0	0	XXX	0
J0696		E	Ceftriaxone sodium injection	0	0	0	0	XXX	0
J0697		E	Sterile cefuroxime injection	0	0	0	0	XXX	0
J0698		E	Cefotaxime sodium injection	0	0	0	0	XXX	0
J0700		D	Betamethasone injection	0	0	0	0	XXX	0
J0702		E	Betamethasone acet&sod phosp	0	0	0	0	XXX	0
J0704		E	Betamethasone sod phosp/4 MG	0	0	0	0	XXX	0
J0710		E	Cephapirin sodium injection	0	0	0	0	XXX	0
J0715		E	Ceftizoxime sodium / 500 MG	0	0	0	0	XXX	0
J0720		E	Chloramphenicol sodium injec	0	0	0	0	XXX	0
J0725		E	Chorionic gonadotropin/1000u	0	0	0	0	XXX	0
J0730		E	Chlorpheniramin maleate inj	0	0	0	0	XXX	0
J0743		E	Cilastatin sodium injection	0	0	0	0	XXX	0
J0745		E	Inj codeine phosphate /30 MG	0	0	0	0	XXX	0
J0760		E	Colchicine injection	0	0	0	0	XXX	0
J0770		E	Colistimethate sodium inj	0	0	0	0	XXX	0
J0780		E	Prochlorperazine injection	0	0	0	0	XXX	0
J0790		D	Nikethamide injection	0	0	0	0	XXX	0
J0800		E	Corticotropin injection	0	0	0	0	XXX	0
J0810		E	Cortisone injection	0	0	0	0	XXX	0
J0820		E	Cortigel 40 injection	0	0	0	0	XXX	0
J0830		D	Cotrophin zinc hydroxid inj	0	0	0	0	XXX	0
J0835		E	Inj cosyntropin per 0.25 MG	0	0	0	0	XXX	0

CPT codes and descriptions only, © 1994 American Medical Association. Reimbursement information, © 1995 McGraw-Hill Inc.

Code/ CPT	Mod- ifier	Status	Description	Work value	Practice expense	Mal- practice	Total value	Global period	Up- date
J0840		D	Warfarin sodium injection	0	0	0	0	XXX	0
J0850		E	Cytomegalovirus imm IV /vial	0	0	0	0	XXX	0
J0895		E	Deferoxamine mesylate inj	0	0	0	0	XXX	0
J0900		E	Testosterone enanthate inj	0	0	0	0	XXX	0
J0945		E	Brompheniramine maleate inj	0	0	0	0	XXX	0
J0970		E	Estradiol valerate injection	0	0	0	0	XXX	0
J1000		E	Depo-estradiol cypionate inj	0	0	0	0	XXX	0
J1020		E	Methylprednisolone 20 MG inj	0	0	0	0	XXX	0
J1030		E	Methylprednisolone 40 MG inj	0	0	0	0	XXX	0
J1040		E	Methylprednisolone 80 MG inj	0	0	0	0	XXX	0
J1050		E	Medroxyprogesterone inj	0	0	0	0	XXX	0
J1055		E	Medrxyprogester acetate inj	0	0	0	0	XXX	0
J1060		E	Testosterone cypionate 1 ML	0	0	0	0	XXX	0
J1070		E	Testosterone cypionat 100 MG	0	0	0	0	XXX	0
J1080		E	Testosterone cypionat 200 MG	0	0	0	0	XXX	0
J1090		E	Testosterone cypionate 50 MG	0	0	0	0	XXX	0
J1100		E	Dexamethosone sodium phos	0	0	0	0	XXX	0
J1110		E	Dehydroergotamine injection	0	0	0	0	XXX	0
J1120		E	Acetazolamid sodium injectio	0	0	0	0	XXX	0
J1155		D	Digitoxin injection	0	0	0	0	XXX	0
J1160		E	Digoxin injection	0	0	0	0	XXX	0
J1165		E	Phenytoin sodium injection	0	0	0	0	XXX	0
J1170		E	Hydromorphone injection	0	0	0	0	XXX	0
J1180		E	Dyphylline injection	0	0	0	0	XXX	0
J1200		E	Diphenhydramine hcl injectio	0	0	0	0	XXX	0
J1205		E	Chlorothiazide sodium inj	0	0	0	0	XXX	0
J1212		E	Dimethyl sulfoxide 50% 50 ML	0	0	0	0	XXX	0
J1230		E	Methadone injection	0	0	0	0	XXX	0
J1240		E	Dimenhydrinate injection	0	0	0	0	XXX	0
J1245		E	Dipyridamole injection	0	0	0	0	XXX	0
J1320		E	Amitriptyline injection	0	0	0	0	XXX	0
J1330		E	Ergonovine maleate injection	0	0	0	0	XXX	0
J1340		E	Aqueous/saline placebo inj	0	0	0	0	XXX	0
J1350		D	Erythromycin-im inj	0	0	0	0	XXX	0
J1360		D	Erythromycin-iv inj	0	0	0	0	XXX	0
J1362		E	Erythromycin glucep / 250 MG	0	0	0	0	XXX	0
J1364		E	Erythro lactobionate /500 MG	0	0	0	0	XXX	0
J1380		E	Estradiol valerate 10 MG inj	0	0	0	0	XXX	0
J1390		E	Estradiol valerate 20 MG inj	0	0	0	0	XXX	0
J1410		E	Inj estrogen conjugate 25 MG	0	0	0	0	XXX	0
J1435		E	Injection estrone per 1 MG	0	0	0	0	XXX	0
J1436		E	Etidronate disodium inj	0	0	0	0	XXX	0
J1440		E	Filgrastim 300 mcg injeciton	0	0	0	0	XXX	0
J1441		E	Filgrastim 480 mcg injection	0	0	0	0	XXX	0
J1455		E	Foscarnet sodium injection	0	0	0	0	XXX	0
J1460		E	Gamma globulin 1 CC inj	0	0	0	0	XXX	0
J1470		E	Gamma globulin 2 CC inj	0	0	0	0	XXX	0
J1480		E	Gamma globulin 3 CC inj	0	0	0	0	XXX	0
J1490		E	Gamma globulin 4 CC inj	0	0	0	0	XXX	0
J1500		E	Gamma globulin 5 CC inj	0	0	0	0	XXX	0

CPT codes and descriptions only, © 1994 American Medical Association. Reimbursement information, © 1995 McGraw-Hill Inc.

Code/ CPT	Mod- ifier	Status	Description	Work value	Practice expense	Mal- practice	Total value	Global period	Up- date
J1510		E	Gamma globulin 6 CC inj	0	0	0	0	XXX	0
J1520		E	Gamma globulin 7 CC inj	0	0	0	0	XXX	0
J1530		E	Gamma globulin 8 CC inj	0	0	0	0	XXX	0
J1540		E	Gamma globulin 9 CC inj	0	0	0	0	XXX	0
J1550		E	Gamma globulin 10 CC inj	0	0	0	0	XXX	0
J1560		E	Gamma globulin 10 CC inj	0	0	0	0	XXX	0
J1561		E	Immune globulin injection	0	0	0	0	XXX	0
J1562		E	Immune globulin 10% /5 grams	0	0	0	0	XXX	0
J1570		E	Ganciclovir sodium injection	0	0	0	0	XXX	0
J1580		E	Garamycin gentamicin inj	0	0	0	0	XXX	0
J1600		E	Gold sodium thiomaleate inj	0	0	0	0	XXX	0
J1610		E	Glucagon hydrochloride/1 MG	0	0	0	0	XXX	0
J1620		E	Gonadorelin hydroch/ 100 mcg	0	0	0	0	XXX	0
J1625		E	Granisetron hydrochlor/1 MG	0	0	0	0	XXX	0
J1630		E	Haloperidol injection	0	0	0	0	XXX	0
J1631		E	Haloperidol decanoate inj	0	0	0	0	XXX	0
J1640		D	Heparin sodium injection	0	0	0	0	XXX	0
J1642		E	Inj heparin sodium per 10 u	0	0	0	0	XXX	0
J1644		E	Inj heparin sodium per 1000u	0	0	0	0	XXX	0
J1660		E	Histamine injection	0	0	0	0	XXX	0
J1670		E	Tetanus immune globulin inj	0	0	0	0	XXX	0
J1690		E	Prednisolone tebutate inj	0	0	0	0	XXX	0
J1700		E	Hydrocortisone acetate inj	0	0	0	0	XXX	0
J1710		E	Hydrocortisone sodium ph inj	0	0	0	0	XXX	0
J1720		E	Hydrocortisone sodium succ i	0	0	0	0	XXX	0
J1730		E	Diazoxide injection	0	0	0	0	XXX	0
J1739		E	Hydroxyprogesterone cap 125	0	0	0	0	XXX	0
J1741		E	Hydroxyprogesterone cap 250	0	0	0	0	XXX	0
J1760		E	Iron dextran 2 CC inj	0	0	0	0	XXX	0
J1770		E	Iron dextran 5 CC inj	0	0	0	0	XXX	0
J1780		E	Iron dextran 10 CC inj	0	0	0	0	XXX	0
J1785		E	Injection imiglucerase /unit	0	0	0	0	XXX	0
J1790		E	Droperidol injection	0	0	0	0	XXX	0
J1800		E	Propranolol injection	0	0	0	0	XXX	0
J1810		E	Droperidol/fentanyl inj	0	0	0	0	XXX	0
J1820		E	Insulin injection	0	0	0	0	XXX	0
J1830		E	Interferon beta-1b / .25 MG	0	0	0	0	XXX	0
J1840		E	Kanamycin sulfate 500 MG inj	0	0	0	0	XXX	0
J1850		E	Kanamycin sulfate 75 MG inj	0	0	0	0	XXX	0
J1885		E	Ketorolac tromethamine inj	0	0	0	0	XXX	0
J1890		E	Cephalothin sodium injection	0	0	0	0	XXX	0
J1910		E	Kutapressin injection	0	0	0	0	XXX	0
J1930		E	Propiomazine injection	0	0	0	0	XXX	0
J1940		E	Furosemide injection	0	0	0	0	XXX	0
J1950		E	Leuprolide acetate /3.75 MG	0	0	0	0	XXX	0
J1960		E	Levorphanol tartrate inj	0	0	0	0	XXX	0
J1970		E	Methotrimeprazine injection	0	0	0	0	XXX	0
J1980		E	Hyoscyamine sulfate inj	0	0	0	0	XXX	0
J1990		E	Chlordiazepoxide injection	0	0	0	0	XXX	0
J2000		E	Lidocaine injection	0	0	0	0	XXX	0

CPT codes and descriptions only, © 1994 American Medical Association. Reimbursement information, © 1995 McGraw-Hill Inc.

Code/ CPT	Mod- ifier	Status	Description	Work value	Practice expense	Mal- practice	Total value	Global period	Up- date
J2010		E	Lincomycin injection	0	0	0	0	XXX	0
J2050		E	Liver injection	0	0	0	0	XXX	0
J2060		E	Lorazepam injection	0	0	0	0	XXX	0
J2100		E	Luminal sodium injection	0	0	0	0	XXX	0
J2150		E	Mannitol injection	0	0	0	0	XXX	0
J2160		D	Cyclizine lactate injection	0	0	0	0	XXX	0
J2175		E	Meperidine hydrochl /100 MG	0	0	0	0	XXX	0
J2180		E	Meperidine/promethazine inj	0	0	0	0	XXX	0
J2190		E	Mersalyl & theophylline inj	0	0	0	0	XXX	0
J2210		E	Methylergonovin maleate inj	0	0	0	0	XXX	0
J2240		E	Metocurine iodide injection	0	0	0	0	XXX	0
J2260		E	Inj milrinone lactate / 5 ML	0	0	0	0	XXX	0
J2270		E	Morphine sulfate injection	0	0	0	0	XXX	0
J2275		E	Morphine sulfate injection	0	0	0	0	XXX	0
J2320		E	Nandrolone decanoate 50 MG	0	0	0	0	XXX	0
J2321		E	Nandrolone decanoate 100 MG	0	0	0	0	XXX	0
J2322		E	Nandrolone decanoate 200 MG	0	0	0	0	XXX	0
J2330		E	Thiothixene injection	0	0	0	0	XXX	0
J2350		E	Niacinamide/niacin injection	0	0	0	0	XXX	0
J2360		E	Orphenadrine injection	0	0	0	0	XXX	0
J2370		E	Phenylephrine hcl injection	0	0	0	0	XXX	0
J2400		E	Chloroprocaine hcl injection	0	0	0	0	XXX	0
J2405		E	Ondansetron hcl injection	0	0	0	0	XXX	0
J2410		E	Oxymorphone hcl injection	0	0	0	0	XXX	0
J2430		E	Pamidronate disodium /30 MG	0	0	0	0	XXX	0
J2440		E	Papaverin hcl injection	0	0	0	0	XXX	0
J2460		E	Oxytetracycline injection	0	0	0	0	XXX	0
J2480		E	Hydrochlorides of opium inj	0	0	0	0	XXX	0
J2490		D	Paraldehyde injection	0	0	0	0	XXX	0
J2495		E	Tridihexethyl chloride inj	0	0	0	0	XXX	0
J2510		E	Penicillin g procaine inj	0	0	0	0	XXX	0
J2512		E	Inj pentagastrin per 2 ML	0	0	0	0	XXX	0
J2515		E	Pentobarbital sodium inj	0	0	0	0	XXX	0
J2520		D	Thiopental sodium injection	0	0	0	0	XXX	0
J2540		E	Penicillin g potassium inj	0	0	0	0	XXX	0
J2545		E	Pentamidine isethionte/300mg	0	0	0	0	XXX	0
J2550		E	Promethazine hcl injection	0	0	0	0	XXX	0
J2560		E	Phenobarbital sodium inj	0	0	0	0	XXX	0
J2590		E	Oxytocin injection	0	0	0	0	XXX	0
J2595		D	Vasopressin tannate inj	0	0	0	0	XXX	0
J2600		D	Posterior pituitary inj	0	0	0	0	XXX	0
J2640		E	Prednisolone sodium ph inj	0	0	0	0	XXX	0
J2650		E	Prednisolone acetate inj	0	0	0	0	XXX	0
J2670		E	Totazoline hcl injection	0	0	0	0	XXX	0
J2672		D	Propantheline bromide inj	0	0	0	0	XXX	0
J2675		E	Inj progesterone per 50 MG	0	0	0	0	XXX	0
J2680		E	Fluphenazine decanoate 25 MG	0	0	0	0	XXX	0
J2690		E	Procainamide hcl injection	0	0	0	0	XXX	0
J2700		E	Oxacillin sodium injeciton	0	0	0	0	XXX	0
J2710		E	Neostigmine methylslfte inj	0	0	0	0	XXX	0

CPT codes and descriptions only, © 1994 American Medical Association. Reimbursement information, © 1995 McGraw-Hill Inc.

Code/ CPT	Mod- ifier	Status	Description	Work value	Practice expense	Mal- practice	Total value	Global period	Up- date
J2720		E	Inj protamine sulfate/10 MG	0	0	0	0	XXX	0
J2725		E	Inj protirelin per 250 mcg	0	0	0	0	XXX	0
J2730		E	Pralidoxime chloride inj	0	0	0	0	XXX	0
J2760		E	Phentolaine mesylate inj	0	0	0	0	XXX	0
J2765		E	Metoclopramide hcl injection	0	0	0	0	XXX	0
J2790		E	Rho d immune globulin inj	0	0	0	0	XXX	0
J2800		E	Methocarbamol injection	0	0	0	0	XXX	0
J2810		E	Inj theophylline per 40 MG	0	0	0	0	XXX	0
J2820		E	Sargramostim injection	0	0	0	0	XXX	0
J2825		D	Sarracenia purpurea injecito	0	0	0	0	XXX	0
J2860		E	Secobarbital sodium inj	0	0	0	0	XXX	0
J2910		E	Aurothioglucose injeciton	0	0	0	0	XXX	0
J2912		E	Sodium chloride injection	0	0	0	0	XXX	0
J2914		E	Sodium salicylate injection	0	0	0	0	XXX	0
J2920		E	Methylprednisolone injection	0	0	0	0	XXX	0
J2930		E	Methylprednisolone injection	0	0	0	0	XXX	0
J2950		E	Promazine hcl injeciton	0	0	0	0	XXX	0
J2970		E	Methicillin sodium injection	0	0	0	0	XXX	0
J2995		E	Inj streptokinase /250000 IU	0	0	0	0	XXX	0
J2996		E	Alteplase recombinant inj	0	0	0	0	XXX	0
J3000		E	Streptomycin injection	0	0	0	0	XXX	0
J3005		E	Strontium-89 chloride /10 ML	0	0	0	0	XXX	0
J3010		E	Fentanyl citrate injeciton	0	0	0	0	XXX	0
J3030		E	Sumatriptan succinate / 6 MG	0	0	0	0	XXX	0
J3050		D	Decamethonium bromide inj	0	0	0	0	XXX	0
J3070		E	Pentazocine hcl injeciton	0	0	0	0	XXX	0
J3080		E	Chlorprothixene injection	0	0	0	0	XXX	0
J3105		E	Terbutaline sulfate inj	0	0	0	0	XXX	0
J3120		E	Testosterone enanthate inj	0	0	0	0	XXX	0
J3130		E	Testosterone enanthate inj	0	0	0	0	XXX	0
J3140		E	Testosterone suspension inj	0	0	0	0	XXX	0
J3150		E	Testosteron propionate inj	0	0	0	0	XXX	0
J3180		D	Tetanus toxoid injection	0	0	0	0	XXX	0
J3230		E	Chlorpromazine hcl injection	0	0	0	0	XXX	0
J3240		E	Thyrotropin injection	0	0	0	0	XXX	0
J3250		E	Trimethobenzamide hcl inj	0	0	0	0	XXX	0
J3260		E	Tobramycin sulfate injection	0	0	0	0	XXX	0
J3270		E	Imipramine hcl injection	0	0	0	0	XXX	0
J3280		E	Thiethylperazine maleate inj	0	0	0	0	XXX	0
J3301		E	Triamcinolone acetonide inj	0	0	0	0	XXX	0
J3302		E	Triamcinolone diacetate inj	0	0	0	0	XXX	0
J3303		E	Triamcinolone hexacetonl inj	0	0	0	0	XXX	0
J3310		E	Perphenazine injeciton	0	0	0	0	XXX	0
J3320		E	Spectinomycn di-hcl inj	0	0	0	0	XXX	0
J3340		E	Cryptenamine acetate inj	0	0	0	0	XXX	0
J3350		E	Urea injection	0	0	0	0	XXX	0
J3360		E	Diazepam injection	0	0	0	0	XXX	0
J3364		E	Urokinase 5000 IU injection	0	0	0	0	XXX	0
J3365		E	"Urokinase 250,000 IU inj"	0	0	0	0	XXX	0
J3370		E	Vancomycin hcl injeciton	0	0	0	0	XXX	0

CPT codes and descriptions only, © 1994 American Medical Association. Reimbursement information, © 1995 McGraw-Hill Inc.

Code/ CPT	Mod- ifier	Status	Description	Work value	Practice expense	Mal- practice	Total value	Global period	Up- date
J3380		E	Isoxsuprine hcl injection	0	0	0	0	XXX	0
J3390		E	Methoxamine injection	0	0	0	0	XXX	0
J3400		E	Triflupromazine hcl inj	0	0	0	0	XXX	0
J3410		E	Hydroxyzine hcl injeciton	0	0	0	0	XXX	0
J3420		E	Vitamin b12 injection	0	0	0	0	XXX	0
J3430		E	Vitamin k phytonadione inj	0	0	0	0	XXX	0
J3450		E	Mephentermine sulfate inj	0	0	0	0	XXX	0
J3470		E	Hyaluronidase injection	0	0	0	0	XXX	0
J3490		E	Drugs unclassified injection	0	0	0	0	XXX	0
J3500		E	Vitamin therapy	0	0	0	0	XXX	0
J3520		N	Endrate ethyl-tetra-acet inj	0	0	0	0	XXX	0
J3530		E	Nasal vaccine inhalation	0	0	0	0	XXX	0
J3535		E	Metered dose inhaler drug	0	0	0	0	XXX	0
J3540		E	Autogenous blood extract	0	0	0	0	XXX	0
J3550		E	Intra-arterial oxygen inj	0	0	0	0	XXX	0
J3560		E	Adrenal cortex extract	0	0	0	0	XXX	0
J3570		N	Laetrile amygdalin vit b17	0	0	0	0	XXX	0
J6015		N	Typhus immun/injection	0	0	0	0	XXX	0
J7010		D	Vl allergy vac sing dos inj	0	0	0	0	XXX	0
J7020		D	Multiple dose vial allrgy va	0	0	0	0	XXX	0
J7030		E	Normal saline solution infus	0	0	0	0	XXX	0
J7040		E	Normal saline solution infus	0	0	0	0	XXX	0
J7042		E	5% dextrose/normal saline	0	0	0	0	XXX	0
J7050		E	Normal saline solution infus	0	0	0	0	XXX	0
J7051		E	Sterile saline/water	0	0	0	0	XXX	0
J7060		E	5% dextrose/water	0	0	0	0	XXX	0
J7070		E	D5w infusion	0	0	0	0	XXX	0
J7080		E	5% albumisol infusion	0	0	0	0	XXX	0
J7090		E	25% albumisol infusion	0	0	0	0	XXX	0
J7100		E	Dextran 40 infusion	0	0	0	0	XXX	0
J7110		E	Dextran 75 infusion	0	0	0	0	XXX	0
J7120		E	Ringers lactate infusion	0	0	0	0	XXX	0
J7130		E	Hypertonic saline solution	0	0	0	0	XXX	0
J7140		N	Prescription oral drug	0	0	0	0	XXX	0
J7150		N	Prescription oral chemo drug	0	0	0	0	XXX	0
J7190		X	Factor viii	0	0	0	0	XXX	0
J7192		X	Factor viii recombinant	0	0	0	0	XXX	0
J7194		X	Factor ix complex	0	0	0	0	XXX	0
J7196		X	Othr hemophilia clot factors	0	0	0	0	XXX	0
J7197		X	Antithrombin iii injection	0	0	0	0	XXX	0
J7300		E	Intraut copper contraceptive	0	0	0	0	XXX	0
J7500		X	Azathiop po tab 50mg 100s ea	0	0	0	0	XXX	0
J7501		X	Azathioprine parenteral	0	0	0	0	XXX	0
J7502		X	Cyclosporine oral solution	0	0	0	0	XXX	0
J7503		X	Cyclosporine parenteral	0	0	0	0	XXX	0
J7504		X	Lymphocyte immune globulin	0	0	0	0	XXX	0
J7505		X	Monoclonal antibodies	0	0	0	0	XXX	0
J7506		X	Prednisone	0	0	0	0	XXX	0
J7507		E	Tacrolimus oral per 1 MG	0	0	0	0	XXX	0
J7508		E	Tacrolimus oral per 5 MG	0	0	0	0	XXX	0

CPT codes and descriptions only, © 1994 American Medical Association. Reimbursement information, © 1995 McGraw-Hill Inc.

Code/ CPT	Mod- ifier	Status	Description	Work value	Practice expense	Mal- practice	Total value	Global period	Up- date
J7610		E	Acetylcysteine 10% injection	0	0	0	0	XXX	0
J7615		E	Acetylcysteine 20% injection	0	0	0	0	XXX	0
J7620		E	Albuterol sulfate .083% inj	0	0	0	0	XXX	0
J7625		E	Albuterol sulfate .5% inj	0	0	0	0	XXX	0
J7627		E	Bitolterolmesylate inhal sol	0	0	0	0	XXX	0
J7630		E	Cromolyn sodium injeciton	0	0	0	0	XXX	0
J7640		E	Epinephrine injection	0	0	0	0	XXX	0
J7645		E	Ipratropium bromide .02%/ml	0	0	0	0	XXX	0
J7650		E	Isoetharine hcl .1% inj	0	0	0	0	XXX	0
J7651		E	Isoetharine hcl .125% inj	0	0	0	0	XXX	0
J7652		E	Isoetharine hcl .167% inj	0	0	0	0	XXX	0
J7653		E	Isoetharine hcl .2%/ inj	0	0	0	0	XXX	0
J7654		E	Isoetharine hcl .25% inj	0	0	0	0	XXX	0
J7655		E	Isoetharine hcl 1% inj	0	0	0	0	XXX	0
J7660		E	Isoproterenol hcl .5% inj	0	0	0	0	XXX	0
J7665		E	Isoproterenol hcl 1% inj	0	0	0	0	XXX	0
J7670		E	Metaproterenol sulfate .4%	0	0	0	0	XXX	0
J7672		E	Metaproterenol sulfate .6%	0	0	0	0	XXX	0
J7675		E	Metaproterenol sulfate 5%	0	0	0	0	XXX	0
J7699		E	Inhalation solution for DME	0	0	0	0	XXX	0
J7799		E	Non-inhalation drug for DME	0	0	0	0	XXX	0
J8499		E	Oral prescrip drug non chemo	0	0	0	0	XXX	0
J8530		E	Cyclophosphamide oral 25 MG	0	0	0	0	XXX	0
J8560		E	Etoposide oral 50 MG	0	0	0	0	XXX	0
J8600		E	Melphalan oral 2 MG	0	0	0	0	XXX	0
J8610		E	Methotrexate oral 2.5 MG	0	0	0	0	XXX	0
J8999		E	Oral prescription drug chemo	0	0	0	0	XXX	0
J9000		E	Doxorubic hcl 10 MG vl chemo	0	0	0	0	XXX	0
J9010		E	Doxorubicin hcl 50 MG inj	0	0	0	0	XXX	0
J9020		E	Asparaginase injection	0	0	0	0	XXX	0
J9031		E	Bcg live intravesical vac	0	0	0	0	XXX	0
J9040		E	Bleomycin sulfate injection	0	0	0	0	XXX	0
J9045		E	Carboplatin injection	0	0	0	0	XXX	0
J9050		E	Carmus bischl nitro inj	0	0	0	0	XXX	0
J9060		E	Cisplatin 10 MG injeciton	0	0	0	0	XXX	0
J9062		E	Cisplatin 50 MG injeciton	0	0	0	0	XXX	0
J9065		E	Inj cladribine per 1 MG	0	0	0	0	XXX	0
J9070		E	Cyclophosphamide 100 MG inj	0	0	0	0	XXX	0
J9080		E	Cyclophosphamide 200 MG inj	0	0	0	0	XXX	0
J9090		E	Cyclophosphamide 500 MG inj	0	0	0	0	XXX	0
J9091		E	Cyclophosphamide 1.0 grm inj	0	0	0	0	XXX	0
J9092		E	Cyclophosphamide 2.0 grm inj	0	0	0	0	XXX	0
J9093		E	Cyclophosphamide lyophilized	0	0	0	0	XXX	0
J9094		E	Cyclophosphamide lyophilized	0	0	0	0	XXX	0
J9095		E	Cyclophosphamide lyophilized	0	0	0	0	XXX	0
J9096		E	Cyclophosphamide lyophilized	0	0	0	0	XXX	0
J9097		E	Cyclophosphamide lyophilized	0	0	0	0	XXX	0
J9100		E	Cytarabine hcl 100 MG inj	0	0	0	0	XXX	0
J9110		E	Cytarabine hcl 500 MG inj	0	0	0	0	XXX	0
J9120		E	Dactinomycin actinomycin d	0	0	0	0	XXX	0

CPT codes and descriptions only, © 1994 American Medical Association. Reimbursement information, © 1995 McGraw-Hill Inc.

Code/ CPT	Mod- ifier	Status	Description	Work value	Practice expense	Mal- practice	Total value	Global period	Up- date
J9130		E	Dacarbazine 10 MG inj	0	0	0	0	XXX	0
J9140		E	Dacarbazine 200 MG inj	0	0	0	0	XXX	0
J9150		E	Daunorubicin hcl injection	0	0	0	0	XXX	0
J9165		E	Diethylstilbestrol injection	0	0	0	0	XXX	0
J9181		E	Etoposide 10 MG inj	0	0	0	0	XXX	0
J9182		E	Etoposide 100 MG inj	0	0	0	0	XXX	0
J9185		E	Fludarabine phosphate inj	0	0	0	0	XXX	0
J9190		E	Fluorouracil injection	0	0	0	0	XXX	0
J9200		E	Floxuridine injection	0	0	0	0	XXX	0
J9202		E	Goserelin acetate implant	0	0	0	0	XXX	0
J9208		E	Ifosfomide injection	0	0	0	0	XXX	0
J9209		E	Mesna injection	0	0	0	0	XXX	0
J9211		E	Idarubicin hcl injeciton	0	0	0	0	XXX	0
J9213		E	Interferon alfa-2a inj	0	0	0	0	XXX	0
J9214		E	Interferon alfa-2b inj	0	0	0	0	XXX	0
J9215		E	Interferon alfa-n3 inj	0	0	0	0	XXX	0
J9216		E	Interferon gamma 1-b inj	0	0	0	0	XXX	0
J9217		E	Leuprolide acetate suspnsion	0	0	0	0	XXX	0
J9218		E	Leuprolide acetate injeciton	0	0	0	0	XXX	0
J9230		E	Mechlorethamine hcl inj	0	0	0	0	XXX	0
J9245		E	Inj melphalan hydrochl 50 MG	0	0	0	0	XXX	0
J9250		E	Methotrexate sodium inj	0	0	0	0	XXX	0
J9260		E	Methotrexate sodium inj	0	0	0	0	XXX	0
J9265		E	Paclitaxel injection	0	0	0	0	XXX	0
J9268		E	Pentostatin injection	0	0	0	0	XXX	0
J9270		E	Plicamycin (mithramycin) inj	0	0	0	0	XXX	0
J9280		E	Mitomycin 5 MG inj	0	0	0	0	XXX	0
J9290		E	Mitomycin 20 MG inj	0	0	0	0	XXX	0
J9291		E	Mitomycin 40 MG inj	0	0	0	0	XXX	0
J9293		E	Mitoxantrone hydrochl / 5 MG	0	0	0	0	XXX	0
J9295		E	Polyestradiol phosphate inj	0	0	0	0	XXX	0
J9320		E	Streptozocin injection	0	0	0	0	XXX	0
J9340		E	Thiotepa injection	0	0	0	0	XXX	0
J9360		E	Vinblastine sulfate inj	0	0	0	0	XXX	0
J9370		E	Vincristine sulfate 1 MG inj	0	0	0	0	XXX	0
J9375		E	Vincristine sulfate 2 MG inj	0	0	0	0	XXX	0
J9380		E	Vincristine sulfate 5 MG inj	0	0	0	0	XXX	0
J9999		E	Chemotherapy drug	0	0	0	0	XXX	0
M0005		A	Off visit 2/more modalities	0.76	0.31	0.03	1.10	XXX	N
M0006		A	One phys therapy modality	0.50	0.15	0.02	0.67	XXX	N
M0007		A	Combined phys ther mod & tx	1.01	0.35	0.04	1.40	XXX	N
M0008		A	Combined phys ther mod & tx	0.50	0.11	0.01	0.62	XXX	N
M0064		A	Visit for drug monitoring	0.37	0.19	0.03	0.59	XXX	N
M0075		N	Cellular therapy	0	0	0	0	XXX	0
M0076		N	Prolotherapy	0	0	0	0	XXX	0
M0100		N	Intragastric hypothermia	0	0	0	0	XXX	0
M0101		A	Cutting or removal of corns	0.37	0.35	0.03	0.75	XXX	S
M0300		N	Iv chelationtherapy	0	0	0	0	XXX	0
M0301		N	Fabric wrapping of aneurysm	0	0	0	0	XXX	0
M0302		N	Assessment of cardiac output	0	0	0	0	XXX	0

CPT codes and descriptions only, © 1994 American Medical Association. Reimbursement information, © 1995 McGraw-Hill Inc.

Code/ CPT	Mod-ifier	Status	Description	Work value	Practice expense	Mal-practice	Total value	Global period	Up-date
M0702		X	Osteopathic thera off-2 regn	0	0	0	0	XXX	0
M0704		X	Osteopathic ther offc 4 regi	0	0	0	0	XXX	0
M0706		X	Osteopathic ther offc 6 regi	0	0	0	0	XXX	0
M0708		X	Osteopathic ther offc 8 regi	0	0	0	0	XXX	0
M0710		X	Osteopathic ther offc 10 reg	0	0	0	0	XXX	0
M0722		X	Osteopathic ther hosp 2 regi	0	0	0	0	XXX	0
M0724		X	Osteopathic ther hosp 4 regi	0	0	0	0	XXX	0
M0726		X	Osteopathic ther hosp 6 regi	0	0	0	0	XXX	0
M0728		X	Osteopathic ther hosp 8 regi	0	0	0	0	XXX	0
M0730		X	Osteopathic therhosp 10 regi	0	0	0	0	XXX	0
M0900		D	Excision/rev a-v shunt anast	0	0	0	0	XXX	0
P2028		X	Cephalin floculation test	0	0	0	0	XXX	0
P2029		X	Congo red blood test	0	0	0	0	XXX	0
P2031		N	Hair analysis	0	0	0	0	XXX	0
P2033		X	Blood thymol turbidity	0	0	0	0	XXX	0
P2038		X	Blood mucoprotein	0	0	0	0	XXX	0
P3000		X	Screen pap by tech w md supv	0	0	0	0	XXX	0
P3001		X	Screening pap smear by phys	0	0	0	0	XXX	0
P3001	26	A	Screening pap smear by phys	0.42	0.32	0.04	0.78	XXX	N
P7001		X	Culture bacterial urine	0	0	0	0	XXX	0
P9010		E	Whole blood for transfusion	0	0	0	0	XXX	0
P9011		E	Blood split unit	0	0	0	0	XXX	0
P9012		E	Cryoprecipitate each unit	0	0	0	0	XXX	0
P9013		E	Unit/s blood fibrinogen	0	0	0	0	XXX	0
P9014		E	Gamma globulin 1 ML	0	0	0	0	XXX	0
P9015		E	Rh immune globulin 1 ML	0	0	0	0	XXX	0
P9016		E	"Leukocyte poor blood, unit"	0	0	0	0	XXX	0
P9017		E	One donor fresh frozn plasma	0	0	0	0	XXX	0
P9018		E	"Plasma protein fract, unit"	0	0	0	0	XXX	0
P9019		E	Platelet concentrate unit	0	0	0	0	XXX	0
P9020		E	Plaelet rich plasma unit	0	0	0	0	XXX	0
P9021		E	Red blood cells unit	0	0	0	0	XXX	0
P9022		E	Washed red blood cells unit	0	0	0	0	XXX	0
P9603		X	One-way allow prorated miles	0	0	0	0	XXX	0
P9604		X	One-way allow prorated trip	0	0	0	0	XXX	0
P9605		X	Routine venipuncture	0	0	0	0	XXX	0
P9610		X	Urine specimen collect singl	0	0	0	0	XXX	0
P9615		X	Urine specimen collect mult	0	0	0	0	XXX	0
Q0034		X	Admin of influenza vaccine	0	0	0	0	XXX	0
Q0035	26	A	Cardiokymography	0.17	0.12	0.01	0.30	XXX	N
Q0035	TC	A	Cardiokymography	0	0.37	0.03	0.40	XXX	N
Q0035		A	Cardiokymography	0.17	0.49	0.04	0.70	XXX	N
Q0068		A	Extracorpeal plasmapheresis	1.67	1.27	0.16	3.10	0	N
Q0091		A	Obtaining screen pap smear	0.37	0.28	0.03	0.68	XXX	N
Q0092		A	Set up port xray equipment	0	0.30	0.01	0.31	XXX	N
Q0103		A	Physical therapy evaluation	1.01	0.35	0.11	1.47	XXX	N
Q0104		A	Phys therapy re-evaluation	0.50	0.04	0.01	0.55	XXX	N
Q0109		A	Occupational therapy eval	1.01	0.35	0.11	1.47	XXX	N
Q0110		A	Occupational therap re-eval	0.50	0.04	0.01	0.55	XXX	N
Q0111		X	Wet mounts/ w preparations	0	0	0	0	XXX	0

CPT codes and descriptions only, © 1994 American Medical Association. Reimbursement information, © 1995 McGraw-Hill Inc.

Code/ CPT	Mod-ifier	Status	Description	Work value	Practice expense	Mal-practice	Total value	Global period	Up-date
Q0112		X	Potassium hydroxide preps	0	0	0	0	XXX	0
Q0113		X	Pinworm examinations	0	0	0	0	XXX	0
Q0114		X	Fern test	0	0	0	0	XXX	0
Q0115		X	Post-coital mucous exam	0	0	0	0	XXX	0
Q0116		X	Hemoglbn sngle analyte exam	0	0	0	0	XXX	0
Q0117		D	"Diabetic shoe, depth-inlay"	0	0	0	0	XXX	0
Q0118		D	"Diabetic shoe, custom moled"	0	0	0	0	XXX	0
Q0119		D	Diabetic shoe density insert	0	0	0	0	XXX	0
Q0120		D	Diabetic shoe roller/rocker	0	0	0	0	XXX	0
Q0121		D	Diabetic shoe with wedge	0	0	0	0	XXX	0
Q0122		D	Diabetic shoe metatarsal bar	0	0	0	0	XXX	0
Q0123		D	Diabetic shoe off-set heel	0	0	0	0	XXX	0
Q0124		D	"Admin/pneumococcal, flu vac"	0	0	0	0	XXX	0
Q0126		X	Immunoassay inf agnt antigen	0	0	0	0	XXX	0
Q0132		X	Dispensing fee DME neb drug	0	0	0	0	XXX	0
Q0134		D	Collagen implant 2.5 CC syrg	0	0	0	0	XXX	0
Q0135		D	High dose inj contrast MRI	0	0	0	0	XXX	0
Q0136		X	Non esrd epoetin alpha inj	0	0	0	0	XXX	0
Q9920		E	Epoetin with hct = 20	0	0	0	0	XXX	0
Q9921		E	Epoetin with hct = 21	0	0	0	0	XXX	0
Q9922		E	Epoetin with hct = 22	0	0	0	0	XXX	0
Q9923		E	Epoetin with hct = 23	0	0	0	0	XXX	0
Q9924		E	Epoetin with hct = 24	0	0	0	0	XXX	0
Q9925		E	Epoetin with hct = 25	0	0	0	0	XXX	0
Q9926		E	Epoetin with hct = 26	0	0	0	0	XXX	0
Q9927		E	Epoetin with hct = 27	0	0	0	0	XXX	0
Q9928		E	Epoetin with hct = 28	0	0	0	0	XXX	0
Q9929		E	Epoetin with hct = 29	0	0	0	0	XXX	0
Q9930		E	Epoetin with hct = 30	0	0	0	0	XXX	0
Q9931		E	Epoetin with hct = 31	0	0	0	0	XXX	0
Q9932		E	Epoetin with hct = 32	0	0	0	0	XXX	0
Q9933		E	Epoetin with hct = 33	0	0	0	0	XXX	0
Q9934		E	Epoetin with hct = 34	0	0	0	0	XXX	0
Q9935		E	Epoetin with hct = 35	0	0	0	0	XXX	0
Q9936		E	Epoetin with hct = 36	0	0	0	0	XXX	0
Q9937		E	Epoetin with hct = 37	0	0	0	0	XXX	0
Q9938		E	Epoetin with hct = 38	0	0	0	0	XXX	0
Q9939		E	Epoetin with hct = 39	0	0	0	0	XXX	0
Q9940		E	Epoetin with hct = 40	0	0	0	0	XXX	0
R0070		C	Transport portable x-ray	0	0	0	0	XXX	N
R0075		C	Transport port x-ray multipl	0	0	0	0	XXX	N
R0076		C	Transport portable EKG	0	0	0	0	XXX	N
V2020		X	Vision svcs frames purchases	0	0	0	0	XXX	0
V2025		N	Eyeglasses delux frames	0	0	0	0	XXX	0
V2100		X	Lens spher single plano 4.00	0	0	0	0	XXX	0
V2101		X	Single visn sphere 4.12-7.00	0	0	0	0	XXX	0
V2102		X	Singl visn sphere 7.12-20.00	0	0	0	0	XXX	0
V2103		X	Spherocylindr 4.00d/12-2.00d	0	0	0	0	XXX	0
V2104		X	Spherocylindr 4.00d/2.12-4d	0	0	0	0	XXX	0
V2105		X	Spherocylinder 4.00d/4.25-6d	0	0	0	0	XXX	0

CPT codes and descriptions only, © 1994 American Medical Association. Reimbursement information, © 1995 McGraw-Hill Inc.

Code/ CPT	Mod- ifier	Status	Description	Work value	Practice expense	Mal- practice	Total value	Global period	Up- date
V2106		X	Spherocylinder 4.00d/6.00d	0	0	0	0	XXX	0
V2107		X	Spherocylinder 4.25d/12-2d	0	0	0	0	XXX	0
V2108		X	Spherocylinder 4.25d/2.12-4d	0	0	0	0	XXX	0
V2109		X	Spherocylinder 4.25d/4.25-6d	0	0	0	0	XXX	0
V2110		X	Spherocylinder 4.25d/over 6d	0	0	0	0	XXX	0
V2111		X	Spherocylindr 7.25d/.25-2.25	0	0	0	0	XXX	0
V2112		X	Spherocylindr 7.25d/2.25-4d	0	0	0	0	XXX	0
V2113		X	Spherocylindr 7.25d/4.25-6d	0	0	0	0	XXX	0
V2114		X	Spherocylinder over 12.00d	0	0	0	0	XXX	0
V2115		X	Lens lenticular bifocal	0	0	0	0	XXX	0
V2116		X	Nonaspheric lens bifocal	0	0	0	0	XXX	0
V2117		X	Aspheric lens bifocal	0	0	0	0	XXX	0
V2118		X	Lens aniseikonic single	0	0	0	0	XXX	0
V2199		X	Lens single vision not oth c	0	0	0	0	XXX	0
V2200		X	Lens spher bifoc plano 4.00d	0	0	0	0	XXX	0
V2201		X	Lens sphere bifocal 4.12-7.0	0	0	0	0	XXX	0
V2202		X	Lens sphere bifocal 7.12-20.	0	0	0	0	XXX	0
V2203		X	Lens sphcyl bifocal 4.00d/.1	0	0	0	0	XXX	0
V2204		X	Lens sphcy bifocal 4.00d/2.1	0	0	0	0	XXX	0
V2205		X	Lens sphcy bifocal 4.00d/4.2	0	0	0	0	XXX	0
V2206		X	Lens sphcy bifocal 4.00d/ove	0	0	0	0	XXX	0
V2207		X	Lens sphcy bifocal 4.25-7d/.	0	0	0	0	XXX	0
V2208		X	Lens sphcy bifocal 4.25-7/2.	0	0	0	0	XXX	0
V2209		X	Lens sphcy bifocal 4.25-7/4.	0	0	0	0	XXX	0
V2210		X	Lens sphcy bifocal 4.25-7/ov	0	0	0	0	XXX	0
V2211		X	Lens sphcy bifo 7.25-12/.25-	0	0	0	0	XXX	0
V2212		X	Lens sphcyl bifo 7.25-12/2.2	0	0	0	0	XXX	0
V2213		X	Lens sphcyl bifo 7.25-12/4.2	0	0	0	0	XXX	0
V2214		X	Lens sphcyl bifocal over 12.	0	0	0	0	XXX	0
V2215		X	Lens lenticular bifocal	0	0	0	0	XXX	0
V2216		X	Lens lenticular nonaspheric	0	0	0	0	XXX	0
V2217		X	Lens lenticular aspheric bif	0	0	0	0	XXX	0
V2218		X	Lens aniseikonic bifocal	0	0	0	0	XXX	0
V2219		X	Lens bifocal seg width over	0	0	0	0	XXX	0
V2220		X	Lens bifocal add over 3.25d	0	0	0	0	XXX	0
V2299		X	Lens bifocal speciality	0	0	0	0	XXX	0
V2300		X	Lens sphere trifocal 4.00d	0	0	0	0	XXX	0
V2301		X	Lens sphere trifocal 4.12-7.	0	0	0	0	XXX	0
V2302		X	Lens sphere trifocal 7.12-20	0	0	0	0	XXX	0
V2303		X	Lens sphcy trifocal 4.0/.12-	0	0	0	0	XXX	0
V2304		X	Lens sphcy trifocal 4.0/2.25	0	0	0	0	XXX	0
V2305		X	Lens sphcy trifocal 4.0/4.25	0	0	0	0	XXX	0
V2306		X	Lens sphcyl trifocal 4.00/6	0	0	0	0	XXX	0
V2307		X	Lens sphcy trifocal 4.25-7/.	0	0	0	0	XXX	0
V2308		X	Lens sphc trifocal 4.25-7/2.	0	0	0	0	XXX	0
V2309		X	Lens sphc trifocal 4.25-7/4.	0	0	0	0	XXX	0
V2310		X	Lens sphc trifocal 4.25-7/6	0	0	0	0	XXX	0
V2311		X	Lens sphc trifo 7.25-12/.25-	0	0	0	0	XXX	0
V2312		X	Lens sphc trifo 7.25-12/2.25	0	0	0	0	XXX	0
V2313		X	Lens sphc trifo 7.25-12/4.25	0	0	0	0	XXX	0

CPT codes and descriptions only, © 1994 American Medical Association. Reimbursement information, © 1995 McGraw-Hill Inc.

Code/ CPT	Mod- ifier	Status	Description	Work value	Practice expense	Mal- practice	Total value	Global period	Up- date
V2314		X	Lens sphcyl trifocal over 12	0	0	0	0	XXX	0
V2315		X	Lens lenticular trifocal	0	0	0	0	XXX	0
V2316		X	Lens lenticular nonaspheric	0	0	0	0	XXX	0
V2317		X	Lens lenticular aspheric tri	0	0	0	0	XXX	0
V2318		X	Lens aniseikonic trifocal	0	0	0	0	XXX	0
V2319		X	Lens trifocal seg width 28	0	0	0	0	XXX	0
V2320		X	Lens trifocal add over 3.25d	0	0	0	0	XXX	0
V2399		X	Lens trifocal speciality	0	0	0	0	XXX	0
V2410		X	Lens variab asphericity sing	0	0	0	0	XXX	0
V2430		X	Lens variable asphericity bi	0	0	0	0	XXX	0
V2499		X	Variable asphericity lens	0	0	0	0	XXX	0
V2500		X	Contact lens pmma spherical	0	0	0	0	XXX	0
V2501		X	Cntct lens pmma-toric/prism	0	0	0	0	XXX	0
V2502		X	Contact lens pmma bifocal	0	0	0	0	XXX	0
V2503		X	Cntct lens pmma color vision	0	0	0	0	XXX	0
V2510		X	Cntct gas permeable sphericl	0	0	0	0	XXX	0
V2511		X	Cntct toric prism ballast	0	0	0	0	XXX	0
V2512		X	Cntct lens gas permbl bifocl	0	0	0	0	XXX	0
V2513		X	Contact lens extended wear	0	0	0	0	XXX	0
V2520		P	Contact lens hydrophilic	0	0	0	0	XXX	0
V2521		X	Cntct lens hydrophilic toric	0	0	0	0	XXX	0
V2522		X	Cntct lens hydrophil bifocl	0	0	0	0	XXX	0
V2523		X	Cntct lens hydrophil extend	0	0	0	0	XXX	0
V2530		X	Contact lens/es scleral	0	0	0	0	XXX	0
V2599		X	Contact lens/es other type	0	0	0	0	XXX	0
V2600		X	Hand held low vision aids	0	0	0	0	XXX	0
V2610		X	Single lens spectacle mount	0	0	0	0	XXX	0
V2615		X	Telescop/othr compound lens	0	0	0	0	XXX	0
V2623		X	Plastic eye prosth custom	0	0	0	0	XXX	0
V2624		X	Polishing artifical eye	0	0	0	0	XXX	0
V2625		X	Enlargemnt of eye prosthesis	0	0	0	0	XXX	0
V2626		X	Reduction of eye prosthesis	0	0	0	0	XXX	0
V2627		X	Scleral cover shell	0	0	0	0	XXX	0
V2628		X	Fabrication & fitting	0	0	0	0	XXX	0
V2629		X	Prosthetic eye other type	0	0	0	0	XXX	0
V2630		X	Anter chamber intraocul lens	0	0	0	0	XXX	0
V2631		X	Iris support intraoclr lens	0	0	0	0	XXX	0
V2632		X	Post chmbr intraocular lens	0	0	0	0	XXX	0
V2700		X	Balance lens	0	0	0	0	XXX	0
V2710		X	Glass/plastic slab off prism	0	0	0	0	XXX	0
V2715		X	Prism lens/es	0	0	0	0	XXX	0
V2718		X	Fresnell prism press-on lens	0	0	0	0	XXX	0
V2730		X	Special base curve	0	0	0	0	XXX	0
V2740		X	Rose tint plastic	0	0	0	0	XXX	0
V2741		X	Non-rose tint plastic	0	0	0	0	XXX	0
V2742		X	Rose tint glass	0	0	0	0	XXX	0
V2743		X	Non-rose tint glass	0	0	0	0	XXX	0
V2744		X	Tint photochromatic lens/es	0	0	0	0	XXX	0
V2750		X	Anti-reflective coating	0	0	0	0	XXX	0
V2755		X	U-v lens/es	0	0	0	0	XXX	0

CPT codes and descriptions only, © 1994 American Medical Association. Reimbursement information, © 1995 McGraw-Hill Inc.

Code/ CPT	Mod- ifier	Status	Description	Work value	Practice expense	Mal- practice	Total value	Global period	Up- date
V2760		X	Scratch resistant coating	0	0	0	0	XXX	0
V2770		X	Occluder lens/es	0	0	0	0	XXX	0
V2780		X	Oversize lens/es	0	0	0	0	XXX	0
V2785		X	Corneal tissue processing	0	0	0	0	XXX	0
V2799		X	Miscellaneous vision service	0	0	0	0	XXX	0
V5008		N	Hearing screening	0	0	0	0	XXX	0
V5010		N	Assessment for hearing aid	0	0	0	0	XXX	0
V5011		N	Hearing aid fitting/checking	0	0	0	0	XXX	0
V5014		N	Hearing aid repair/modifying	0	0	0	0	XXX	0
V5020		N	Conformity evaluation	0	0	0	0	XXX	0
V5030		N	Body-worn hearing aid air	0	0	0	0	XXX	0
V5040		N	Body-worn hearing aid bone	0	0	0	0	XXX	0
V5050		N	Body-worn hearing aid in ear	0	0	0	0	XXX	0
V5060		N	Behind ear hearing aid	0	0	0	0	XXX	0
V5070		N	Glasses air conduction	0	0	0	0	XXX	0
V5080		N	Glasses bone conduction	0	0	0	0	XXX	0
V5090		N	Hearing aid dispensing fee	0	0	0	0	XXX	0
V5100		N	Body-worn bilat hearing aid	0	0	0	0	XXX	0
V5110		N	Hearing aid dispensing fee	0	0	0	0	XXX	0
V5120		N	Body-worn binaur hearing aid	0	0	0	0	XXX	0
V5130		N	In ear binaural hearing aid	0	0	0	0	XXX	0
V5140		N	Behind ear binaur hearing ai	0	0	0	0	XXX	0
V5150		N	Glasses binaural hearing aid	0	0	0	0	XXX	0
V5160		N	Dispensing fee binaural	0	0	0	0	XXX	0
V5170		N	Within ear cros hearing aid	0	0	0	0	XXX	0
V5180		N	Behind ear cros hearing aid	0	0	0	0	XXX	0
V5190		N	Glasses cros hearing aid	0	0	0	0	XXX	0
V5200		N	Cros hearing aid dispens fee	0	0	0	0	XXX	0
V5210		N	In ear bicros hearing aid	0	0	0	0	XXX	0
V5220		N	Behind ear bicros hearing ai	0	0	0	0	XXX	0
V5230		N	Glasses bicros hearing aid	0	0	0	0	XXX	0
V5240		N	Dispensing fee bicros	0	0	0	0	XXX	0
V5299		R	Hearing service	0	0	0	0	XXX	N
V5336		N	Repair communication device	0	0	0	0	XXX	0
V5362		R	Speech screening	0	0	0	0	XXX	N
V5363		R	Language screening	0	0	0	0	XXX	N
V5364		R	Dysphagia screening	0	0	0	0	XXX	N

CPT codes and descriptions only, © 1994 American Medical Association. Reimbursement information, © 1995 McGraw-Hill Inc.

CHAPTER 8

Geographic Practice Cost Indices

1995 GEOGRAPHIC PRACTICE COST INDICES BY MEDICARE CARRIER AND LOCALITY

Carrier number	Locality number	Locality name	Work	Practice expense	Malpractice
00510	05	Birmingham, AL	0.988	0.912	0.876
00510	04	Mobile, AL	0.970	0.884	0.876
00510	02	North Central AL	0.972	0.858	0.876
00510	01	Northwest AL	0.988	0.871	0.876
00510	06	Rest Of AL	0.970	0.834	0.876
00510	03	Southeast AL	0.971	0.864	0.876
01020	01	Alaska	1.085	1.205	1.330
01030	05	Flagstaff, AZ	0.977	0.924	1.288
01030	01	Phoenix, AZ	1.004	0.990	1.288
01030	07	Prescott, AZ	0.977	0.912	1.288
01030	99	Rest Of AZ	0.988	0.946	1.288
01030	02	Tucson, AZ	0.982	0.966	1.288
01030	08	Yuma, AZ	0.984	0.918	1.288
00520	13	Arkansas	0.957	0.854	0.364

Note: Work GPCI is the 1/4 work GPCI required by Section 1848 (e)(1)(A)(iii) of the Social Security Act. GPCIs rescaled by the following factors to assure budget neutrality: Work=1.00073; Practice expense=1.00125; Malpractice=1.02307.

CPT codes and descriptions only, © 1994 American Medical Association. Reimbursement information, © 1995 McGraw-Hill Inc.

Carrier number	Locality number	Locality name	Work	Practice expense	Malpractice
02050	26	Anaheim/Santa Ana, CA	1.042	1.212	1.061
00542	14	Bakersfield , CA	1.026	1.021	1.028
00542	11	Fresno/Madera, CA	1.003	0.993	0.983
00542	13	Kings/Tulare, CA	0.993	0.978	0.983
02050	18	Los Angeles (1st Of 8)	1.058	1.202	1.061
02050	19	Los Angeles (2nd Of 8)	1.058	1.202	1.061
02050	20	Los Angeles (3rd Of 8)	1.058	1.202	1.061
02050	21	Los Angeles (4th Of 8)	1.058	1.202	1.061
02050	22	Los Angeles (5th Of 8)	1.058	1.202	1.061
02050	23	Los Angeles (6th Of 8)	1.058	1.202	1.061
02050	24	Los Angeles (7th Of 8)	1.058	1.202	1.061
02050	25	Los Angeles (8th Of 8)	1.058	1.202	1.061
00542	03	Marin/Napa/Solano, CA	1.014	1.189	0.983
00542	10	Merced/Surr.Cntys, CA	1.010	0.998	0.983
00542	12	Monterey/Santa Cruz, CA	1.016	1.126	0.983
00542	01	N. Coastal Cntys, CA	1.003	1.081	0.983
00542	02	Ne Rural, CA	0.992	0.972	0.983
00542	07	Oakland/Berkley, CA	1.035	1.236	0.983
00542	27	Riverside, CA	1.018	1.070	1.018
00542	04	Sacramento/Surr. Cntys, CA	1.023	1.078	0.983
00542	15	San Bernadino/E.Ctrl Cntys CA	1.020	1.066	1.060
02050	28	San Diego/Imperial, CA	1.022	1.084	0.994
00542	05	San Francisco, CA	1.053	1.316	0.983
00542	06	San Mateo, CA	1.044	1.302	0.983
02050	16	Santa Barbara, CA	1.014	1.096	1.028
00542	09	Santa Clara, CA	1.056	1.288	0.983
00542	08	Stockton/Surr. Cntys, CA	1.010	1.034	0.983
02050	17	Ventura, CA	1.031	1.162	1.028
00824	01	Colorado	0.994	0.970	0.755
10230	04	Eastern CT	1.016	1.092	1.018
10230	01	Nw And N. Cntrl CT	1.026	1.115	1.013
10230	03	S. Cntrl CT	1.037	1.164	1.094
10230	02	Sw CT	1.054	1.207	1.116
00570	01	Delaware	1.024	1.025	0.728
00580	01	DC + MD/VA Suburbs	1.055	1.180	0.964
00590	03	Fort Lauderdale, FL	0.996	1.008	1.622
00590	04	Miami, FL	1.025	1.056	2.049
00590	02	N/Nc FL Cities	0.976	0.942	1.262
00590	01	Rest Of Florida	0.968	0.892	1.262
01040	01	Atlanta, GA	0.991	1.026	0.827
01040	04	Rest Of GA	0.960	0.848	0.827
01040	02	Small GA Cities 02	0.972	0.906	0.827
01040	03	Small GA Cities 03	0.964	0.876	0.827
01120	01	Hawaii/Guam	1.001	1.157	0.973
05130	12	North Idaho	0.961	0.890	0.738
05130	11	South Idaho	0.965	0.912	0.738
00621	10	Champaign-Urbana, IL	0.958	0.902	1.072
00621	16	Chicago, IL	1.036	1.097	1.578
00621	03	De Kalb, IL	0.966	0.899	0.958
00621	11	Decatur, IL	0.972	0.896	1.008

CPT codes and descriptions only, © 1994 American Medical Association. Reimbursement information, © 1995 McGraw-Hill Inc.

Carrier number	Locality number	Locality name	Work	Practice expense	Malpractice
00621	12	East St. Louis, IL	0.988	0.944	1.390
00621	06	Kankakee, IL	0.966	0.903	1.019
00621	08	Normal, IL	0.983	0.930	0.934
00621	01	Northwest, IL	0.962	0.869	0.934
00621	05	Peoria, IL	0.994	0.968	0.934
00621	07	Quincy, IL	0.960	0.860	0.934
00621	04	Rock Island, IL	0.984	0.908	0.934
00621	02	Rockford, IL	0.994	0.980	0.975
00621	13	Southeast IL	0.960	0.855	0.934
00621	14	Southern IL	0.960	0.859	0.980
00621	09	Springfield, IL	0.988	0.951	1.042
00621	15	Suburban Chicago, IL	1.014	1.095	1.148
00630	01	Metropolitan IN	0.994	0.950	0.455
00630	03	Rest Of IN	0.976	0.884	0.431
00630	02	Urban IN	0.977	0.900	0.431
00640	00	Iowa	0.968	0.898	0.672
00740	05	Kansas City, Kansas	0.984	0.956	1.162
00650	01	Rest Of Kansas	0.956	0.885	1.162
00740	04	Suburban Kansas City, Kansas	0.984	0.956	1.162
00660	01	Lexington & Louisville, KY	0.986	0.910	0.743
00660	03	Rest Of Kentucky	0.966	0.848	0.743
00660	02	Sm Cities (City Limits) KY	0.968	0.874	0.743
00528	07	Alexandria, LA	0.972	0.876	0.860
00528	03	Baton Rouge, LA	0.988	0.930	0.860
00528	06	Lafayette, LA	0.976	0.892	0.860
00528	04	Lake Charles, LA	0.974	0.904	0.860
00528	05	Monroe, LA	0.968	0.874	0.860
00528	01	New Orleans, LA	0.996	0.974	1.091
00528	50	Rest Of LA	0.968	0.865	0.868
00528	02	Shreveport, LA	0.987	0.914	0.860
21200	02	Central Maine	0.952	0.916	0.738
21200	01	Northern Maine	0.956	0.916	0.738
21200	03	Southern Maine	0.968	1.007	0.738
00901	01	Baltimore/Surr. Cntys, MD	1.024	1.038	1.021
00901	03	South & E. Shore MD	0.998	0.991	0.841
00901	02	Western MD	0.994	0.972	0.852
00700	02	MA Suburbs/Rural Cities	1.006	1.086	0.916
00700	01	Urban MA	1.016	1.149	0.916
00623	01	Detroit, MI	1.051	1.064	2.394
00623	02	Michigan, Not Detroit	1.004	0.953	1.520
00720	00	Minnesota (Blue Shield)	0.994	0.968	0.671
10240	00	Minnesota (Travelers)	0.994	0.968	0.671
10250	01	Rest Of Mississippi	0.955	0.826	0.688
10250	02	Urban Mississippi	0.965	0.885	0.688
00740	03	K.C. (Jackson Cnty), MO	0.984	0.956	1.193
00740	02	N K.C. (Clay/Platte), MO	0.984	0.956	1.192
11260	03	Rest Of MO	0.947	0.828	1.169
00740	06	Rural Nw Counties, MO	0.952	0.850	1.169
11260	02	Sm E. Cities, MO	0.947	0.824	1.169
00740	01	St Joseph, MO	0.951	0.858	1.169

CPT codes and descriptions only, © 1994 American Medical Association. Reimbursement information, © 1995 McGraw-Hill Inc.

Carrier number	Locality number	Locality name	Work	Practice expense	Malpractice
11260	01	St. Louis/Lg E. Cities, MO	0.986	0.942	1.272
00751	01	Montana	0.960	0.895	0.737
00655	00	Nebraska	0.956	0.878	0.440
01290	03	Elko & Ely (Cities), NV	0.984	1.006	1.016
01290	01	Las Vegas, Et Al. (Cities), NV	1.024	1.052	1.016
01290	02	Reno, Et Al. (Cities), NV	1.002	1.095	1.016
01290	99	Rest Of Nevada	1.008	1.046	1.016
00780	40	New Hampshire	0.975	1.022	0.759
00860	02	Middle NJ	1.033	1.104	0.958
00860	01	Northern NJ	1.050	1.173	0.958
00860	03	Southern NJ	1.020	1.056	0.958
01360	05	New Mexico	0.978	0.914	0.780
00801	01	Buffalo/Surr. Cntys, NY	1.004	0.939	0.892
00803	01	Manhattan, NY	1.077	1.307	1.596
00801	03	N. Central Cities, NY	1.001	0.960	0.892
00803	02	Nyc Suburbs/Long I., NY	1.064	1.232	1.844
00803	03	Poughkpsie/N Nyc Suburbs, NY	1.008	1.050	1.272
14330	04	Queens, NY	1.058	1.248	1.774
00801	04	Rest Of New York	0.988	0.936	0.892
00801	02	Rochester/Surr. Cntys, NY	1.016	1.004	0.892
05535	00	North Carolina	0.970	0.910	0.406
00820	01	North Dakota	0.958	0.878	0.652
16360	00	Ohio	0.992	0.946	0.984
01370	00	Oklahoma	0.970	0.896	0.498
01380	02	Eugene, Et Al. (Cities), OR	0.964	0.973	0.794
01380	01	Portland, Et Al. (Cities), OR	0.995	1.016	0.794
01380	99	Rest Of Oregon	0.970	0.952	0.794
01380	03	Salem, Et Al. (Cities), OR	0.970	0.960	0.794
01380	12	Sw OR Cities (City Limits)	0.970	0.971	0.794
00865	02	Lg PA Cities	1.007	1.002	1.188
00865	01	Philly/Pitt Med Shcls/Hosps, PA	1.020	1.027	1.382
00865	04	Rest Of PA	0.974	0.914	0.852
00865	03	Sm PA Cities	0.984	0.931	0.861
00973	20	Puerto Rico	0.882	0.751	0.367
00870	01	Rhode Island	1.014	1.036	1.152
00880	01	South Carolina	0.974	0.886	0.404
00820	02	South Dakota	0.944	0.856	0.566
05440	35	Tennessee	0.972	0.898	0.466
00900	29	Abilene, TX	0.966	0.870	0.666
00900	26	Amarillo, TX	0.974	0.892	0.666
00900	31	Austin, TX	0.978	0.977	0.666
00900	20	Beaumont, TX	0.996	0.924	0.966
00900	09	Brazoria, TX	1.009	0.960	0.966
00900	10	Brownsville, TX	0.968	0.868	0.666
00900	24	Corpus Christi, TX	0.980	0.921	0.666
00900	11	Dallas, TX	1.004	0.992	0.698
00900	12	Denton, TX	0.982	0.962	0.666
00900	14	El Paso, TX	0.984	0.894	0.698
00900	28	Fort Worth, TX	0.981	0.954	0.698
00900	15	Galveston, TX	0.986	0.967	0.966

CPT codes and descriptions only, © 1994 American Medical Association. Reimbursement information, © 1995 McGraw-Hill Inc.

Carrier number	Locality number	Locality name	Work	Practice expense	Malpractice
00900	16	Grayson, TX	0.962	0.888	0.666
00900	18	Houston, TX	1.018	0.994	1.042
00900	33	Laredo, TX	0.962	0.854	0.666
00900	17	Longview, TX	0.970	0.896	0.666
00900	21	Lubbock, TX	0.952	0.888	0.666
00900	19	Mc Allen, TX	0.953	0.855	0.666
00900	23	Midland, TX	1.007	0.949	0.666
00900	02	Northeast Rural TX	0.964	0.870	0.666
00900	13	Odessa, TX	1.000	0.936	0.666
00900	25	Orange, TX	0.996	0.924	0.666
00900	30	San Angelo, TX	0.951	0.873	0.666
00900	07	San Antonio, TX	0.976	0.928	0.666
00900	03	Southeast Rural TX	0.968	0.884	0.696
00900	06	Temple, TX	0.968	0.885	0.666
00900	08	Texarkana, TX	0.954	0.878	0.666
00900	27	Tyler, TX	0.978	0.912	0.666
00900	32	Victoria, TX	0.980	0.920	0.666
00900	22	Waco, TX	0.974	0.874	0.666
00900	04	Western TX	0.958	0.835	0.666
00900	34	Wichita Falls, TX	0.960	0.876	0.666
00910	09	Utah	0.986	0.922	0.692
00780	50	Vermont	0.958	0.964	0.492
00973	50	Virgin Islands	0.983	0.989	1.012
10490	04	Rest Of VA	0.972	0.882	0.513
10490	01	Richmond & Charlottesville, VA	0.990	0.972	0.486
10490	03	Sm Town/Industrial VA	0.972	0.894	0.524
10490	02	Tidewater & N VA Cntys	0.990	0.980	0.616
01390	03	E Cntrl & Ne WA	0.990	0.969	0.906
01390	02	Seattle (King Cnty), WA	1.012	1.063	0.906
01390	01	W & Se WA (Excl Seattle)	0.995	0.980	0.906
16510	16	Charleston, WV	0.984	0.922	0.846
16510	18	Eastern Valley, WV	0.961	0.890	0.846
16510	19	Ohio River Valley, WV	0.960	0.857	0.846
16510	20	Southern Valley, WV	0.956	0.846	0.846
16510	17	Wheeling, WV	0.966	0.870	0.846
00951	13	Central WI	0.960	0.868	0.961
00951	40	Green Bay (Northeast), WI	0.978	0.904	0.961
00951	54	Janesville (S Cntrl), WI	0.968	0.900	0.961
00951	19	La Crosse (W Cntrl), WI	0.974	0.899	0.961
00951	15	Madison (Dane Cnty), WI	0.984	0.990	0.961
00951	46	Milwaukee Surburbs (Se), WI	1.000	0.984	0.961
00951	04	Milwaukee, WI	1.004	0.994	0.961
00951	12	Northwest WI	0.964	0.874	0.961
00951	60	Oshkosh (E Cntrl), WI	0.974	0.898	0.961
00951	14	Southwest WI	0.960	0.869	0.961
00951	36	Wausau (N Cntrl), WI	0.966	0.882	0.961
00825	21	Wyoming	0.978	0.910	0.726

CPT codes and descriptions only, © 1994 American Medical Association. Reimbursement information, © 1995 McGraw-Hill Inc.

Procedural Index

This index is intended to direct the user to a general area. Please refer to your CPT index for a more specific procedural description and/or code reference.

CPT codes and descriptions only, © 1994 American Medical Association. Reimbursement information, © 1995 McGraw-Hill Inc.

CPT codes and descriptions only, © 1994 American Medical Association. Reimbursement information, © 1995 McGraw-Hill Inc.

CPT codes and descriptions only, © 1994 American Medical Association. Reimbursement information, © 1995 McGraw-Hill Inc.

CPT codes and descriptions only, © 1994 American Medical Association. Reimbursement information, © 1995 McGraw-Hill Inc.

CPT codes and descriptions only, © 1994 American Medical Association. Reimbursement information, © 1995 McGraw-Hill Inc.

CPT codes and descriptions only, © 1994 American Medical Association. Reimbursement information, © 1995 McGraw-Hill Inc.

CPT codes and descriptions only, © 1994 American Medical Association. Reimbursement information, © 1995 McGraw-Hill Inc.